THE NETTER COLLECTION
of Medical Illustrations
2nd Edition

Reproductive System
Endocrine System
Respiratory System
Integumentary System
Urinary System
Musculoskeletal System
Digestive System
Nervous System
Cardiovascular System

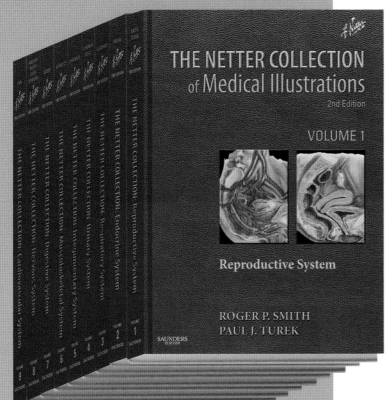

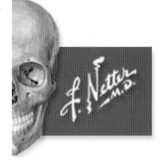
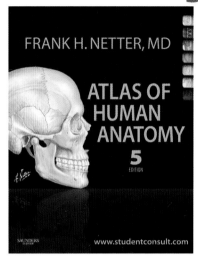
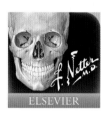
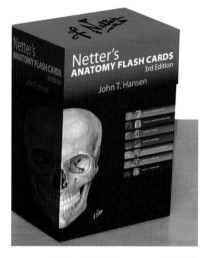

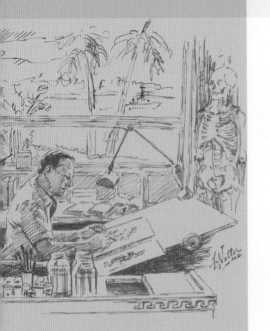

The Netter Collection
OF MEDICAL ILLUSTRATIONS
Musculoskeletal System
Part III—Biology and Systemic Diseases

2nd Edition

A compilation of paintings prepared by
FRANK H. NETTER, MD

Edited by

Joseph P. Iannotti MD, PhD

Maynard Madden Professor and Chairman
Orthopaedic and Rheumatologic Institute
Cleveland Clinic Lerner College of Medicine
Cleveland, Ohio

Richard D. Parker, MD

Professor and Chairman
Department of Orthopaedic Surgery
Orthopaedic and Rheumatologic Institute
Cleveland Clinic Lerner College of Medicine
Cleveland, Ohio

Additional Illustrations by Carlos A. G. Machado, MD

CONTRIBUTING ILLUSTRATORS
John A. Craig, MD
Tiffany S. DaVanzo, MA, CMI
Kristen Wienandt Marzejon, MS, MFA
James A. Perkins, MS, MFA

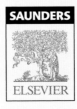

SAUNDERS

ELSEVIER

ELSEVIER
SAUNDERS

1600 John F. Kennedy Blvd.
Ste. 1800
Philadelphia, PA 19103-2899

THE NETTER COLLECTION OF MEDICAL ILLUSTRATIONS: ISBN: 978-1-4160-6379-7
MUSCULOSKELETAL SYSTEM, PART III: BIOLOGY AND SYSTEMIC DISEASES,
Volume 6, Second Edition

Notices

Knowledge and best practice in this field are constantly changing. As new research and experience
broaden our understanding, changes in research methods, professional practices, or medical
treatment may become necessary.

Practitioners and researchers must always rely on their own experience and knowledge in
evaluating and using any information, methods, compounds, or experiments described herein. In
using such information or methods they should be mindful of their own safety and the safety of
others, including parties for whom they have a professional responsibility.

With respect to any drug or pharmaceutical products identified, readers are advised to check the
most current information provided (i) on procedures featured or (ii) by the manufacturer of each
product to be administered, to verify the recommended dose or formula, the method and duration of
administration, and contraindications. It is the responsibility of practitioners, relying on their own
experience and knowledge of their patients, to make diagnoses, to determine dosages and the best
treatment for each individual patient, and to take all appropriate safety precautions.

To the fullest extent of the law, neither the Publisher nor the authors, contributors, or editors,
assume any liability for any injury and/or damage to persons or property as a matter of products
liability, negligence or otherwise, or from any use or operation of any methods, products,
instructions, or ideas contained in the material herein.

ISBN: 978-1-4160-6379-7

Senior Content Strategist: Elyse O'Grady
Content Development Manager: Marybeth Thiel
Publishing Services Manager: Patricia Tannian
Senior Project Manager: John Casey
Senior Design Manager: Lou Forgione

Printed in China

Last digit is the print number: 9 8 7 6

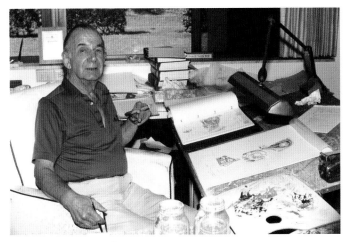

Dr. Frank Netter at work.

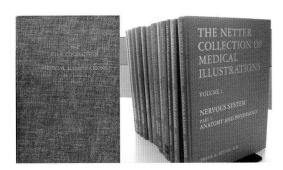

The single-volume "blue book" that paved the way for the multivolume *Netter Collection of Medical Illustrations* series affectionately known as the "green books."

D r. Frank H. Netter exemplified the distinct vocations of doctor, artist, and teacher. Even more important— he unified them. Netter's illustrations always began with meticulous research into the forms of the body, a philosophy that steered his broad and deep medical understanding. He often said: "Clarification is the goal. No matter how beautifully it is painted, a medical illustration has little value if it does not make clear a medical point." His greatest challenge and greatest success was charting a middle course between artistic clarity and instructional complexity. That success is captured in this series, beginning in 1948, when the first comprehensive collection of Netter's work, a single volume, was published by CIBA Pharmaceuticals. It met with such success that over the following 40 years the collection was expanded into an 8-volume series—each devoted to a single body system.

In this second edition of the legendary series, we are delighted to offer Netter's timeless work, now arranged and informed by modern text and radiologic imaging contributed by field-leading doctors and teachers from world-renownedmedical institutions, and supplemented with new illustrations created by artists working in the Netter tradition. Inside the classic green covers, students and practitioners will find hundreds of original works of art—the human body in pictures—paired with the latest in expert medical knowledge and innovation and anchored in the sublime style of Frank Netter.

Noted artist-physician, Carlos Machado, MD, the primary successor responsible for continuing the Netter tradition, has particular appreciation for the Green Book series. "*The Reproductive System* is of special significance for those who, like me, deeply admire Dr. Netter's work. In this volume, he masters the representation of textures of different surfaces, which I like to call 'the rhythm of the brush,' since it is the dimension, the direction of the strokes, and the interval separating them that create the illusion of given textures: organs have their external surfaces, the surfaces of their cavities, and texture of their parenchymas realistically represented. It set the style for the subsequent volumes of Netter's Collection—each an amazing combination of painting masterpieces and precise scientific information."

Though the science and teaching of medicine endures changes in terminology, practice, and discovery, some things remain the same. A patient is a patient. A teacher is a teacher. And the pictures of Dr. Netter—he called them pictures, never paintings—remain the same blend of beautiful and instructional resources that have guided physicians' hands and nurtured their imaginations for more than half a century.

The original series could not exist without the dedication of all those who edited, authored, or in other ways contributed, nor, of course, without the excellence of Dr. Netter. For this exciting second edition, we also owe our gratitude to the Authors, Editors, Advisors, and Artists whose relentless efforts were instrumental in adapting these timeless works into reliable references for today's clinicians in training and in practice. From all of us with the Netter Publishing Team at Elsevier, we thank you.

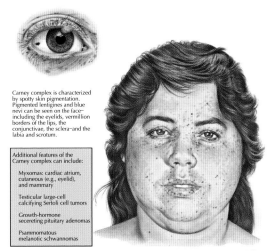

CUSHING'S SYNDROME IN A PATIENT WITH THE CARNEY COMPLEX

Carney complex is characterized by spotty skin pigmentation. Pigmented lentigines and blue nevi can be seen on the face— including the eyelids, vermillion borders of the lips, the conjunctivae, the sclera–and the labia and scrotum.

Additional features of the Carney complex can include:

Myxomas: cardiac atrium, cutaneous (e.g., eyelid), and mammary

Testicular large-cell calcifying Sertoli cell tumors

Growth-hormone secereting pituitary adenomas

Psammomatous melanotic schwannomas

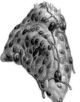

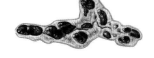

PPNAD adrenal glands are usually of normal size and most are studded with black, brown, or red nodules. Most of the pigmented nodules are less than 4 mm in diameter and interspersed in the adjacent atrophic cortex.

A brand new illustrated plate painted by Carlos Machado, MD, for *The Endocrine System*, Volume 2, 2nd ed.

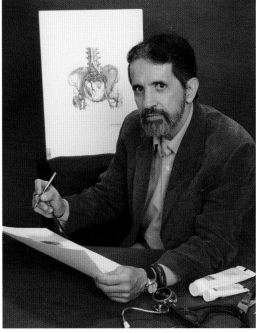

Dr. Carlos Machado at work.

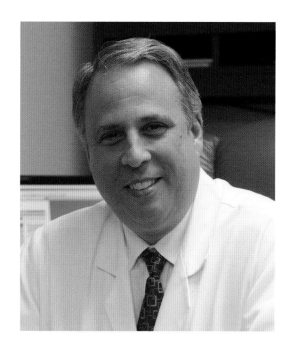

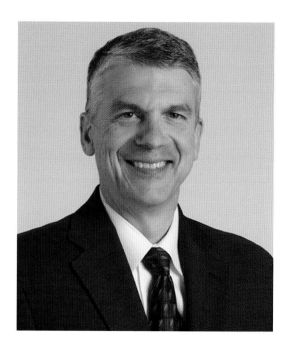

Joseph P. Iannotti, MD, PhD, is Maynard Madden Professor of Orthopaedic Surgery at the Cleveland Clinic Lerner College of Medicine and Chairman of the Orthopaedic and Rheumatologic Institute at the Cleveland Clinic. He is Medical Director of the Orthopaedic Clinical Research Center and has a joint appointment in the department of bioengineering.

Dr. Iannotti joined the Cleveland Clinic in 2000 from the University of Pennsylvania, leaving there as a tenured professor of orthopaedic surgery and Head of the Shoulder and Elbow Service. Dr. Iannotti received his medical degree from Northwestern University in 1979, completed his orthopaedic residency training at the University of Pennsylvania in 1984, and earned his doctorate in cell biology from the University of Pennsylvania in 1987.

Dr. Iannotti has a very active referral surgical practice that is focused on the treatment of complex and revision problems of the shoulder, with a primary interest in the management of complex shoulder problems in joint replacement and reconstruction.

Dr. Iannotti's clinical and basic science research program focuses on innovative treatments for tendon repair and tendon tissue engineering, prosthetic design, software planning, and patient-specific instrumentation. Dr. Iannotti has had continuous extramural funding for his research since 1981. He has been the principal or co-principal investigator of 31 research grants totaling $9.4 million. He has been a co-investigator on 13 other research grants. Dr. Iannotti has been an invited lecturer and visiting professor to over 70 national and international academic institutions and societies, delivering over 600 lectures both nationally and internationally.

Dr. Iannotti has published two textbooks on the shoulder, one in its second edition and the other in its third edition. He has authored over 250 original peer-reviewed articles, review articles, and book chapters. Dr. Iannotti has over 13 awarded patents and 40 pending patent applications related to shoulder prosthetics, surgical instruments, and tissue-engineered implants.

He has received awards for his academic work from the American Orthopaedic Association, including the North American and ABC traveling fellowships and the Neer research award in 1996 and 2001 from the American Shoulder and Elbow Surgeons. He has won the orthopaedic resident teaching award in 2006 for his role in research education. He was awarded the Mason Sones Innovator of the Year award in 2012 from the Cleveland Clinic.

He has served in many leadership roles at the national level that includes past Chair of the Academic Affairs Council and the Board of Directors of the American Academy of Orthopaedic Surgery. In addition he has served and chaired several committees of the American Shoulder and Elbow Surgeons and was President of this International Society of Shoulder and Elbow Surgeons in 2005-2006. He is now Chairman of the Board of Trustees of the *Journal of Shoulder and Elbow Surgery*.

Richard D. Parker, MD, is Chairman of the Department of Orthopaedic Surgery at the Cleveland Clinic and Professor of Surgery at the Cleveland Clinic Lerner College of Medicine. Dr. Parker is an expert of the knee, ranging from nonoperative treatment to all aspects of surgical procedures including articular cartilage, meniscus, ligament, and joint replacement. He has published more than 120 peer-reviewed manuscripts, numerous book chapters, and has presented his work throughout the world. Dr. Parker received his undergraduate degree at Walsh College in Canton, Ohio, his medical education at The Ohio State University College of Medicine, and completed his orthopaedic residency at The Mt. Sinai Medical Center in Cleveland, Ohio. He received his fellowship training with subspecialization in sports medicine through a clinical research fellowship in sports medicine, arthroscopy, knee and shoulder surgery in Salt Lake City, Utah. He obtained his CSS (Certificate of Subspecialization) in orthopaedic sports medicine in 2008 which was the first year it was available.

Prior to joining Cleveland Clinic in 1993, Dr. Parker acted as head of the section of sports medicine at The Mt. Sinai Medical Center. His current research focuses on clinical outcomes focusing on articular cartilage, meniscal transplantation, PCL, and the MOON (Multicenter Orthopaedic Outcomes Network) ACL registry. In addition to his busy clinical and administrative duties he also serves as the head team physician for the Cleveland Cavaliers, is currently President of the NBA Physician Society, and serves as a knee consultant to the Cleveland Browns and Cleveland Indians. He lives in the Chagrin Falls area with his wife, Jana, and enjoys biking, golfing, and swimming in his free time.

Frank Netter produced nearly 20,000 medical illustrations spanning the entire field of medicine over a five-decade career. There is not a physician that has not used his work as part of his or her education. Many educators use his illustrations to teach others. One of the editors of this series had the privilege and honor to be an author of portions of the original "Green Book" of musculoskeletal medical illustrations as a junior faculty, and it is now a special honor to be part of this updated series.

Many of Frank Netter's original illustrations have stood the test of time. His work depicting basic musculoskeletal anatomy and relevant surgical anatomy and exposures have remained unaltered in the current series. His illustrations demonstrated the principles of treatment or the manifestation of musculoskeletal diseases and were rendered in a manner that only a physician-artist could render.

This edition of musculoskeletal illustrations has been updated with modern text and our current understanding of the pathogenesis, diagnosis, and treatment of a wide array of diseases and conditions. We have added new illustrations and radiographic and advanced imaging to supplement the original art. We expect that this series will prove to be useful to a wide spectrum of both students and teachers at every level.

Part I covers specific disorders of the upper limb including anatomy, trauma, and degenerative and acquired disorders. Part II covers these same areas in the lower limb and spine. Part III covers the basic science of the musculoskeletal system, metabolic bone disease, rheumatologic diseases, musculoskeletal tumors, the sequelae of trauma, and congenital deformities.

The series is jointly produced by the clinical and research staff of the Orthopaedic and Rheumatologic Institute of the Cleveland Clinic and Elsevier. The editors thank each of the many talented contributors to this three-volume series. Their expertise in each of their fields of expertise has made this publication possible. We are both very proud to work with these colleagues. We are thankful to Elsevier for the opportunity to work on this series and for their support and expertise throughout the long development and editorial process.

Joseph P. Iannotti
Richard D. Parker

INTRODUCTIONS TO THE FIRST EDITION

INTRODUCTION TO PART I—ANATOMY, PHYSIOLOGY, AND METABOLIC DISORDERS

I had long looked forward to undertaking this volume on the musculoskeletal system. It deals with the most humanistic, the most soul-touching, of all the subjects I have portrayed in THE CIBA COLLECTION OF MEDICAL ILLUSTRATIONS. People break bones, develop painful or swollen joints, are handicapped by congenital, developmental, or acquired deformities, metabolic abnormalities, or paralytic disorders. Some are beset by tumors of bone or soft tissue; some undergo amputations, either surgical or traumatic; some occasionally have reimplantation; and many have joint replacement. The list goes on and on. These are people we see about us quite commonly and are often our friends, relatives, or acquaintances. Significantly, such ailments lend themselves to graphic representation and are stimulating subject matter for an artist.

When I undertook this project, however, I grossly underestimated its scope. This was true also in regard to the previous volumes of the CIBA COLLECTION, but in the case of this book, it was far more marked. When we consider that this project involves every bone, joint, and muscle of the body, as well as all the nerves and blood vessels that supply them and all the multitude of disorders that may affect each of them, the magnitude of the project becomes enormous. In my naiveté, I originally thought I could cover the subject in a single book, but it soon became apparent that this was impossible. Even two books soon proved inadequate for such an extensive undertaking and, accordingly, three books are now planned. This book, Part I, Volume 8 of the CIBA COLLECTION, covers basic gross anatomy, embryology, physiology, and histology of the musculoskeletal system, as well as its metabolic disorders. Part II, now in press, covers rheumatic and other arthritic disorders, as well as their conservative and surgical management (including joint replacement), congenital and developmental disorders, and both benign and malignant neoplasms of bones and soft tissues. Part III, on which I am still at work, will include fractures and dislocations and their emergency and definitive care, amputations (both surgical and traumatic) and prostheses, sports injuries, infections, peripheral nerve and plexus injuries, burns, compartment syndromes, skin grafting, arthroscopy, and care and rehabilitation of handicapped patients.

But classification and organization of this voluminous material turned out to be no simple matter, since many disorders fit equally well into several of the above groups. For example, osteogenesis imperfecta might have been classified as metabolic, congenital, or developmental. Baker's cyst, ganglion, bursitis, and villonodular synovitis might have been considered with rheumatic, developmental, or in some instances even with traumatic disorders. Pathologic fractures might be covered with fractures in general or with the specific underlying disease that caused them. In a number of instances, therefore, empiric decisions had to be made in this connection, and some subjects were covered under several headings. I hope that the reader will be considerate of these problems. In addition, there is much overlap between the fields of orthopedics, neurology, and neurosurgery, so that the reader may find it advantageous to refer at times to my atlases on the nervous system.

I must express herewith my thanks and appreciation for the tremendous help which my very knowledgeable collaborators gave to me so graciously. In this Part I, there was first of all Dr. Russell Woodburne, a truly great anatomist and professor emeritus at the University of Michigan. It is interesting that during our long collaboration I never actually met with Dr. Woodburne, and all our communications were by mail or phone. This, in itself, tells of what a fine understanding and meeting of the minds there was between us. I hope and expect that in the near future I will have the pleasure of meeting him in person.

Dr. Edmund S. Crelin, professor at Yale University, is a long-standing friend (note that I do not say "old" friend because he is so young in spirit) with whom I have collaborated a number of times on other phases of embryology. He is a profound student and original investigator of the subject, with the gift of imparting his knowledge simply and clearly, and is in fact a talented artist himself.

Dr. Frederick Kaplan (now Freddie to me), assistant professor of orthopaedics at the University of Pennsylvania, was invaluable in guiding me through the difficult subjects of musculoskeletal physiology and metabolic bone disease. I enjoyed our companionship and friendship as much as I appreciated his knowledge and insight into the subject.

I was delighted to have the cooperation of Dr. Henry Mankin, the distinguished chief of orthopaedics at Massachusetts General Hospital and professor at Harvard University, for the complex subject of rickets in its varied forms—nutritional, renal, and metabolic. He is a great but charming and unassuming man.

There were many others, too numerous to mention here individually, who gave to me of their knowledge and time. They are all credited elsewhere in this book but I thank them all very much herewith. I will write about the great people who helped me with other parts of Volume 8 when those parts are published.

Finally, I give great credit and thanks to the personnel of the CIBA-GEIGY Company and to the company itself for having done so much to ease my burden in producing this book. Specifically, I would like to mention Mr. Philip Flagler, Dr. Milton Donin, Dr. Roy Ellis, and especially Mrs. Regina Dingle, all of whom did so much more in that connection than I can tell about here.

Frank H. Netter, 1987

INTRODUCTION TO PART II—
DEVELOPMENTAL DISORDERS, TUMORS, RHEUMATIC DISEASES, AND JOINT REPLACEMENT

In my introduction to Part I of this atlas, I wrote of how awesome albeit fascinating I had found the task of pictorializing the fundamentals of the musculoskeletal system, both its normal structure as well as its multitudinous disorders and diseases. As compactly, simply, and succinctly as I tried to present the subject matter, it still required three full books (Parts I, II, and III of Volume 8 of THE CIBA COLLECTION OF MEDICAL ILLUSTRATIONS). Part I of this trilogy covered the normal anatomy, embryology, and physiology of the musculoskeletal system as well as its diverse metabolic diseases, including the various types of rickets. This book, Part II, portrays its congenital and developmental disorders, neoplasms—both benign and malignant—of bone and soft tissue, and rheumatic and other arthritic diseases, as well as joint replacement. Part III, on which I am still at work, will cover trauma, including fractures and dislocations of all the bones and joints, soft-tissue injuries, sports injuries, bums, infections including osteomyelitis

and hand infections, compartment syndromes, amputations, both traumatic and surgical, replantation of limbs and digits, prostheses, and rehabilitation, as well as a number of related subjects.

As I stated in my above-mentioned previous introduction, some disorders, however, do not fit exactly into a precise classification and are therefore covered piecemeal herein under several headings. Furthermore, a considerable number of orthopedic ailments involve also the fields of neurology and neurosurgery, so readers may find it helpful to refer in those instances to my atlases on the anatomy and pathology of the nervous system (Volume 1, Parts I and II of THE CIBA COLLECTION OF MEDICAL ILLUSTRATIONS).

Most meaningfully, however, I herewith express my sincere appreciation of the many great physicians, surgeons, orthopedists, and scientists who so graciously shared with me their knowledge and supplied me with so much material on which to base my illustrations. Without their help I could not have created this atlas. Most of these wonderful people are credited elsewhere in this book under the heading of "Acknowledgments" but I must nevertheless specifically mention a few who

were not only collaborators and consultants in this undertaking but who have become my dear and esteemed friends. These are Dr. Bob Hensinger, my consulting editor, who guided me through many puzzling aspects of the organization and subject matter of this atlas; Drs. Alfred and Genevieve Swanson, pioneers in the correction of rheumatically deformed hands with Silastic implants, as well as in the classification and study of congenital limb deficits; Dr. William Enneking, who has made such great advances in the diagnosis and management of bone tumors; Dr. Ernest ("Chappy") Conrad III; the late Dr. Charley Frantz, who first set me on course for this project, and Dr. Richard Freyberg, who became the consultant on the rheumatic diseases plates; Dr. George Hammond; Dr. Hugo Keim; Dr. Mack Clayton; Dr. Philip Wilson; Dr. Stuart Kozinn; and Dr. Russell Windsor.

Finally, I also sincerely thank Mr. Philip Flagler, Ms. Regina Dingle, and others of the CIBA-GEIGY organization who helped in more ways than I can describe in producing this atlas.

Frank H. Netter, MD, 1990

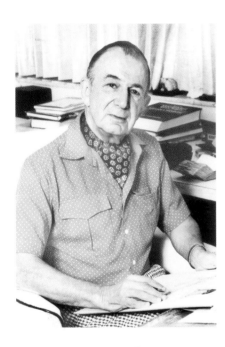

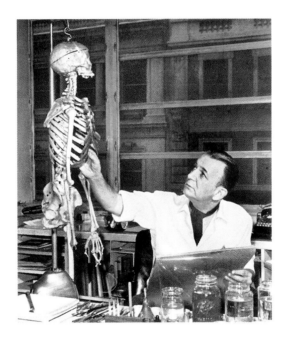

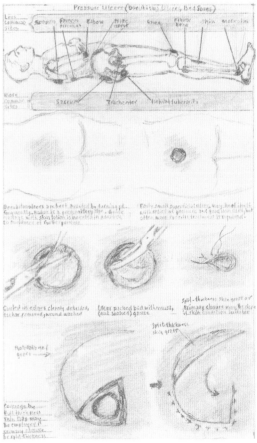

Sketch appearing in the front matter of Part III of the first edition.

ADVISORY BOARD

Prof. Dr. Sergio Checchia, MD
Professor
Shoulder and Elbow Service
Santa Casa Hospitals and School of Medicine
Sao Paulo, Brazil

Myles Coolican, MBBS, FRACS, FA Orth A
Director
Sydney Orthopaedic Research Institute
Sydney, Australia

Roger J. Emery, MBBS
Professor of Orthopaedic Surgery
Department of Surgery and Cancer
Imperial College
London, UK

Prof. Eugenio Gaudio, MD
Professor, Dipartimento di Anatomia Umana
Università degli Studi di Roma "La Sapienza"
Rome, Italy

Jennifer A. Hart, MPAS, ATC, PA-C
Physician Assistant
Department of Orthopaedic Surgery
Sports Medicine Division
University of Virginia
Charlottesville, Virginia

Miguel A. Khoury, MD
Medical Director
Cleveland Sports Institute
Associate Professor
University of Buenos Aires
Buenos Aires, Argentina

Dr. Santos Guzmán López, MD
Head of the Department of Anatomy
Faculty of Medicine
Universidad Autónoma de Nuevo León
Nuevo León, Mexico

June-Horng Lue, PhD
Associate Professor
Department of Anatomy and Cell Biology
College of Medicine
National Taiwan University
Taipei, Taiwan

Dr. Ludwig Seebauer, MD
Chief Physician, Medical Director
Center for Orthopaedics, Traumatology, and Sports
  Medicine
Bogenhausen Hospital
Munich, Germany

Prof. David Sonnabend, MBBS, MD, BSC(Med), FRACS, FA Orth A
Orthopaedic Surgeon
Shoulder Specialist
Sydney Shoulder Specialists
St. Leonards, NSW, Australia

Dr. Gilles Walch, MD
Orthopedic Surgery
Department of Shoulder Pathology
Centre Orthopédique Santy
Hôpital Privé Jean Mermoz
Lyon, France

EDITORS-IN-CHIEF

Joseph P. Iannotti, MD, PhD
Maynard Madden Professor and Chairman
Orthopaedic and Rheumatologic Institute
Cleveland Clinic Lerner College of Medicine
Cleveland, Ohio

Richard D. Parker, MD
Professor and Chairman
Department of Orthopaedic Surgery
Orthopaedic and Rheumatologic Institute
Cleveland Clinic Lerner College of Medicine
Cleveland, Ohio
Plates 8-1–8-9

SECTION EDITORS

Chad Deal, MD
Department of Rheumatic and Immunologic Diseases
Director, Center for Osteoporosis and Metabolic
  Bone Diseases
Cleveland Clinic
Cleveland, Ohio
*Sections 3 and 5; Plates 3-25–3-29, 3-34–3-36,
  3-43–3-47*

David P. Gurd, MD
Pediatric Orthopaedic and Scoliosis Surgeon
Director of Pediatric Spinal Deformity
Department of Orthopaedic Surgery
Cleveland Clinic
Cleveland, Ohio
Section 4; Plates 4-1–4-19

Ronald J. Midura, PhD
Staff
Department of Biomedical Engineering
Lerner Research Institute
Cleveland Clinic
Cleveland, Ohio
Sections 1 and 2; Plates 2-1–2-40, Plate 3-1

CONTRIBUTORS

Abby Abelson, MD
Chair, Department of Rheumatic and Immunologic
  Diseases
Orthopaedic and Rheumatologic Institute
Cleveland Clinic
Cleveland, Ohio
Plates 3-26–3-29, 3-34–3-36, 3-43–3-46

Suneel Apte, MBBS, DPhil
Department of Biomedical Engineering
Lerner Research Institute
Cleveland Clinic
Cleveland, Ohio
Plates 1-1–1-21

Robert Tracy Ballock, MD
Director, Center for Pediatric Orthopaedic Surgery
Department of Orthopaedic Surgery
Orthopaedic and Rheumatologic Institute
Professor of Surgery
Cleveland Clinic Lerner College of Medicine
Cleveland, Ohio
Plates 4-32–4-36

Thomas Bauer, MD, PhD
Staff, Departments of Pathology, Orthopaedic
  Surgery, and the Center for Spine Health
Cleveland Clinic
Cleveland, Ohio
Plate 3-33

Matthew P. Bunyard, MD
Staff Physician
Department of Rheumatic and Immunologic Diseases
Cleveland Clinic
Cleveland, Ohio
Plates 5-10–5-12

Scott R. Burg, DO
Clinical Assistant Professor of Medicine
Rheumatologic and Immunologic Disease
Cleveland Clinic Lerner College of Medicine
Clinical Associate Professor of Medicine
Ohio College of Osteopathic Medicine
Cleveland, Ohio
Plate 5-41

Leonard H. Calabrese, DO
R.J. Fasenmyer Chair of Clinical Immunology
Professor of Medicine
Department of Rheumatic and Immunologic Diseases
Cleveland Clinic
Cleveland, Ohio
Plate 5-60

Andrew C. Calabria, MD
Attending Physician
Division of Endocrinology and Diabetes
The Children's Hospital of Philadelphia
Assistant Professor of Pediatrics
Perelman School of Medicine at the University of
  Pennsylvania
Philadelphia, Pennsylvania
Plates 3-5–3-10

Soumya Chatterjee, MD, MS, FRCP
Staff, Department of Rheumatic and Immunologic
  Diseases
Cleveland Clinic
Cleveland, Ohio

Clemencia Colmenares, PhD
Staff, Department of Cancer Biology
Lerner Research Institute
Associate Director, Research Education
Cleveland Clinic Lerner College of Medicine
Cleveland, Ohio
Plates 2-1–2-40

Nicholas C. Frisch, MD
Resident Physician
Department of Orthopaedic Surgery
Cleveland Clinic
Cleveland, Ohio
Plates 9-1–9-16

Carmen E. Gota, MD
Staff
Orthopaedic and Rheumatologic Institute
Center for Vasculitis Care and Research
Cleveland Clinic
Cleveland, Ohio
Plates 5-51–5-53

Manjula K. Gupta, PhD
Professor of Pathology and Medicine [Endocrinology,
  Diabetes, and Metabolism]
Cleveland Clinic Lerner College of Medicine
Director of Endo/Immunology Labs
Department of Clinical Pathology
Cleveland Clinic
Cleveland, Ohio
Plates 3-11, 3-12, 3-24

Rula A. Hajj-Ali, MD
Assistant Professor of Medicine
Center of Vasculitis Care and Research
Cleveland Clinic Lerner College of Medicine
Cleveland Clinic
Cleveland, Ohio
Plate 5-60–5-62

Vincent C. Hascall, PhD
Department of Biomedical Engineering
Lerner Research Institute
Cleveland Clinic
Cleveland, Ohio
Plates 2-1–2-40

Gary S. Hoffman, MD, MS, MACR
Professor of Medicine
Center for Vasculitis Care and Research
Cleveland Clinic Lerner College of Medicine
Cleveland, Ohio
Plates 5-42, 5-43

M. Elaine Husni, MD, MPH
Assistant Professor of Medicine
Cleveland Clinic Lerner College of Medicine
Department Vice Chair, Arthritis Center
Department of Rheumatic and Immunologic Diseases
Cleveland Clinic
Cleveland, Ohio
Plates 5-29–5-33

Atul A. Khasnis, MD, MS
Staff, Department of Rheumatic and Immunologic
  Diseases
Cleveland Clinic
Cleveland, Ohio
Plate 5-54

Carol A. Langford, MD, MHS
Harold C. Schott Chair in Rheumatic and
   Immunologic Diseases
Director, Center for Vasculitis Care and Research
Cleveland Clinic
Cleveland, Ohio
Plates 5-48, 5-50

Michael A. Levine, MD
Lester Baker Chair in Diabetes
Chief, Division of Endocrinology and Diabetes
Director, Center for Bone Health
The Children's Hospital of Philadelphia
Professor of Pediatrics and Medicine
Perelman School of Medicine at the University of
   Pennsylvania
Philadelphia, Pennsylvania
Plates 3-5–3-10

Angelo Licata, MD, PhD, FACP, FACE
Consultant, Director, Center for Space Medicine
Department of Biomedical Engineering and Calcium
   Unit, Endocrine Metabolism Institute
Cleveland Clinic
Cleveland, Ohio
Plates 3-2–3-4

Steven A. Lietman, MD
Co-Director, Musculoskeletal Tumor and Trauma
   Center
Orthopaedic and Rheumatologic Institute
Cleveland Clinic
Associate Professor of Surgery
Cleveland Clinic Lerner College of Medicine
Cleveland, Ohio
Plates 6-1–6-33

Yih Chang Lin, MD
Fellow, Rheumatology and Immunology
Orthopaedic and Rheumatologic Institute
Cleveland Clinic Lerner College of Medicine
Cleveland, Ohio
Plate 5-60

Bruce D. Long, MD
Department of Rheumatic and Immunologic Diseases
Orthopaedic and Rheumatologic Institute
Cleveland Clinic Lerner College of Medicine
Cleveland, Ohio
Plates 5-36, 5-37

Brian F. Mandell, MD, PhD, FACR, MACP
Professor and Chairman of Medicine
Department of Rheumatic and Immunologic Diseases
Cleveland Clinic Lerner College of Medicine
Cleveland, Ohio
Plates 5-13–5-15, 5-34, 5-35, 5-38–5-40

Adam F. Meisel, MD
Orthopaedic Resident
Department of Orthopaedic Surgery
Orthopaedic and Rheumatologic Institute
Cleveland Clinic Lerner College of Medicine
Cleveland, Ohio
Plates 7-1–7-26

Nathan W. Mesko, MD
Orthopaedic Resident
Department of Orthopaedic Surgery
Orthopaedic and Rheumatologic Institute
Cleveland Clinic Lerner College of Medicine
Cleveland, Ohio
Plates 4-20–4-27, 4-30, 4-31

Paul D. Miller, MD
Program Chair
Distinguished Clinical Professor of Medicine
University of Colorado Health Sciences Center
Denver, Colorado;
Medical Director
Colorado Center for Bone Research
Lakewood, Colorado
Plates 3-13–3-23

Justin S. Mitchell, DO
Chief Resident, Orthopedic Surgery
Cleveland Clinic / South Pointe Hospital
Cleveland, Ohio
Plates 4-28, 4-29

Roland W. Moskowitz, MD, MS (Med)
Clinical Professor of Medicine
University Hospitals Case Medical Center
Cleveland, Ohio
Plates 5-22–5-28

Marvin R. Natowicz, MD, PhD
Staff
Genomic Medicine Institute and Institutes of
   Pathology and Laboratory Medicine, Neurology,
   and Pediatrics
Cleveland Clinic
Cleveland, Ohio
Plates 3-37–3-42

Bradford J. Richmond, MD, MS, FACR
Associate Professor of Radiology
Cleveland Clinic Lerner College of Medicine
Musculoskeletal Radiology
Cleveland Clinic
Cleveland, Ohio
Plates 3-30–3-32

Steven Spalding, MD
Director, Center for Pediatric Rheumatology
Cleveland Clinic Children's Hospital
Cleveland, Ohio
Plates 5-16–5-21, 5-45–5-47

Jason Springer, MD
Rheumatology Fellow
Center of Vasculitis Research and Care
Cleveland Clinic
Cleveland, Ohio
Plate 5-61, 5-62

Christopher J. Utz, MD
Chief Resident
Department of Orthopaedic Surgery
Cleveland Clinic Lerner College of Medicine
Cleveland, Ohio
Plates 4-37–4-50

Alexandra Villa-Forte, MD, MPH
Staff Physician
Center for Vasculitis Care and Research
Department of Rheumatic and Immunologic Diseases
Cleveland Clinic Lerner College of Medicine
Cleveland, Ohio
Plates 5-58, 5-59

William S. Wilke, MD
Senior Staff
Orthopaedic and Rheumatologic Institute
Cleveland Clinic (retired)
Consultant, Crescendo Bioscience
Cleveland, Ohio
Plate 5-44

Qingping Yao, MD, PhD
Senior Staff Rheumatologist
Department of Rheumatic and Immunologic Diseases
Cleveland Clinic
Cleveland, Ohio
Plates 5-1–5-9

CONTENTS OF COMPLETE VOLUME 6, MUSCULOSKELETAL SYSTEM: THREE-PART SET

Cleveland Clinic

Joseph P. Iannotti ● Richard D. Parker

CONTENTS

SECTION 5—RHEUMATIC DISEASES

SECTION 6—TUMORS OF MUSCULOSKELETAL SYSTEM

EMBRYOLOGY

Plate 1-1

Musculoskeletal System: PART III

DEVELOPMENT OF MUSCULOSKELETAL SYSTEM

EVOLUTION

The development of the human musculoskeletal system is an interesting demonstration of ontogeny recapitulating phylogeny. The genetic code that guides the continually changing body plan of the developing human results in a résumé of body plans of the various forms of our vertebrate ancestors from which fish, amphibians, reptiles, and mammals evolved. In their adult state, a number of living animals resemble some of the ancient ancestors of the central stem line. The knowledge of the fossil record of extinct forms and the comparative anatomy and physiology of living animals makes rational so many aspects of human development that would otherwise have to be regarded as completely wasteful and nonsensical, or both.

AMPHIOXUS

The extant adult amphioxus, or lancelet, is considered to resemble an ancient ancestor of the vertebrates (see Plate 1-1). It is a fishlike animal, about 2 inches long, that has the basic body plan of the early human embryo. The central nervous system consists of a nerve cord resembling the portion of the human embryonic neural tube that becomes the spinal cord. The digestive, respiratory, excretory, and circulatory systems of the amphioxus also closely resemble those of the early human embryo. As in the early human embryo, the skeleton of the amphioxus consists of a notochord, a slender rod of turgid cells that runs the length of the body directly beneath the nerve cord, or neural tube. The muscular system of the amphioxus consists of individual muscle segments on each side of the body, known as myotomes or myomeres, which are similar in appearance to the myotomes of the early human embryo. The nerve cord of the amphioxus gives off a pair of nerves to each myotome, and the striated muscle fibers of the myotomes contract to produce the lateral bending movements of swimming.

AXIAL SKELETON

The axial skeleton includes the vertebrae, ribs, sternum, and skull. The first structure of the future axial skeleton to form is the notochord (see Plate 1-1). It appears in the midline of the embryonic disc at 15 days of development as a cord of cells budding off from a mass of ectoderm known as Hensen's node. The notochordal cells become temporarily intercalated in the endoderm, which forms the roof of the yolk sac. After separating from the endoderm, the notochord becomes a slender rod of cells running the length of the embryo between the neural tube and the developing gut.

The dorsal mesoderm on either side of the notochord becomes thickened and arranged into 42 to 44 pairs of cell masses known as somites (4 occipital, 8 cervical, 12 thoracic, 5 lumbar, 5 sacral, 8 to 10 coccygeal) between the 19th and 32nd day of development. The formation of these primitive segments, or somites, reflects the serial repetition of homologous parts known as metamerism, which is retained in many adult prevertebrates. The vertebrate embryo is fundamentally metameric, even though much of its segmentation is lost as development proceeds to the adult form. The first significant change in the somite of the human embryo is the formation of a cluster of mesenchymal cells, the

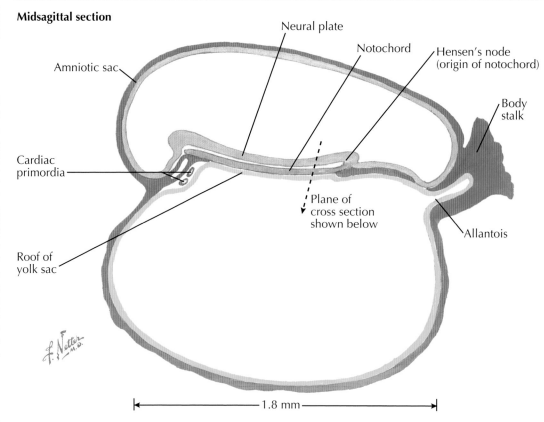

Amphioxus (left half of anterior part of body wall excised)

Nerve cord with central canal exposed (right half)
Notochord (right half)
Dorsal nerve
Segmented myotomes
Dorsal fin
Tail
Mouth
Gill slits of pharynx
Ventral nerve
Anus

Human embryo at 16 days

Midsagittal section

Neural plate
Notochord
Hensen's node (origin of notochord)
Amniotic sac
Body stalk
Cardiac primordia
Plane of cross section shown below
Allantois
Roof of yolk sac
|—————— 1.8 mm ——————|

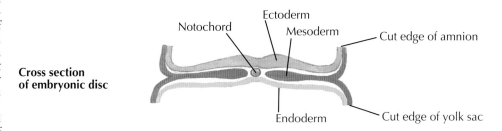

Ectoderm
Notochord
Mesoderm
Cut edge of amnion
Cross section of embryonic disc
Endoderm
Cut edge of yolk sac

sclerotome, on the ventromedial border of the somite (see Plate 1-2). The sclerotomal cells migrate from the somites and become aggregated about the notochord to ultimately give rise to the vertebral column and ribs (see Plate 1-3).

VERTEBRAL COLUMN AND RIBS

During the fourth week of development, a clustering of sclerotomal cells derived from two adjacent somites on either side of the notochord becomes the primordium of the body, or centrum, of a vertebra. Soon after the body takes shape, paired concentrations of mesenchymal cells extend dorsally and laterally from the body to form the primordia of the neural arches and the costal processes. The costal process becomes a rib that articulates with the body and transverse process of the neural arch of the thoracic vertebrae (see Plate 1-4). The costal process becomes the anterior part of the transverse foramen of the cervical vertebrae, the transverse process

Plate 1-2

Embryology

DEVELOPMENT OF MUSCULOSKELETAL SYSTEM
(Continued)

of the lumbar vertebrae, and the lateral part of the sacrum. Occasionally, the costal process of the seventh cervical or the first lumbar vertebra becomes a supernumerary rib. Failure of fusion of the neural folds results in various types of spina bifida.

The vertebrae and ribs in the mesenchymal, or blastemal, stage are one continuous mass of cells. This stage is quickly followed by the cartilage stage, when the mesenchymal cells become chondrocytes and produce cartilage matrix during the seventh week, beginning in the upper vertebrae. By the time ossification begins at 9 weeks, the rib cartilages have become separated from the vertebrae.

The clustering of sclerotomal cells to form the bodies of the vertebrae establishes intervertebral fissures that fill with mesenchymal cells to become the intervertebral discs (see Plate 1-3). The notochord in the center of the developing intervertebral disc expands as its cells produce a large amount of mucoid semifluid matrix to form the nucleus pulposus. The mesenchymal cells surrounding the nucleus pulposus produce proteoglycans and collagen fibers to become the fibrocartilage anulus fibrosus of the intervertebral disc. At birth, the nucleus pulposus makes up the bulk of an intervertebral disc. From birth to adulthood, it serves as a shock-absorbing mechanism, but by 10 years of age the notochordal cells have disappeared and the surrounding fibrocartilage begins to gradually replace the mucoid matrix. The water-binding capacity and elasticity of the matrix are also gradually reduced.

The portion of the notochord surrounded by the developing body of a vertebra usually disappears completely before maturity. This is also true of the portions that become incorporated into the body of the sphenoid and the basilar part of the occipital bone. However, the portion of the notochord that normally becomes the nucleus pulposus in the intervertebral discs becomes the apical dental ligament, connecting the dens of the axis with the occipital bone. The dens evolved as an addition to the body of the first cervical vertebra, the atlas, in those reptiles that gave rise to mammals. The most primitive of mammals, the duck-billed platypus and the spiny anteater, have a large atlas body and a dens. In the human embryo, the atlas body and dens become dissociated as a unit from the rest of the atlas and fuse with the body of the second cervical vertebra, the axis (see Plate 1-5). This fusion results in a mature ring-shaped atlas with an anterior arch lacking a body.

At 5 weeks, a prominent tail containing coccygeal vertebrae is present in the human embryo (see Plate 1-3). A free-moving tail is characteristic of most adult vertebrates. However, the human tail is concealed by the growing buttocks and actually regresses to become the coccyx, which consists of four or five rudimentary vertebrae fused together.

STERNUM

At 6 weeks, a pair of bands of mesenchymal cells, the sternal bars, appear ventrolaterally in the body wall (see Plate 1-5). They have no connection with the ribs or with each other, and their formation is independent of any sclerotomal derivatives. After the attachment of the upper ribs to the sternal bars, they fuse together progressively in a craniocaudal direction. At 9 weeks, the

union of the bars, which have become cartilaginous, is complete. At the cranial end of the sternal bars, two suprasternal masses form and fuse with the future manubrium to serve as sites where the clavicles articulate. Influenced by the ribs, the cartilaginous body of the sternum becomes secondarily segmented into six sternebrae. Faulty fusion of the sternal bars in the midline results either in a cleft or perforated sternum or in a bifid xiphoid process.

DIFFERENTIATION OF SOMITES INTO MYOTOMES, SCLEROTOMES, AND DERMATOMES

Cross section of human embryos

A. At 19 days

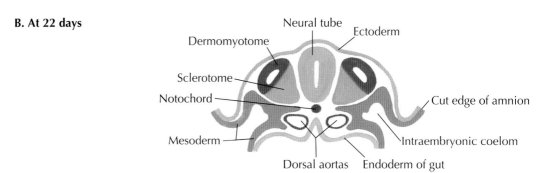

Somite — Neural groove — Ectoderm of embryonic disc
Cut edge of amnion
Mesoderm — Intraembryonic coelom
Notochord — Endoderm (roof of yolk sac)

B. At 22 days

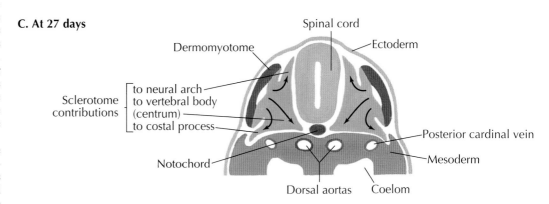

Neural tube
Dermomyotome — Ectoderm
Sclerotome
Notochord — Cut edge of amnion
Mesoderm — Intraembryonic coelom
Dorsal aortas — Endoderm of gut

C. At 27 days

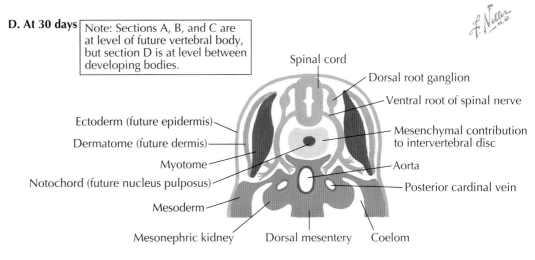

Spinal cord
Dermomyotome — Ectoderm
Sclerotome contributions: to neural arch / to vertebral body (centrum) / to costal process
Posterior cardinal vein
Notochord — Mesoderm
Dorsal aortas — Coelom

D. At 30 days

Note: Sections A, B, and C are at level of future vertebral body, but section D is at level between developing bodies.

Spinal cord
Dorsal root ganglion
Ventral root of spinal nerve
Ectoderm (future epidermis)
Dermatome (future dermis) — Mesenchymal contribution to intervertebral disc
Myotome — Aorta
Notochord (future nucleus pulposus) — Posterior cardinal vein
Mesoderm
Mesonephric kidney — Dorsal mesentery — Coelom

SKULL

The skeleton of the head consists of three primary components: (1) the capsular investments of the sense organs, (2) the brain case, and (3) the branchial arch skeleton (see Plate 1-6). Other than some exceptions of the branchial arch skeleton, these three primary components unite into a composite mammalian skull.

The notochord originally extends into the head of the embryo as far as the oropharyngeal membrane. Its

Plate 1-3

Musculoskeletal System: PART III

DEVELOPMENT OF MUSCULOSKELETAL SYSTEM
(Continued)

termination later shifts to the caudal border of the hypophyseal fossa of the sphenoid bone. (The replacement of the notochord in the head region during evolution involved the formation of a cartilaginous cranium similar to that in the primitive fish of the shark type, which had a skeleton composed of only cartilage.) The earliest indication of skull formation in the human embryo is the concentration of mesenchyme about the notochord at the level of the hindbrain during the fifth and sixth weeks (see Plate 1-3). This mesenchymal skull formation extends forward to form a floor for the developing brain. By the seventh week, the skull begins to become cartilaginous as it completely or incompletely encapsulates the organs of olfaction (nasal capsule), vision (orbitosphenoid), and audition and equilibrium (otic capsule). This chondrocranium is essentially roofless.

As the evolving brain increased in size, additional rudiments were acquired to form a top to the braincase—the calvaria (skullcap). In bony fish, these were derived from the enlarged scales of the head region, which sank into the head and sheathed the chondrocranium to become the bones of the top and sides of the skull and the jaws. These encasing bones derived from the skin are known as dermal, or membrane, bones. In the human embryo, the mesenchymal membrane bone rudiments form the top and sides of the skull and the bones of the face and jaws. They never transform into cartilage; therefore, bone forms directly within the membranous tissue. Most of the membrane bone rudiments become independent bones, but a few become parts of bones formed in the chondrocranium.

The branchial arch skeleton is derived from the embryonic counterparts of the gill arches that support the mouth and pharynx of present-day adult fish and tailed amphibians. The most primitive skeletal rudiments of the branchial arches develop from neural crest cells that migrate into the arches, not from the mesoderm of the arches. The neural crest rudiments become cartilaginous and are retained as cartilage in present-day adult cartilaginous fish, such as the shark, to support the jaw and aqueous respiratory system. In the evolutionary transformation from water breathing to air breathing, much of the skeleton of the aqueous respiratory system was modified to become parts of the air respiratory system, as well as of the modified acoustic apparatus. The human embryo goes through the essential structural stages of this evolutionary water-breathing to air-breathing transformation. Some of the cartilages remain in the adult human (laryngeal cartilages), whereas others become bone (hyoid, styloid process, and ossicles of the middle ear). The branchial arch components originally subserved the function of mastication as well as that of respiration. Although the primitive cartilages of the first branchial arches become the skeletons of the upper and lower jaws in cartilaginous fish, they do not do so in humans, in whom the maxillae and mandible are derived from membrane bones.

Because the brain grows large before birth, the calvaria is much larger than the facial skeleton in the neonate with a ratio of 8:1, compared with a ratio of 2:1 in the adult (see Plate 1-7).

Progressive stages in formation of vertebral column, dermatomes, and myotomes

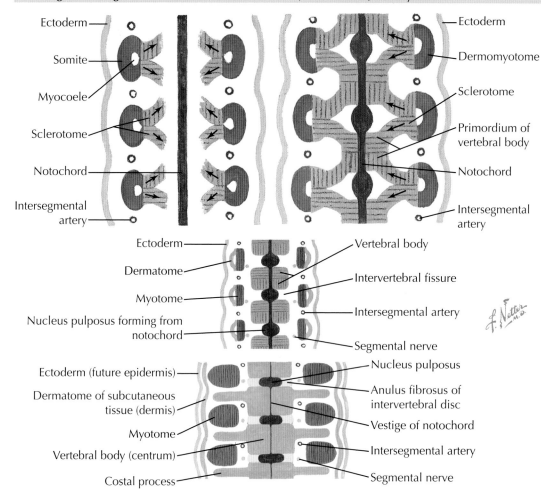

Mesenchymal precartilage primordia of axial and appendicular skeletons at 5 weeks

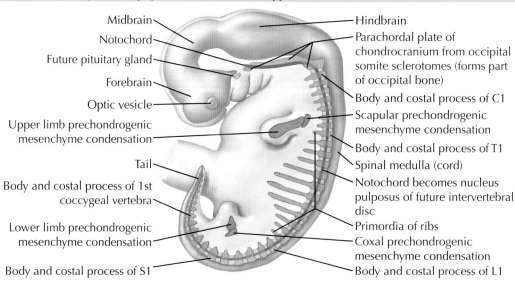

APPENDICULAR SKELETON

The appendicular skeleton consists of the pectoral and pelvic girdles and the bones of the free appendages attached to them. The paired appendages of land vertebrates evolved from the paired fins of fish. The development of the human limbs is a résumé of their evolution.

The upper limb buds appear first, differentiate sooner, and attain their final relative size earlier than the lower limbs (see Plates 1-3, 1-8, and 1-9). Not until birth do the lower limbs equal the upper limbs in length (see Plate 1-7). However, throughout childhood, the lower limbs elongate faster than the upper limbs. In essence, an upper limb was never a lower limb, and vice versa; each has its own unique evolutionary and developmental history. Even so, it is interesting that the structures of the mature upper and lower limbs have a number of similarities. They are most similar during the earliest stages of development, when both sets of

Plate 1-4   Embryology

DEVELOPMENT OF MUSCULOSKELETAL SYSTEM
(Continued)

finlike appendages point caudally. They then become paddle-like and project outward almost at right angles to the body wall. After this, they bend at the elbow and knee directly anteriorly, so that the elbow and knee point laterally, or outward, and the palm and sole face the trunk. Then a series of major changes occurs that causes the upper and lower limbs to differ markedly both structurally and functionally (see Plate 1-8). By the seventh week, both undergo a 90-degree torsion about their long axes, but in opposite directions, so that the elbow points caudally and the knee points cranially. Accompanying this torsion is a permanent twisting of the entire lower limb, which results in its cutaneous innervation assuming a twisted, "barber pole" arrangement (see Plate 1-9). This would be similar to twisting the upper limb so that the forearm and hand become fully and permanently pronated.

The limb buds appear during the fourth week and consist of a core of condensed mesenchyme covered with an epidermal cap, the apical ectodermal ridge. They are functionally related in a two-way process of induction: the mesenchyme induces the development and maintenance of the ridge, which in turn gives the mesenchymal cells the "competence" to form the skeletal rudiments. Any genetic breakdown of differentiating cells or the presence of a teratogenetic substance that interferes with this two-way process of induction results in various limb malformations, such as amelia (total failure of limb development), hemimelia (failure of development of distal parts of limbs), or phocomelia (failure of development of the bulk of the limb but not of its distal part).

Once the appendicular skeleton starts to develop, the progress is rapid. Early in the sixth week, only vague concentrations of mesenchyme represent the primordia of future bones. By the end of the sixth week, these cellular concentrations are sufficiently molded so that some of the larger future bones can be detected. During the seventh week, the primordia of many of the smaller bones of the hand and foot are present.

By the eighth week, well-molded cartilage rudiments represent all the major future bones of the appendicular skeleton.

BONE FORMATION

Bone forms in areas occupied by either connective tissue or cartilage. Bone formed in connective tissue is of intramembranous origin and is called membrane bone. Most of the bones of the calvaria, the facial bones, and, in part, the clavicle and mandible, are membrane bones. All the other bones of the body form in areas occupied by cartilage, which they gradually replace. These bones are of endochondral origin and are called cartilage bones. The terms *membrane bone* and *cartilage bone* merely describe the environment in which a bone forms, not the microscopic structure once the bone is completely developed.

Membrane Bone. The cells of the mesenchymal rudiment of a membrane bone begin to produce a mucoprotein matrix in which collagen fibers are embedded (see Plate 1-10). Within this organic matrix, which is known as osteoid, inorganic crystals of calcium phosphate are deposited between, on, and within the collagen fibers. This mineralization of the osteoid is

FATE OF BODY, COSTAL PROCESS, AND NEURAL ARCH COMPONENTS OF VERTEBRAL COLUMN, WITH SITES AND TIME OF APPEARANCE OF OSSIFICATION CENTERS

Cervical vertebra

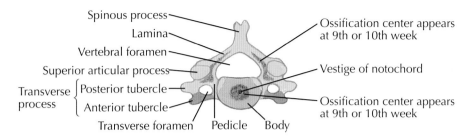

Thoracic vertebra

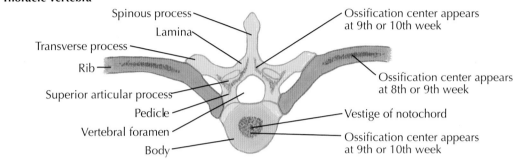

Lumbar vertebra

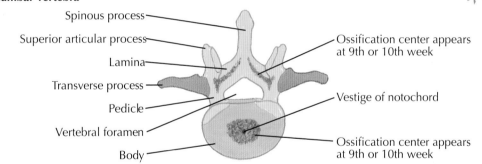

Sacrum

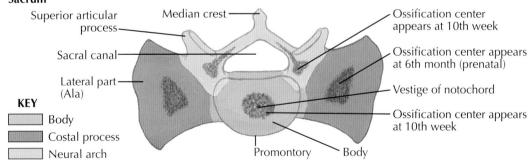

KEY
- Body
- Costal process
- Neural arch

known as ossification. The calcium-to-phosphate ratio increases in the bone matrix as ossification proceeds before birth, chiefly in the form of a series of minerals known as apatites. As development proceeds to the time of birth, hydroxyapatite emerges as the dominant component of bone mineral. Hydroxyapatite is the basic inorganic constituent of mature bone, and its hydroxyl groups are partially substituted by other chemical elements and radicals, such as fluoride or carbonate.

The mesenchymal cells involved in bone formation become known as osteoblasts. As bone formation proceeds, the osteoblasts divide and some become completely surrounded by osteoid. The trapped osteoblasts, then known as osteocytes, send out long, thin extensions of their cell bodies in all directions, which make contact with the cellular extensions of adjacent osteocytes also laying down osteoid (see Plate 1-10). When bone mineral is deposited in the osteoid, the

Plate 1-5

Musculoskeletal System: PART III

DEVELOPMENT OF MUSCULOSKELETAL SYSTEM
(Continued)

space in the matrix housing the portion of the osteocyte containing its nucleus is known as a lacuna, and the tiny, tubular spaces radiating out from the lacuna containing the extensions of the osteocyte are known as canaliculi (see Plate 1-11).

Once the matrix is ossified, diffusion of nutrients to sustain the osteocytes and transport of ions through it cannot occur. Therefore, the canaliculi are the transport channels that interconnect the bone spaces containing blood capillaries and the lacunae surrounding the part of the osteocyte in which the nucleus is located. Because the extensions of the osteocytes fill the canaliculi, the passage of material through the canaliculi is via cell transport.

In the formation of membrane bone, individual shafts of bone, known as trabeculae, are laid down (see Plate 1-10). Trabeculae increase in length and thickness and join each other at various points to produce a lattice framework of primary trabecular bone. At the outer surface of the bone rudiment, the dense sheath of connective tissue acquires an inner layer of osteoblasts to become the periosteum. The osteoblastic layer lays down bone in the form of subperiosteal layers, or lamellae. The coalescing trabeculae in the deeper parts of the rudiment surround capillaries and nerves. Bone is laid down in layers on these trabeculae to constitute the lamellae of primary trabecular bone. Up to the time of birth, the bones of the fetal skeleton are made up chiefly of this type of bone, but near the time of birth, this primary trabecular bone begins to transform into compact bone (see Plate 1-11).

The transformation from trabecular to compact bone is essentially the reduction in the size of the marrow spaces containing mesenchymal cells, capillaries, and nerve fibers. The relatively large marrow spaces with their surrounding bony trabeculae are known as primary osteons. The osteoblasts lining the trabeculae surrounding a marrow space (which contains one or two capillaries, some perivascular cells, and a non-myelinated and occasionally a myelinated nerve fiber) lay down bone in concentric layers, or lamellae. This process continues until the marrow space is nearly obliterated, leaving a small central osteonal, or haversian, canal. The canal is about 50 μm in diameter and usually contains a single capillary and nerve fiber and some perivascular cells in the center of what is known as a secondary osteon (haversian system). There are from 4 to 20 (usually 6 or less) concentric lamellae that are each 3 to 7 μm thick. The formation of many such adjacent secondary osteons converts what was originally trabecular bone into compact bone. In the central core of a membrane bone, the marrow cavities persist and their mesenchymal tissue develops into hematopoietic red bone marrow. Thus, in a fully formed, flat bone of the calvaria, there is an inner and outer table of compact bone, between which is trabecular bone surrounding a marrow cavity, the diploë.

The secondary osteons of compact bone usually run the length of a bone. In cross section, the outer limit of each osteon is clearly demarcated by a narrow refractile ring known as a cement line, which lacks collagen fibrils and is highly mineralized. The central haversian canals are connected to one another and communicate with the periosteal surface as well as with the marrow cavity via transverse and oblique channels known as Volkmann's canals. The blood flows through the

compact bone from the inner marrow cavity via vessels in Volkmann's and haversian canals until it emerges at the periosteal surface.

Cartilage Bone. The cartilage rudiments of bones of endochondral origin are temporary miniatures of the future adult bone. With the exception of the clavicle, the long bones are of endochondral origin. The first of two or more ossification centers of a long bone appears in the shaft, or diaphysis (see Plate 1-12). Diaphyseal

ossification is actually a form of intramembranous ossification, because bone is laid down by the connective tissue outer sheath of the cartilage rudiment known as the perichondrium. The perichondrium becomes known as the periosteum once it starts to lay down bone in the form of a delicate collar surrounding the center of the diaphysis of the cartilage rudiment. Deep to this collar of bone, the cartilage matrix becomes calcified and the chondrocytes hypertrophy.

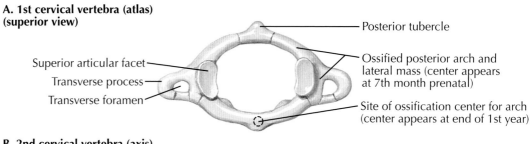

First and second cervical vertebrae at birth

A. 1st cervical vertebra (atlas)
(superior view)

Posterior tubercle

Superior articular facet

Ossified posterior arch and lateral mass (center appears at 7th month prenatal)

Transverse process

Transverse foramen

Site of ossification center for arch (center appears at end of 1st year)

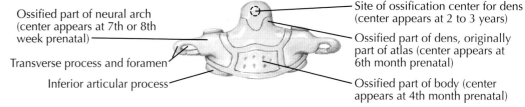

B. 2nd cervical vertebra (axis)
(anterior view)

Ossified part of neural arch (center appears at 7th or 8th week prenatal)

Site of ossification center for dens (center appears at 2 to 3 years)

Ossified part of dens, originally part of atlas (center appears at 6th month prenatal)

Transverse process and foramen

Inferior articular process

Ossified part of body (center appears at 4th month prenatal)

Development of sternum

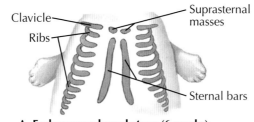

Clavicle

Suprasternal masses

Ribs

Sternal bars

A. Early mesenchymal stage (6 weeks)

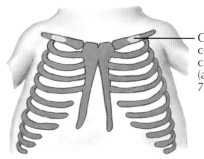

Ossification center for clavicle (appears at 7th week)

B. Late mesenchymal stage (8 weeks)

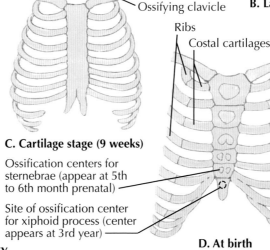

Ossifying clavicle

Ribs

Costal cartilages

Sternal angle (other sternal joints disappear between puberty and 25th year)

Manubrium

Body

C. Cartilage stage (9 weeks)

Ossification centers for sternebrae (appear at 5th to 6th month prenatal)

Site of ossification center for xiphoid process (center appears at 3rd year)

D. At birth

Xiphoid process (still largely cartilage)

E. Young adulthood

KEY

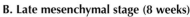

- Mesenchyme
- Cartilage
- Bone

Plate 1-6

Embryology

DEVELOPMENT OF MUSCULOSKELETAL SYSTEM
(Continued)

Irruption canals appear in the bony collar through which vascular buds of capillaries and mesenchymal cells pass from the periosteum to the calcified cartilage, which undergoes a breakdown. Most of the chondrocytes within this degrading matrix die via programmed cell death mechanisms. This process brings into existence primordial marrow cavities, which contain osteoblasts, and vascular marrow tissue, which is derived from the irruption canal cells. The osteoblasts initially lay down bone along the remaining spicules of calcified cartilage matrix. As a result, the endochondral bone becomes trabecular. As the periosteal and the endochondral bone formation occurring at the center of the diaphysis extends toward each end of the long bone, a large central medullary (marrow) cavity arises in the trabecular bone of the diaphysis. Toward the end of fetal life and continuing into puberty, ossification centers appear in the two cartilaginous ends, or epiphyses, of the long bone (see Plate 1-12). Between the bone formed in the diaphysis and that formed in the epiphysis is the epiphyseal plate, a circular mass of cartilage in a region of the long bone known as the metaphysis. It is at the epiphyseal plate that the diaphysis continues to grow in length.

BONE GROWTH

Cartilage grows continually on the side of the epiphyseal plate facing the epiphysis of a long bone, while on the opposite side of the plate facing the diaphysis, cartilage breaks down continually and is replaced by bone (see Plate 1-12). These epiphyseal growth plates persist during the entire postnatal growth period. The plates are finally resorbed and replaced by bone that joins the epiphyses permanently to the diaphysis when the skeleton has acquired its adult size. The epiphyses unite with the diaphysis sooner in females than in males, so that growth in length ceases about 2 years earlier in females. In males, most fusions of the epiphyses with the diaphyses end at about age 20. Interference with the normal growth occurring at the epiphyseal plates of the appendicular skeleton results in abnormally short limbs, such as those of an achondroplastic dwarf who may have a head and body of normal length.

Peripheral growth of a typical flat bone of membrane origin occurs at the margins that articulate via connective tissue with other flat bones. At first, these articulations are broad. At certain intervals between the growing skull bones, even wider gaps known as fonticuli, or fontanels, occur (see Plate 1-7). Of these large, soft spots, the two sphenoid fonticuli may become nearly obliterated as early as 6 months after birth, whereas the two mastoid fonticuli and the single anterior fonticulus are nearly obliterated by age 2. Obliteration of the narrow intervals between the bones of the calvaria, the sutures, does not begin until about age 30.

Growth in width of a flat membrane bone and a long endochondral bone is similar. The osteoblasts of the periosteum of both the outer and inner tables of a flat bone and of the surface of a long bone lay down bone in the form of subperiosteal circumferential layers, or lamellae, that are parallel to the bone surface (see Plate 1-13). To prevent an overly thick mass of compact bone from forming as the bone grows in width, bone is resorbed concomitantly at the endosteal surface bordering the marrow cavity. This laying down of bone at the surface involves a peripheral shift of osteons that retains the necessary distance between the intrinsic blood supply and the osteocytes of the bone. There is an eccentric resorption of osteons on the side facing the outer surface of the widening bone. The bone resorption is the result of progenitor cells within the central haversian canal modulating into osteoclasts, as well as osteoclastic activity of the osteocytes within the lacunae of the circular lamellae in the path of bone erosion. The dissolution of their surrounding matrix by individual osteocytes is known as osteocytic osteolysis. When these osteoclastic osteocytes are released from their lacunae, they may fuse with each other to form multinucleated osteoclasts. Plate 1-13 shows the sequence of events in this destruction of osteons and the formation of new ones.

EARLY DEVELOPMENT OF SKULL

Chondrocranium at 9 weeks

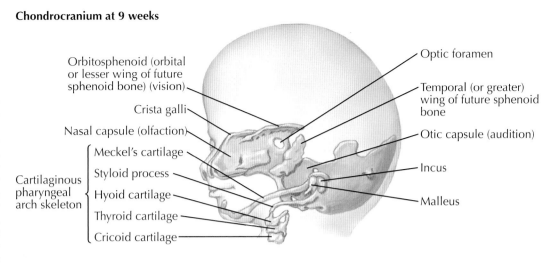

Orbitosphenoid (orbital or lesser wing of future sphenoid bone) (vision)
Crista galli
Nasal capsule (olfaction)
Cartilaginous pharyngeal arch skeleton
Meckel's cartilage
Styloid process
Hyoid cartilage
Thyroid cartilage
Cricoid cartilage
Optic foramen
Temporal (or greater) wing of future sphenoid bone
Otic capsule (audition)
Incus
Malleus

Membrane bones at 9 weeks

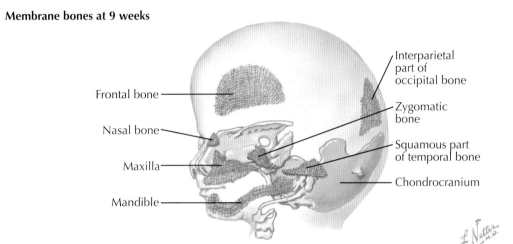

Frontal bone
Nasal bone
Maxilla
Mandible
Interparietal part of occipital bone
Zygomatic bone
Squamous part of temporal bone
Chondrocranium

Membrane bones at 12 weeks

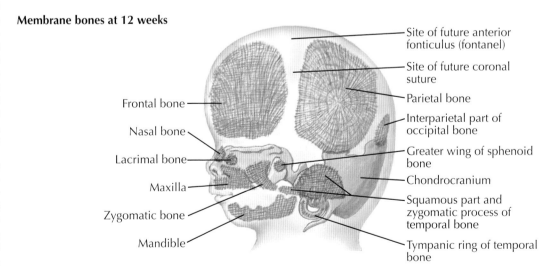

Frontal bone
Nasal bone
Lacrimal bone
Maxilla
Zygomatic bone
Mandible
Site of future anterior fonticulus (fontanel)
Site of future coronal suture
Parietal bone
Interparietal part of occipital bone
Greater wing of sphenoid bone
Chondrocranium
Squamous part and zygomatic process of temporal bone
Tympanic ring of temporal bone

Plate 1-7

Musculoskeletal System: PART III

DEVELOPMENT OF MUSCULOSKELETAL SYSTEM
(Continued)

BONE REMODELING

For a bone to maintain its proper form and proportions while it lengthens and thickens, the growth process must involve more than merely bone formation at the periosteal surface and concomitant bone resorption at the endosteal surface (see Plate 1-14). Progressive remodeling, with formation and resorption (or a reversal of this process), must occur at all parts of the bone as its dimensions alter. At times, all activity ceases.

Although bone remodeling begins during the fetal period, it is not very active before birth but accelerates during the first year after birth. The annual rate of bone renewal during the first 2 years after birth is 50%, compared with a rate of 5% in the adult. During the first 2 years after birth, the infant progresses from an essentially helpless state to an erect walking individual.

At birth, the ossification centers present in the skeleton are, with few exceptions, primary centers (see Plate 1-7). The exceptions are the secondary, or epiphyseal, centers in the distal condyle of the femur in the proximal condyle of the tibia and possibly in the head of the humerus; numerous primary centers do not form until a number of years after birth. The mechanical stresses on the skeleton, as the infant begins to acquire increasing voluntary neuromuscular function during its first 2 years, serve to stimulate skeletal growth, ossification, and especially remodeling. During bone remodeling, the attachments of muscles and ligaments are also shifted and modified. Bone remodeling is most active during the growing period but continues throughout life in response to stresses created by an individual's ever-changing type of physical activity.

DEVELOPMENTAL HISTORY OF BONES

Each of the more than 200 bones of the skeleton has its own developmental history. Some bones have a simple history, whereas others have quite a complicated one. The history of the clavicle and mandible is unique. The clavicle is the first bone in the entire skeleton to ossify (during the 7th week), followed shortly thereafter by the mandible (see Plates 1-5 and 1-6). Both the clavicle and the mandible are originally membrane bones that secondarily develop growth cartilage. The temporal bone is a good example of a bone with a complicated developmental history. It is a composite bone that forms initially as the otic capsule enclosing the organ for audition and equilibrium (inner ear) of the primitive chondrocranium, which then acquires secondary additions. Its squamous part, zygomatic process, and tympanic ring are derived from membrane bones, whereas its styloid process and ear ossicles are derived from the branchial arch skeleton. Although the overall size of the temporal bone is less than half its adult size at birth, the bony labyrinth of the inner ear, the middle ear cavity, the ear ossicles, and the eardrum have attained their adult size at birth. In contrast, the articular tubercle and mastoid process are absent at birth (see Plates 1-6 and 1-7).

HOMEOSTASIS

Homeostasis is the maintenance of constant conditions in the internal environment of the body. There is a constant turnover of bone mineral throughout life in

response to mechanical stresses exerted on the skeleton. The bones of athletes become considerably heavier than those of nonathletes. Owing to the atrophy of disuse, the bones of a limb immobilized in a cast become thin and demineralized. In astronauts, a general demineralization of the entire skeleton occurs in response to the weightlessness caused by the lack of gravity in outer space. These alterations in the mineral content of bones allow the skeleton to serve as a dynamic structural

support of the body. However, this support function is not really significant until the end of the first year after birth when the child starts to walk. Long before that time, the alterations in the mineral content of the bones are a part of another function of the skeleton related to the homeostasis of the body.

About 56% of the adult human body consists of fluid. There is intracellular fluid within the 75 trillion cells of the body and extracellular fluid outside the cells. The

SKELETON OF FULL-TERM NEWBORN
Time of appearance of ossification centers (primary unless otherwise indicated)

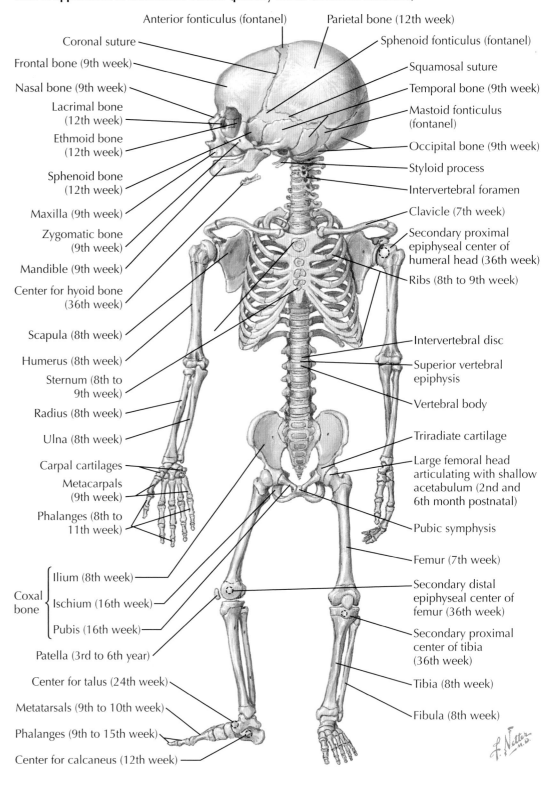

- Anterior fonticulus (fontanel)
- Coronal suture
- Frontal bone (9th week)
- Nasal bone (9th week)
- Lacrimal bone (12th week)
- Ethmoid bone (12th week)
- Sphenoid bone (12th week)
- Maxilla (9th week)
- Zygomatic bone (9th week)
- Mandible (9th week)
- Center for hyoid bone (36th week)
- Scapula (8th week)
- Humerus (8th week)
- Sternum (8th to 9th week)
- Radius (8th week)
- Ulna (8th week)
- Carpal cartilages
- Metacarpals (9th week)
- Phalanges (8th to 11th week)
- Coxal bone
  - Ilium (8th week)
  - Ischium (16th week)
  - Pubis (16th week)
- Patella (3rd to 6th year)
- Center for talus (24th week)
- Metatarsals (9th to 10th week)
- Phalanges (9th to 15th week)
- Center for calcaneus (12th week)

- Parietal bone (12th week)
- Sphenoid fonticulus (fontanel)
- Squamosal suture
- Temporal bone (9th week)
- Mastoid fonticulus (fontanel)
- Occipital bone (9th week)
- Styloid process
- Intervertebral foramen
- Clavicle (7th week)
- Secondary proximal epiphyseal center of humeral head (36th week)
- Ribs (8th to 9th week)
- Intervertebral disc
- Superior vertebral epiphysis
- Vertebral body
- Triradiate cartilage
- Large femoral head articulating with shallow acetabulum (2nd and 6th month postnatal)
- Pubic symphysis
- Femur (7th week)
- Secondary distal epiphyseal center of femur (36th week)
- Secondary proximal center of tibia (36th week)
- Tibia (8th week)
- Fibula (8th week)

Plate 1-8   Embryology

DEVELOPMENT OF MUSCULOSKELETAL SYSTEM
(Continued)

cells are capable of living, growing, and providing their special functions as long as proper concentrations of oxygen, glucose, ions, amino acids, and fatty substances are available in the internal environment. The skeleton plays a vital role in the regulation of calcium metabolism, which is fully described in Section 3, Metabolic Diseases.

BLOOD SUPPLY

Hematopoiesis, or the formation of blood cells, begins before birth. The first hematopoietic cells to appear are erythrocytes, or red blood cells. They are derived from the extraembryonic mesoderm of the yolk sac during the third week. During the fifth week, the erythrocytes are derived primarily from the liver and secondarily from the spleen. The myeloid, or bone marrow, period of hematopoiesis begins during the fourth month. Chiefly, granulocytes, or white blood cells, are initially derived from the bone marrow, while the liver and spleen continue to give rise to only erythrocytes. The marrow tissue also gives rise to the lymphoid stem cells that migrate both to the thymus to induce differentiation of T cells involved in cellular immunity and to the intestinal walls to induce differentiation of B cells involved in antibody production. During the fifth month, the liver erythropoiesis begins to diminish, while the bone marrow, in addition to granulocytes, begins to give rise to erythrocytes. The bone marrow is the principal site of all blood cell formation during the last 3 months before birth. At birth, hematopoiesis occurs almost exclusively in the bone marrow, because only residual hematopoiesis occurs in the liver and spleen.

During the first 3 or 4 years after birth, almost all the bones of the body contain hematopoietic marrow, although regression of hematopoiesis begins in the distal phalanges of the digits before birth, and the red marrow of the phalanges of the toes is completely replaced by yellow, fatty marrow by 1 year of age. Shortly before puberty, yellow marrow appears in the distal ends of the long bones of the forearm, arm, leg, and thigh and gradually extends proximally until 20 years of age, by which age only the upper end of the humerus and femur still contain red marrow.

The other bones in which hematopoiesis occurs in the skeleton of the young adult are the vertebrae, ribs, sternum, clavicles, scapulae, coxal (hip) bones, and skull.

Blood reaches the marrow cavity of the diaphysis of a long bone via one or two relatively large diaphyseal nutrient arteries. The nutrient artery passes obliquely through the nutrient foramen of the bone, without branching and in a direction that usually points away from the end of the bone, where the greatest amount of growth is occurring at the epiphyseal plate. Once the nutrient artery enters the marrow cavity, it sends off branches that pass toward the two ends of the bone to anastomose with a number of branches of small metaphyseal arteries that pass directly through the bone into the marrow cavity at the two metaphyses. The arteries of the metaphysis supply the metaphyseal side of the epiphyseal growth plate of cartilage.

Numerous small epiphyseal arteries pass directly through the bone into the marrow cavity of the epiphyses at each end of the bone. The epiphyseal arteries

Changes in position of limbs before birth

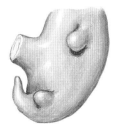
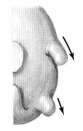
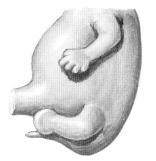
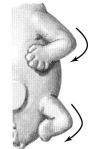

At 5 weeks. Upper and lower limbs have formed as finlike appendages pointing laterally and caudally.

At 6 weeks. Limbs bend anteriorly, so elbows and knees point laterally, palms and soles face trunk.

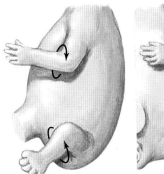
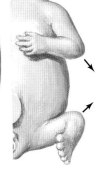
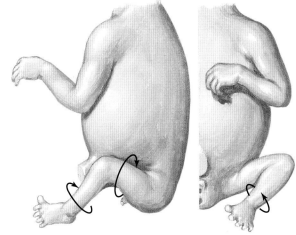

At 7 weeks. Upper and lower limbs have undergone 90-degree torsion about their long axes, but in opposite directions, so elbows point caudally and knees cranially.

At 8 weeks. Torsion of lower limbs results in twisted or "barber pole" arrangement of their cutaneous innervation.

Precartilage mesenchymal cell concentrations of appendicular skeleton at 6th week

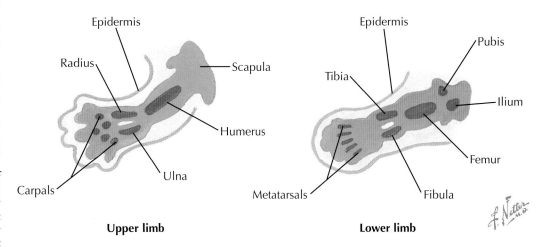

Upper limb

Epidermis
Radius
Scapula
Humerus
Ulna
Carpals

Lower limb

Epidermis
Pubis
Tibia
Ilium
Femur
Fibula
Metatarsals

supply the deep part of the articular cartilage and the epiphyseal side of the epiphyseal growth plate. In a growing bone with a relatively thick growth plate, there are few, if any, anastomoses between the epiphyseal and metaphyseal vessels. The growth plate also receives a blood supply from a collar of periosteal arteries adjacent to the periphery of the plate.

The branches of the diaphyseal nutrient arteries, which pass to each end of the bone to anastomose with the metaphyseal arteries, give off two sets of branches

along the way, one peripheral and one central. The peripheral set passes directly to the bone as arterioles that give off the capillaries that enter Volkmann's canals and branch to supply the central haversian canals, ultimately emerging at the outer surface of the bone and anastomosing with the periosteal vessels. The direction of the blood flow in these capillaries is from within the bone outward; thus, the blood flow through the canal system of the bony wall is relatively slow and at a low pressure.

Plate 1-9   Musculoskeletal System: PART III

DEVELOPMENT OF MUSCULOSKELETAL SYSTEM

(Continued)

The central set of branches given off by the diaphyseal nutrient arteries become arterioles that join plexuses of large irregularly shaped capillaries known as sinusoids. In a young child, sinusoids, which are the sites of hematopoiesis, are found throughout the marrow cavity. An extensive, delicate meshwork of reticular fibers containing hematopoietic cells, fibroblasts, and occasional fat cells surrounds the single-celled endothelial wall of the sinusoids; this constitutes red marrow. The newly formed blood cells eventually pass out of the sinusoids into large veins that directly pierce the diaphyseal bony shaft, without branching, as the venae comitantes of the nutrient diaphyseal arteries. Others pass directly through the bony wall, without branching, as independent emissary veins.

The myeloid, or bone marrow, period of hematopoiesis begins during the fourth month. The bone marrow is the principal site of all blood cell formation during the last 3 months before birth, at which time only residual hematopoiesis occurs in the liver and spleen.

SYMPHYSEAL JOINTS

In the first vertebrates, the skeleton evolved as an axial skeleton, the vertebral column. The segmentation that evolved in the increasingly substantial column allowed the necessary swimming movements that the flexible notochord afforded the prevertebrates. Intervening regions between the firmer segments of the column became pliable cartilage that allowed very limited and yet every possible type of motion between the firmer segments. Thus, in humans, intervertebral discs between the vertebral bodies allow a limited degree of twisting and bending in all directions. However, the sum total of a given motion occurring between the vertebral bodies throughout the column is considerable.

The multiaxial joint between the vertebral bodies is known as a symphysis because of its structure. A central portion of fibrocartilage, including the nucleus pulposus, blends with a layer of hyaline cartilage lining the surface of each of the two vertebral bodies bordering the joint. The only symphysis of the appendicular skeleton is the pubic symphysis (see Plate 1-7).

Because a symphyseal joint has limited motion, it is an amphiarthrosis. A central cleft containing fluid occurs in some symphyses, such as the pubic and manubriosternal (sternal angle) joints, but true gliding surfaces do not develop (see Plate 1-5). This is an intermediate phase in the evolution of synovial joints.

Although the majority of articulations of the appendicular skeleton are synovial joints, many of the articulations of the axial skeleton are also typical synovial joints. For example, the numerous joints between the articular processes of the vertebral arches are synovial joints of the plane variety in that their apposed articular surfaces are fairly flat (see Plate 1-4).

SYNOVIAL JOINTS

Synovial, or diarthrodial, joints have a wide range of motion; they link cartilaginous bones with one another and with certain membrane bones, such as the mandible and clavicle.

The earliest mesenchymal rudiments of long bones are essentially continuous. As the rudiments pass into

the precartilage stage, the sites of the future joints can be discerned as intervals of less concentrated mesenchyme (see Plate 1-15). When the mesenchymal rudiments transform into cartilage, the mesenchymal cells in the future joint region become flattened in the center. At the periphery of the future joint, these flattened cells are continuous with the investing perichondrium; this perichondral investment becomes the joint capsule.

During the third month, the joint cavity arises from a cleft that appears in the circumferential part of the mesenchyme. The mesenchymal cells in the center of the developing joint disappear, allowing the cartilage rudiments to come into direct contact with each other, and, for a time, a transitory fusion may result in a small area of direct cartilaginous union. Soon, all the remaining mesenchymal cells undergo dissolution and a distinct joint cavity is formed. The surrounding joint

CHANGES IN VENTRAL DERMATOME PATTERN (CUTANEOUS SENSORY NERVE DISTRIBUTION) DURING LIMB DEVELOPMENT

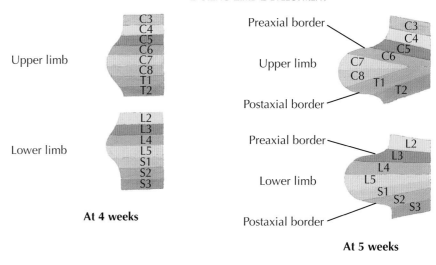

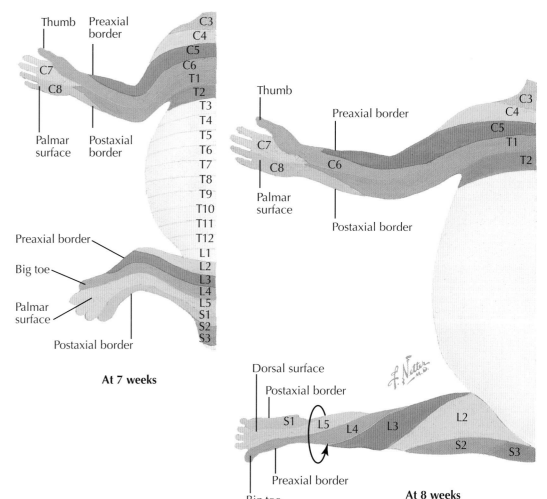

Plate 1-10

Embryology

DEVELOPMENT OF MUSCULOSKELETAL SYSTEM
(Continued)

capsule maintains its continuity with the perichondrium when it becomes transformed into periosteum as the cartilage rudiments become bones. The original cartilage of the rudiment forming the joint surface is retained as the articular hyaline cartilage.

Deep to the articular cartilage, epiphyseal bone is laid down. Because the articular cartilage was never actually lined with perichondrium, it grows in thickness by intrinsic, or interstitial, growth. Some perichondrium is retained at the periphery of the articular cartilage, which continues to form cartilage until the articular surface of the joint attains adult size. Once full growth is attained, the chondrocytes normally do not undergo division.

Articular cartilage, especially that found in weight-bearing joints, is uniquely structured to withstand tremendous abuse. It can resist crushing by static loads considerably greater than those required to break a bone. No painful sensations are elicited in traumatized cartilage because it lacks nerves. The chondrocytes in weight-bearing joints are genetically programmed to tolerate crushing forces without overreacting, such as by inducing their surrounding matrix to undergo extensive dissolution or by laying down excessive amounts of matrix. Such responses would markedly alter the surface contour of the cartilage in a manner that would interfere with the normal joint motion.

As soon as the joint cavity appears during development, it contains watery fluid. The joint capsule develops an outer fibrous portion that is lined with an inner, more highly vascularized synovial membrane. Although this membrane lines the fibrous capsule as well as any bony surfaces, ligaments, and tendons within the joint, it does not line the surfaces of the joint discs, menisci, or articular cartilage.

The synovial membrane is the site of formation of the synovial fluid that fills the joint cavity. This fluid is similar to that found in bursae and tendon sheaths. Before birth, it is sticky, viscous, and much like egg white in consistency. Only a small amount of the fluid is normally present in a joint cavity, where it forms a sticky film that lines all the surfaces of the joint cavity (for example, the adult knee joint contains only a little more than 1 mL of synovial fluid). Even so, before birth and thereafter, the fluid is the chief source of nourishment of the chondrocytes of the articular cartilage, which lacks blood and lymphatic vessels.

The articular cartilage is never very thick, averaging 1 to 2 mm in thickness in the adult and reaching a maximum of 5 to 7 mm in the larger joints of young individuals. However, compared with cells in the vascularized tissue of the body, which are not more than 25 to 50 μm from a capillary, the chondrocytes are at an enormous distance from their source of nourishment. Joint activity enhances both the diffusion of nutrients through the cartilage matrix to the chondrocytes and the diffusion of metabolic waste products away from them. The alternating compression and decompression of the cartilage during joint activity produce a pumping action that enhances the exchange

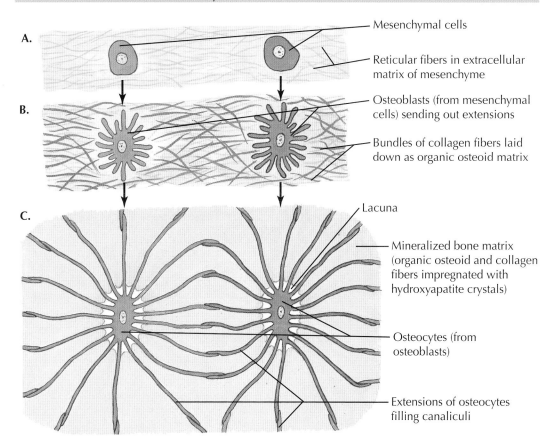

Initial bone formation in mesenchyme

A. — Mesenchymal cells
— Reticular fibers in extracellular matrix of mesenchyme

B. — Osteoblasts (from mesenchymal cells) sending out extensions
— Bundles of collagen fibers laid down as organic osteoid matrix

C. — Lacuna
— Mineralized bone matrix (organic osteoid and collagen fibers impregnated with hydroxyapatite crystals)
— Osteocytes (from osteoblasts)
— Extensions of osteocytes filling canaliculi

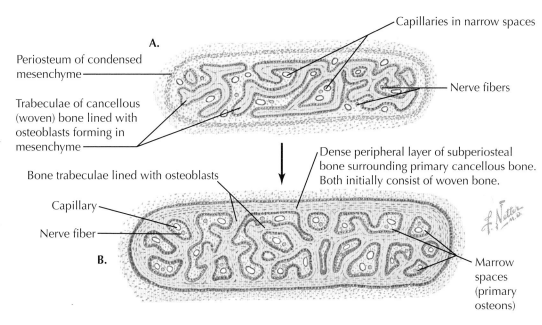

Early stages of flat (membrane or dermal) bone formation

A. — Capillaries in narrow spaces
Periosteum of condensed mesenchyme —
— Nerve fibers
Trabeculae of cancellous (woven) bone lined with osteoblasts forming in mesenchyme —

Bone trabeculae lined with osteoblasts —
— Dense peripheral layer of subperiosteal bone surrounding primary cancellous bone. Both initially consist of woven bone.
Capillary —
Nerve fiber —
B. — Marrow spaces (primary osteons)

of nutrients and waste products between the cartilage matrix and the synovial fluid.

In some developing joints, the mesenchymal tissue between the cartilage rudiments, instead of disappearing, gives rise to a fibrous sheet that completely divides the joint into two separate compartments. The sheet develops into an intra-articular disc, which is made up of fibrous connective tissue and, possibly, a small amount of fibrocartilage. A separate synovial cavity develops on each side of the disc, as found in the temporomandibular joint.

In other developing joints, the mesenchymal tissue between the cartilage rudiments gives rise to a fibrous sheet that is incomplete centrally. This fibrous sheet projects from the joint capsule into a single joint cavity and gives rise to articular menisci consisting of fibrous tissue and possibly a small amount of fibrocartilage, such as found in the knee joint.

Plate 1-11

Musculoskeletal System: PART III

DEVELOPMENT OF MUSCULOSKELETAL SYSTEM
(Continued)

After the synovial joint cavity is established during the third month, the muscles that move the joint begin to undergo contractions. This movement is essential for the normal development of the synovial joints, because it not only enhances the nutrition of the articular cartilage but also prevents fusion between the apposed articular cartilages.

Restriction of joint motion by permanent paralysis early in development can result in the loss of the joint cavity by having a permanent fusion occur between the apposed surfaces of the articular cartilage. If the restriction of joint movement occurs later in development, the joint space may be present but the associated soft tissues of the joint are abnormal. An example is the nongenetic form of clubfoot (talipes varus) caused by the severe restriction of movement of the ankle joint before birth. The normal positioning of the fetus in the uterus allows a fair degree of movement of the upper limbs, but the lower limbs are folded together and pressed firmly against the body. The hip and knee joints are flexed and the feet are inverted in the pigeon-toed position. The ankle joint may become fixed in this inverted position because of the abnormal shortening of the muscles that invert the foot and the lengthening of their antagonists. Also, the ligaments on the medial side of the ankle joint may become abnormally shortened.

HIP JOINT

The upper limbs are far more functionally advanced at birth than are the lower limbs. The neonate can reflexly grasp objects firmly with the hands. In contrast, the underdeveloped lower limbs are reflexly maintained in the position they were held in before birth and in fact their straightening is strongly resisted. Relative to this, the very underdeveloped hip joint is prone to dislocation when the limbs are shortened. The hip socket, or acetabulum, is normally very small compared with the relatively large head of the femur (see Plate 1-7). When the lower limbs arc in the fetal position, the firm ligament of the head of the femur, by virtue of its attachments, strongly prevents the hip joint from becoming dislocated posterosuperiorly. However, if the ligament is abnormally long, it will not prevent a posterosuperior dislocation.

Normally, the ligament does not function to prevent hip dislocation in any limb position other than the fetal one. The thin, flimsy joint capsule is the chief resistance to dislocation when the limbs are not held in the fetal position. Once the infant tends to maintain the lower limbs in extension in the months after birth, the hip joint becomes secure and the ligament of the head of the femur serves no further useful function.

ERECT POSTURE

During the evolution of the human erect posture, the lumbar joints and especially the lumbosacral joint

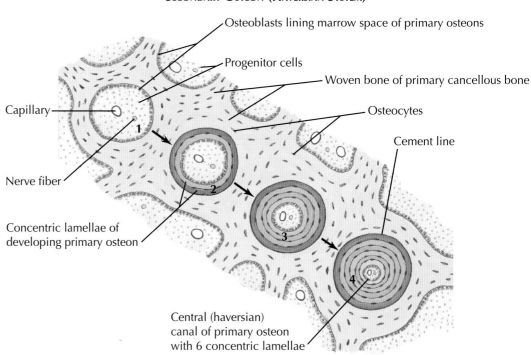

Osteoblasts lining marrow space of primary osteons

Progenitor cells

Woven bone of primary cancellous bone

Capillary

Osteocytes

Cement line

Nerve fiber

Concentric lamellae of developing primary osteon

Central (haversian) canal of primary osteon with 6 concentric lamellae

A. Successive stages in formation of primary osteon (haversian system) during transformation of cancellous to compact bone (schematic)

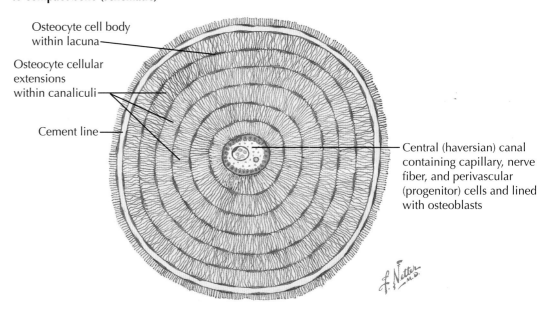

Osteocyte cell body within lacuna

Osteocyte cellular extensions within canaliculi

Cement line

Central (haversian) canal containing capillary, nerve fiber, and perivascular (progenitor) cells and lined with osteoblasts

B. Diagram of primary osteon (haversian system) with 6 concentric lamellae (greatly enlarged)

acquired the ability to undergo a pronounced extension that allows a marked lumbar curvature, or lordosis, of the vertebral column. Except for the fixed sacral curve, the vertebral column at birth has no curves. The thoracic part of the spine gradually develops a relatively fixed curve in the young child. A flexible cervical curve appears when the infant is able to raise the head, and a flexible lumbar curve appears at the end of the first year when the child starts to walk. The lumbar curve is

necessary to attain the erect posture, because the pelvis remains essentially in the same position as that in a standing quadruped.

The fact that the pelvis did not shift from its quadruped position during evolution of the erect posture also necessitated placing the hip and knee joints into full extension. In addition, the arch of the foot evolved so that the bones were structurally arranged to bear the body weight with a minimum of muscular activity.

Plate 1-12

Embryology

DEVELOPMENT OF MUSCULOSKELETAL SYSTEM
(Continued)

Therefore, in the human, the passive ligaments of the foot bones and those of the fully extended hip and knee joints bear the brunt of the forces involved in standing erect.

Only humans stand perfectly erect. Quadrupeds, including the knuckle-walking apes, can only mimic the erect human posture. They do it with a great expenditure of muscular energy because their hip and knee joints cannot be fully extended so that the passive ligaments of the joints can withstand the brunt of the forces involved in standing erect. This same expenditure of energy is made when a child first starts to stand with the hip and knee joints partially flexed. The erect human posture may appear to be a most awkward position compared with the normal standing posture of quadrupeds, but it is the most efficient and economical posture that ever evolved. Once a person rises by muscular activity to the fully erect position, only occasional brief contractions of postural muscles are required to keep the head, trunk, and limbs aligned with the vertical line of the center of gravity. The upper limbs are included in the economics of the erect posture because the passive ligaments of the joints, not the muscles of the upper limbs, bear the brunt of supporting the limbs as they hang at the sides of the body.

MUSCLES

Characteristically, all living cells, including protozoa and slime molds, contain the contractile proteins actin and myosin. Thus, actin and myosin are present in all the cells of the human body—from the most highly differentiated nerve cells to the shed fragments of megakaryocyte cytoplasm, the platelets, which are important in the formation of blood clots. Actin and myosin are arranged in the cytoplasm of a cell to interact and slide in relationship to one another to produce contraction of the cell when driven by the energy supplied by the hydrolysis of adenosine triphosphate.

During the evolution of single-celled protozoa into metazoa, or multicellular organisms, cells became specialized to perform specific functions. Certain cells accumulated larger than usual amounts of actin and myosin in their cytoplasm to become muscle cells scattered throughout the body of the primitive metazoan. As the higher forms developed distinct organ systems, the muscle cells grouped together to become the smooth (involuntary, visceral, nonsegmental) muscles of the viscera and blood vessels.

SMOOTH AND CARDIAC MUSCLE

All the smooth and cardiac muscle cells in the human embryo arise from mesoderm, except the sphincter and dilator smooth muscles of the iris of the eye and the myoepithelial cells of the sweat and mammary glands, which arise from ectoderm. Both smooth and cardiac muscle cells have a centrally placed nucleus. During development, numerous smooth muscle cells become elongated in the same direction and form layers, such as the circular and longitudinal smooth muscle layers of the small intestine.

For a time during evolution, a simple layer of smooth muscle surrounding the vessels of the circulatory system was also sufficient for the demands of function. However, as organisms became larger and increasingly complex, the need arose for the system to have a strong pump—the heart. In the human embryo, two endothelial tubes fuse to become one vessel, which then becomes surrounded with mesenchyme that differentiates into cardiac. The muscle cells surrounding the developing heart accumulated a larger amount of more compactly and more orderly arranged actin and myosin molecules than did simple smooth muscle cells. Despite undergoing repeated mitotic divisions, they remained attached to one another in such a manner that they formed long tubes of cells known as fibers.

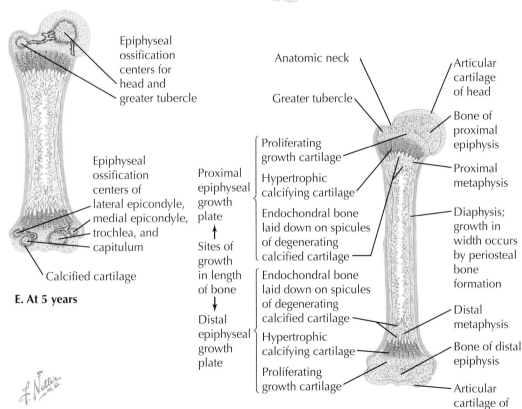

GROWTH AND OSSIFICATION OF LONG BONES (HUMERUS, MIDFRONTAL SECTIONS)

A. At 8 weeks

Perichondrium

Periosteum

Proliferating small cell hyaline cartilage

Hypertrophic calcifying cartilage

Thin collar of cancellous bone from periosteum around diaphysis

B. At 9 weeks

Canals, containing capillaries, periosteal mesenchymal cells, and osteoblasts, passing through periosteal bone into calcified cartilage (primary ossification center)

C. At 10 weeks

Epiphyseal capillaries

Cancellous endochondral bone laid down on spicules of calcified cartilage

Primordial marrow cavities

D. At birth

Calcified cartilage

Epiphysial (secondary) ossification center for head

Outer part of periosteal bone beginning to transform into compact bone

Central marrow (medullary) cavity

Epiphyseal capillary

E. At 5 years

Epiphyseal ossification centers for head and greater tubercle

Epiphyseal ossification centers of lateral epicondyle, medial epicondyle, trochlea, and capitulum

Calcified cartilage

F. At 10 years

Anatomic neck

Greater tubercle

Proliferating growth cartilage

Hypertrophic calcifying cartilage

Endochondral bone laid down on spicules of degenerating calcified cartilage

Endochondral bone laid down on spicules of degenerating calcified cartilage

Hypertrophic calcifying cartilage

Proliferating growth cartilage

Proximal epiphyseal growth plate

Sites of growth in length of bone

Distal epiphyseal growth plate

Articular cartilage of head

Bone of proximal epiphysis

Proximal metaphysis

Diaphysis; growth in width occurs by periosteal bone formation

Distal metaphysis

Bone of distal epiphysis

Articular cartilage of condyles

Plate 1-13

Musculoskeletal System: PART III

DEVELOPMENT OF MUSCULOSKELETAL SYSTEM
(Continued)

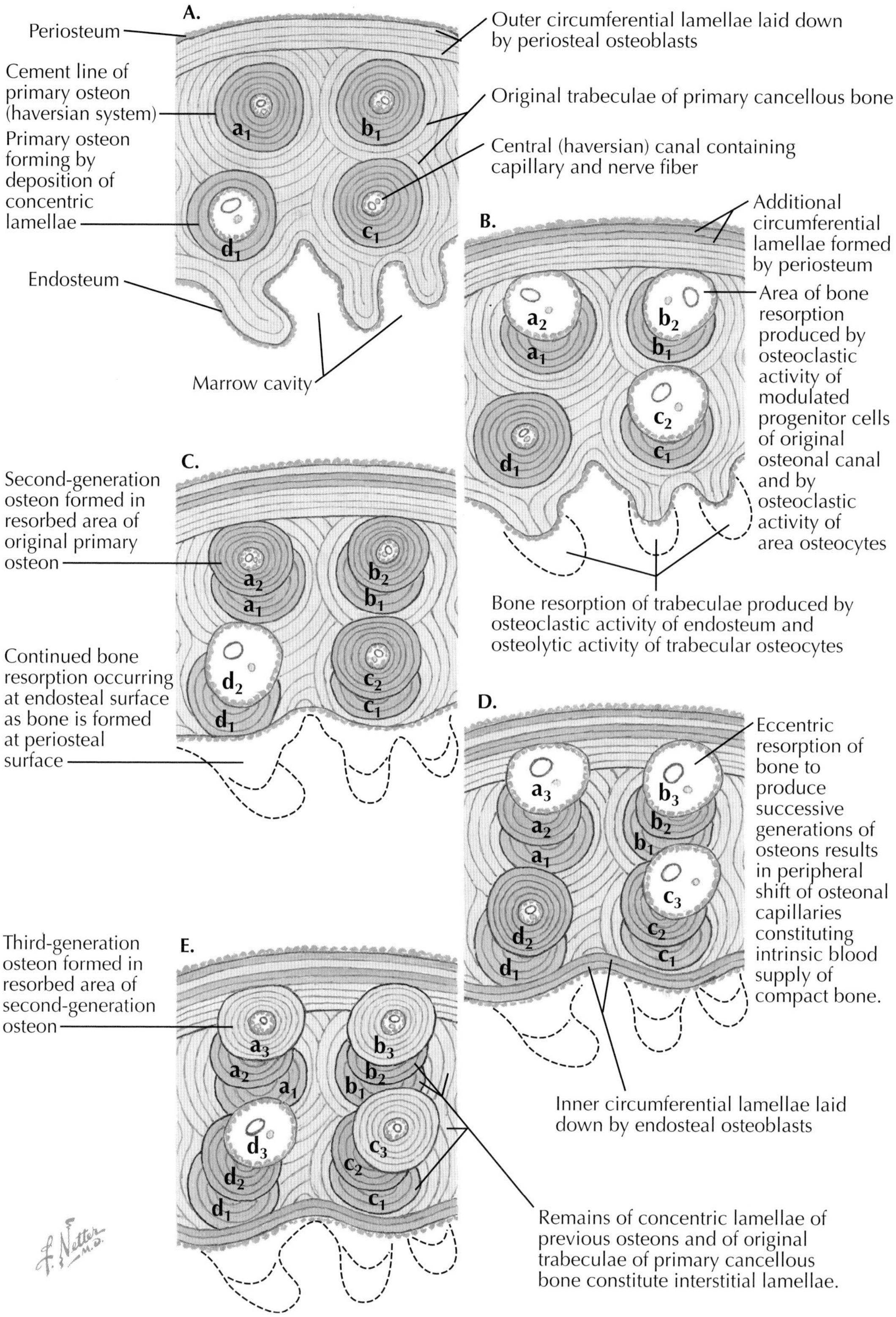

Within each cell of the fibers, the myosin formed thick myofilaments and the actin formed thin myofilaments that ran parallel to the longitudinal axis of the cell. The myofilaments became identically aligned and organized within the cell into larger longitudinal bundles, the myofibrils, which in turn became aligned with the adjacent myofibrils. Mitochondria were interspersed between the myofibrils. This identical, side-by-side alignment coincided with that of the cells of adjacent fibers, resulting in the cross-banded, or striated, appearance of longitudinally sectioned cardiac muscle at the microscopic level.

The dense concentration in cardiac muscle of orderly arrangements of interdigitating actin and myosin molecules, which could synchronously slide across each other throughout the atrial or ventricular muscle, resulted in an organ that could make strong, quick contractions of short duration. And so, between the third and fourth week, the cardiac muscle of the single-tube heart begins to contract. The bundles, nodes, and Purkinje fibers, which are the components of the conducting system of the heart, are merely modified cardiac muscle fibers.

If damaged, smooth muscle is able to regenerate to a limited degree by division of preexisting muscle cells and by division and differentiation of nearby connective tissue cells of the mesenchymal type. However, there is no regeneration of damaged cardiac muscle; repair of damaged myocardium is by means of fibrous scar tissue.

SKELETAL MUSCLE

Skeletal muscle is also known as voluntary, striated, striped, or segmental muscle. The last term refers to the origin of most of the skeletal muscles of the vertebrate body from the segmented paraxial mesoderm, the somites.

In the adult prevertebrate amphioxus, there are, according to the species, from 50 to 85 muscle segments known as myotomes, or myomeres (see Plate 1-1). The V-shaped myotomes are dovetailed into one another along the length of the body. The individual striated muscle fibers of each myotome run parallel to the long axis of the body, and each myotome receives a pair of nerves from the dorsal nerve cord. The original myotomic segments are retained in a similar fashion throughout the trunk of adult fish. However, each myotome is divided into a dorsal, or epaxial, and a ventral, or hypaxial, portion, which are separated in fish by the transverse processes of the vertebral column and a fibrous septum extending from these processes to the lateral body line. Each myotome is supplied by a spinal nerve, with a dorsal ramus innervating the epaxial portion and a ventral ramus innervating the hypaxial portion.

In the human embryo, the maximum number of 42 to 44 somites is attained during the fifth week, after which the first of the four occipital and the last seven or eight coccygeal somites regress and disappear. In addition to the somites, there are three masses of mesenchyme on each side of the embryonic head that are anterior to the otic vesicles—the future membranous

GROWTH IN WIDTH OF A BONE AND OSTEON REMODELING

A.
Periosteum
Cement line of primary osteon (haversian system)
Primary osteon forming by deposition of concentric lamellae
Endosteum
Marrow cavity

Outer circumferential lamellae laid down by periosteal osteoblasts
Original trabeculae of primary cancellous bone
Central (haversian) canal containing capillary and nerve fiber

B.
Additional circumferential lamellae formed by periosteum
Area of bone resorption produced by osteoclastic activity of modulated progenitor cells of original osteonal canal and by osteoclastic activity of area osteocytes
Bone resorption of trabeculae produced by osteoclastic activity of endosteum and osteolytic activity of trabecular osteocytes

C.
Second-generation osteon formed in resorbed area of original primary osteon
Continued bone resorption occurring at endosteal surface as bone is formed at periosteal surface

D.
Eccentric resorption of bone to produce successive generations of osteons results in peripheral shift of osteonal capillaries constituting intrinsic blood supply of compact bone

E.
Third-generation osteon formed in resorbed area of second-generation osteon
Inner circumferential lamellae laid down by endosteal osteoblasts
Remains of concentric lamellae of previous osteons and of original trabeculae of primary cancellous bone constitute interstitial lamellae.

labyrinths of the inner ears—which represent the three pairs of preotic somites found in primitive vertebrate embryos that give rise to the striated extrinsic muscles of the eye. The three preotic mesenchymal masses in the human embryo aggregate into one mass around the developing eyeball during the fifth week, giving rise to the extrinsic ocular muscles that become innervated by the initially nearby oculomotor (III), trochlear (IV), and abducens (VI) nerves (see Plate 1-16).

In the human embryo, the early differentiation of all the persisting *somites* (the second occipital to the third or fourth coccygeal) is similar: the ventromedial portion of the somite becomes the *sclerotome*; the sclerotomal cells migrate toward the notochord to give rise to the vertebral column and ribs, and the remaining portion of the somite is then called the *dermomyotome* (a fluid-filled cavity, the myocoele, appears in the somite but is soon obliterated); the cells of the dermomyotome then

Plate 1-14   Embryology

REMODELING: MAINTENANCE OF BASIC FORM AND PROPORTIONS OF BONE DURING GROWTH

DEVELOPMENT OF MUSCULOSKELETAL SYSTEM
(Continued)

proliferate to form a medial mass, the *myotome*, which can be distinguished from the less proliferative lateral portion, the *dermatome* (see Plates 1-2 and 1-3). Finally, the cells of the dermatome spread beneath the overlying ectoderm to give rise to the subcutaneous fascia and the dermis of the skin. The segmental dermatome distribution of the embryo is reflected in the innervation of the skin of the trunk and limbs of the adult. The area of skin supplied by a single spinal nerve in the adult constitutes a dermatome.

In fish, the myotome stays in place and occupies the equivalent position of its parent somite, giving rise to a segmental muscle that attaches to the vertebral column. This prevents the sclerotome portion of the somite from also retaining its original position and giving rise to only a single vertebra. If this had happened, each muscle would attach to only a single vertebra, and then the vertebral column could not move when the muscle contracted. The process of establishing an overlapping arrangement between myotomes and vertebrae is recapitulated in the human embryo.

The cells of the myotome, the mononucleated myoblasts, elongate in a direction parallel to the long axis of the embryo (see Plate 1-17) and undergo repeated mitotic divisions, subsequently fusing with each other to form syncytia. Each syncytium becomes a tube with continuous cytoplasm, and the numerous nuclei within it are centrally located. The process is similar to the formation of the tubular cardiac muscle fiber except that in the latter each centrally located nucleus is within a separate cell.

The syncytial myotubes of skeletal muscle become muscle fibers as myofilaments of actin and myosin are laid down within the cytoplasm. The thin actin and the thick myosin polypeptide myofilaments become strung out parallel to the long axis of the fiber and are arranged in a side-by-side, interdigitating relationship so that they can slide past each other to cause muscle contraction. The cross-banded, or striated, appearance of skeletal muscle at the microscopic level reflects this relationship between the two types of submicroscopic filaments. The myofilaments group together into numerous longitudinal bundles known as myofibrils, which occupy the bulk of the fiber; the nuclei and nearly all the mitochondria are relocated to the periphery, where they are in contact with the outer membrane of the fiber, the sarcolemma (see Plate 1-17).

The myotube stage of fiber formation begins at about the fifth week. Subsequent generations of myotubes develop from the persisting population of myoblasts found in close relationship to muscle fibers. The nuclei of the muscle fibers themselves, once in place, do not divide mitotically or amitotically; consequently, in order to increase their number, the incorporation of new myoblasts into the syncytia is required, especially when the fibers grow in length.

The growth of skeletal muscles is the result of an increase in both the number of muscle fibers and the size of the individual fibers. The greatest increase in the number of fibers occurs before birth, after which time both the number and size of the fibers increase. In the male, there is a fourteen-fold increase in fiber number

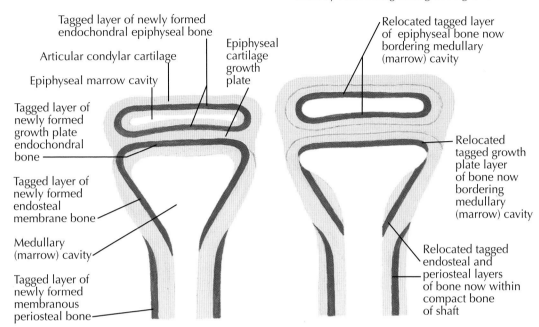

Proximal end of growing tibia with newly formed bone tagged by incorporation of radioactive material

Same segment of bone 1 week after newly formed bone was radioactively tagged, showing relocation of tagged bone by remodeling during bone growth

Tagged layer of newly formed endochondral epiphyseal bone

Articular condylar cartilage

Epiphyseal marrow cavity

Epiphyseal cartilage growth plate

Tagged layer of newly formed growth plate endochondral bone

Tagged layer of newly formed endosteal membrane bone

Medullary (marrow) cavity

Tagged layer of newly formed membranous periosteal bone

Relocated tagged layer of epiphyseal bone now bordering medullary (marrow) cavity

Relocated tagged growth plate layer of bone now bordering medullary (marrow) cavity

Relocated tagged endosteal and periosteal layers of bone now within compact bone of shaft

Diagram shows how change occurred through bone formation and bone resorption in remodeling process.

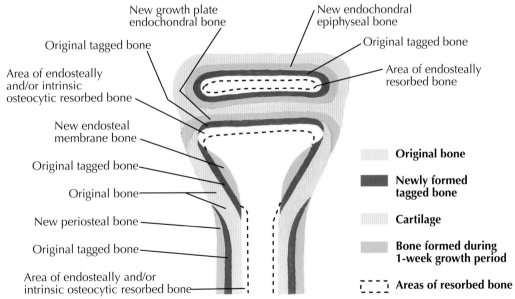

New growth plate endochondral bone

New endochondral epiphyseal bone

Original tagged bone

Original tagged bone

Area of endosteally and/or intrinsic osteocytic resorbed bone

Area of endosteally resorbed bone

New endosteal membrane bone

Original tagged bone

Original bone

New periosteal bone

Original tagged bone

Area of endosteally and/or intrinsic osteocytic resorbed bone

Original bone

Newly formed tagged bone

Cartilage

Bone formed during 1-week growth period

Areas of resorbed bone

from 2 months to age 16, with a rapid spurt at age 2, and a maximum rate of increase from ages 10 to 16, during which time the fibers double in number. There is also a steady linear increase in the size of muscle fibers from infancy to adolescence and beyond in the male. In the female, the increase in fiber number is more linear than in the male, with an overall tenfold postnatal increase. However, in the female, the increase in fiber size is more rapid than in the male after age $3\frac{1}{2}$,

reaching a plateau at age $10\frac{1}{2}$. After age $14\frac{1}{2}$, fiber size in males exceeds that in females. Fiber numbers increase steadily in both sexes up to about age 50, after which there is a steady decline.

Muscle fibers are very fine threads, up to 30 cm in length but less than 0.1 mm in width, which contract to about 57% of their resting length. Only the largest muscle fibers in an adult would be visible to the naked eye if they could be individually excised. Muscles will

Plate 1-15   Musculoskeletal System: PART III

DEVELOPMENT OF MUSCULOSKELETAL SYSTEM
(Continued)

develop completely in the absence of an innervation that is due to a congenital nervous system abnormality. Thus, nerves do not supply a necessary organizing stimulus, and gross muscle morphogenesis will go to completion with function never having occurred. However, a muscle that never had a nerve supply does not attain its full differentiation at the fiber level and disappears with time.

Skeletal muscles make up the bulk of the adult body and comprise about 45% of its total weight. There are over 650 named muscles, and nearly all are paired. Each has a characteristic shape that is circumscribed by a connective tissue sheath.

During vertebrate evolution, the head underwent changes related to the development of the special senses. The anterior end of the nerve cord became a brain, and the nerves passing to and from the brain became the cranial nerves. In the prevertebrate amphioxus, which has no brain, muscle is present in the region of the mouth of the digestive system (see Plate 1-1). In the vertebrate fish, the gills have a branchial arch musculature that arises from the mesoderm associated with the developing pharyngeal region of the foregut. Therefore, this musculature can properly be called visceral musculature, even though it is voluntary and striated. A better term is *branchial*, or *branchiomeric*, musculature because it represents a serial division, or metamerism, of the lateral (gill or branchial) mesoderm that does not segment in its counterpart in the trunk.

In the human embryo, the branchial arches and their contained structures initially develop as if the aqueous gill-slit type of breathing apparatus were going to be retained. Instead of disappearing, most of the branchial arch structures are gradually modified and incorporated into the permanent acoustic and air-breathing respiratory systems. The branchiomeric musculature that develops from the mesoderm of the series of branchial arches on each side of the embryonic head becomes innervated by cranial nerves. Most of these muscles ultimately attach to the skull.

In addition to the skeletal muscles derived from the myotome and branchial arch, there are those that arise, in situ, directly from the local mesenchyme. Some of these locally derived muscles are the result of the slurring over of the sequence of evolutionary events during development, so that their derivation from myotome or branchial arch mesenchyme is obscured. Others, such as the limb muscles, appear relatively late in evolution and development. In the human embryo, the muscles of the limbs that evolved from fins appear after the myotomic and branchial arch musculature formation is well under way. The muscles of the pelvic diaphragm, perineum, and external genitalia also appear relatively late in development.

A developing skeletal muscle normally provides attractive forces that serve to guide a nerve to it. With only a few exceptions, the muscles retain their original innervation throughout life, no matter how far they may migrate from their site of origin during development; this is true whether a muscle is of myotomic origin and innervated by a spinal nerve or of branchial arch origin and innervated by a cranial nerve. Therefore, the innervation of adult muscles can be used as a clue to determine their embryonic origin. Embryonic muscle masses receive their motor innervation very early at or near their midpoint.

If a nerve supplies more than one muscle, it can be assumed that the muscles are subdivisions of an original myotome. Thus, the developmental histories of adult muscles formed by early fusion, splitting, migration, or other modifications can be reconstructed with considerable certainty.

Nearly all the skeletal muscles are present and, in essence, have their mature form in a fetus of 8 weeks with a crown-to-rump length of about 30 mm (see Plate 1-16). From the time the first myotomes begin to differentiate into skeletal muscles early in the fifth week, six fundamental processes that occur up to the eighth week are involved in the gross development of the muscles. Frequently, the formation of a muscle is the result of more than one of these processes.

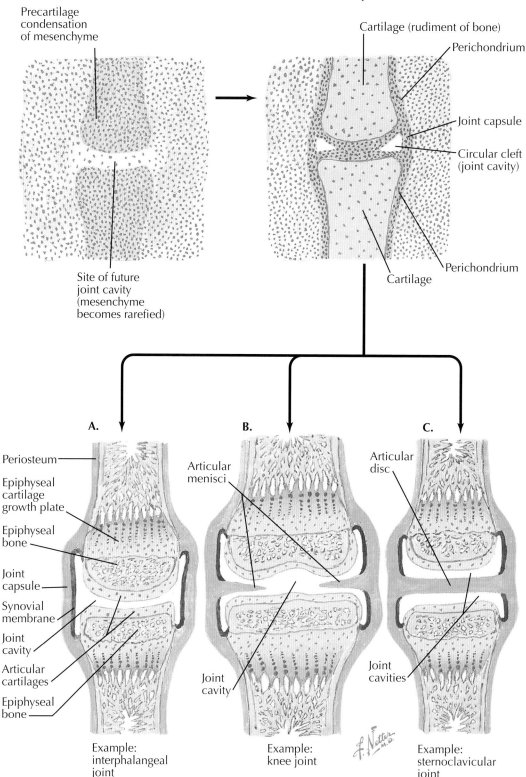

DEVELOPMENT OF THREE TYPES OF SYNOVIAL JOINTS

Precartilage condensation of mesenchyme

Cartilage (rudiment of bone)

Perichondrium

Joint capsule

Circular cleft (joint cavity)

Site of future joint cavity (mesenchyme becomes rarefied)

Cartilage

Perichondrium

A.

Periosteum

Epiphyseal cartilage growth plate

Epiphyseal bone

Joint capsule

Synovial membrane

Joint cavity

Articular cartilages

Epiphyseal bone

Example: interphalangeal joint

B.

Articular menisci

Joint cavity

Example: knee joint

C.

Articular disc

Joint cavities

Example: sternoclavicular joint

Plate 1-16

Embryology

DEVELOPMENT OF MUSCULOSKELETAL SYSTEM
(Continued)

1. The direction of the muscle fibers may change from the original craniocaudal orientation in the myotome. Only a few muscles retain their initial fiber orientation parallel to the long axis of the body (the rectus abdominis, erector spinae, and some small vertebral column muscles). Good examples of muscles that undergo a directional change are the flat muscles of the abdominal wall—the external and internal abdominal oblique muscles and especially the transverse abdominal muscle.

2. Portions of successive myotomes commonly fuse to form a composite single muscle (the erector spinae and rectus abdominis muscles). The latter is formed by the fusion of the ventral portions of the last six or seven thoracic myotomes. Only a few muscles are derivatives of single myotomes (the intercostals and some deep, short vertebral column muscles).

3. A myotome, or branchial arch muscle primordium, may split longitudinally into two or more parts that become separate muscles (the sternohyoid and omohyoid muscles and the trapezius and sternocleidomastoid muscles).

4. The original myotome masses may split tangentially into two or more layers (the external and internal intercostal and abdominal oblique and transverse abdominal muscles).

5. A portion or all of a muscle segment may degenerate. The degenerated muscle leaves connective tissue that becomes a sheet known as an aponeurosis (the epicranial aponeurosis [galea aponeurotica], which connects the frontal and occipital portions of the occipitofrontalis muscle).

6. Finally, muscle primordia may migrate, wholly or in part, to regions more or less remote from their original site of formation. An example is the formation of certain muscles of the upper limb that arise from cervical myotomes. The serratus anterior muscle migrates to the thoracic region, to attach ultimately to the scapula and the upper eight or nine ribs, taking along its fifth, sixth, and seventh cervical spinal nerve innervation. The trapezius muscle, along with the upper five cervical spinal nerves, migrates to attach ultimately to the skull, the nuchal ligament, and the spinous processes of the seventh cervical to twelfth thoracic vertebrae. The migration of the latissimus dorsi muscle is even more extensive; it carries with it its seventh and eighth cervical spinal nerve innervation to attach ultimately to the humerus, the lower thoracic and lumbar vertebrae, the last three or four ribs, and the iliac crest of the pelvis.

As these migrating upper limb muscles acquire their attachments to the trunk, they are all superficial to the underlying muscles of the body wall. The muscles of facial expression are also good examples of muscle migration. They arise from the mesenchyme of the second or hyoid branchial arch of the future neck and migrate with their facial (VII) nerve innervation to their final positions around the mouth, nose, and eyes.

A wide range of normal variations in skeletal muscle morphology result from one or more of the six fundamental processes going awry. Usually, the variations do not interfere with an individual's normal functional ability, except when a greater part or all of a muscle is absent due to an initial failure to form, or when the usual amount of degeneration of a muscle segment is excessive. Some unusual muscle variations can be explained as genetic atavisms or muscles that were typical in one of the human's vertebrate ancestors.

Skeletal muscle can undergo limited regeneration. When damaged, macrophages enter the necrotic area and remove the dead material. The damaged muscle fibers on each side of the necrotic area, which are actually open-ended syncytial tubes, form growth buds on their ends that grow toward each other, meet, and fuse. This reestablishes muscle fiber continuity across the damaged area and may be sufficient for the repair of a small muscle injury. When there is more extensive damage, the repair process is similar to the embryologic process of muscle fiber formation. Undifferentiated mononucleated cells normally present within the damaged muscle (named satellite cells) become

Segmental distribution of myotomes in fetus of 6 weeks

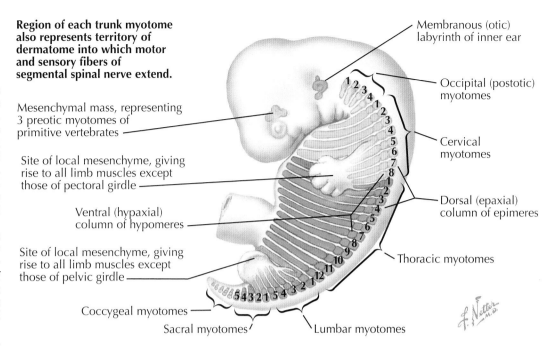

Region of each trunk myotome also represents territory of dermatome into which motor and sensory fibers of segmental spinal nerve extend.

Mesenchymal mass, representing 3 preotic myotomes of primitive vertebrates

Site of local mesenchyme, giving rise to all limb muscles except those of pectoral girdle

Ventral (hypaxial) column of hypomeres

Site of local mesenchyme, giving rise to all limb muscles except those of pelvic girdle

Coccygeal myotomes

Sacral myotomes

Lumbar myotomes

Membranous (otic) labyrinth of inner ear

Occipital (postotic) myotomes

Cervical myotomes

Dorsal (epaxial) column of epimeres

Thoracic myotomes

Developing skeletal muscles at 8 weeks (superficial dissection)

Orbicularis oculi
Zygomatic
Orbicularis oris
Brachioradialis
Extensor carpi radialis longus
Extensor digitorum
Extensor carpi ulnaris
Flexor carpi ulnaris
Rectus abdominis
Tendinous intersection
Tibialis anterior
Extensor hallucis longus
Extensor digitorum longus
Peroneus longus
Biceps femoris
Fibula
Femur

Temporalis
Masseter
Deltoid
Brachialis
Triceps brachii
Teres minor
Teres major
Trapezius
Serratus anterior
Latissimus dorsi
Rib
External abdominal oblique
Thoracolumbar fascia covering erector spinae
Developing vertebral neural arches
Quadriceps femoris
Tensor fasciae latae
Spinal medulla (cord)
Gluteus medius
Gluteus maximus

Plate 1-17

Musculoskeletal System: PART III

DEVELOPMENT OF MUSCULOSKELETAL SYSTEM
(Continued)

myoblasts that divide and then fuse together to become new multinucleated syncytial myotubes go on to differentiate into typical muscle fibers. Even so, when large areas are damaged, the muscle regeneration may be so limited that the missing muscle is replaced chiefly with connective tissue.

TRUNK MUSCLES

Between the fifth and sixth weeks, the myotomes of the trunk of the human embryo become divided by a slight longitudinal constriction into a dorsal epaxial column of *epimeres* and a more ventral hypaxial column of *hypomeres* (see Plates 1-16 and 1-18). The original spinal nerve to the myotome that gives rise to an epimere and a hypomere also divides into dorsal and ventral rami. Thus, the epimeres and hypomeres are innervated, respectively, by the dorsal and ventral rami of the serially repeated spinal nerves, just as in adult primitive fish. In addition, the developing transverse processes of the vertebrae serve to help separate the epaxial and hypaxial columns. The mesenchyme between the two columns attaches to the transverse processes and becomes a connective tissue sheet or intermuscular septum, the rudiment of the thoracolumbar fascia, which permanently separates the two columns.

After the transverse processes appear, the ribs form in the sclerotomal tissue that extends by differentiation into the ventral portions of the original clefts between the somites. The maximum development of the ribs is in the thoracic region; consequently, of all the muscles in the adult, the intercostal muscles retain to the greatest degree the original segmental pattern of the hypaxial musculature.

The epaxial column of epimeres divides further into a medial, or deep, and a lateral, or superficial, group of muscles that eventually give rise to the extensors of the vertebral column. The medial group of muscles, supplied by the medial branches of the posterior primary rami of the spinal nerves, retains a resemblance to the primitive segmental arrangement by arising from the fusion of only a few consecutive segments. By subsequent longitudinal and tangential splitting, they become the short oblique muscles of the vertebral column (the semispinalis, multifidus, and rotatores muscles and a longer muscle, the spinalis division of the erector spinae muscle). The lateral, more superficial group of muscles, which is supplied by the lateral branches of the posterior primary rami of the spinal nerves, arises by the fusion of a larger number of consecutive segments and subsequent splitting to become the long extensor muscles of the back (the iliocostalis and longissimus divisions of the erector spinae muscle).

The hypaxial column of hypomeres invades the region ventral to the vertebrae to give rise to the psoas and quadratus lumborum muscles (see Plate 1-18). The hypomeres also extend into the lateral and ventral body wall to form the layered muscles of the thorax and abdomen (see Plate 1-16). In the thorax, they are the intercostals; in the abdomen, they are the external and internal oblique, transverse abdominal, and rectus abdominis muscles (see Plate 1-18). The rectus abdominis muscle develops from the most ventral extension of the lower thoracic and first abdominal hypomeres that fuse in a cephalocaudal direction to become a single

DEVELOPMENT OF SKELETAL MUSCLE FIBERS

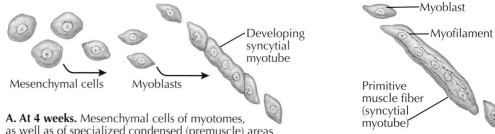

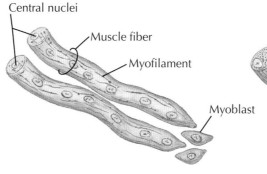

A. At 4 weeks. Mesenchymal cells of myotomes, as well as of specialized condensed (premuscle) areas of mesenchyme, in limb buds and branchial region and in somatic mesoderm of body wall modulate into myoblasts, which begin to aggregate into syncytial tubes.

B. At 5 weeks. Syncytial myotubes have formed primitive muscle fibers in which longitudinal myofilaments appear. Myotubes grow in length by incorporating additional myoblasts.

C. At 9 weeks. More myofilaments have appeared, but nuclei are still centralized. Growth in length continues through addition of myoblasts.

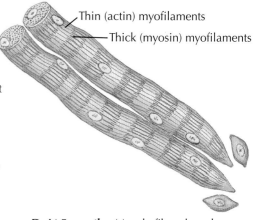

D. At 5 months. Muscle fibers have become thicker as myofilaments have multiplied and differentiated into thin (actin) and thick (myosin) myofilaments arranged in alternate overlapping bands, giving a cross-striated appearance. Nuclei move peripherally. Growth in length continues through addition of myoblasts.

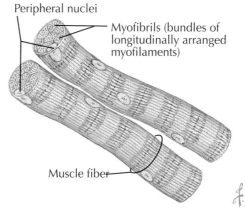

E. At birth. Myofilaments have aggregated into bundles to form myofibrils, as muscle fibers have grown in length and thickness and nuclei have shifted to periphery of muscle fibers.

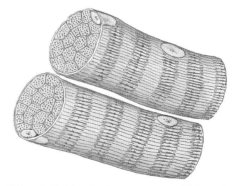

F. In adult. Muscle fibers are now thick and mature, consisting of alternating thin (actin) and thick (myosin) myofilaments aggregated into longitudinal bundles as myofibrils, with nuclei located at periphery.

longitudinal muscle on either side of the midline of the body, which is separated in the abdomen by the linea alba of dense connective tissue. The tendinous intersections (inscriptions) are indicative of the original segmental character of the rectus abdominis muscle (see Plate 1-16). Also, the fibers of this muscle retain the cephalocaudal orientation of the original myotomic fibers. In the upper thoracic region, there is also a longitudinal muscle sheet that is continuous with the sheet that gives rise to the rectus abdominis muscle.

It normally disappears but is occasionally retained as the sternalis muscle. All muscles derived from the hypomeres are primarily flexors of the vertebral column.

PERINEAL MUSCLES

The formation of the muscles derived from both the epimeres and the hypomeres is well advanced by the seventh week, except for the muscles of the pelvic diaphragm, perineum, and external genitalia (see Plate

Plate 1-18

Embryology

DEVELOPMENT OF MUSCULOSKELETAL SYSTEM
(Continued)

1-19). These muscles develop later because of the late division of the single cloacal opening into a urethral and anal opening in the male and female and the acquisition of an additional opening in the female—the vagina.

This late development is a reflection of the more recent changes occurring in the evolution of the urogenital system. A single cloacal opening is characteristic of all adult fish, amphibians, reptiles, birds, and the primitive egg-laying mammals. In all mammals higher up the phylogenetic ladder than egg layers, there are separate anal and urogenital openings; however, it is only in female primates that the urethra and vagina are completely separate and have separate openings to the exterior.

In humans, a striated cloacal sphincter muscle and levator ani muscle (pelvic diaphragm) arise from the third sacral to the first coccygeal myotomic hypomeres and are well developed by the eighth week. The striated external anal sphincter, perineal, and external genital muscles arise from the cloacal sphincter muscle by its rearrangements and additions during the establishment of the urogenital and anal openings. The deep, or inner, fibers of the cloacal sphincter muscle give rise to the urethral sphincter muscle. Although the muscles of the external genitalia are the same in both sexes, they, of necessity, must undergo a different arrangement in each sex. The mature pelvic muscle arrangement in the two sexes is present by the 16th week of development. However, not until sometime during the second year after birth do the urethral and external anal sphincter muscles come under voluntary control.

LIMB MUSCLES

During their early development, the limbs are literally ectodermal sacs that become stuffed with mesenchyme. As the limb buds grow, the proliferating local somatic mesenchyme eventually gives rise to all skeletal rudiments. Myotome cells from the adjacent somites invade the limb buds to give rise to all the skeletal muscles. When the ingrowth of myotome cells, nerve fibers, neurilemmal cells, pigment cells, and, possibly, the endothelium of the blood and lymphatic systems are excluded, the limb buds would still have the capacity for self-differentiation to become limbs containing all the normal skeletal rudiments. The muscles of the pectoral and pelvic girdles are also of myotomic origin.

Early in the seventh week, the mesenchymal premuscle masses of the girdle musculature are formed in the human embryo. As the rudiments of the appendicular skeleton become differentiated within the developing limb, the mesenchyme from which the limb muscles arise is aggregated into masses grouped dorsal and ventral to the developing skeletal parts. The progressive formation of distinct muscles reaches the level of the hand and foot during the seventh week. The muscles of the upper limb develop slightly ahead of those of the lower limb.

The early limbs are flattened dorsoventrally and look like paddles projecting straight out from the body. They each have a cephalic (preaxial) border and a caudal (postaxial) border, as well as a craniocaudal attachment to the body opposite a number of myotomes (see Plate 1-9). Each upper limb bud lies opposite the lower five cervical and the first thoracic myotomes. Each lower

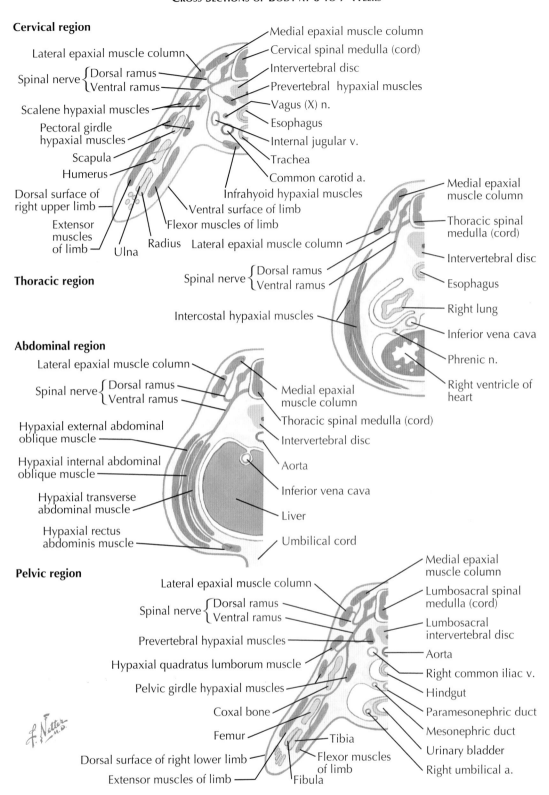

CROSS SECTIONS OF BODY AT 6 TO 7 WEEKS

Cervical region
Lateral epaxial muscle column
Spinal nerve { Dorsal ramus / Ventral ramus
Scalene hypaxial muscles
Pectoral girdle hypaxial muscles
Scapula
Humerus
Dorsal surface of right upper limb
Extensor muscles of limb
Ulna
Medial epaxial muscle column
Cervical spinal medulla (cord)
Intervertebral disc
Prevertebral hypaxial muscles
Vagus (X) n.
Esophagus
Internal jugular v.
Trachea
Common carotid a.
Infrahyoid hypaxial muscles
Ventral surface of limb
Flexor muscles of limb
Radius   Lateral epaxial muscle column

Thoracic region
Medial epaxial muscle column
Thoracic spinal medulla (cord)
Intervertebral disc
Esophagus
Right lung
Inferior vena cava
Phrenic n.
Right ventricle of heart
Spinal nerve { Dorsal ramus / Ventral ramus
Intercostal hypaxial muscles

Abdominal region
Lateral epaxial muscle column
Spinal nerve { Dorsal ramus / Ventral ramus
Hypaxial external abdominal oblique muscle
Hypaxial internal abdominal oblique muscle
Hypaxial transverse abdominal muscle
Hypaxial rectus abdominis muscle
Medial epaxial muscle column
Thoracic spinal medulla (cord)
Intervertebral disc
Aorta
Inferior vena cava
Liver
Umbilical cord

Pelvic region
Lateral epaxial muscle column
Spinal nerve { Dorsal ramus / Ventral ramus
Prevertebral hypaxial muscles
Hypaxial quadratus lumborum muscle
Pelvic girdle hypaxial muscles
Coxal bone
Femur
Dorsal surface of right lower limb
Extensor muscles of limb
Medial epaxial muscle column
Lumbosacral spinal medulla (cord)
Lumbosacral intervertebral disc
Aorta
Right common iliac v.
Hindgut
Paramesonephric duct
Mesonephric duct
Urinary bladder
Right umbilical a.
Tibia
Flexor muscles of limb
Fibula

limb bud is opposite the second and fifth lumbar and the upper three sacral myotomes. The branches of the spinal nerves supplying these myotomes reach the base of their respective limb bud. As the bud elongates to form a limb, the nerves grow into it in such a manner that the group of limb muscles along the preaxial border of the upper limb becomes innervated by the fourth to the seventh cervical nerves, and those of the postaxial border, by the eighth cervical and the first thoracic

nerves. In the lower limb, the group of muscles along the preaxial border receives innervation from the second to the fifth lumbar nerves and the group of muscles along the postaxial border receives innervation from the first to the third sacral nerves.

The preaxial and postaxial groups of developing muscles become split and rearranged. In so doing, they both contribute to the formation of the ventral, or anterior, limb-flexor group of muscles and a dorsal, or

Plate 1-19

Musculoskeletal System: PART III

DEVELOPMENT OF MUSCULOSKELETAL SYSTEM
(Continued)

posterior, limb-extensor group (see Plate 1-18). The original preaxial and postaxial nerves of the limbs are similarly divided into anterior and posterior divisions, supplying the flexors and extensors, respectively. Thus, the ulnar and median nerves in the upper limb, which contain both preaxial and postaxial nerve fibers, are branches of the anterior divisions of the trunks of the brachial plexus and innervate flexor muscles. Likewise, the radial nerve, containing both preaxial and postaxial nerve fibers, is derived from the posterior divisions of the trunks of the brachial plexus and innervates extensor muscles.

In the lower limb, the tibial part of the sciatic nerve, which contains both preaxial and postaxial nerve fibers, arises from the anterior divisions of the sacral plexus and innervates flexor muscles via branches of the sciatic and tibial nerves. The femoral nerve, containing only preaxial nerve fibers, arises from the posterior divisions of the lumbar plexus and innervates the extensor muscles. The peroneal part of the sciatic nerve and its peroneal branch, which contains both preaxial and postaxial nerve fibers, arise from the posterior divisions of the sacral plexus and also innervate the extensor muscles.

At 6 weeks, the flexed limbs have not yet rotated out of their primary position (see Plate 1-8). Because the upper and lower limbs later undergo opposite rotations to reach their definitive positions, the eventual anterior, or ventral, flexor muscle compartment of the mature arm corresponds to the posterior, or dorsal, flexor muscle compartment of the mature thigh. Also, the eventual anterior, or ventral, flexor muscle compartment of the mature forearm corresponds to the posterior, or dorsal, flexor muscle compartment (calf) of the mature leg. Because of the twist of the lower limb during development that results in permanent pronation of the foot, extension of the mature wrist corresponds to the so-called dorsiflexion of the ankle that is actually its extension.

HEAD AND NECK MYOTOMIC MUSCLES

The formation of the three preotic somites is slurred over in the human embryo. What would have been their myotomes appear as three closely apposed aggregations of mesenchyme in the region of the developing eye that give rise to the extrinsic ocular muscles (see Plate 1-20). The three surviving postotic occipital somites of the original four give rise to typical myotomes.

Comparative anatomy indicates that during evolution, the tongue muscles first appeared in amphibian forms because, in fish, the tongue is a membranous sac lacking muscle. In ancestral forms, the tongue muscles are derived from the occipital myotomes that are innervated exclusively by the hypoglossal (XII) nerves.

In the human embryo, the origin of the tongue muscles is abbreviated and slurred over. The muscles arise directly from an ill-defined mass of mesenchyme located adjacent to the pharynx in the region of the branchial arch mesenchyme from which the

branchiomeric skeletal muscles arise (see Plate 1-20). However, because of the close relationship of the hypoglossal nerves to the occipital somites when they first form in the human embryo, the tongue muscles are regarded as being derived from occipital myotomes even though they appear to arise directly from mesenchyme in the region of the tongue rudiment.

Another muscle mass that has slurred-over development gives rise to the trapezius and

sternocleidomastoid muscles. It forms in mesenchyme situated between the occipital myotomes and the branchiomeric mesenchyme of the most caudal branchial arch. The innervation of the muscle mass is unique because it arises as a number of motor roots from the side of the upper five segments of the cervical spinal medulla (cord) between the dorsal and ventral roots of the cervical spinal nerves, which eventually become the spinal part of the accessory (XI) nerve.

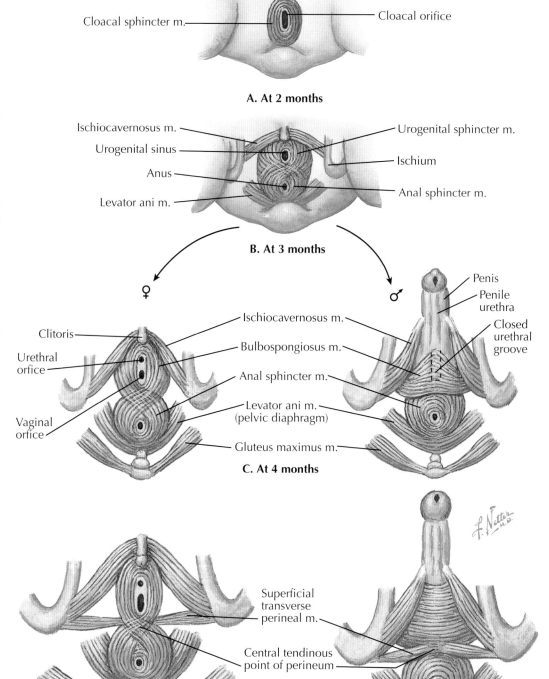

PRENATAL DEVELOPMENT OF PERINEAL MUSCULATURE

Genital tubercle
Cloacal sphincter m.
Cloacal orifice

A. At 2 months

Ischiocavernosus m.
Urogenital sinus
Anus
Levator ani m.
Urogenital sphincter m.
Ischium
Anal sphincter m.

B. At 3 months

♀

Clitoris
Urethral orfice
Vaginal orfice

Ischiocavernosus m.
Bulbospongiosus m.
Anal sphincter m.
Levator ani m. (pelvic diaphragm)
Gluteus maximus m.

♂
Penis
Penile urethra
Closed urethral groove

C. At 4 months

Superficial transverse perineal m.
Central tendinous point of perineum

D. At 5 months

Plate 1-20

Embryology

DEVELOPMENT OF MUSCULOSKELETAL SYSTEM
(Continued)

The epaxial column of epimeres derived from the cervical myotomes becomes the extensor musculature of the neck in the same manner as that in the trunk. However, the neck musculature is more elaborately developed than that of the thorax. The medial, or deep, group of muscles derived from the epaxial column are the short oblique muscles of the vertebral column—the multifidus and rotatores muscles—and some longer muscles—the spinalis and semispinalis muscles that also attach to the skull. The lateral, or superficial, group of muscles derived from the epaxial column are the long extensor muscles of the vertebral column—the iliocostalis cervicis, longissimus cervicis, and capitis divisions of the erector spinae muscle and the splenius capitis muscle.

The formation of muscles from the cervical hypaxial column of hypomeres, however, is quite different from what happens in the thorax; this is due to the development of the adjacent upper limbs, to the caudal recession of the coelomic, or body, cavity that originally extended into the head region, and to the presence of the branchial arches. It is interesting that the muscle mass giving rise to the infrahyoid muscles is continuous with the mass giving rise to the tongue muscles and that the infrahyoid muscle mass is also continuous caudally with the muscle mass that becomes the diaphragmatic striated muscle.

The diaphragm is originally located in the neck region. Because of its caudal migration, mainly due to differential growth, its cervical spinal innervation via the phrenic nerves has to elongate markedly.

HEAD AND NECK BRANCHIOMERIC MUSCLES

During evolution, the switch from water breathing to air breathing resulted in the loss of the branchial arch, gill slit, and aqueous respiratory apparatus and the acquisition of a definitive face and neck. Many of the branchial arch structures, especially the skeleton, underwent modification and were retained in the resulting air-breathing upper respiratory system and acoustic system. A résumé of these modifications is recapitulated in the human embryo. Of the six branchial arches of primitive vertebrates, the fifth and sixth arches are completely rudimentary in humans. Even so, the deep tissue in the territories of the fifth and sixth arches gives rise to certain primitive structures that undergo modifications and are retained in the adult. The four definitive arches are present by the fifth week.

During the fifth week, condensations of mesoderm appear in the dorsal end of each of the four branchial arches, including the territories of the fifth and sixth arches. In the development of primitive vertebrates, there is continuity between the mesodermal condensations of each arch and one of the head somites, indicating that the condensations represent the hypaxial portion of the head somites. However, in the human embryo, this phase of development is slurred over because no such continuity occurs between the condensations and the somites. Therefore, the myoblasts that

ORIGINS AND INNERVATIONS OF PHARYNGEAL ARCH AND SOMITE MYOTOME MUSCLES

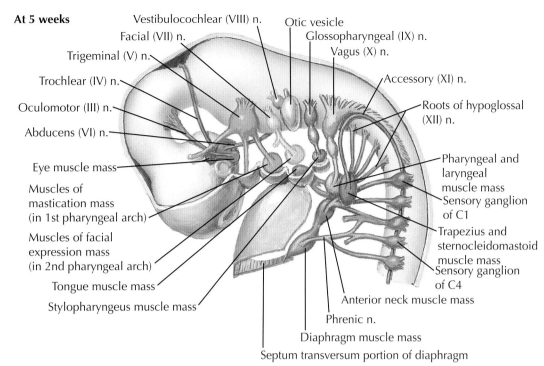

At 5 weeks

Vestibulocochlear (VIII) n. — Otic vesicle
Facial (VII) n. — Glossopharyngeal (IX) n.
Trigeminal (V) n. — Vagus (X) n.
Trochlear (IV) n. — Accessory (XI) n.
Oculomotor (III) n. — Roots of hypoglossal (XII) n.
Abducens (VI) n.
Eye muscle mass — Pharyngeal and laryngeal muscle mass
Muscles of mastication mass (in 1st pharyngeal arch) — Sensory ganglion of C1
Muscles of facial expression mass (in 2nd pharyngeal arch) — Trapezius and sternocleidomastoid muscle mass
Tongue muscle mass — Sensory ganglion of C4
Stylopharyngeus muscle mass — Anterior neck muscle mass
Phrenic n.
Diaphragm muscle mass
Septum transversum portion of diaphragm

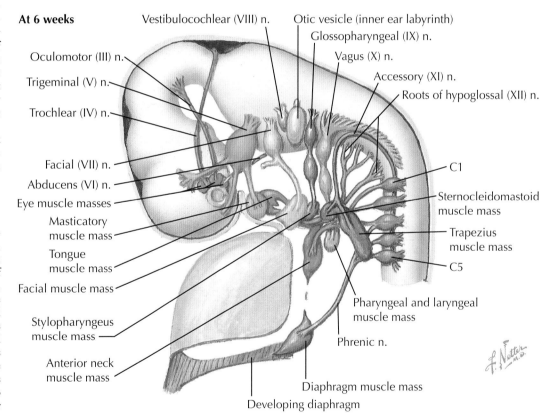

At 6 weeks

Vestibulocochlear (VIII) n. — Otic vesicle (inner ear labyrinth)
Glossopharyngeal (IX) n.
Oculomotor (III) n. — Vagus (X) n.
Trigeminal (V) n. — Accessory (XI) n.
Trochlear (IV) n. — Roots of hypoglossal (XII) n.
Facial (VII) n. — C1
Abducens (VI) n. — Sternocleidomastoid muscle mass
Eye muscle masses — Trapezius muscle mass
Masticatory muscle mass — C5
Tongue muscle mass — Pharyngeal and laryngeal muscle mass
Facial muscle mass
Stylopharyngeus muscle mass — Phrenic n.
Anterior neck muscle mass
Diaphragm muscle mass
Developing diaphragm

differentiate directly from the mesodermal condensations of the arches give rise to skeletal striated muscles that are regarded as branchiomeric in origin. The voluntary motor part of a special visceral cranial nerve grows into each of the muscle rudiments of the arches, including those of the territories of the fifth and sixth arches.

The muscles of branchiomeric origin retain their original cranial nerve innervation as they migrate to

their final destinations (see Plates 1-20 and 1-21). The muscles that arise from the primordial mesenchymal mass of the first or mandibular branchial arch become innervated by the motor neurons of the trigeminal (V) nerve. These muscles become the masticatory muscles (the temporal, masseter, and pterygoid muscles) as well as the mylohyoid, anterior belly of the digastric, tensor veli palatini, and tensor tympani muscles. The muscles arising in the region of the second, or hyoid, branchial

Plate 1-21

Musculoskeletal System: PART III

BRANCHIOMERIC AND ADJACENT MYOTOMIC MUSCLES AT BIRTH

DEVELOPMENT OF MUSCULOSKELETAL SYSTEM
(Continued)

arch become the muscles of facial expression and receive their motor innervation from the facial (VII) nerve. Other muscles arising from the second arch mesenchyme and innervated by the facial nerve are the posterior belly of the digastric, stylohyoid, and stapedius muscles. The glossopharyngeal (IX) nerve supplies motor innervation to the muscle mass of the third branchial arch, which becomes the stylopharyngeus muscle.

The muscles arising in the fourth arch and in the territories of the fifth and sixth branchial arches become those of the soft palate (the levator veli palatini, uvulae, and palatoglossus muscles); those of the pharynx (the pharyngeal constrictor, palatopharyngeus, and salpingopharyngeus muscles); and all the intrinsic muscles of the larynx. The innervation of all these muscles derived from the fourth arch and the fifth and sixth arch territories is actually from the vagus (X) nerve. However, the rootlets containing the axons of the motor neurons leave the side of the medulla oblongata portion of the brainstem to become what is named the cranial part of the accessory (XI) nerve. The cranial part, after being attached by connective tissue to the spinal part of the accessory nerve as they pass through the jugular foramen of the skull, separates from the spinal part in the neck to join the main trunk of the vagus nerve. Its motor neurons to the striated muscles of the soft palate and pharynx pass via the pharyngeal branches of the vagus nerve, whereas those to the intrinsic muscles of the larynx pass via the superior and recurrent laryngeal branches.

SKELETAL MUSCLE INNERVATION

The establishment of neural contacts with developing skeletal muscle fibers is a critical developmental stage. The contacts enhance muscle development and are important for the complete differentiation and function of the fibers. The motor nerve axons make contact with the masses of myoblasts constituting the developing muscles as early as between the 5th and 6th week if they are trunk muscles. However, it is between this time and the 10th week that the branches of the large somatic (alpha) motor neurons begin to ramify among the developing motor fibers of the muscles and to establish the formation of neuromuscular junctions. Muscle spindles (proprioceptors) can be distinguished at about the 12th week. They become innervated by the small gamma motor nerves.

Movements of the mother, and especially of the uterus, serve as stimuli to induce muscular activity to occur in the fetus before the 4th month, although the mother is not aware of it until the "quickening" at about the 4th month. Long before birth, the diaphragm contracts periodically in response to phrenic nerve activity (hiccups). The fetus begins to swallow amniotic fluid at 12½ weeks; before birth, it may at times suck the fingers. Therefore, the phrenic nerves and the muscular

Superficial muscles

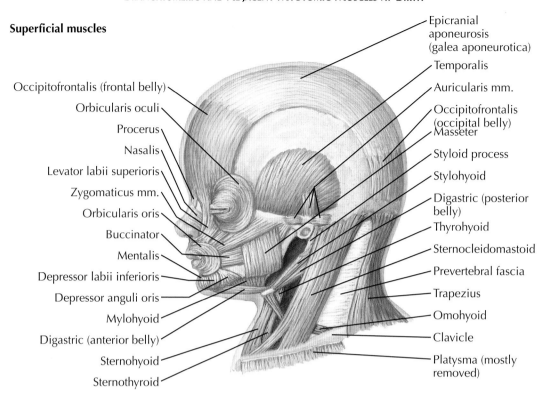

Occipitofrontalis (frontal belly)
Orbicularis oculi
Procerus
Nasalis
Levator labii superioris
Zygomaticus mm.
Orbicularis oris
Buccinator
Mentalis
Depressor labii inferioris
Depressor anguli oris
Mylohyoid
Digastric (anterior belly)
Sternohyoid
Sternothyroid

Epicranial aponeurosis (galea aponeurotica)
Temporalis
Auricularis mm.
Occipitofrontalis (occipital belly)
Masseter
Styloid process
Stylohyoid
Digastric (posterior belly)
Thyrohyoid
Sternocleidomastoid
Prevertebral fascia
Trapezius
Omohyoid
Clavicle
Platysma (mostly removed)

Deep muscles

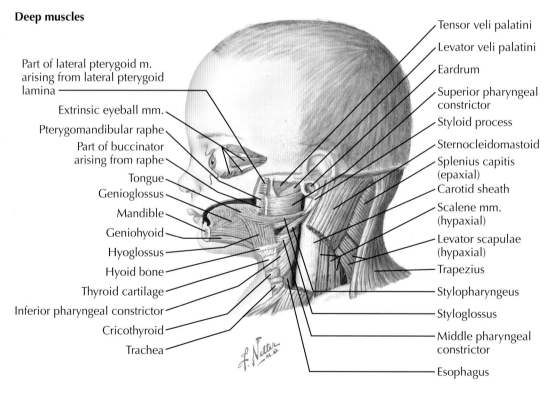

Part of lateral pterygoid m. arising from lateral pterygoid lamina
Extrinsic eyeball mm.
Pterygomandibular raphe
Part of buccinator arising from raphe
Tongue
Genioglossus
Mandible
Geniohyoid
Hyoglossus
Hyoid bone
Thyroid cartilage
Inferior pharyngeal constrictor
Cricothyroid
Trachea

Tensor veli palatini
Levator veli palatini
Eardrum
Superior pharyngeal constrictor
Styloid process
Sternocleidomastoid
Splenius capitis (epaxial)
Carotid sheath
Scalene mm. (hypaxial)
Levator scapulae (hypaxial)
Trapezius
Stylopharyngeus
Styloglossus
Middle pharyngeal constrictor
Esophagus

diaphragm used for breathing, and the sensory nerves of the lips, mouth, and throat, as well as the striated muscle with their motor nerves of the lips, tongue, jaws, and throat used for the complicated reflex functions of suckling and swallowing, are functionally well developed at birth. In contrast, the trunk and limb muscles at birth are uniformly slow in contracting.

Voluntary control of the skeletal muscles cannot occur in the neonate because of the lack of dendritic

development of the cerebral neurons, especially those of the motor cortex, and the fact that the fibers of the upper motor neurons of the corticobulbar and corticospinal tracts have only begun to be myelinated. It is not until the end of the first year after birth that the myelination of the nerve fibers of the corticospinal tract is nearly completed. This is about the time when the child has sufficient voluntary control over the skeletal muscles to be able to stand and walk.

PHYSIOLOGY

Plate 2-1

Physiology

MICROSCOPIC APPEARANCE OF SKELETAL MUSCLE FIBERS

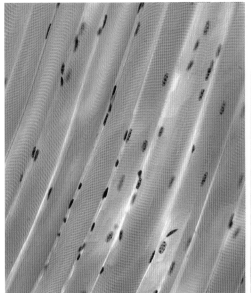

Skeletal muscle tissue section stained with hematoxylin and eosin

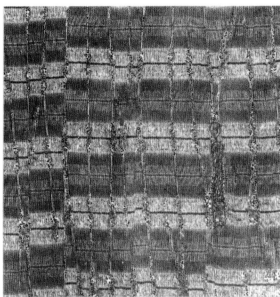

On electron microscopy, banding pattern is seen to result from overlap of regularly arranged thick and thin filaments. Above: longitudinal section stained with lead, x9,800. Below: transverse section stained with lead, x66,000

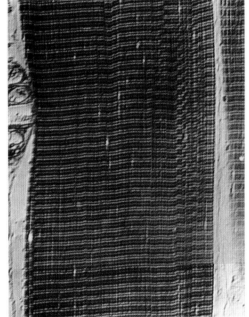

On light microscopy, skeletal muscle fibers have a strikingly regular banding pattern (longitudinal section of frog skeletal muscle under differential interference microscopy, x1,280).

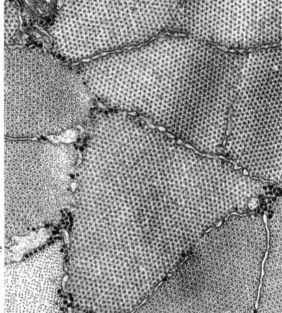

STRUCTURAL ORGANIZATION OF SKELETAL MUSCLE

The principal function of skeletal muscles is to move the limbs, trunk, head, respiratory apparatus, and eyes. Most skeletal muscles are under voluntary control. They are composed of long multinucleated cells called muscle fibers, which are derived by fusion of many embryonic cells called *myoblasts* to form *myotubes* during development. The ends of the muscle fibers insert into tendons that, in turn, attach to bones across the joints. The entire muscle is surrounded by a connective tissue sheath, the *epimysium*. The connective tissue extends into the muscle as the *perimysium*, which divides the muscle into a number of fascicles, each containing several muscle fibers. Within the fascicle, muscle fibers are separated from one another by the *endomysium*.

Each muscle fiber is invested by a thin layer of connective tissue called the basal lamina, or *basement membrane*. It is now believed that the basement membrane contains molecules important to the development and differentiation of the neuromuscular apparatus. Satellite cells, enclosed between the basement membrane and the sarcolemma, are believed to derive from undifferentiated myoblasts and are considered the skeletal muscle stem cell niche, capable of fusing with damaged muscle fibers in a regenerative process.

A muscle fiber exerts force by contracting. The microscopic structure of the muscle fiber gives a great deal of information about the way it functions. The contractile apparatus of each muscle fiber is subdivided into *myofibrils*, which are longitudinally oriented bundles of thick and thin filaments. The thick and thin filaments provide the mechanical force of contraction by sliding past one another. A myofibril measures about 1 μm in diameter and extends the entire length of the fiber. The thin filaments of the myofibril are anchored at one end to a meshlike lattice structure made up largely of protein and oriented at right angles to the filaments. Seen from the side, this lattice appears narrow and dense. The resulting image in a longitudinal section observed on light microscopy is called the *Z band* (Zwischenscheibe). Z bands occur at very regular intervals along the length of the myofibril. The stretch of myofibril between two adjacent Z bands is called a *sarcomere*, which can be considered the unit of

Plate 2-2

Musculoskeletal System: PART III

ORGANIZATION OF SKELETAL MUSCLE

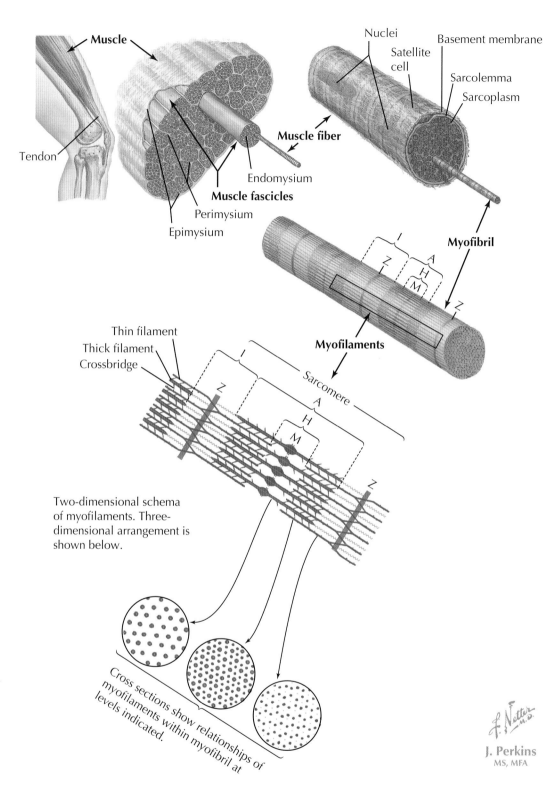

Two-dimensional schema of myofilaments. Three-dimensional arrangement is shown below.

Cross sections show relationships of myofilaments within myofibril at levels indicated.

J. Perkins
MS, MFA

STRUCTURAL ORGANIZATION OF SKELETAL MUSCLE (Continued)

contractile action. Thus, myofibrils are made up of many sarcomeres linked end to end. The thick filaments are disposed in the center of the sarcomere. Because they strongly rotate polarized light, the thick filaments are responsible for the appearance of the anisotropic bands, or *A bands*, on longitudinal section.

The contractile filaments slide past one another by a grappling action. The thick filaments are linked to the thin filaments by *crossbridges*, which are part of the structure of the thick filaments (see Plate 2-4). Electron microscopy reveals that, except at the middle portion, the crossbridges are located along the length of the thick filament. The crossbridges slant away from the middle portions of the filament toward the Z band closest to them. Thick filaments widen slightly at their middle portions, and the widened middle portions of adjacent thick filaments are in register, thus creating the appearance of the *M band*. The protein composition of these ultrastructural features is detailed in Plate 2-4.

Most of the time, the sarcomere is in a state of relaxation. Because it is longer than a thick filament, there is a region at either end of the sarcomere that contains only thin filaments. The thin filaments rotate polarized light very little; therefore, the region of the sarcomere on either side of the Z band where thin filaments are not overlapped by thick filaments is called the isotropic band, or *I band*. In the relaxed state, the thin filaments of a single sarcomere that are attached to

adjacent Z bands point toward each other but do not touch. Thus, there is a region in the middle of the sarcomere where thick filaments are not overlapped by thin filaments, which is called Hensen's disk, or the *H zone*.

The three-dimensional structure of the sarcomere is very regular. On cross section, each thick filament is surrounded by six thin filaments and each thin filament is equidistant to three thick filaments.

Plate 2-3

Physiology

INTRINSIC BLOOD AND NERVE SUPPLY OF SKELETAL MUSCLE

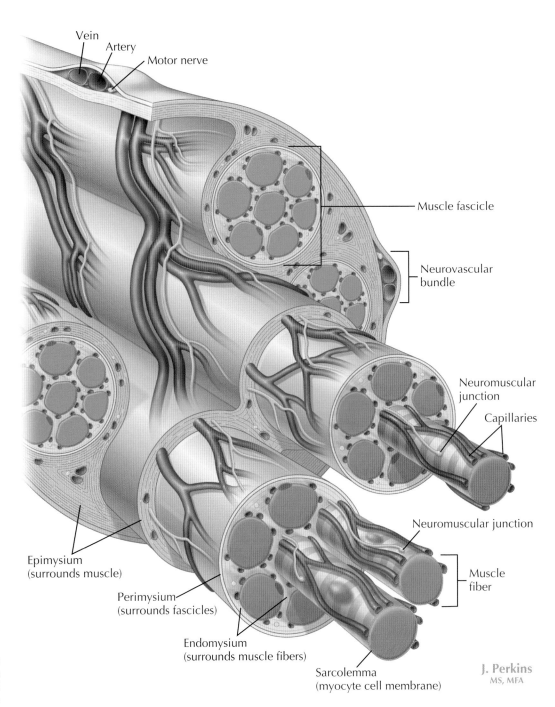

Vein
Artery
Motor nerve

Muscle fascicle

Neurovascular bundle

Neuromuscular junction

Capillaries

Neuromuscular junction

Muscle fiber

Epimysium (surrounds muscle)

Perimysium (surrounds fascicles)

Endomysium (surrounds muscle fibers)

Sarcolemma (myocyte cell membrane)

J. Perkins
MS, MFA

INTRINSIC BLOOD SUPPLY OF SKELETAL MUSCLE

Muscles use a great deal of energy and therefore require a rich blood supply. Arteries and veins usually enter the muscle together with the nerve. This grouping, termed a *neurovascular bundle*, is a common anatomic organization in many organs of the body. The main arteries supplying muscles run longitudinally within the connective tissue perimysium. They give rise to smaller branches, or *arterioles*, which penetrate the endomysium of the fascicle. These endomysial arterioles give rise to capillaries that nourish the muscle fibers. Other branches of the main arteries are transversely oriented and remain within the epimysium and perimysium. Because these branches give rise to only a few capillaries, they do not serve to nourish the muscle fibers; instead, they form non-nutritive connections, or

anastomoses, with other arteries, or they form shunts directly to the veins.

During muscle contraction, the shortened muscle fibers bulge, squeezing against the surrounding connective tissue and one another. During very vigorous contraction, the blood vessels within the endomysium can be choked off completely. Arterial blood would back up and the blood pressure would rise excessively were it not for the fact that the anastomotic channels permit

blood to bypass the nutritive circulation. Muscles that need to generate a lot of force (e.g., muscles used during sprinting) work much of the time without a supply of oxygen, because their nutritive blood supply is closed off while they are contracting. These muscles are specialized to function anaerobically, but in so doing they rapidly use up their energy stores. The so-called oxygen debt is repaid when the muscle stops working and the nutritive arterioles open once again.

Plate 2-4

Musculoskeletal System: PART III

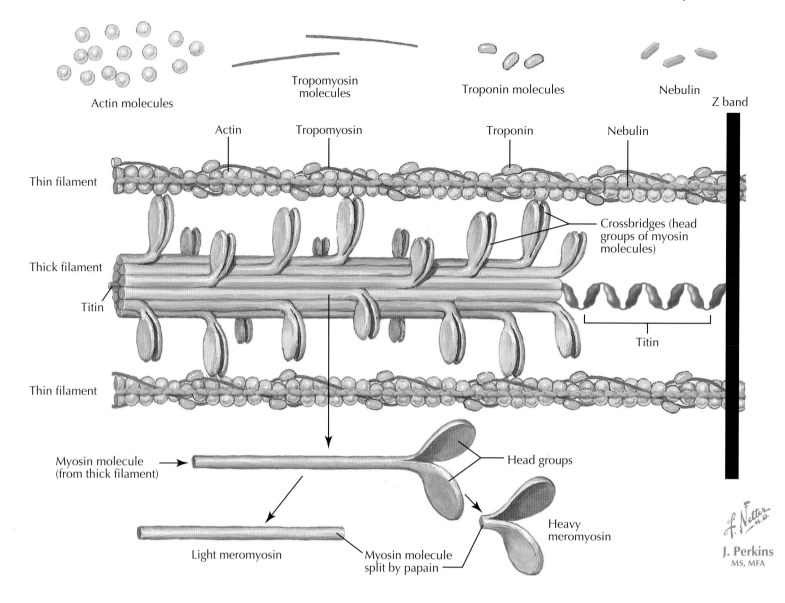

Actin molecules

Tropomyosin molecules

Troponin molecules

Nebulin

Z band

Actin
Tropomyosin
Troponin
Nebulin

Thin filament

Crossbridges (head groups of myosin molecules)

Thick filament

Titin

Titin

Thin filament

Myosin molecule (from thick filament)

Head groups

Heavy meromyosin

Light meromyosin

Myosin molecule split by papain

J. Perkins
MS, MFA

COMPOSITION AND STRUCTURE OF MYOFILAMENTS

Thick filaments are composed primarily of a protein called myosin, which can be extracted from muscle by treating it with concentrated salt solutions. *Myosin* is a large protein with a molecular weight of approximately 500,000 daltons. On electron microscopy, a myosin molecule looks like a long rod with two paddles attached to one end. Actually, a myosin molecule consists of a pair of long filaments, each coiled in a configuration called an α-helix, a pattern of protein folding frequently seen in nature. Although wound around each other, the two filaments can be separated by treatment with high concentrations of urea or detergent. This procedure reveals that each filament has a globular enlargement, or *head group*, at one end; that is, each paddle is associated with one filament. These paddles form the *crossbridges* between the thick and thin filaments. The angle between the crossbridges and the rod portion of the myosin molecule becomes more acute during muscle contraction. This change of angle occurs when the end of the paddle is bound to a nearby thin filament, which provides the mechanical force for pulling the thin filaments past the thick filaments. This, in turn, results in a shortening of the sarcomere and therefore in muscle contraction.

The structure of myosin has also been studied by breaking it down into smaller pieces with enzymatic digestion. For example, the enzyme papain splits off the head groups and a small portion of the rod from the rest of the myosin molecule. The portion with the head groups is called *heavy meromyosin*, whereas the rod portion is called *light meromyosin*. With further digestion, the two head groups can be separated from each other. As far as is known, the head groups are identical, each weighing about 120,000 daltons. In the muscle, the myosin molecules are arranged with the head groups slanting away from the middle of the thick filament. In the middle of the thick filament, the tails of the myosin molecules overlap one another end to end, creating a region devoid of head groups and with a smooth appearance on electron microscopy. A structural protein called titin acts as a central scaffold for properly arranging myosin molecules into thick filaments and provides anchoring points for the thick filaments at each opposing Z band within a sarcomere. It extends from the Z line of the sarcomere to the M band and its coiled domains provide for elastic deformation during sarcomere contraction. It functions as a sarcomeric ruler and as a template for sarcomere assembly.

Thin filaments consist chiefly of a protein called fibrous actin, or *F-actin*, which is in the form of a double helix. In very dilute salt solutions, F-actin breaks down into globular protein molecules called globular actin, or *G-actin*. These molecules are much smaller than myosin, with molecular weights of about 42,000 daltons. If the concentration of salt in the solution is increased, the G-actin molecules repolymerize end to end into their normal chainlike configuration. Thus, the actin filament is like a double string of G-actin "pearls" wound around each other. One turn of the helix contains 13.5 molecules of G-actin.

Although G-actin is the largest constituent of thin filaments, three other proteins form part of the structure and play important roles in muscle contraction. Along the notches between the two strands of actin subunits lie molecules of a globular protein, *troponin*. (Actually, this is a complex of three polypeptide subunits—troponin I, troponin C, and troponin T—each of which plays an important role in muscle contraction.) Attached to each troponin (at the T subunit) is a molecule of a thin, fibrous protein, *tropomyosin*, which lies along the grooves in the double helix. The precise disposition of tropomyosin along the F-actin chain probably varies importantly during the contraction-relaxation cycle. A third structural protein called nebulin extends along the length of thin filaments and the entire I band. Analogous to titin's role in the thick filaments, nebulin acts as a templating scaffold for thin filament assembly.

Plate 2-5   Physiology

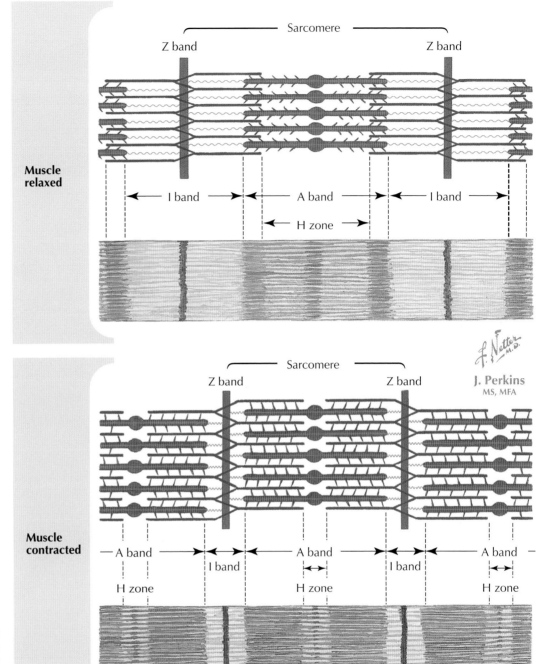

MUSCLE CONTRACTION AND RELAXATION

Under normal conditions, the arrival of a nerve impulse at the neuromuscular junction causes muscle fibers to contract. Usually, the amount of the neurotransmitter *acetylcholine (ACh)* released at the nerve terminal is sufficient to evoke a rapidly conducting electric impulse, or *action potential*, in the muscle fiber. This impulse is transmitted into the depth of the fiber and triggers the mechanical contraction. A single impulse in the motor nerve results in contraction of the muscle fiber in an all-or-nothing fashion. This is because the muscle action potential is propagated along the entire length of the fiber and thus activates the entire contractile machinery almost simultaneously.

The contraction of a muscle fiber in response to a single nerve impulse is called a *twitch*. Under a given set of starting conditions, the force of a single fiber's twitch is fixed and the strength of a muscular contraction is therefore determined by the number of muscle fibers contracting at the same time. Most skeletal muscle contraction is under voluntary control of the central nervous system.

Muscle contraction thus results from the simultaneous shortening of all the sarcomeres in all the activated muscle fibers. It is brought about by the increase in overlap between the thick and thin filaments within

During muscle contraction, thin filaments of each myofibril slide deeply between thick filaments, bringing Z bands closer together and shortening sarcomeres. A bands remain same width, but I bands are narrowed. H zones also are narrowed or disappear as thin filaments encroach upon them. Myofibrils and, consequently, muscle fibers (muscle cells), fascicles, and muscle as a whole grow thicker. During relaxation, the reverse occurs.

each sarcomere. The increase in overlap is accomplished by a cycle of making and breaking crossbridge linkages between the thick and thin filaments.

The head groups of the myosin molecules alternately flex and extend to interact with successive actin subunits on the thin filaments, which are brought progressively closer to the opposite Z band.

This "rowing" action slides the thin filaments past the thick filaments, narrowing the I band. As the ends of the actin filaments get closer to the M band, the I

band appears denser and the H zone becomes narrower. The force of the contraction depends on the number of crossbridges linking the thick and the thin filaments at the same time.

Muscle relaxation occurs when the crossbridge linkages are broken, allowing the thick and thin filaments to slide in the reverse direction. The elastic properties of the muscle and the tension on the ends of the muscle (e.g., due to the weight of the limb) determine the muscle length during relaxation.

Plate 2-6   Musculoskeletal System: PART III

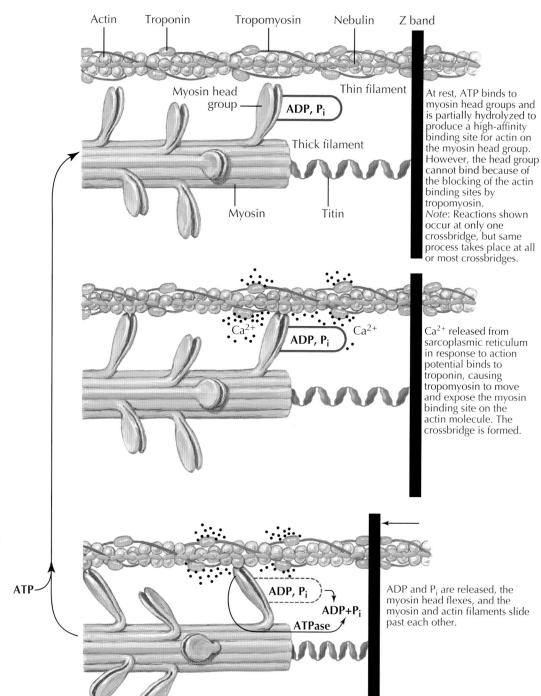

At rest, ATP binds to myosin head groups and is partially hydrolyzed to produce a high-affinity binding site for actin on the myosin head group. However, the head group cannot bind because of the blocking of the actin binding sites by tropomyosin.
Note: Reactions shown occur at only one crossbridge, but same process takes place at all or most crossbridges.

Ca^{2+} released from sarcoplasmic reticulum in response to action potential binds to troponin, causing tropomyosin to move and expose the myosin binding site on the actin molecule. The crossbridge is formed.

ADP and P_i are released, the myosin head flexes, and the myosin and actin filaments slide past each other.

BIOCHEMICAL MECHANICS OF MUSCLE CONTRACTION

In the process of making crossbridge linkages, the thick filaments "grip" the thin filaments, producing the force for muscle contraction. The energy needed for this process is provided in the form of adenosine triphosphate (ATP). Crossbridges are formed by the globular head groups of the myosin molecules of the thick filament, which interact with the actin thin filaments. For the cross bridges to occur, ATP must bind to the myosin head groups, forming a charged myosin-ATP intermediate. This charged intermediate is not capable of tightly binding to an appropriate site on the actin subunit until the enzymatic ATPase activity of the myosin head groups partially hydrolyzes ATP into adenosine diphosphate (ADP) and inorganic phosphate (P_i). In the resting state, binding sites for the myosin heads on the thin actin filaments are also blocked by tropomyosin molecules.

When the muscle fiber is electrically excited, calcium (Ca^{2+}) ions released from the sarcoplasmic reticulum bind to the troponin C subunit of the troponin molecules on the actin filaments, with four calcium ions binding to each troponin molecule. Calcium binding causes allosteric changes in the configuration of troponin molecules that affect both the troponin T and I subunits, and subsequent changes in the troponin-tropomyosin-actin interactions ultimately allow tropomyosin to "unblock" the actin-binding sites for the myosin crossbridges. These sites are then bound by the closest myosin head groups, with the attached ADP and P_i. At this point, the thick and thin filaments are mechanically connected but no movement has occurred. Movement requires the head groups to change their angle and drag the thick and thin filaments past one another, and this process involves another conformational change of the myosin head groups that is tightly

A new molecule of ATP binds to the myosin head, causing it to release from the actin molecule. Partial hydrolysis of this ATP (ADP, P_i) will "recock" the myosin head and produce a high-affinity binding site for actin. If Ca^{2+} levels are still elevated, the crossbridge will quickly re-form, causing further sliding of the actin and myosin filaments past each other. If Ca^{2+} is no longer elevated, the muscle relaxes.

coupled to release of the P_i ion, followed by release of ADP. This results in a change in the angle of the head group, tightly bound to actin, causing the thin filament to be pulled toward the middle of the sarcomere, and the sarcomere is shortened.

The flexed position of the myosin head groups bound to the actin of the thin filament is called the *rigor complex.* It is so named after the term *rigor mortis,* because, after death, muscle fibers run out of ATP and

all the myosin and actin molecules are tightly cross-linked in this configuration. However, in healthy muscle, ATP rapidly binds to myosin, causing release of the actin filament and the beginning of a new cycle. When electric activity ceases, excess calcium is rapidly taken up by the sarcoplasmic reticulum. Without calcium bound to the troponin, the head groups cannot bind actin. The cycle is interrupted, the sarcomeres lengthen, and the muscle once again relaxes.

J. Perkins
MS, MFA

Plate 2-7

Physiology

SARCOPLASMIC RETICULUM

Segment of muscle fiber greatly enlarged to
show sarcoplasmic structures and inclusions

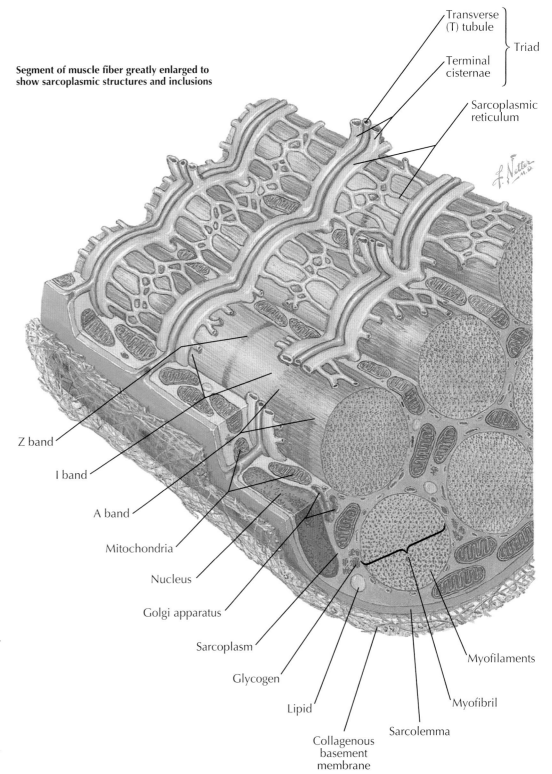

Transverse
(T) tubule
Terminal
cisternae
Triad

Sarcoplasmic
reticulum

Z band

I band

A band

Mitochondria

Nucleus

Golgi apparatus

Sarcoplasm

Glycogen

Lipid

Collagenous
basement
membrane

Sarcolemma

Myofibril

Myofilaments

SARCOPLASMIC RETICULUM AND INITIATION OF MUSCLE CONTRACTION

An impulse in the motor nerve releases the neurotransmitter substance acetylcholine at the neuromuscular junction (also called the motor end plate). Acetylcholine excites the muscle fiber membrane, or *sarcolemma*, causing an electric impulse to spread over the surface of the muscle. The electric impulse is coupled to the activation of the muscle's contractile mechanism, and some aspects of this process are described next (see Plates 2-7 and 2-8).

The immediate trigger for muscular contraction is a sudden increase in the concentration of calcium ions in the cytoplasm of the muscle fiber, the *sarcoplasm*. To prevent the muscle from being in a continual state of contraction, the calcium is stored in a system of intracellular membrane-bound channels. This system, called the *sarcoplasmic reticulum*, permeates the entire muscle fiber, so that each sarcomere is surrounded by it.

The membranes of the sarcoplasmic reticulum contain a calcium pump that uses the energy stored in ATP to transport calcium ions from the sarcoplasm, where the calcium concentration is maintained at a very low level, into the sarcoplasmic reticulum, where the calcium concentration is very high. The pump contains an enzyme that catalyzes the splitting of ATP into adenosine diphosphate ADP and P_i. This converting enzyme requires calcium and magnesium ions for its operation and thus is called calcium-magnesium ATPase. During the cleavage of one ATP molecule, two calcium ions are transported into the sarcoplasmic reticulum. The capacity of the sarcoplasmic reticulum to store calcium is enhanced by the existence of a special calcium-binding protein called calsequestrin, which has been identified in purified preparations of sarcoplasmic reticulum. It is estimated that when the muscle is at rest,

the calcium concentration in the sarcoplasmic reticulum is more than 100 mmol/kg of dry weight.

Maintenance of the steep concentration gradient for calcium across the membranes of the sarcoplasmic reticulum and activation of the contractile mechanism use up ATP, which must be replenished quickly. ATP is most efficiently replenished by the oxidative pathway. Because of their high energy requirements, muscle fibers are rich in mitochondria, which contain

the enzymatic machinery for oxidative metabolism. Mitochondria are most heavily concentrated near the sarcolemma, close to the capillaries that supply them with oxygen.

The muscle action potential is propagated from the region of the neuromuscular junction along the entire length of the muscle fiber. The electric impulse of muscle is similar to that of most nerve fibers. The sarcolemma contains voltage-dependent sodium channels

Plate 2-8

Musculoskeletal System: PART III

SARCOPLASMIC RETICULUM AND INITIATION OF MUSCLE CONTRACTION (Continued)

that open in response to an injection of depolarizing (positive) into the muscle fiber. Because the action of acetylcholine is to depolarize the sarcolemma at the neuromuscular junction, sodium channels open in the neighboring area of sarcolemma. The concentration of sodium ions inside the muscle fiber is kept very low by a pump consisting of a sodium/potassium–activated ATPase. The cleavage of one ATP molecule into ADP and phosphate is accompanied by the transport of three sodium ions out of the fiber and two potassium ions into the fiber. Because the intracellular sodium concentration is so low (about 10 mmol/L), when sodium channels open, sodium ions move into the muscle fiber from the extracellular fluid, where the concentration is much higher (about 110 mmol/L). The inward movement of these positively charged ions further depolarizes the sarcolemma, opening more sodium channels in a cycle of depolarization and increase in sodium conductance until the membrane potential reaches almost +50 mV.

This process turns itself off by two mechanisms. First, the sodium conductance channels are not only voltage dependent, they are also time dependent: they close if the depolarization of the sarcolemma is maintained for longer than a few milliseconds. Second, the sarcolemma also contains voltage-dependent potassium channels. The depolarization associated with the muscle action potential opens these channels, allowing the positively charged potassium ions to escape from the muscle fiber. This causes the sarcolemma to be repolarized (the inside becomes negative again), thereby closing the sodium channels. Thus, immediately before contraction, the sarcolemma undergoes a large depolarization lasting only 1 or 2 msec. This electric impulse is in some way responsible for the sudden release of large amounts of calcium from the sarcoplasmic reticulum. This calcium release from a storage site within the muscle fiber triggers the contraction of the muscle fiber.

However, for the action potential to affect the sarcoplasmic reticulum deep within the muscle fiber, it must be propagated inward as well as along the surface. This is accomplished through invaginations of the sarcolemma called the transverse tubules, or T tubules. In mammalian skeletal muscle, T tubules occur in register with the junction between the A bands and the I bands. Thus, each sarcomere is associated with two systems of T tubules, one at each end of the A band. (This is not true throughout the animal kingdom. In frogs, from which we have derived much of our knowledge about the structure and function of skeletal muscle, the T tubules occur in register with the Z band; thus, there is only one system of T tubules per sarcomere.)

Flanking the T tubules are paired dilatations of the sarcoplasmic reticulum called cisternae, or cisterns. On electron microscopy, the characteristic grouping of one

INITIATION OF MUSCLE CONTRACTION BY ELECTRIC IMPULSE AND CALCIUM MOVEMENT

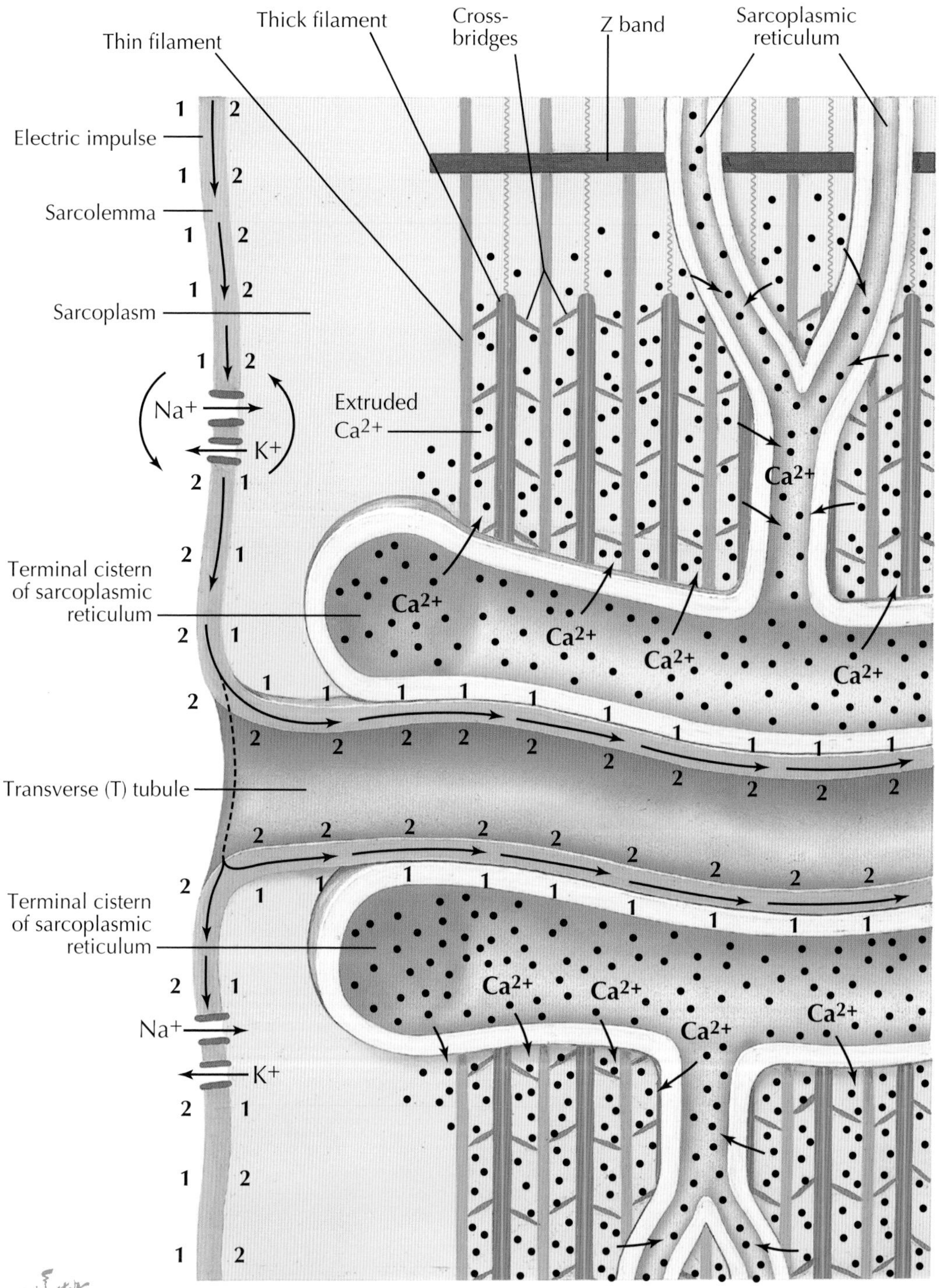

Electric impulse traveling along muscle cell membrane (sarcolemma) from motor end plate (neuromuscular junction) and then along transverse tubules affects sarcoplasmic reticulum, causing extrusion of Ca^{2+} to initiate contraction by "rowing" action of crossbridges, sliding filaments past one another.

J. Perkins
MS, MFA

T tubule and two cisterns seen in cross sections is called the triad. Thus, the action potential is propagated into the depths of the muscle fiber very close to elements of the sarcoplasmic reticulum. A protein in the T-tubule membrane called the dihydropyridine receptor functions as a voltage sensor and undergoes a conformational change as a result of the action potential. This change is transmitted to another adjacent large protein, the ryanodine receptor, which is located between the sarcoplasmic reticulum and the T tubules. The ryanodine receptor functions as a calcium channel and leads to a release of calcium from the sarcoplasmic reticulum, where calcium is bound to calsequestrin. Note that in skeletal muscle, influx of extracellular calcium is not required for muscle contraction, unlike the case for motor nerve terminals.

Plate 2-9

Physiology

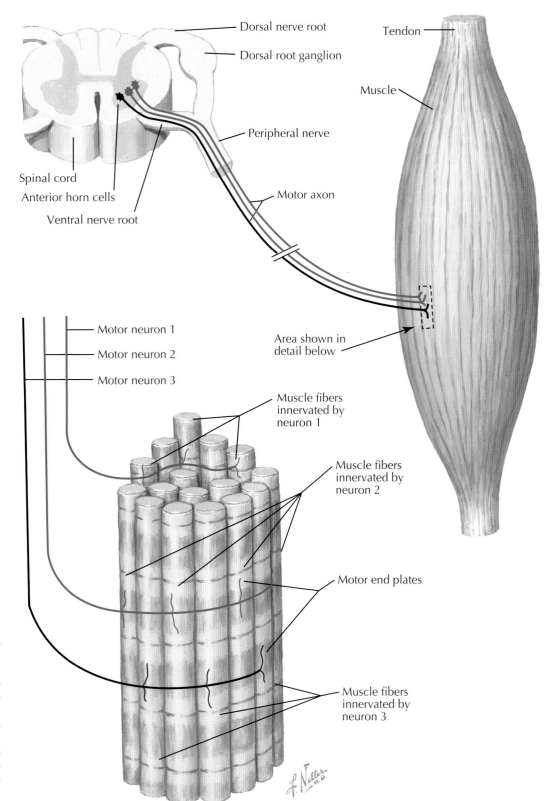

MOTOR UNIT

Muscle fibers are innervated by neurons whose cell bodies are located in the anterior (ventral) horn of the spinal cord gray matter and in the motor nuclei of the brainstem. The nerve fibers, or *axons*, of these motor neurons leave the spinal cord via the ventral roots and are distributed to the motor nerves. They enter the muscle at a region called the *end plate zone*. Each motor axon branches several times and innervates many muscle fibers.

In mammalian skeletal muscle, each muscle fiber is innervated by only one motor neuron. The combination of a single motor neuron and all the muscle fibers it innervates is called a *motor unit*. Although the muscle fibers of a given motor unit tend to be located near one another, motor units have overlapping territories.

The strength of muscle contraction depends on the number of muscle fibers active at the same time. However, the central nervous system cannot control each individual muscle fiber. It can only activate the motor neurons and therefore the motor units. The degree of control that can be exerted on the strength of contraction depends on the number of muscle fibers in a motor unit. Motor units of large muscles such as the gastrocnemius, which exert a great deal of power, may contain more than 2,000 muscle fibers. Motor units of small muscles such as the extraocular muscles, which exert very fine control but not much power, may contain as few as six muscle fibers.

Even within a given muscle, the motor units are not equal in size. In general, small motor neurons innervate fewer muscle fibers (they have smaller motor units). Small motor neurons are also more easily activated by synaptic inputs than are large motor neurons. Therefore, when signals from the brain initiate a movement, the smallest motor neurons and motor units are usually activated first. If only a small fine movement is required, the smallest motor units alone can be activated. As more power and less fine control is needed, the larger motor units are progressively recruited. This process is called the size principle of motor control.

The mechanical properties of the muscle fibers are also matched to the size of their motor unit. Because the muscle fibers of the smallest motor units are those most often activated, they must be relatively resistant to fatigue (see Plate 2-15).

Plate 2-10   Musculoskeletal System: PART III

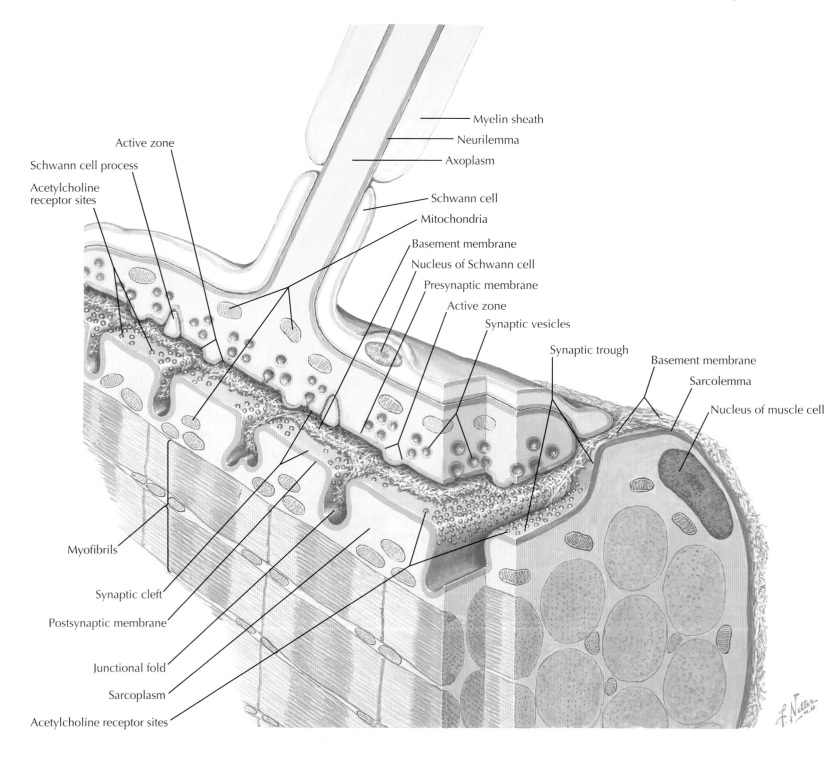

Myelin sheath
Neurilemma
Axoplasm
Schwann cell
Mitochondria
Basement membrane
Nucleus of Schwann cell
Presynaptic membrane
Active zone
Synaptic vesicles
Synaptic trough
Basement membrane
Sarcolemma
Nucleus of muscle cell

Active zone
Schwann cell process
Acetylcholine receptor sites

Myofibrils
Synaptic cleft
Postsynaptic membrane
Junctional fold
Sarcoplasm
Acetylcholine receptor sites

STRUCTURE OF NEUROMUSCULAR JUNCTION

Motor axons are generally large myelinated fibers. The terminals, although unmyelinated, are invested by a Schwann cell, which projects finger-like processes between the membranes of the nerve and the muscle. The nerve terminal lies in a trough within the muscle fiber membrane (sarcolemma); it is rich in mitochondria and contains numerous synaptic vesicles about 50 nm in diameter. These vesicles, which contain the neurotransmitter acetylcholine, are clustered around nipple-shaped active zones located at regular intervals along the terminal membrane. Acetylcholine is released by exocytosis of vesicles lying adjacent to both sides of the active zone. Opposite each active zone, the sarcolemma is invaginated by junctional folds. The presynaptic and postsynaptic membranes are separated by a space approximately 50 nm wide. Freeze-fracture electron microscopy reveals granular structures embedded in the postsynaptic membrane. These structures, which are concentrated on the banks of the junctional folds opposite the sites of acetylcholine release, are acetylcholine receptors that mediate the action of the transmitter. They are sparse in regions of the sarcolemma not close to the neuromuscular junction.

The muscle fiber is surrounded by a connective tissue basement membrane that continues into the synaptic cleft, sending extensions into the junctional folds. The basement membrane contains a large amount of collagen as well as most of the acetylcholinesterase (AChE) in the neuromuscular junction (see Plate 2-11). It also contains other important molecules that help guide the growth of the nerve terminal during development and regeneration, determine the locations of the presynaptic active zones, and induce the clumping of acetylcholine receptors opposite the synaptic vesicle.

Plate 2-11

Physiology

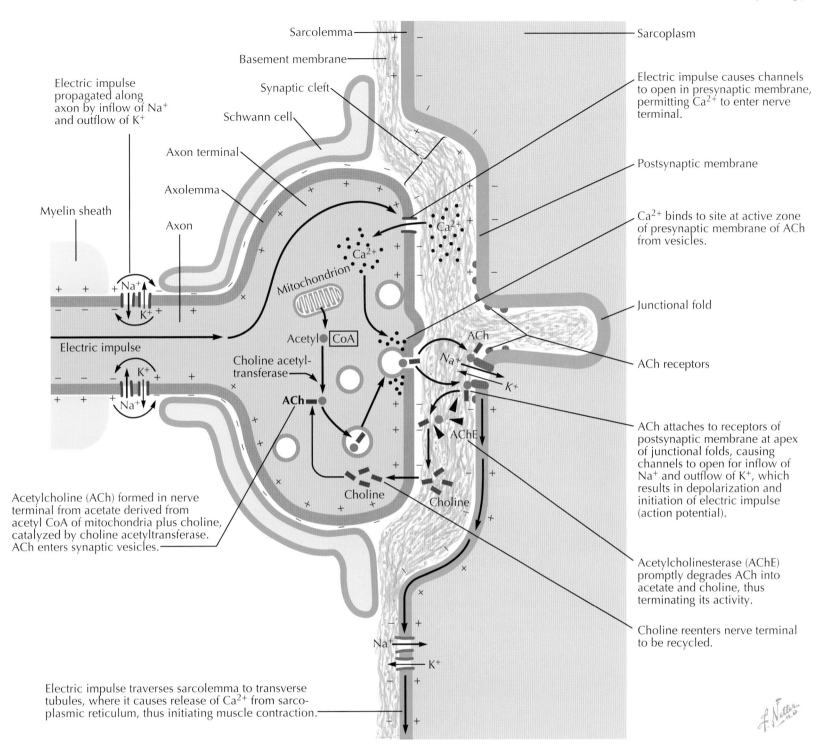

Sarcolemma

Basement membrane

Synaptic cleft

Schwann cell

Axon terminal

Axolemma

Myelin sheath

Axon

Electric impulse propagated along axon by inflow of Na$^+$ and outflow of K$^+$

Electric impulse

Mitochondrion

Acetyl CoA

Choline acetyl-transferase

ACh

Acetylcholine (ACh) formed in nerve terminal from acetate derived from acetyl CoA of mitochondria plus choline, catalyzed by choline acetyltransferase. ACh enters synaptic vesicles.

Choline

Sarcoplasm

Electric impulse causes channels to open in presynaptic membrane, permitting Ca^{2+} to enter nerve terminal.

Postsynaptic membrane

Ca^{2+} binds to site at active zone of presynaptic membrane of ACh from vesicles.

Junctional fold

ACh receptors

ACh attaches to receptors of postsynaptic membrane at apex of junctional folds, causing channels to open for inflow of Na$^+$ and outflow of K$^+$, which results in depolarization and initiation of electric impulse (action potential).

Acetylcholinesterase (AChE) promptly degrades ACh into acetate and choline, thus terminating its activity.

Choline reenters nerve terminal to be recycled.

Electric impulse traverses sarcolemma to transverse tubules, where it causes release of Ca^{2+} from sarco-plasmic reticulum, thus initiating muscle contraction.

PHYSIOLOGY OF NEUROMUSCULAR JUNCTION

Electric impulses are propagated along the motor axon by the inward movement of positively charged sodium ions through depolarization-activated channels located at the nodes of Ranvier. The insulating properties of myelin prevent leakage of current. Adjacent nodes are thus depolarized, and the nerve impulse is regenerated. The axon is repolarized by the outward movement of potassium ions through other depolarization-activated channels, which are thought to be located in the paranodal membrane.

The membrane of the nerve terminal has a different assortment of ion channels: fewer sodium channels, several types of potassium channels, and, most important, voltage-dependent calcium channels. When an action potential arrives at the nerve terminal, it opens the calcium channels and calcium ions move from the extracellular fluid, where the concentration is about 2.5 mmol/L, into the nerve terminal. There, active pumping of calcium ions across the nerve membrane into intracellular organelles (especially the endoplasmic reticulum and the mitochondria) keeps the concentration at about 1 mmol/L. The sudden increase in intraterminal concentration of calcium ions is linked to the release of acetylcholine by exocytosis at the synaptic vesicle release sites. The acetylcholine binds to receptor molecules on the postsynaptic membrane, opening channels that permit the influx of sodium ions and efflux of potassium ions. The net effect is a depolarization of the muscle membrane and a triggering of the muscle action potential. The acetylcholine is then rapidly hydrolyzed by acetylcholinesterase (AChE) into choline and acetate. The choline is conserved by active uptake into the nerve terminal, where it is reconverted into acetylcholine by the enzyme choline acetyltransferase.

Plate 2-12   Musculoskeletal System: PART III

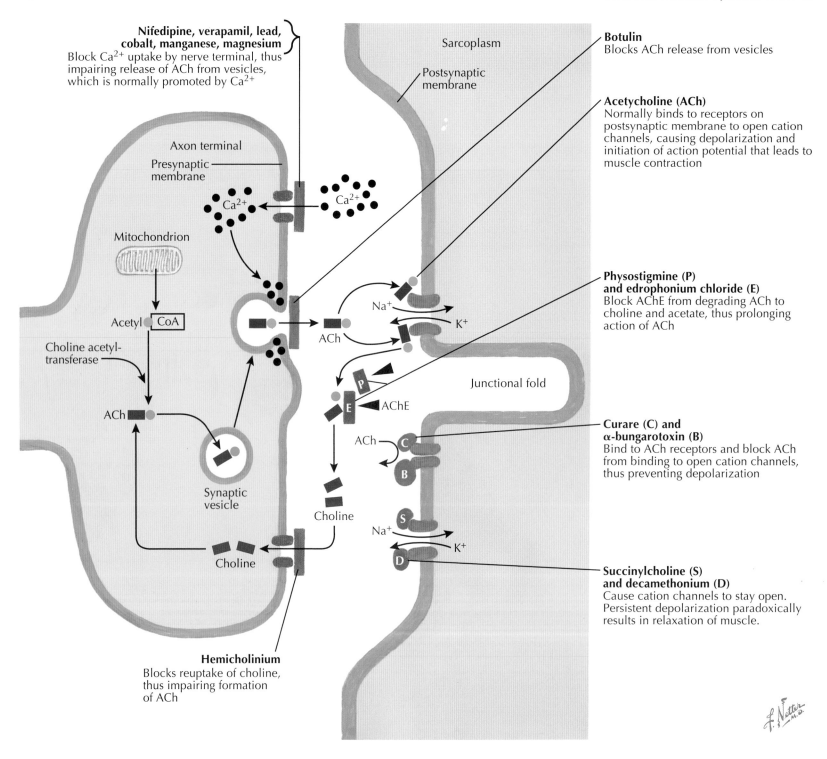

Nifedipine, verapamil, lead, cobalt, manganese, magnesium
Block Ca²⁺ uptake by nerve terminal, thus impairing release of ACh from vesicles, which is normally promoted by Ca²⁺

Sarcoplasm

Postsynaptic membrane

Botulin
Blocks ACh release from vesicles

Acetycholine (ACh)
Normally binds to receptors on postsynaptic membrane to open cation channels, causing depolarization and initiation of action potential that leads to muscle contraction

Axon terminal
Presynaptic membrane

Mitochondrion

Ca²⁺   Ca²⁺

Acetyl   CoA

Na⁺

K⁺

ACh

Physostigmine (P) and edrophonium chloride (E)
Block AChE from degrading ACh to choline and acetate, thus prolonging action of ACh

Choline acetyl-transferase

ACh

P

Junctional fold

E   AChE

ACh

Curare (C) and α-bungarotoxin (B)
Bind to ACh receptors and block ACh from binding to open cation channels, thus preventing depolarization

C

B

Synaptic vesicle

Choline

S

Na⁺

K⁺

D

Succinylcholine (S) and decamethonium (D)
Cause cation channels to stay open. Persistent depolarization paradoxically results in relaxation of muscle.

Choline

Hemicholinium
Blocks reuptake of choline, thus impairing formation of ACh

PHARMACOLOGY OF NEUROMUSCULAR TRANSMISSION

Neuromuscular transmission can be interrupted by many drugs. Organic calcium channel blockers, such as verapamil, and divalent cations, such as lead, prevent calcium ions from entering the nerve terminal and thus block release of the neurotransmitter acetylcholine. The neurotoxin botulin blocks acetylcholine release more directly by a mechanism that is still unknown. Some drugs block the acetylcholine receptors either reversibly (curare) or irreversibly (α-bungarotoxin).

Succinylcholine and decamethonium produce muscle relaxation not by preventing the opening of the acetylcholine-activated channels but by keeping them open too long.

The voltage-dependent sodium channel, which mediates the muscle action potential, is also time dependent: prolonged depolarization inactivates the action potential. This can be reversed only by a repolarization of the membrane. By keeping the acetylcholine channel open, the just-mentioned depolarizing blockers keep the muscle membrane depolarized and refractory to impulse initiation. Hemicholinium weakens neuromuscular transmission by blocking the

reuptake of choline, thus reducing the synthesis of acetylcholine.

Some drugs strengthen neuromuscular transmission. Acetylcholine agonists, such as nicotine, react directly with the acetylcholine receptor. Others, such as physostigmine, pyridostigmine bromide, and edrophonium chloride, inhibit acetylcholinesterase and strengthen transmission by delaying the breakdown of acetylcholine. The action of physostigmine and pyridostigmine bromide persists for hours, and these agents are used to treat the neuromuscular disease myasthenia gravis; edrophonium chloride, on the other hand, is short acting and is used in diagnosing the disease.

Plate 2-13

Physiology

Muscle response to nerve stimuli

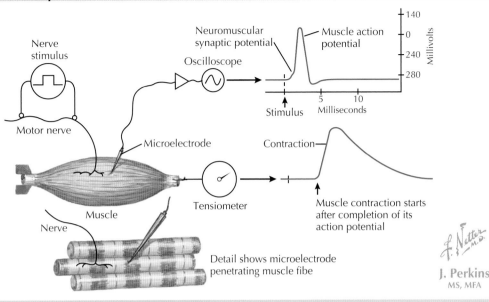

Neuromuscular synaptic potential • Muscle action potential

Nerve stimulus
Oscilloscope
Motor nerve
Microelectrode
Muscle
Nerve
Tensiometer
Contraction

Stimulus
Milliseconds

Muscle contraction starts after completion of its action potential

Detail shows microelectrode penetrating muscle fibe

J. Perkins
MS, MFA

Summation of muscle response with progressive frequency of stimulation

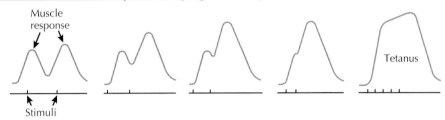

Muscle response

Tetanus

Stimuli

Muscle length–muscle tension relationships

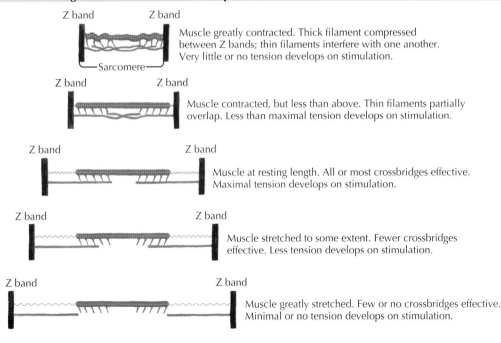

Z band   Z band

Muscle greatly contracted. Thick filament compressed between Z bands; thin filaments interfere with one another. Very little or no tension develops on stimulation.

Sarcomere

Z band   Z band

Muscle contracted, but less than above. Thin filaments partially overlap. Less than maximal tension develops on stimulation.

Z band   Z band

Muscle at resting length. All or most crossbridges effective. Maximal tension develops on stimulation.

Z band   Z band

Muscle stretched to some extent. Fewer crossbridges effective. Less tension develops on stimulation.

Z band   Z band

Muscle greatly stretched. Few or no crossbridges effective. Minimal or no tension develops on stimulation.

PHYSIOLOGY OF MUSCLE CONTRACTION

Muscle Response to Nerve Stimuli. The amount of transmitter released at the nerve terminal of the skeletal neuromuscular junction is sufficient to produce an end plate potential that always reaches the threshold required to activate a muscle action potential. This is not the case in certain pathologic conditions, such as myasthenia gravis or the Lambert-Eaton (myasthenic) syndrome. The muscle action potential is propagated along the entire length of the muscle fiber and deep into the fiber through the transverse (T) tubules. Calcium ions are released almost synchronously from the entire sarcoplasmic reticular system, which elicits a contraction, or twitch.

The tension of the twitch can be measured under conditions in which the muscle is not allowed to shorten (isometric contraction). Because all the sarcomeres are activated, the single-twitch strength of a fiber tends to be the same each time, providing the muscle remains the same length. If a second twitch is elicited before the first has relaxed, the maximum tension achieved is increased. If the muscle is activated at a high enough frequency, the twitches fuse into a continuous smooth contraction (tetanus) of even greater tension.

Muscle Length-Muscle Tension Relationships. The tension developed by a tetanically stimulated muscle depends on the final length the muscle fibers are permitted to reach. Maximum tension is exerted when the length of the sarcomere allows activation of all the crossbridges between the thick and the thin filaments. This occurs at the normal resting length of the muscle fiber. If the muscle is contracted too far, the thin filaments overlap, which interferes with their interactions with the thick filaments, reducing the maximum attainable tension.

On the other hand, if the muscle is stretched, the thin filaments do not have access to all of the available myosin head groups and fewer than the maximum number of crossbridges are formed. If the muscle is greatly stretched, the thick and thin filaments may not overlap at all and no additional tension can develop in response to stimulation.

Plate 2-14

Musculoskeletal System: PART III

REGENERATION OF ATP FOR SOURCE OF ENERGY IN MUSCLE CONTRACTION

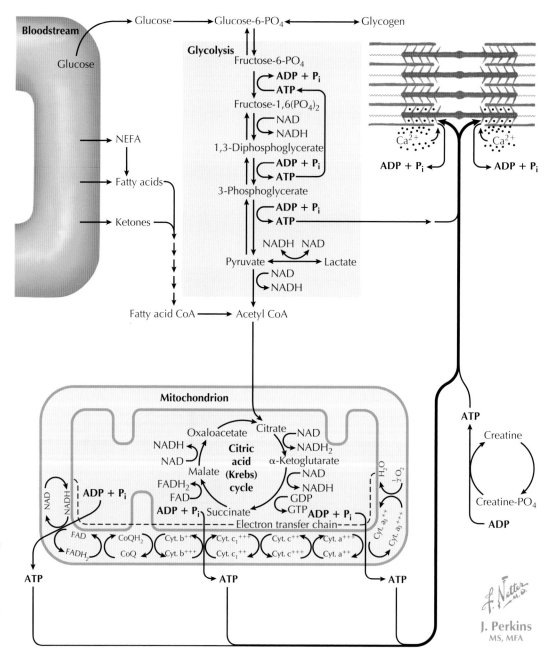

ENERGY METABOLISM OF MUSCLE

The immediate source of energy for muscle contraction is adenosine triphosphate (ATP) generated in the mitochondria by glycolysis and the oxidative metabolism of carbohydrates and fats. The economy of ATP can be understood by counting all the points of its synthesis and breakdown in these metabolic pathways.

In glycolysis, glucose-6-phosphate, derived either from the degradative phosphorylation of glycogen or from the phosphorylation of glucose in serum, is broken down into two molecules of acetyl coenzyme A (CoA). This process may take place in the absence of oxygen, yet three molecules of ATP are generated for each molecule of glucose used. Acetyl CoA enters the citric acid (Krebs) cycle, which generates the reduced forms of flavin adenine dinucleotide ($FADH_2$) and nicotinamide adenine dinucleotide (NADH). Both of these can fuel the conversion of adenosine diphosphate (ADP) into ATP only through the cytochrome oxidative pathway, which involves the reduction of oxygen to water. (The glycolytic pathway also generates NADH, whereas the citric acid cycle generates guanosine triphosphate [GTP], which can contribute a high-energy phosphate

to ADP and thus make ATP.) Thus, whereas only 3 molecules of ATP are generated under anaerobic conditions, 35 molecules of ATP are generated by oxygen-requiring steps in the metabolism of one molecule of glucose derived from glycogen.

The level of ATP in muscle must remain high; it does not decrease substantially, even during continuous

contraction, because muscle fibers have a built-in ATP-buffering system. Energy is stored as creatine phosphate. If the ATP level falls, a small amount of creatine phosphate transfers a phosphate into ADP, forming creatine and regenerating ATP. However, even this reserve pool is not unlimited and can be depleted by intense exercise.

Plate 2-15

Physiology

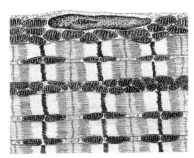

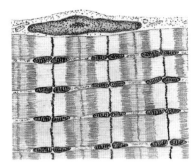

Type I: Dark or red fiber. Large profuse mitochondria beneath sarcolemma and in rows as well as paired in interfibrillar regions. Z lines are wider than in type II.

Type II: Light or white skeletal muscle fiber in longitudinal section on electron microscopy. Small, relatively sparse mitochondria are chiefly paired in interfibrillar spaces at Z lines.

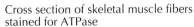

Histochemical classification		
Fiber type	ATPase stain	SDH stain
1. Fast-twitch, fatigable (IIb) Stain deeply for ATPase, poorly for succinic acid dehydrogenase (SDH), a mitochondrial enzyme active in citric acid cycle. Therefore, fibers rapidly release energy from ATP but poorly regenerate it, thus becoming fatigued.		
2. Fast-twitch, fatigue-resistant (IIa) Stain deeply for both ATPase and SDH. Therefore, fibers rapidly release energy from ATP and also rapidly regenerate ATP in citric acid cycle, thus resisting fatigue.		
3. Slow-twitch, fatigue-resistant (I) Stain poorly for ATPase but deeply for SDH. Therefore, fibers only slowly release energy from ATP but regenerate ATP rapidly, thus resisting fatigue.		

MUSCLE FIBER TYPES

For a short time, muscles are able to function without oxygen by using the glycolytic pathway to generate ATP. Muscle fibers specialized for a high-power output over a short time (type II or fast-twitch fibers) make extensive use of this pathway; however, carbohydrates are utilized rather inefficiently in the production of energy, thus the carbohydrate store is depleted rapidly.

Muscle fibers that must remain active over a long time (type I or slow-twitch fibers) are rich in mitochondria, whose iron-containing cytochrome oxidase enzymes and abundant myoglobin content give the fibers their red appearance. These type I fibers stain darkly for enzymes of the oxidative pathway, such as succinic acid dehydrogenase (SDH), but they do not have to generate high tensions and thus do not stain deeply for myofibrillar adenosine triphosphatase (ATPase) and glycolytic enzymes. Type I fibers, which tend to be small, are used in fine manipulations. They are the first fibers in any muscle to be activated when a low level of power is required. Because of their mechanical properties, they are called *slow-twitch, fatigue-resistant (S) fibers.* Energy is conserved by S fibers by a slow rate of relaxation following a twitch, and thus they require a low frequency of stimulation for the twitches to fuse into a sustained contraction (tetanus).

Compared with type I fibers, type II fibers, which must generate high tensions rapidly but need not remain active for prolonged periods, are relatively poor in mitochondrial enzymes and are white in appearance. On the other hand, they are rich in ATPase and glycolytic enzymes. Because of the mechanical properties, they are called *fast-twitch, fatigable (FF) or type 2b fibers.*

In recent years, it has become clear that some fibers have mechanical properties intermediate between those of S and FF fibers. They can generate a relatively fast twitch but are still fatigue resistant and are therefore called *fatigue-resistant (FR) or type 2a fibers.* Most muscles consist of a mixture of these three types of fibers, but the proportions vary depending on each muscle's function and pattern of stimulation (i.e., training).

Muscles can respond to exercise patterns by an appropriate shift in their metabolic characteristics. Isometric, anaerobic exercise results in an increase in the number of myofibrils and in the amount of contractile protein per fiber. Either other fiber types are converted to FF fibers or a higher actomyosin ATPase and glycolytic enzyme activity occurs for all fiber types in the muscle. Thus, muscles of weight lifters and sprinters contain a high proportion of FF fibers. In contrast, aerobic exercise such as long-distance running and swimming induces the reverse enzymatic pattern and increases the muscle's ability to use oxygen. The proportion of FR and S fibers is larger in marathon runners than in other athletes. It is still unclear whether the fiber types actually change as a consequence of training or whether marathon runners choose this sport because of their muscle fiber composition.

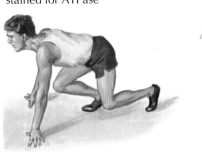

Cross section of skeletal muscle fibers stained for ATPase

Identical section stained for SDH

Sprinter
Training induces a greater proportion of type IIb fibers relative to type IIa.

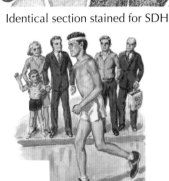

Marathon runner
Type IIa fiber is increased relative to type IIb.

Plate 2-16   Musculoskeletal System: PART III

STRUCTURE, PHYSIOLOGY, AND PATHOPHYSIOLOGY OF GROWTH PLATE

Zones / Structures	Histology	Functions	Blood supply	Po_2	Cell (chondrocyte) health	Cell respiration	Cell glycogen
Secondary bony epiphysis — Epiphyseal artery	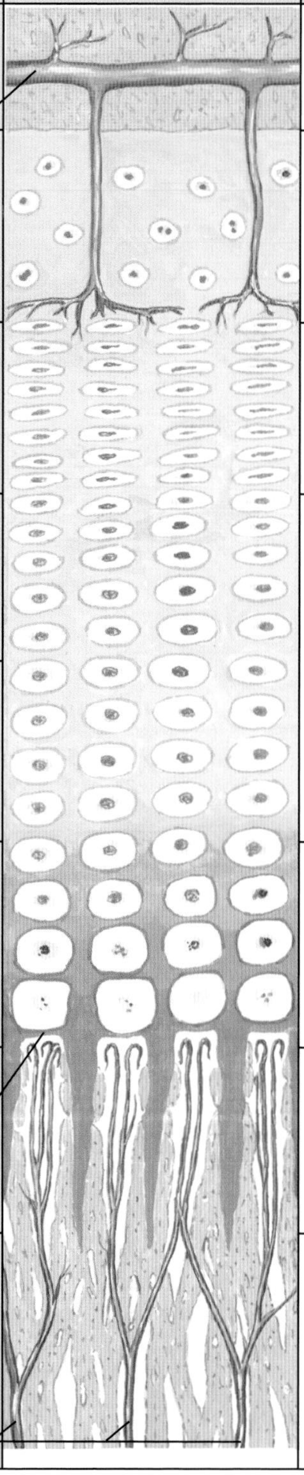						
Reserve zone		Matrix production / Storage	Vessels pass through, do not supply this zone	Poor (low)	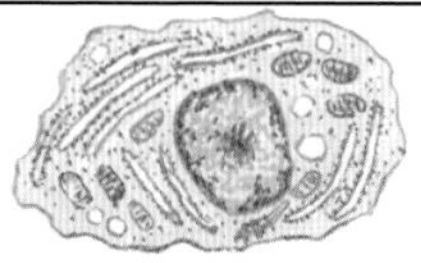 Good, active. Much endoplasmic reticulum, vacuoles, mitochondria	Anaerobic	High concentration
Proliferative zone		Matrix production / Cellular proliferation (longitudinal growth)	Excellent	Excellent / Fair	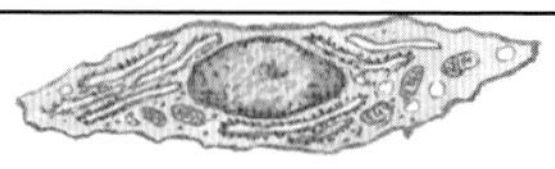 Excellent. Much endoplasmic reticulum, ribosomes, mitochondria. Intact cell membrane	Aerobic	High concentration (less than in above)
Hypertrophic zone — **Maturation zone**		Matrix production persists / Preparation of matrix for calcification		Poor (low)	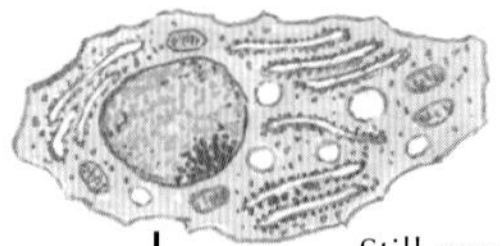 Still good	Progressive change to anaerobic	Glycogen consumed until depleted
Degenerative zone			Progressive decrease	Progressive decrease	Progressive deterioration	Anaerobic glycolysis	
Zone of provisional calcification		Calcification of matrix	Nil	Poor (very low)	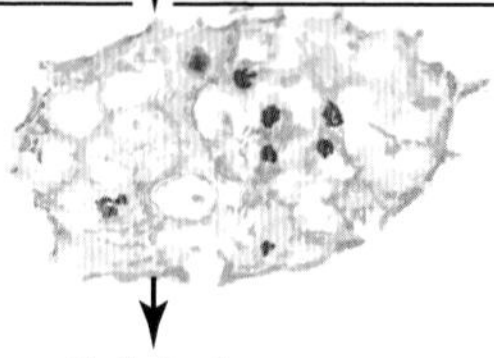 Cell death	Anaerobic glycolysis	Nil
Metaphysis — Last intact transverse septum / **Primary spongiosa**		Vascular invasion and resorption of transverse septa / Bone formation on calcified cartilage remnants	Closed capillary loops / Good	Poor / Good		Progressive reversion to aerobic	?
Secondary spongiosa — Branches of metaphyseal and nutrient arteries		Remodeling Internal: removal of cartilage bars, replacement of woven-fiber bone with lamellar bone / External: funnelization	Excellent	Excellent		Aerobic	?

GROWTH PLATE

The growth plate is an organ composed of cartilage, bone, and fibrous components. The two growth plates in a typical long bone are peripheral extensions of the primary center of ossification in the midportion of the fetal cartilaginous anlage of the bone. The primary center of ossification grows and expands centrifugally in all directions until it eventually becomes confined to two platelike structures at each end of the bone (see Plates 2-16 to 2-18).

STRUCTURE, BLOOD SUPPLY, AND PHYSIOLOGY

The growth plate may be divided into three anatomic components: a cartilaginous component with various histologic zones; a bony component, or metaphysis; and a fibrous component that surrounds the periphery of the plate and consists of the ossification groove of Ranvier and the perichondral ring of La Croix. Each of the three components of the growth plate has its own distinct blood supply. Their vascular differences influence their metabolic activity levels (see Plate 2-17).

Reserve Zone. This zone contains chondroprogenitor cells and exhibits a relatively low level of matrix production. It lies immediately adjacent to the secondary ossification center and comprises cells that appear to be storing lipid and other materials. The cells are

Plate 2-16　　　　　　　　　　　　　　　　　　　　　　　　　Physiology

STRUCTURE, PHYSIOLOGY, AND PATHOPHYSIOLOGY OF GROWTH PLATE (CONTINUED)

Proteoglycans in matrix	Mitochondrial activity	Matrix calcification	Matrix vesicles	Exemplary diseases	Defect (if known)
Aggregated proteoglycans inhibit calcification.	High Ca^{2+} content	Ca^{2+} intracellular	Few vesicles, contain little Ca^{2+}	Diastrophic dwarfism (also, defects in other zones)	Defective type II collagen synthesis
				Pseudoachondroplasia (also, defects in other zones)	Defective processing and transport of proteoglycans
				Kniest syndrome (also, defects in other zones)	Defective processing of proteoglycans
	ATP made	Ca^{2+} intracellular	Few vesicles, contain little Ca^{2+}	Gigantism	Increased cell proliferation (growth hormone increased)
				Achondroplasia	Deficiency of cell proliferation
				Hypochondroplasia	Less severe deficiency of cell proliferation
Progressively disaggregated	Ca^{2+} uptake, no ATP made	Ca^{2+} intracellular	Contain little Ca^{2+}	Malnutrition, irradiation injury, glucocorticoid excess	Decreased cell proliferation and/or matrix synthesis
	Ca^{2+} release begins	Ca^{2+} passes into matrix	Begin Ca^{2+} uptake	Mucopolysaccharidosis (Morquio syndrome, Hurler syndrome)	Deficiencies of specific lysosomal acid hydrolases, with lysosomal storage of mucopolysaccharides
Disaggregated proteoglycans are broken down and removed in order to permit calcification.	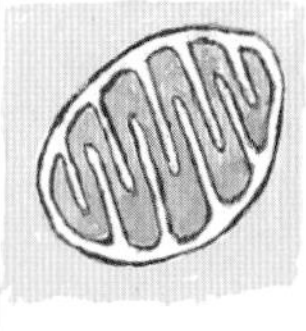 Ca^{2+} released	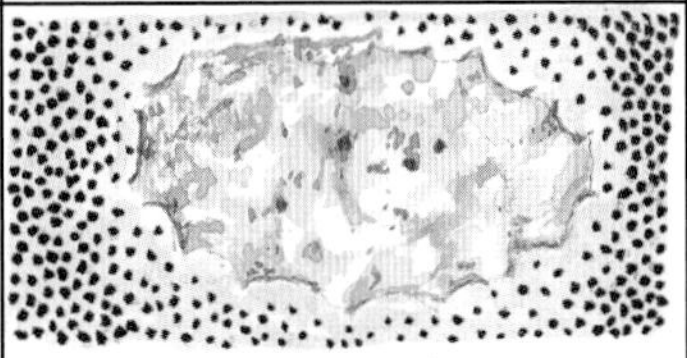 Matrix calcified	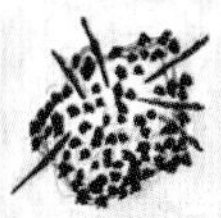 Crystals in and on vesicles	Rickets, osteomalacia (also, defects in metaphysis)	Insufficiency of Ca^{2+} and/or P$_i$ for normal calcification of matrix
				Metaphyseal chondro-dysplasia (Jansen and Schmid types)	Extension of hypertrophic cells into metaphysis
				Acute hematogenous osteomyelitis	Flourishing of bacteria due to sluggish circulation, low Po$_2$, reticuloendothelial deficiency
				Osteopetrosis	Abnormality of osteoclasts (internal remodeling)
				Osteogenesis imperfecta	Abnormality of osteoblasts and collagen synthesis
				Scurvy	Inadequate collagen formation
				Metaphyseal dysplasia (Pyle disease)	Abnormality of funnelization (external remodeling)

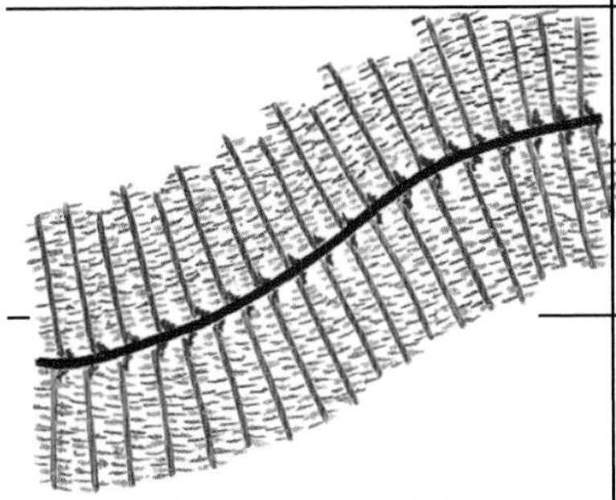

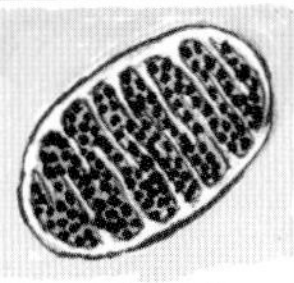

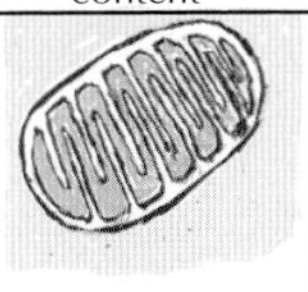

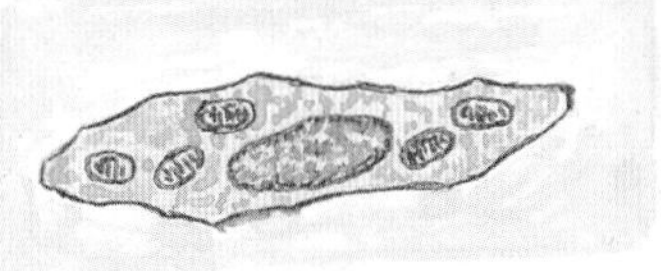

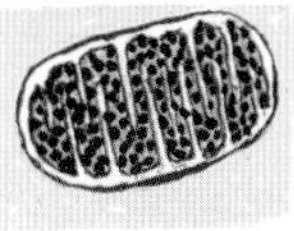

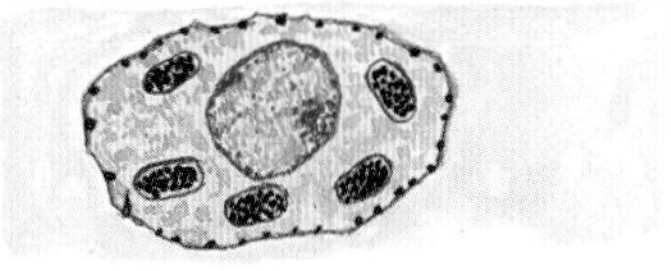

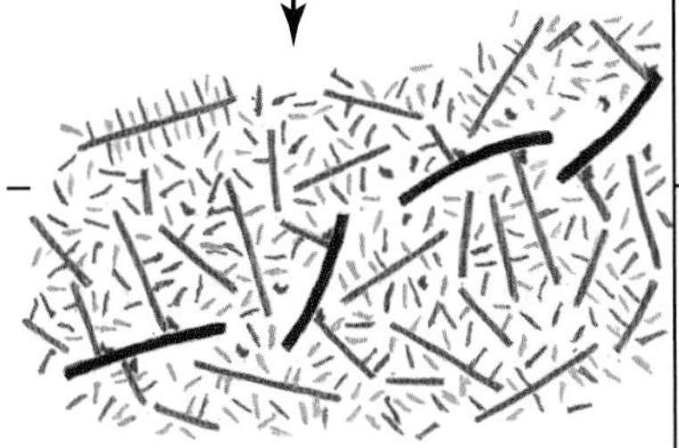

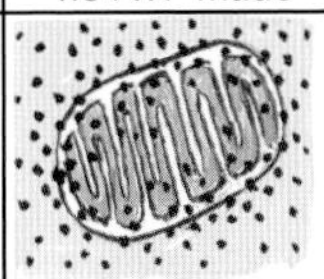

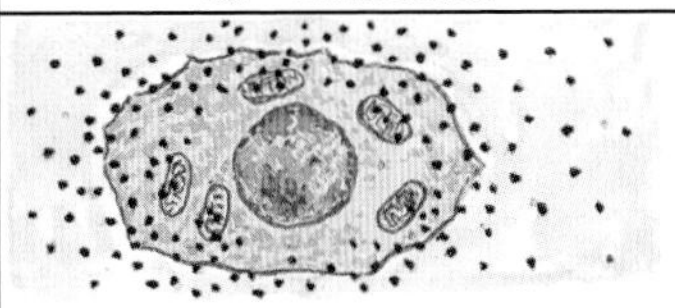

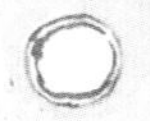

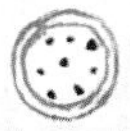

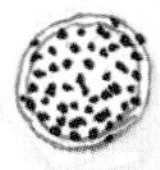

Labels in figures: Mito-chondria; Cell membrane

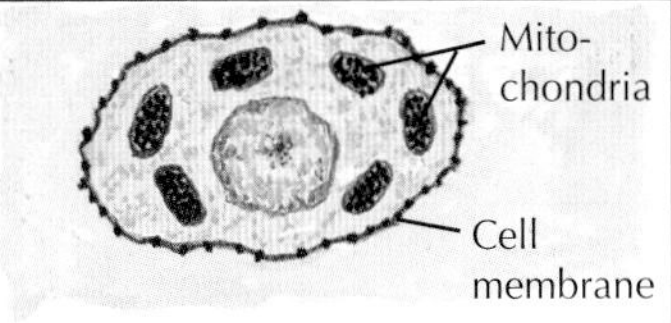

GROWTH PLATE (Continued)

spherical and may exist singly or in pairs. They are relatively few in number, with more extracellular matrix between them than between cells in any other zone.

The matrix shows a positive histochemical reaction for the presence of a hyaluronan and an aggrecan proteoglycan aggregate. The cytoplasm exhibits a positive stain for glycogen. Electron microscopy reveals that these cells contain abundant endoplasmic reticulum, a clear indication that they are actively synthesizing protein.

Oxygen tension (Po$_2$) is low, which suggests that blood vessels passing through the reserve zone in cartilage canals do not readily exchange nutrients with it (see Plate 2-16). Chondrocytes in the reserve zone do not proliferate or do so only sporadically.

Proliferative Zone. This zone exhibits higher levels of cellular proliferation and matrix production, which together contribute to longitudinal growth. These chondrocytes are flattened and aligned in longitudinal columns, with the long axis of the cells lying perpendicular to the long axis of the bone; they are packed with endoplasmic reticulum. The cytoplasm stains positively for glycogen.

With few exceptions, chondrocytes in the proliferative zone are the principal cells in the cartilaginous portion of the growth plate that divide. With the boundary between the reserve zone and the top of the proliferative zone being the true germinal layer of the growth plate, the top cell of each column represents the "mother" cartilage cell for each column.

Plate 2-17

Musculoskeletal System: PART III

GROWTH PLATE (Continued)

Longitudinal growth in the growth plate equals the rate of production of new chondrocytes at the top of the proliferative zone multiplied by the maximum size of the chondrocytes at the bottom of the hypertrophic zone.

Because of the rich vascular supply to the top of the proliferative zone, Po_2 is highest in this region of the growth plate. The high Po_2 coupled with the presence of glycogen in the chondrocytes suggests that aerobic metabolism with glycogen storage is taking place.

Hypertrophic Zone. The functions of this zone are preparation of the matrix for expansion, degradation, and matrix calcification. Chondrocytes in this zone progressively become more spherical and greatly enlarged along their vertical axis. By the bottom of the zone, they have enlarged to five times their size in the proliferative zone. The cytoplasm of chondrocytes in the top half of the zone stains positively for glycogen; near the middle of the zone it abruptly loses all glycogen-staining ability.

On electron microscopy, chondrocytes in the top half of the hypertrophic zone appear normal and contain the full complement of cytoplasmic components, but in the bottom half of the zone the cytoplasm contains numerous vacuoles that can occupy over 85% of the total cytoplasmic volume.

The last cell at the base of each cell column is clearly nonviable and shows extensive fragmentation of the cell membrane and the nuclear envelope, with loss of all cytoplasmic components except a few mitochondria and scattered remnants of endoplasmic reticulum. Mitochondria and cell membranes of chondrocytes in the top half of the hypertrophic zone are loaded with calcium. Toward the middle of the zone, mitochondria rapidly lose calcium, and at the bottom of the zone, both mitochondria and cell membranes have no calcium. These findings suggest that mitochondrial calcium may be involved in cartilage calcification.

The hypertrophic zone is avascular, and Po_2 is therefore low. In the bottom half of the zone, glycogen is completely depleted. There is no other source of nutrition to serve as an energy source for the mitochondria. Because calcium uptake and retention require energy, as soon as the chondrocytes' glycogen supplies are exhausted, mitochondria release calcium, a factor that may play a role in matrix calcification.

The metabolic events in the proliferative and hypertrophic zones can be summarized as follows. In the proliferative zone, Po_2 is high, aerobic metabolism occurs, glycogen is stored, and mitochondria form ATP. In the hypertrophic zone, Po_2 is low, anaerobic metabolism occurs, and glycogen is consumed until near the middle of the zone, where mitochondria switch from forming ATP to accumulating calcium. ATP formation and calcium accumulation cannot take place simultaneously. Both processes require energy, which comes from the respiratory chain in the mitochondria. In addition, ATP formation requires the presence of ADP, whereas calcium accumulation does not. Possibly, in the hypertrophic zone, there is insufficient ADP for significant ATP formation.

The matrix of the hypertrophic zone shows positive histochemical reactions for hyaluronan and proteoglycan degradation products (see Plate 2-25). From the reserve zone through the hypertrophic zone there is a progressive decrease in the length of proteoglycan aggregates and in the number of aggregate subunits in the matrix. The distance between the subunits also increases.

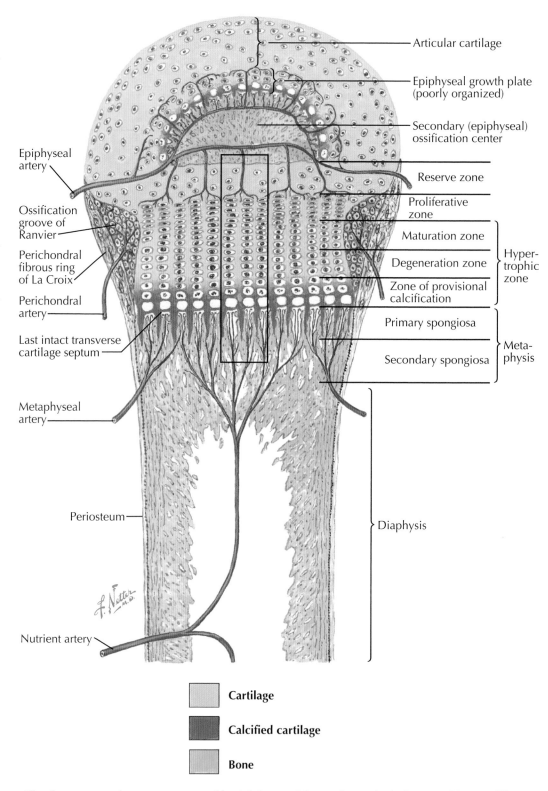

Cartilage

Calcified cartilage

Bone

The large proteoglycan aggregates with tightly packed subunits suppress mineralization and its spread, whereas smaller aggregates with widely spaced subunits at the bottom of the hypertrophic zone tend to be less effective in preventing mineral growth. In any event, proteoglycan disaggregation and degradation must take place before significant mineralization occurs.

The initial calcification (seeding, or nucleation) in the bottom of the hypertrophic zone, called the *zone of provisional calcification*, occurs within or on vesicles in the longitudinal septa of the matrix (see Plate 2-16). Matrix

vesicles are densest in the hypertrophic zone. They are small, trilamellar membrane structures (100 to 150 nanometers in diameter) released by chondrocytes. Matrix vesicles are rich in various phosphatases, some of which act as a pyrophosphatase to destroy pyrophosphate, another inhibitor of calcium-phosphate precipitation. Matrix vesicles begin to accumulate calcium at the same level in the hypertrophic zone at which mitochondria begin to lose it. This suggests that mitochondrial calcium is involved in the initial calcification in the growth plate. Initial calcification, whether it is within

Plate 2-18

Physiology

GROWTH PLATE *(Continued)*

or on matrix vesicles or collagen fibers, may be in the form of amorphous calcium phosphate, but this mineral phase rapidly transitions to hydroxyapatite crystal formation. With continued crystal growth and confluence, the longitudinal septa become gradually calcified.

Matrix calcification in the zone of provisional calcification makes the extracellular matrix less permeable to metabolites. The hypertrophic zone has the lowest diffusion coefficient in the entire growth plate, primarily because of its high mineral content.

Metaphysis. The three functions of the metaphysis are vascular invasion of the transverse septa at the bottom of the cartilaginous portion of the growth plate, bone formation, and bone remodeling (see Plate 2-17). The metaphysis begins just distal to the last intact transverse septum at the base of each cell column of the cartilaginous portion of the growth plate and ends at the junction with the diaphysis. In the first part of the metaphysis, Po_2 is low, which, together with the rouleaux formation frequently seen just distal to the last intact transverse septum, indicates that this is a region of vascular stasis.

Electron microscopy shows capillary sprouts, which are lined with a layer of endothelial and perivascular cells, invading the base of the cartilaginous portion of the plate. Cytoplasmic processes from these cells push into the transverse septa and through their proteolytic enzyme activities degrade and remove the nonmineralized transverse septa. This region of the metaphysis is known as the *primary spongiosa*. The longitudinal septa are partially or completely calcified, with osteoblasts lining up along the calcified bars. Between this layer of osteoblasts and the capillary sprouts are osteoprogenitor cells that contain little cytoplasm but have a prominent ovoid- to spindle-shaped nucleus.

A short distance down the calcified longitudinal septa is the region called the *secondary spongiosa*. Osteoblasts begin laying down bone by a process called *endochondral ossification*, or bone formation on a cartilage scaffold. The amount of osteoid and bone tissue formed on the calcified longitudinal septa increases downward and into the metaphysis. At the same time, the calcified septa gradually become thinner until they disappear altogether. Still farther down in the metaphysis, the original woven-fiber bone is replaced with lamellar bone. The gradual replacement of the calcified longitudinal septa with newly formed woven bone, as well as the gradual replacement of woven bone with lamellar bone, is called *internal*, or *histologic*, *remodeling*. Large, irregularly shaped osteoclasts are distributed evenly throughout the metaphysis (except in the primary spongiosa) and subperiosteally around the outside of the metaphysis, where it narrows to meet the diaphysis. This narrowing of the metaphysis is called *external*, or *anatomic*, *remodeling*.

PERIPHERAL FIBROCARTILAGINOUS ELEMENT

Encircling the periphery of the growth plate in a typical long bone are two structures: a wedge-shaped groove of cells, the *ossification groove*, first described by Ranvier, and a band of fibrous tissue and bone called the *perichondral fibrous ring*, studied by La Croix (see Plate 2-18). Although both structures are simply different parts of the peripheral fibrocartilaginous element of the growth plate, they can be considered separate entities because of their different functions.

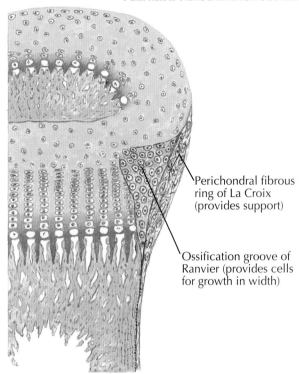

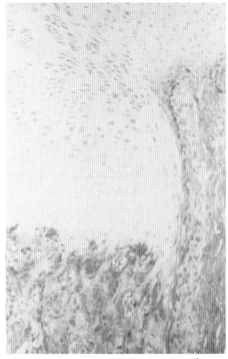

Perichondral fibrous ring of La Croix (provides support)

Ossification groove of Ranvier (provides cells for growth in width)

Microscopic section (H&E) corresponds generally to illustration at left.

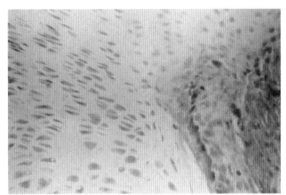

High-power section shows cells of ossification groove of Ranvier apparently "flowing" into cartilage at level of reserve zone, thus contributing to growth in width of growth plate. Note presence of arterioles (cut-in section).

Load

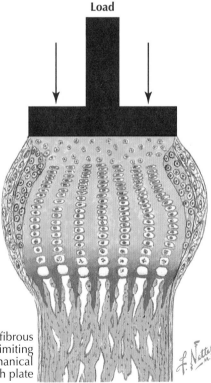

Illustration of how perichondral fibrous ring of La Croix acts as limiting membrane and provides mechanical support to cartilaginous growth plate

The function of the ossification groove of Ranvier appears to be the contribution of chondrocytes for the increase in width of the growth plate. The groove of Ranvier contains round-to-ovoid cells that, on light microscopy, appear to "flow" from the groove into the cartilage at the level of the reserve zone. The perichondral fibrous ring of La Croix acts as a limiting membrane that provides mechanical support for the bone-cartilage junction of the growth plate. It is a dense fibrous band encircling the growth plate, in which collagen fibers run vertically, obliquely, and

circumferentially. The structure is continuous at one end with the ossification groove and at the other end with the periosteum and subperiosteal bone of the metaphysis.

PATHOPHYSIOLOGY

Certain representative disorders whose pathophysiology exemplifies the known functions of the highly synchronized and interrelated zones in the growth plate have been identified and are shown in Plate 2-16.

Plate 2-19

Musculoskeletal System: PART III

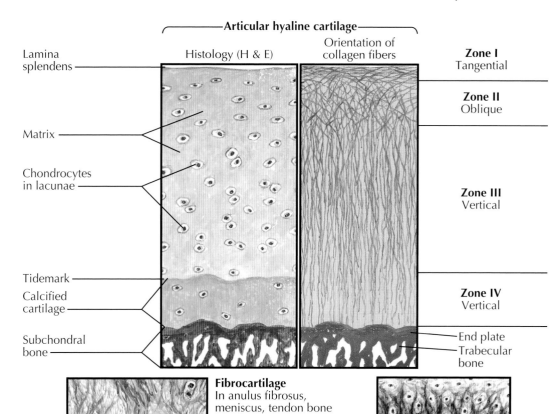

Articular hyaline cartilage

Histology (H & E) — Orientation of collagen fibers

Lamina splendens

Matrix

Chondrocytes in lacunae

Tidemark

Calcified cartilage

Subchondral bone

Zone I — Tangential
Zone II — Oblique
Zone III — Vertical
Zone IV — Vertical

End plate
Trabecular bone

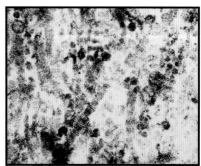

Fibrocartilage
In anulus fibrosus, meniscus, tendon bone interface

Interlacing strands of fibrous tissue throughout matrix (H & E)

Elastic cartilage
In auricle, eustachian tube, nose, epiglottis

Dark-staining elastic fibers between and around lacunae (H & E)

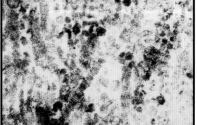

Although hyaline cartilage appears smooth and homogeneous to naked eye, electron microscopy reveals basic structure of network of collagen fibers and proteoglycans (×80,000).

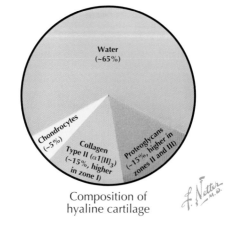

Water (~65%)

Chondrocytes (~5%)

Collagen Type II (α1[II]₃) (~15%, higher in zone I)

Proteoglycans (~15%, higher in zones II and III)

Composition of hyaline cartilage

COMPOSITION AND STRUCTURE OF CARTILAGE

Cartilage is a complex and versatile connective tissue. *Growth plate cartilage* is a hyaline cartilage responsible for much of the shape, growth, and development of the skeleton. *Articular hyaline cartilage* provides the self-lubricating, low-friction gliding and load-distributing surfaces of the synovial (diarthrodial) joints. *Fibrocartilage* attaches tendons and ligaments to bone. *Elastic cartilage* contributes structural integrity to the auricles, nose, eustachian tubes, epiglottis, and trachea. *Fibroelastic cartilage* is responsible for the load-distributing and shock-absorbing properties of the intervertebral discs and intra-articular menisci.

Regardless of its specialized function, all cartilage consists of cells—chondrocytes and chondroblasts. These cells synthesize and deposit around them an elaborate matrix of macromolecules that are some of the largest in nature. The mechanical properties of cartilage tissue are derived primarily from the properties of the complex extracellular matrix.

On gross examination and on light microscopy, all cartilage appears smooth and homogeneous. However, electron microscopy reveals that its basic fibrillar structure consists of a meshwork of collagen fibers and large proteoglycans in approximately equal amounts. In addition, water is a major component of cartilage, contributing 65% to 80% of its weight. Type II collagen, the major fibrillar component of cartilage matrix, contributes tensile strength and form to the tissue. Proteoglycans, by their ability to entrap large amounts of water (tissue fluid) in their macromolecular domains, give cartilage a resiliency and stiffness to compression (see Plate 2-25). The exact mechanisms by which collagen and proteoglycans interact in the various types of

cartilage remain unclear. However, another function of collagen is to trap proteoglycans and restrain their swelling pressure.

In addition to properties shared with other types of hyaline cartilage, articular cartilage has a complex internal structure. Electron microscopy and biochemical studies reveal four poorly demarcated zones: a small superficial, or tangential, zone (I); a larger intermediate, or transitional, zone (II); a deep vertical zone (III), which occupies the greatest volume; and a zone

of calcified cartilage (IV), which lies adjacent to the subchondral bone. On light microscopy, the boundary between zones III and IV is demarcated by an undulating plate, referred to as a tidemark.

The cells in the four zones differ dramatically in size, shape, orientation, and number, as well as in the relative composition, proportion, and orientation of macromolecules in their matrix. Even small differences in the composition and organization of the matrix give each zone slightly different mechanical properties.

Plate 2-20

Physiology

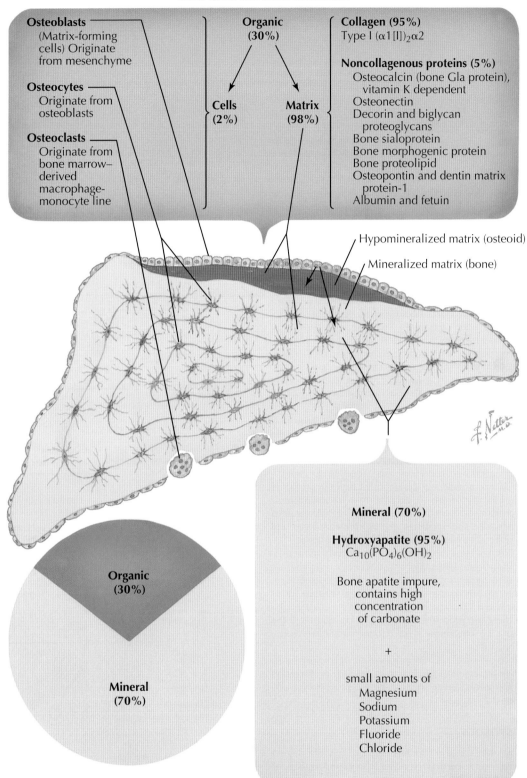

BONE CELLS AND BONE DEPOSITION

Osteoblasts (Matrix-forming cells) Originate from mesenchyme

Osteocytes Originate from osteoblasts

Osteoclasts Originate from bone marrow–derived macrophage-monocyte line

Organic (30%)

Cells (2%)

Matrix (98%)

Collagen (95%) Type I $(\alpha 1 [I])_2 \alpha 2$

Noncollagenous proteins (5%)
Osteocalcin (bone Gla protein), vitamin K dependent
Osteonectin
Decorin and biglycan proteoglycans
Bone sialoprotein
Bone morphogenic protein
Bone proteolipid
Osteopontin and dentin matrix protein-1
Albumin and fetuin

Hypomineralized matrix (osteoid)

Mineralized matrix (bone)

Organic (30%)

Mineral (70%)

Mineral (70%)

Hydroxyapatite (95%) $Ca_{10}(PO_4)_6(OH)_2$

Bone apatite impure, contains high concentration of carbonate

+

small amounts of
Magnesium
Sodium
Potassium
Fluoride
Chloride

COMPOSITION AND STRUCTURE OF BONE

The skeleton is an adaptable and well-articulated frame providing mechanical support for movement and organ protection. It is also a dynamic mineral reserve bank in which the body stores its calcium and phosphate in a metabolically stable and structurally useful manner. The cells of bone—the osteoblasts, osteocytes, and osteoclasts—function in a coordinated manner acting as both construction workers and metabolic bankers, which are dual roles that can sometimes interfere with each other.

The osteoblast, or bone-forming cell, is approximately 20 μm in diameter and contains a single eccentric nucleus. Under the direction of RUNX2 and Osterix transcription factors, osteoblasts arise from osteoprogenitor cells found in the apical cell layers of periosteum and within marrow tissue. Osteoblasts adhere to an organic matrix scaffolding called osteoid (found on periosteal, endosteal, trabecular, and haversian surfaces). Osteoblasts also preside over the mineralization of osteoid, leading to the formation of new bone tissue. The osteoblast phenotype is identified by its large quantities of bone alkaline phosphatase and its production of a bone-specific matrix protein called osteocalcin.

The mature osteocyte, derived from an osteoblast, is an oval cell 20 to 60 μm long and buried within the mineralized bone matrix in a small cavern called a lacuna. Numerous processes extend from its cell surface and leave the lacuna via a network of canals or canaliculi. Many osteocyte processes extend into the canalicular system and contact processes from other osteocytes. This extensive osteocyte-canaliculi network is believed to play a vital role in transportation of cell metabolites, communication between cells, and regulation of mineral homeostasis.

The other major type of bone cell, the osteoclast, resorbs mineralized bone matrix. The osteoclast is a large cell (as great as 100 μm in diameter) containing as many as 100 nuclei per cell (although most osteoclasts contain many fewer nuclei). It is rich in lysosomal enzymes (including acid phosphatase and proteases) and proton pumps and possesses a specialized cell membrane (the ruffled border) at sites where active bone resorption occurs. Unlike the osteoblast and the osteocyte that derive from a mesenchymal progenitor cell, the osteoclast is derived from circulating cells of the monocyte-macrophage lineage that differentiate into preosteoclasts near a bone's surface.

Bone cells account for only a small portion (2%) of the entire organic component of bone, most of which consists of osteoid produced by osteoblasts.

Collagen (predominantly type I) is the major organic component of bone, accounting for a majority of the

Plate 2-21

Musculoskeletal System: PART III

COMPOSITION AND STRUCTURE OF BONE (Continued)

protein in osteoid. Bone collagen is deposited along lines of mechanical stress according to Wolff's law and provides an important template for mineral crystal deposition (see Plate 2-36). Although constituting only a minor portion of osteoid's protein content, noncollagenous bone proteins play important roles in regulating osteoblast proliferation, metabolism, matrix production, and mineralization of bone matrix. Major noncollagenous proteins found in bone include fetuin (α_2-HS-glycoprotein), osteonectin, osteopontin, osteocalcin (bone Gla protein), bone sialoprotein, decorin and biglycan proteoglycans, bone proteolipid, and bone morphogenic proteins.

The organic component of bone (cells plus organic matrix) makes up approximately 30% of bone's dry weight. The inorganic, or mineral, component of bone (70% of dry weight) consists mainly of a carbonate-rich hydroxyapatite analog called bone apatite, which is smaller and less perfect in crystal arrangement than pure hydroxyapatite. Because of its crystalline imperfections, bone apatite is more soluble than pure hydroxyapatite and is therefore more readily available for metabolic activity and for exchange with body fluids. In addition to incorporating carbonate, bone apatite possesses the ability to incorporate magnesium, sodium, potassium, chloride, fluoride, strontium, and other bone-seeking elements.

Mature lamellar bone has the same chemical composition and material properties throughout the skeleton, regardless of its mechanism of formation—intramembranous or endochondral—or its structural organization—cortical (compact) or trabecular bone.

Skeletal growth and development begin in utero and continue for nearly 2 decades in a series of well-orchestrated events. These events are determined genetically and regulated by central endocrine and peripheral biophysical and biochemical processes.

Normal bone forms either by intramembranous ossification from mesenchymal osteoblasts in the absence of cartilage scaffolding or by endochondral ossification using a preexisting calcified cartilage matrix. Long bones and vertebrae increase in size by a combination of these two processes. For example, ossification of the shaft of a long bone is an intramembranous process: subperiosteal deposition of new bone widens the shaft, while endosteal resorption widens the medullary canal. Long bones increase in length by cartilage proliferation at the growth plate in an elaborate process of endochondral ossification.

HISTOLOGY

The adult skeleton contains only two types of mature bone tissue, cortical (compact) bone and trabecular (cancellous or spongy) bone.

Both of these histologic types are represented in a typical long bone such as the femur (see Plate 2-21). Cortical bone forms the wall of the shaft, and trabecular bone is concentrated at each end.

The articular surface of the femur is covered with a cap of hyaline cartilage, which is better suited than bone to withstand the friction and relative motion in the joint. The cartilage cap is continuous with the synovial membrane lining the joint cavity (see Plate 2-26). The rest of the outer surface of the bone is lined with periosteum, a dense fibrous connective tissue. In a growing bone, the inner surface of the periosteum contains

COMPOSITION OF BONE

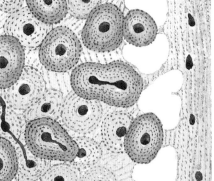

Section of trabecular bone (H & E)

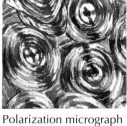

Cross section of cortical (compact) bone

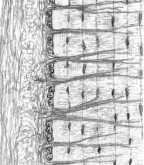

Cambium layer (osteoblasts)

Section of decalcified bone shows attachment of periosteum to bone by perforating (Sharpey's) fibers.

Electron micrograph shows different generations of secondary osteons. New bone (dark) replaces old bone (light) and nonhaversian bone.

Polarization micrograph reveals alternating light and dark rings of mineral hydroxyapatite crystals embedded in osteoid.

osteogenic cells that are actively laying down sheets of bone matrix. The cell morphology ranges from cuboidal-shaped active cells near the bone itself to inactive flattened-appearing cells embedded among dense collagen fibers in the outer edge of the periosteum. As the layers of bone are deposited, perpendicular-arranged bundles of collagen fibers become embedded in them, forming perforating, or Sharpey's, fibers.

The inner layer of the shaft of a long bone is lined with endosteum, a much less substantial layer.

Endosteal cells possess an osteogenic capacity that is expressed during bone remodeling and fracture healing.

STRUCTURE OF CORTICAL (COMPACT) BONE

The fundamental functional unit of adult human cortical bone is the osteon, or haversian system, a cylindrical structure measuring approximately 250 μm in radius and 1 to 5 cm in length. The osteon consists of

Plate 2-22

Physiology

COMPOSITION AND STRUCTURE OF BONE (Continued)

concentric layers of bony lamellae, each 2 to 3 μm thick, which surround a central haversian canal (see Plates 2-21 and 2-22). The haversian canal, first described in 1691 by the English anatomist Clopton Havers, contains blood vessels, nerve supplies, and a supporting extracellular matrix. Lateral branches, called Volkmann's canals, carry blood vessels from one osteon to another. Each cylindrical lamella within the osteon is lined with a sparse population of regularly arranged osteocytes, which communicate with one another by fine cell processes projecting into the lamellae through minute channels or canaliculi. Oxygen and nutrients reach osteocytes in the outer lamellae through these canaliculi by diffusion or convection forces resulting from mechanical motions. In addition to osteons, the compact collar of a long bone contains at its periphery subperiosteal circumferential lamellae, which are deposited by the inner layer of the periosteum.

As the long bone grows in width (or if it is subjected to changing stress patterns), remodeling occurs. The initial step in cortical bone remodeling is the removal of portions of osteons by the activity of tunneling osteoclasts. After the bone is removed, new lamellae are deposited in new concentric layers, from outside inward, until a complete new osteon is formed. In mature bone, extensive remodeling causes the destruction and formation of many generations of osteons. The newest ones can be recognized by their complete outer circumference. In some osteons of earlier generations, a portion of the outer border has been removed and occupied by the outer border of a new osteon. Indeed, in some old osteons, these destructive processes have occurred so frequently that only small portions of the original lamellae remain (see Section 1, Plate 1-13). These remnants, which may also include portions of circumferential lamellae, are called interstitial lamellae.

Cortical bone is remodeled by on the periosteal, endosteal, and haversian canal surfaces. These surfaces are called bone envelopes, or remodeling bays. The periosteal surface is responsible for the growth in bone width. The endosteum, which lines the medullary cavity of long bones, carries out complex metabolic and structural activities throughout life. These activities include phases of bone resorption alternating with phases of bone formation (see Plate 2-40). Endosteal activity determines the diameter of the medullary canal, while the combined activities of the periosteum and endosteum determine the overall thickness of the bone cortex. The haversian canal surface is important in bone remodeling and is responsible for the density of the cortex.

Arterial blood supply to two thirds of the inner bone cortex is predominantly centrifugal and is carried out by nutrient arteries entering from the medullary canal (see Plate 2-22); periosteal arterioles supply approximately one third of the outer cortex of a long bone. A highly developed anastomotic network connects the centripedal periosteal arterial system with the centrifugal endosteal arterial system. Venous drainage of the cortex is predominantly centripedal via a large plexus of veins in the medullary canal. (See pages 9 and 10 in Section 1 for a comprehensive discussion of blood supply to bone.)

STRUCTURE OF TRABECULAR BONE

In contrast to the compact structure of cortical bone, trabecular bone is a complex network of intersecting

STRUCTURE OF CORTICAL (COMPACT) BONE

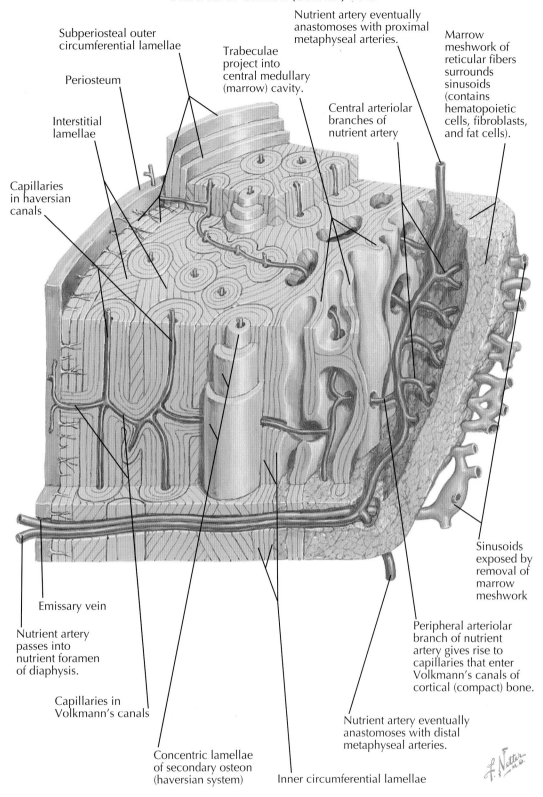

Subperiosteal outer circumferential lamellae

Periosteum

Interstitial lamellae

Capillaries in haversian canals

Trabeculae project into central medullary (marrow) cavity.

Nutrient artery eventually anastomoses with proximal metaphyseal arteries.

Central arteriolar branches of nutrient artery

Marrow meshwork of reticular fibers surrounds sinusoids (contains hematopoietic cells, fibroblasts, and fat cells).

Emissary vein

Nutrient artery passes into nutrient foramen of diaphysis.

Capillaries in Volkmann's canals

Concentric lamellae of secondary osteon (haversian system)

Inner circumferential lamellae

Nutrient artery eventually anastomoses with distal metaphyseal arteries.

Peripheral arteriolar branch of nutrient artery gives rise to capillaries that enter Volkmann's canals of cortical (compact) bone.

Sinusoids exposed by removal of marrow meshwork

curved plates and tubes (see Plate 2-23). The bone within each trabecula is mature lamellar bone; the osteocytes are concentrically oriented and have a well-developed canalicular network.

Trabecular bone is typically located at the ends of a long bone. Here, the well-defined medullary cavity of the shaft gives way to a different organization: bony trabeculae fill the entire cross section of the bone, occupying approximately 20% of its volume. In the proximal end of the femur, the trabeculae are quite regularly

arranged, reflecting the direction of the principal mechanical stresses to which this bone is subjected.

Cortical bone accounts for 80% of skeletal bone mass, whereas trabecular bone constitutes the remaining 20%. However, because of the larger surface area of trabecular bone, its surface-to-volume ratio is approximately 10 times that of cortical bone.

The metabolic activity of trabecular bone is nearly eight times greater than that of cortical bone, which may help to explain why disorders of skeletal

Plate 2-23   Musculoskeletal System: PART III

STRUCTURE OF TRABECULAR BONE

Trabecular bone (schematic)

On cut surfaces (as in sections), trabeculae may appear as discontinuous spicules.

Osteoid (hypomineralized matrix)

Active osteoblasts producing osteoid

Inactive osteoblasts (lining cells)

Marrow spaces (containing hematopoietic cells and fat)

Osteocytes

Osteoclasts (in Howship's lacunae)

Trabeculae

COMPOSITION AND STRUCTURE OF BONE *(Continued)*

homeostasis (metabolic bone diseases) have a greater tendency to effect trabecular bone rather than cortical bone. Observations indicate that the rate of remodeling in trabecular bone may vary greatly in different parts of the skeleton. For example, in adults, trabecular bone at the ends of long bones is in contact with a fatty marrow, whereas in vertebrae of the axial skeleton, it is in contact with a more highly cellular hematopoietic marrow. These differences may help to account for the axial distribution of trabecular osteopenia.

Despite its apparent porosity and relatively small volume, trabecular bone is well adapted to distribute compressive forces, a capacity best exemplified by the vertebral body. In contrast, the structural properties of cortical bone are best suited to resist bending and torsional stresses.

In actively growing, or remodeling, trabecular bone, the direction of deposition can be determined by a row of osteoblasts on one border of the trabecula (see Plate 2-23). The deposition of new bone by these osteoblasts is often counterbalanced by the removal of bone by osteoclasts from the opposite surface of the trabecula. By this means of coordinated resorption and deposition, the position of a trabecula can shift within a bone while still maintaining relative mass homeostasis.

With age, the balance between the rate of bone formation and the rate of bone resorption changes, leading to a progressive decrease in bone mass. Any number of combinations can cause this effect. Evidence from kinetic studies indicates that after age 40, bone formation remains constant whereas bone resorption increases. Over several decades, through age-related bone loss (men and women) and postmenopausal bone loss (women), the skeletal mass may be reduced to 50% of what it was at age 30. If the bone density and structure becomes so depleted that the skeleton can no longer withstand the mechanical stresses of everyday life, pathologic fractures also known as fragility fractures may result. The compressive strength of bone is proportional to the square of its apparent density; thus, if its density decreases by a factor of 2, its compressive strength decreases by a factor of 4. Many other variables

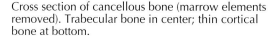

Section of trabecula (schematic)

Active osteoblasts

Osteoid (hypomineralized matrix)

Inactive osteoblasts (lining cells)

Osteocytes

Osteoclast (in Howship's lacuna)

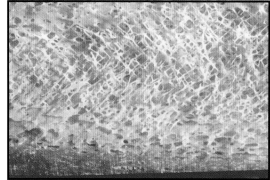

Cross section of cancellous bone (marrow elements removed). Trabecular bone in center; thin cortical bone at bottom.

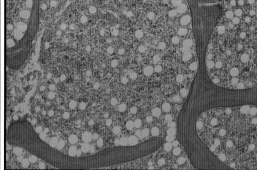

Photomicrograph of decalcified trabecular bone showing relationship of trabeculae to marrow (H & E, x35).

determine the fracture threshold, not the least of which is peak bone density at the time of skeletal maturity.

The biochemical composition and microscopic physical properties are comparable in both cortical and trabecular bone. However, the macroscopic structure of bone produces markedly different physical properties that have broad variations in strength and stiffness to suit local physical requirements. Thus, the thin cortical shell supported by trabecular bone at the ends of long

bones is well suited to distribute the concentrated loads in the joints, whereas the tubular cortical midshaft is better suited to support the large torsional and bending loads applied to this area.

All normal adult bone is lamellar bone, whether it has a cortical or a trabecular structure. In adults, immature woven bone, or fiber bone, is seen only in normal fracture healing or in pathologic conditions such as hyperparathyroidism or Paget disease.

Plate 2-24

Physiology

FORMATION AND COMPOSITION OF COLLAGEN

Collagen is the most abundant and ubiquitous family of proteins in the body, and its members are major constituents of all connective tissues. One of its most amazing biologic properties is the ability to spontaneously self-assemble outside the cell into a variety of fibrillar and nonfibrillar forms. Collagen formation plays a vital role in the process of tissue repair.

Like members of most families, the collagens share certain similarities but also possess characteristic differences. To date, 28 types of collagen macromolecules have been identified. The most abundant, type I collagen, is found in skin, fasciae, tendons, ligaments, and bones. Type II collagen is found in all forms of hyaline cartilage (including growth plate and articular cartilage) and in the nucleus pulposus of the intervertebral disc. Type III collagen is less abundant but is generally found with type I collagen. Type IV collagen, the most abundant nonfibrillar type, is a major constituent of the basement membrane. Type V collagen, the least abundant fibrillar collagen, is found in the placenta and blood vessels. In addition, there is a variety of minor collagens whose distribution and function are still being investigated.

All collagen molecules are composed of three polypeptide α chains wrapped around one another like a three-stranded rope.

Although each collagen type is a unique combination of three α chains (in the form of either a homotrimer or a heterotrimer) and although each α chain is encoded by a unique gene and possesses a unique amino acid sequence, there are many similarities among the various types. Each α chain has a primary structure that is relatively simple and highly repetitive; a good example is glycine-X-Y334. Glycine, the amino acid having the smallest side-chain, occupies every third amino acid position, and X and Y are often proline and hydroxyproline, respectively. This repeating triplet allows the α chains to form a tight helix.

Despite the relatively simple structure of collagen, its biosynthetic pathway is complex and can be divided into intracellular and extracellular events. The intracellular assembly begins with the transcription of messenger ribonucleic acid (mRNA) from collagen genes. The pro-α chains of procollagen are synthesized on the rough endoplasmic reticulum by translation of the corresponding mRNA. Subsequently, many post-translational modifications occur. Hydroxylation of specific proline and lysine residues takes place in the lumen of the rough endoplasmic reticulum while the still-growing α chains are attached to ribosomes. This process requires the presence of vitamin C, oxygen, ferrous iron, α-ketoglutarate, and the appropriate hydroxylation enzymes—prolyl 4-hydroxylase, prolyl 3-hydroxylase, and lysyl hydroxylase. Deficiencies in cofactors or enzymes can lead to deficits in secretion. Other post-translational modifications involve glycosylation of hydroxylysine residues, glycosylation of the carboxyl (C)-terminal propeptide, and formation of disulfide bonds among the C-terminal propeptides of the three α chains. The last process initiates the formation of the triple helix in the lumen of the rough endoplasmic reticulum. Once the triple helix is formed, procollagen is transported from the rough endoplasmic reticulum to the Golgi apparatus and packaged for secretion by exocytosis.

Once outside the cell, the C-terminal and N-terminal propeptides of some collagens are cleaved by

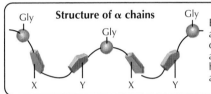

Fibroblast, chondroblast, or osteoblast

Endoplasmic reticulum cistern

Nucleus

Ribosome

Cell membrane

Hydroxylation of certain prolyl and lysyl amino acid residues begins as pre-pro-α chains enter cistern. This requires vitamin C, Fe₂, O₂, and α-ketoglutarate.

Glycosylation involves enzymatic addition of galactose to certain hydroxylysine residues by galactosyltransferase.

Golgi apparatus

Disulfide bonds

Three pro-α chains assemble into triple helix, bonded by OH groups.

Procollagen released to extracellular space by pinocytosis

Terminal propeptides split off by procollagen peptidase

Collagen

Assembly into fibrils (quarter staggered). Cross links formed under influence of lysyl oxidase and copper.

Gal galactose
Glc glucose
Gly glycine

Structure of α chains

Gly   Gly   Gly

X   Y   X   Y

Each α chain comprises about 1,000 amino acids. Every third amino acid in chain is glycine, smallest of amino acids. Glycine has no side chains, which thus permits tight coil. X and Y here indicate other amino acids (X often proline; Y often hydroxyproline). Proline and hydroxyproline, respectively, constitute about 20% and 25% of total amino acids in each α chain.

Types of collagen
(based on a chain composition of fibrils)

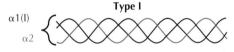

Type I

α1(I)

α2

Two α1(I) chains and one α2 chain = (α1[I])₂ α2; in bone, tendon, ligament, fascia, skin, artery, uterus

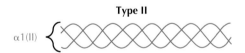

Type II

α1(II)

Three α1(II) chains = (α1[II])₃; in articular cartilage

Type III (α1[III])₃; in skin, artery, uterus, GI tract.
Type IV (α1[IV])₃; in basement membranes, lens capsule.
Type V (αB)₃ or (αB)₂ αA; in basement membranes, other tissues. At least 12 different collagen molecules identified.

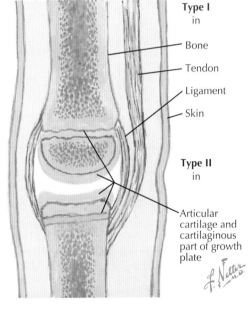

Type I in
- Bone
- Tendon
- Ligament
- Skin

Type II in
- Articular cartilage and cartilaginous part of growth plate

procollagen peptidase C and procollagen peptidase N, respectively. Following cleavage of the terminal propeptides, these collagen molecules spontaneously precipitate as fibrils under physiologic conditions. The 68-nm periodic staining of fibrillar collagen results from the staggered structure of the fibrils. Collagen structures are stabilized by intermolecular crosslinking between lysine or hydroxylysine residues in adjacent collagen molecules.

As the major component of the connective tissue matrix, collagen determines the tensile strength of tissues, provides the framework for tissues, limits the movement of other components of tissue and matrix, induces platelet aggregation and clot formation, regulates the deposition of hydroxyapatite crystals in bone, and plays an important role in the regulation and differentiation of various cells and tissues.

Heritable disorders of collagen metabolism include Ehlers-Danlos syndrome, Marfan syndrome, and osteogenesis imperfecta. Acquired disorders include scurvy, keloid formation, proliferative scar formation, atherosclerosis, pulmonary fibrosis, and cirrhosis.

Plate 2-25

Musculoskeletal System: PART III

FORMATION AND COMPOSITION OF PROTEOGLYCAN

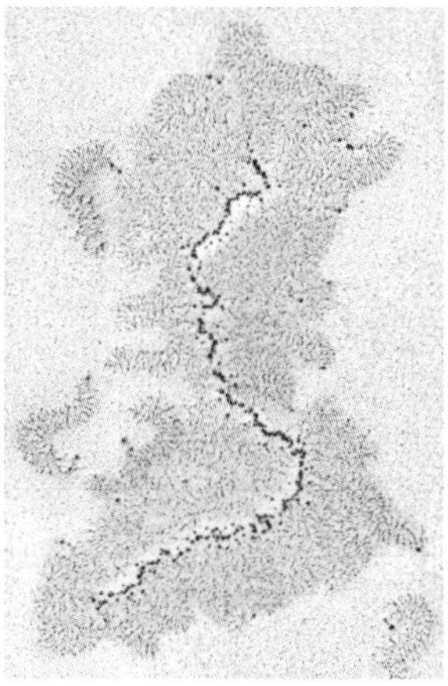

The normal growth and development of cartilage are critically dependent on the presence of proteoglycans in the cartilage matrix. Cartilage proteoglycans are large, complex macromolecules. They are composed of a core protein to which are attached a variable number of two glycosaminoglycan chains (keratan sulfate and chondroitin sulfate) of varying length that consist of repeating, negatively charged disaccharide units. The core protein of aggrecan, the major cartilage proteoglycan monomer, contains more than 2000 amino acids and is divided into five regions, a hyaluronan-binding globular (G1) domain, a keratan sulfate–rich region next to the G1 domain, a second globular (G2) domain, a large chondroitin sulfate-rich region, and a terminal third globular (G3) domain. The average intact aggrecan molecule can contain approximately 100 chondroitin sulfate chains, approximately 60 keratan sulfate chains, and a variable number of smaller N- and O-oligosaccharides. Thus, the total molecular weight of an aggrecan monomer is in the 2 to 3 million dalton range.

To make the situation even more complex, aggrecans form aggregates with two other matrix components—hyaluronan and link proteins. This aggregate consists of a variable number of proteoglycan monomers, depending on the length of the hyaluronan, which are noncovalently attached to a single hyaluronan chain through the hyaluronan-binding G1 domain. This interaction is stabilized by the noncovalent association of link proteins to both the hyaluronan and the G1 domain. The typical molecular weight of such an aggregate can exceed 200 million (see the electron micrograph in Plate 2-25).

All the components of the proteoglycan aggregate are synthesized by chondroblasts and chondrocytes and are then transported by them for extracellular self-assembly. For example, the core protein is synthesized and some oligosaccharides are added in the rough endoplasmic reticulum, whereas the synthesis of remaining oligosaccharides and glycosaminoglycan chains and their subsequent sulfation occur in the Golgi apparatus. While aggrecan proteoglycans and link proteins are being assembled and secreted together, the cartilage cells are also synthesizing hyaluronan macromolecules at their plasma membranes and extruding them extracellularly. Once the aggrecan-link protein interacts with the hyaluronan in the extracellular space, the proteoglycan aggregate forms, resulting in one of the largest molecular complexes in nature.

The proteoglycan contents of articular cartilage, elastic cartilage, and fibrocartilage give these tissues many of their characteristic properties. For example, the critical mechanical properties of hyaline cartilage—resiliency and stiffness to compression—exist because the large bottlebrush macromolecular domains of the aggrecan proteoglycans sequester water. The anionic charges on the sulfated glycosaminoglycan chains cause them to repel one another, which expands the aggrecan domains. The concentration of aggrecan molecules within the collagen matrix prevents them from fully expanding, and they often occupy as little as one fifth of their fully expanded domains. This greatly increases

Electron micrograph of large, aggregated proteoglycan molecule from epiphyseal cartilage. Numerous closely spaced monomers bound to central hyaluronan filament; free monomers surround aggregate (x50,000). (*Courtesy of Matthias Mörgelin, PhD.*)

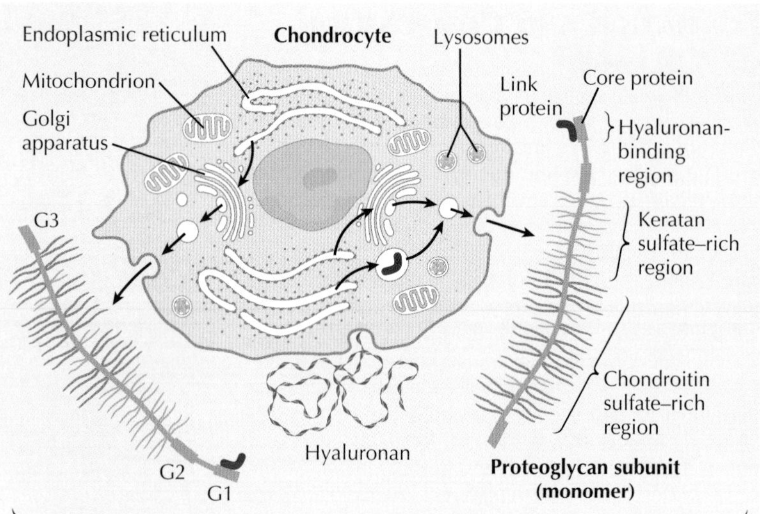

Each component is synthesized separately and transported to the chondrocyte cell surface for assembly into giant aggregated proteoglycan supramolecular structures in the cartilage matrix.

J. Perkins
MS, MFA

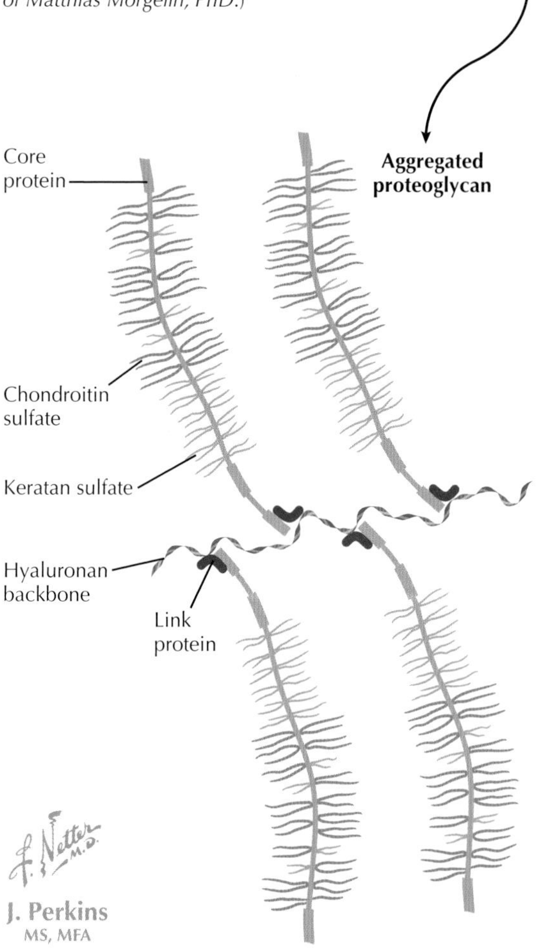

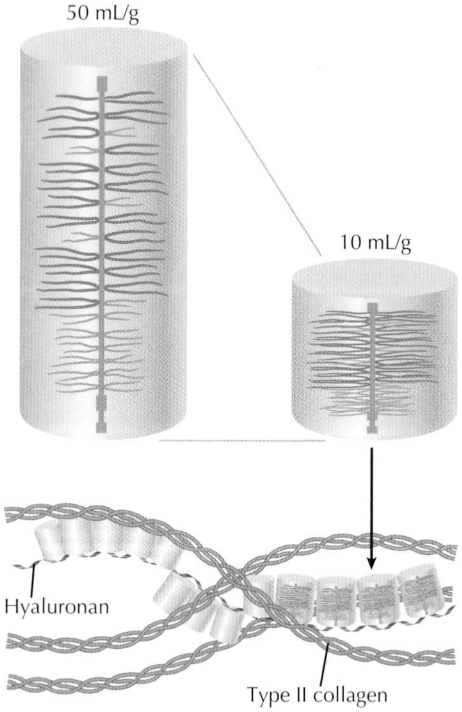

Electronegative charges on chondroitin sulfate and keratan sulfate molecules (SO_4^{2-}) cause side chains to repel each other and to attract and trap electropositive dipoles of water (H^+), thus acting as molecular sponge. Collagen fibers in matrix entangle proteoglycan aggregate, preventing its full extension.

the concentration of negative charges within their domain, which increases their swelling pressure due to anionic charge repulsion. This allows the cartilage to resist compressive loads with less net changes in aggrecan matrix volume per compressive load and to expand to their original compressed volume when the load is released.

The result is an efficient composite structure in which the collagen molecules form a fibrillar network that resists tensile loads and restrains the compressed aggrecan proteoglycans, which in turn resist the variable compressive loads that cartilages undergo during their normal physiological functions. Because cartilage is avascular, diffusion of nutrients and exchange of waste products occur through the tissue fluid that is mostly maintained within the aggrecan domains, which allow relatively free exchanges with the water and solutes of synovial fluid.

Plate 2-26

Physiology

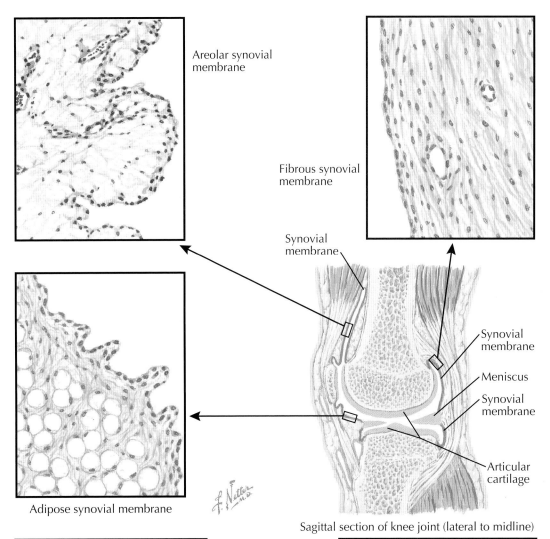

Areolar synovial membrane

Fibrous synovial membrane

Synovial membrane

Synovial membrane

Meniscus

Synovial membrane

Articular cartilage

Sagittal section of knee joint (lateral to midline)

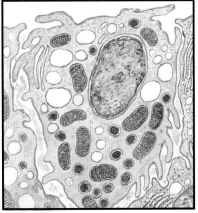

Adipose synovial membrane

STRUCTURE AND FUNCTION OF SYNOVIAL MEMBRANE

The synovial membrane, or synovium, is the vascular mesenchymal tissue that lines the joint space of all synovial (diarthrodial) joints. Only the cartilage and surfaces of the meniscus are not covered by synovial membrane. In normal joints, this tissue serves primarily to produce the joint fluid with its diverse components and to remove cellular and connective tissue debris from the joint space.

On gross examination, the synovial surface appears pale pink and shiny. Although some folds can be seen with the naked eye, the characteristic villi that increase the effective surface area of the synovial membrane are visible only on microscopic examination. One or two layers of cells, with their long axes generally lying parallel to the surface, line the synovial membrane; these lining cells are not joined by intracellular junctions. The deeper tissue consists predominantly of loose connective tissue, fibrous tissue, or fat. Thus, the associated synovial membrane is described as areolar, fibrous, or adipose. Fibrous synovial membrane is found in areas that need more strength but less flexibility.

Capillaries and venules lie immediately beneath the lining cells. Lymphatics, which are difficult to identify with standard light microscopy, are most abundant in areolar synovial membrane. Nonmyelinated nerve fibers extend from the capsule into the adventitia of the synovial blood vessels.

Ultrastructural and immunopathologic studies have added considerably to the understanding of the synovial membrane. The lining cell layer consists of some cells that are rich in rough endoplasmic reticulum. These cells, called type B, are probably related to fibroblasts. Type B cells are most important because of their ability to secrete prostaglandins, collagenase, hyaluronan, and many other components of joint fluid.

Electron micrograph shows type A cell of synovial lining characterized by many vacuoles, lysosomes (dark bodies), mitochondria, and filopodia but little endoplasmic reticulum, all evidence of macrophage and phagocytic function.

Type B cell of synovial lining shows much rough endoplasmic reticulum and pinocytotic vesicles, related to its presumed function of synthesizing and excreting hyaluronic acid and glycoprotein for synovial fluid.

Phagocytic cells (type A), which have prominent lysosomes, are now known to originate from monocytes. They often lie superficially to the type B cells. Some cells, which appear to have features of both type A and type B cells, are less well understood. Mast cells in perivascular areas, easily identified on electron microscopy, are a source of important vasoactive substances. Collagen (types I and III), fibronectin, and proteoglycans are present in the matrix.

Electron microscopic examination reveals that the superficial capillaries and venules have a fenestrated endothelium through which fluid, together with small amounts of low-molecular-weight protein, transudes to form the joint fluid. The addition of hyaluronan by the lining cells gives the joint fluid its characteristic viscosity. The deeper vessels, which have thicker walls, are the vessels through which most inflammatory cells emigrate.

Plate 2-27

Musculoskeletal System: PART III

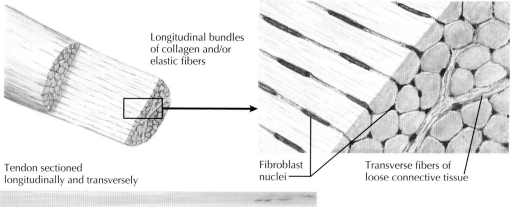

Loose connective tissue

Amorphous matrix

Collegen fibers

Elastic fibers

Reticular fibers (thin, modified collagen fibers)

Fibroblast

Macrophage

Lymphocyte

Monocyte

Mast cell

Fat cells

Macrophage

Eosinophil

Plasma cell

Capillary

Red blood cell

Endothelial cell

Pericyte

HISTOLOGY OF CONNECTIVE TISSUE

Adult connective tissue comprises a family of tissue types that includes connective tissue proper, blood, cartilage, and bone. All tissues in this family originate from embryonic mesenchymal tissue. Connective tissue itself includes a range of recognizable histologic types, which are determined by the proportion of the various components in the tissue. The two extremes of the continuum of connective tissue are *loose connective tissue* and *dense connective tissue*. These two classifications are based on the proportion and density of the fibrous component of the tissue. Connective tissue may have a regular arrangement, as in the tendon, or an irregular arrangement, as in the dermis. Often, one component of the connective tissue predominates, such as the fat cell in adipose tissue.

Regardless of its histologic type, connective tissue is made up of two components, cells and extracellular matrix. Fibroblasts (which synthesize collagen), fat cells, fixed macrophages, mast cells, plasma cells, and some leukocytes are the principal cellular elements of connective tissue. Extracellular matrix consists of collagenous, elastic, or reticular fibers and a variety of glycoproteins and proteoglycans, which are either sulfated or nonsulfated. These are often present as components of gigantic macromolecular assemblies such as aggrecan proteoglycan aggregates (see Plate 2-25). Among the important sulfated compounds are chondroitin sulfate, keratan sulfate, and heparan sulfate. The principal nonsulfated compound is hyaluronan. In addition, connective tissue also contains blood and lymphatic vessels and nerves that vary in number and size.

The composition and organization of a particular connective tissue largely depends on its function. Loose, or areolar, connective tissue is found throughout the body wherever biologic packing material is needed.

Dense connective tissue

Longitudinal bundles of collagen and/or elastic fibers

Tendon sectioned longitudinally and transversely

Fibroblast nuclei

Transverse fibers of loose connective tissue

Light microscopic longitudinal section of tendon shows fascicles (predominantly collagen) and fibroblasts (H & E).

It is well vascularized and highly cellular, with a large proportion of matrix. The fibrous component varies in amount and orientation, depending on the mechanical stresses in the region. Adipose tissue is a specialized form of loose connective tissue in which fat cells predominate. Although the fat cell is sometimes thought of as a type of fibroblast, it is increasingly being regarded as a separate cell type that, when it does not contain lipid, resembles a fibroblast.

Dense connective tissue, found in tendons and ligaments, is poorly vascularized. Parallel bundles of densely packed collagen fibers are the predominant elements. Alongside the bundles of collagen fibers are inactive-appearing fibroblasts with densely staining, elongated nuclei. In some species, the fibroblasts of tendons have the tendency to form nodules of ectopic cartilage and bone after injury. Occasionally, nodules of fibrocartilage are seen in tendons.

Plate 2-28

Physiology

BONE HOMEOSTASIS

The skeleton acts as a dynamic mineral reserve bank in which the body stores its ionized calcium and phosphorus (in the form of phosphate ions) in a metabolically stable and structurally useful way. Although each bone cell population—the osteoblasts, osteoclasts, and osteocytes—is under the direction of numerous endocrine factors and is influenced by various local biochemical and bioelectric factors, the cells themselves are endowed with genetic instructions that determine their ability to form, resorb, or maintain bone (see Plate 2-28).

Calcium Requirements. The body regulates few functions with greater fidelity than the concentration of ionized calcium in the extracellular fluid. Although extracellular calcium represents less than 1% of the body's calcium stores, it is the metabolically active component that is critically important for numerous life-sustaining processes that include enzymatic reactions, mitochondrial function, cell membrane maintenance, intracellular and intercellular communication, inter-neuronal transmission, neuromuscular transmission, muscle contraction, and blood clotting. An elaborate endocrine system maintains the serum calcium concentration within a very narrow physiologic range. When this level falls, even momentarily, it is restored to normal through the parathyroid hormone (PTH)/vitamin D system, which increases calcium absorption in the gastrointestinal tract and reabsorption in the kidneys, and the resorption of bone (see Plate 2-33).

The National Research Council of the National Academy of Sciences has established recommended daily allowances (RDAs) of calcium for all age groups. These values, which may be conservative estimates, reflect the average amount of calcium required to maintain a positive calcium balance and to prevent withdrawal of the mineral stores banked in bone. For young adults, the RDA of calcium is 1000 to 1300 mg. Despite this recommendation, large-scale dietary surveys of women with osteoporosis show that the average American woman consumes less than 500 mg/day. On such a calcium-deficient diet, the body mobilizes calcium from its skeletal reserve for its daily needs by increasing secretion of PTH and 1,25-dihydroxyvitamin D, or 1,25(OH)₂D, the hormonally active metabolite of vitamin D. (Because both D₂ and D₃ isomers are treated identically and act in similar manners, the numeric designator has been omitted.)

Absorption of calcium from the upper gastrointestinal tract becomes less efficient with age because of decreases in baseline levels and secretory reserves of 1,25(OH)₂D; thus, older persons need more dietary calcium to maintain a calcium balance. Healthy premenopausal women older than age 30 may require as much as 1300 mg/day, and pregnant women and women older than age 50 need more than 1500 mg/day. Lactating women need 2000 mg/day to prevent untimely catabolism of bone.

Calcium consumption may be inadequate in persons with lactase deficiency who avoid eating dairy products, the primary source of dietary calcium. Increased protein intake accelerates calcium excretion by the kidney. Therefore, the high-protein diet common in Western industrialized countries may be a contributing factor to accelerated bone loss in these populations.

Vitamin D Requirements. The vitamin D metabolite 1,25(OH)₂D helps to maintain normal serum calcium and phosphate levels by increasing the absorption of these substances from the intestine and the osteoclastic

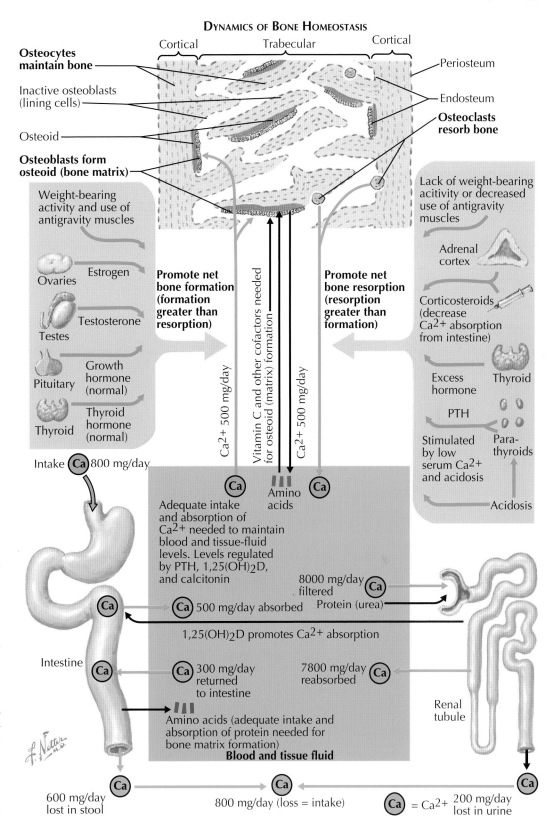

DYNAMICS OF BONE HOMEOSTASIS

resorption of bone. About half of our vitamin D comes from dietary sources (particularly from vitamin D–enriched milk), and the remainder comes from a reaction in the skin stimulated by ultraviolet radiation. Only a few natural foods, such as fish liver oils, contain vitamin D. Elderly persons frequently have a mild vitamin D deficiency because of their meager exposure to sunlight, decreased intake of milk and other dairy products, and decreased intestinal absorption of vitamin

D. The RDA of vitamin D is 600 IU for young adults and 800 IU for elderly persons. Larger amounts may cause hypercalcemia. Premature infants may require 500 to 1000 IU daily.

In addition to age- and sex-related effects on bone loss, endocrine and metabolic changes affect bone homeostasis, leading to osteoporosis. In both osteoporotic and normal elderly women, 1,25(OH)₂D levels are normal. However, in elderly patients, the kidney's

Plate 2-29

Musculoskeletal System: PART III

BONE HOMEOSTASIS *(Continued)*

production of $1,25(OH)_2D$ in response to PTH infusion is impaired. Also, in postmenopausal women, bone-resorbing cells (osteoclasts) appear to be excessively responsive to endogenous PTH. Estrogen receptors have been found in both osteoblasts and osteoclasts. Estrogen decreases the sensitivity of osteoclasts to PTH, making estrogen deficiency the major cause of bone loss in the early postmenopausal period.

REGULATION OF CALCIUM AND PHOSPHATE METABOLISM

Despite considerable daily variations in calcium intake, the body maintains the serum calcium concentration at a remarkably constant level. The primary homeostatic regulation of serum calcium concentration is under the control of the parathyroid gland, which produces PTH; the thyroid gland, which secretes calcitonin; and the kidney, which provides $1,25(OH)_2D$ from less active vitamin D metabolites. Other factors contributing to the regulation of serum calcium levels include hormones (e.g., gonadal steroids, thyroid hormone, growth hormone, glucocorticoids, insulin); vitamins C and D; proteins (e.g., albumin, calcium-binding protein, vitamin D–binding protein); phosphate; small inhibitors of mineralization such as pyrophosphates; and pH of blood (see Plate 2-29).

The exchange of calcium between extracellular fluid and bone can be considered kinetically (see Plate 2-28). Through a slow phase of bone formation and resorption, approximately 1000 mg/day of calcium is exchanged between bone and extracellular fluid; this represents approximately one tenth of 1% of the total calcium reserve (1000 to 1200 g). Most of the calcium in bone does not readily diffuse into the extracellular compartment but must be mobilized by endocrine-regulated, cell-mediated bone resorption. There is no known sustained biologic process by which the body can remove just the mineral component of bone. Thus, when the body needs to withdraw calcium from its mineral reserves, it can do so only by resorbing bone (mineral component plus organic matrix). Through the process of *coupling*, bone formation increases and osteoblasts are stimulated to fill in the resorption defect, although this repair may not be complete in the elderly.

Endocrine-mediated bone formation and bone resorption involve more than the stimulation of existing differentiated bone cells; these processes are dependent on the transformation of undifferentiated stem cells in both osteoblast and osteoclast lineages. Thus, bone formation and bone resorption are contingent not only on the metabolic activity of each cell but also on the recruitment of new cells to the job.

The major function of calcitonin, a hormone secreted by the parafollicular cells of the thyroid gland, is to inhibit osteoclastic bone resorption in response to elevated serum calcium levels. The biologically active vitamin D metabolite $1,25(OH)_2D$ regulates intestinal absorption of calcium and phosphate and activates bone resorption by stimulating the recruitment of osteoclast precursors (preosteoclasts). There is evidence that $1,25(OH)_2D$ also stimulates the recruitment of osteoblast precursors. Conversion of 25-hydroxyvitamin D, or $25(OH)D$, to $1,25(OH)_2D$ in the kidney is controlled by the enzyme 25-hydroxyvitamin D-1α-hydroxylase,

or $25(OH)D-1\alpha-OH_{ase}$, and stimulated maximally by increased serum PTH and decreased serum phosphate levels.

Efficient gastrointestinal absorption of calcium depends primarily on daily calcium intake, vitamin D status, and age. Because the major storage form of vitamin D is $25(OH)D$, the serum level of $25(OH)D$ is an excellent indicator of the body's total vitamin D reserves. With the vitamin D axis intact, efficiency of calcium absorption increases if calcium intake decreases.

Some calcium secreted into the intestine is absorbed, but much of it passes into the stool as unabsorbed calcium.

The kidney filters about 8000 mg of calcium daily and, under the influence of PTH, reabsorbs more than 95%. For each additional gram of calcium ingested, only about 50 mg of additional calcium appears in urine. Thus, the urinary calcium level is better determined by the rate of calcium absorption by the intestine than by the amount of calcium ingested.

REGULATION OF CALCIUM AND PHOSPHATE METABOLISM

	Parathyroid hormone (PTH) (peptide)	$1,25(OH)_2D$ (steroid)	Calcitonin (peptide)
Hormone	From chief cells of parathyroid glands	From proximal tubule of kidney	From parafollicular cells of thyroid gland
Factors stimulating production	Decreased serum Ca^{2+}	Elevated PTH Decreased serum Ca^{2+} Decreased serum P_i	Elevated serum Ca^{2+}
Factors inhibiting production	Elevated serum Ca^{2+} Elevated	Decreased PTH Elevated serum Ca^{2+} Elevated serum P_i	Decreased serum Ca^{2+}
End organs for hormone action — Intestine	No direct effect Acts indirectly on bowel by stimulating production of $1,25(OH)_2D$ in kidney	Strongly stimulates intestinal absorption of Ca^{2+} and P_i	?
Kidney	Stimulates $25(OH)D-1\alpha-OH_{ase}$ in mitochondria of proximal tubular cells to convert $25(OH)D$ to $1,25(OH)_2D$ Increases fractional reabsorption of filtered Ca^{2+} Promotes urinary excretion of P_i	?	?
Bone	Stimulates osteoclastic resorption of bone Stimulates recruitment of preosteoclasts	Strongly stimulates osteoclastic resorption of bone	Inhibits osteoclastic resorption of bone ? Role in normal human physiology
Net effect on calcium and phosphate concentrations in extracellular fluid and serum	Increased serum calcium Decreased serum phosphate	Increased serum calcium Increased serum phosphate	Decreased serum calcium (transient)

Plate 2-30

Physiology

REGULATION OF BONE MASS

EFFECTS OF BONE FORMATION AND RESORPTION ON SKELETAL MASS

Once peak bone mass has been achieved by the middle of the third decade, net bone mass remains relatively constant throughout early adult life until about age 50. However, living bone is never metabolically at rest but constantly remodels and reappropriates its mineral stores along lines of mechanical stress. In the normal adult skeleton, bone formation and resorption processes are balanced in a state called *coupling*, so that net bone formation equals net bone resorption.

Unless a significant metabolic insult occurs to bone early in life, the peak adult bone mass will exceed the threshold for spontaneous fracture. Noninvasive techniques to measure bone density have provided a useful definition of osteoporosis: a mass-per-unit volume of normally mineralized bone that falls below a population-defined threshold for spontaneous fracture. While such bone mineral density assessments do not entirely account for a complete assessment of fracture risk, they do indicate that significant osteoporosis can develop only if there is a net loss of bone mass; in other words, an *uncoupling* of the balance between bone formation and bone resorption processes.

If net bone resorption exceeds net bone formation, bone mass declines with time (see Plate 2-30). Under these conditions, with a rapid rate of bone turnover, the decrease of bone mass is rapid. Conversely, with a slow rate of bone turnover, the decline in mass is correspondingly slow. Similarly, if net bone formation exceeds net bone resorption (as in normal bone growth and even after longitudinal growth ceases), bone mass increases with time.

Some possible combinations of bone formation/resorption are shown in the table in the upper half of Plate 2-30 and graphically presented in the lower half. *Example 8* represents normal bone turnover: bone formation and bone resorption are appropriately coupled, leading to a stable bone mass with no net change (black bar on middle line). *Example 4* represents greatly increased bone turnover rate, but again because formation and resorption are appropriately coupled there is no net change in bone mass. This state of bone remodeling is seen in the active stage of Paget disease (see Section 3, Metabolic Diseases, Plates 3-44 to 3-46).

Example 11 shows decreased bone turnover rate, but here, too, bone formation and resorption are appropriately coupled, with no net change in bone mass. This state of bone remodeling might be seen in the inactive phase of normal bone turnover (see example 8), or it might reflect a decrease in appropriately coupled bone remodeling that represents a normal variation.

Increased Bone Turnover. *Example 1* depicts a state of severe uncoupling (decreased bone formation and increased bone resorption), which causes a net decline in bone mass over time. Such an imbalance in formation and resorption occurs in chronic glucocorticoid excess, which may be endogenous (Cushing syndrome) or iatrogenic (see Section 3, Metabolic Diseases, Plate 3-26).

Example 2 illustrates increased bone turnover rate with a normal rate of bone formation but an increased rate of bone resorption. To use the bank analogy illustrated in Plate 2-31: with time, net withdrawal from the bone bank exceeds net deposition, resulting in a

decreased skeletal reserve (bone mass). This state is represented in the lower half of Plate 2-30 by the black bar below the zero line and by the red dot above the green column, indicating resultant osteoporosis. (An example of this situation is the rapid increase in bone resorption that occurs after menopause.)

In *example 3*, both bone formation and resorption are increased but the rate of resorption is greater than the rate of formation. Thus, there is a net loss of bone mass over a period of time, which leads to osteoporosis. Mild

hyperthyroidism, mild hyperparathyroidism, and a chronic dietary calcium deficiency can cause increased bone turnover, with resorption exceeding formation. In severe hyperthyroidism and hyperparathyroidism, remodeling rates can be even greater than those shown in example 3, with a correspondingly greater difference between formation and resorption and often a greater net loss of bone mass.

Example 5 illustrates a state of increased bone formation and resorption, with formation exceeding

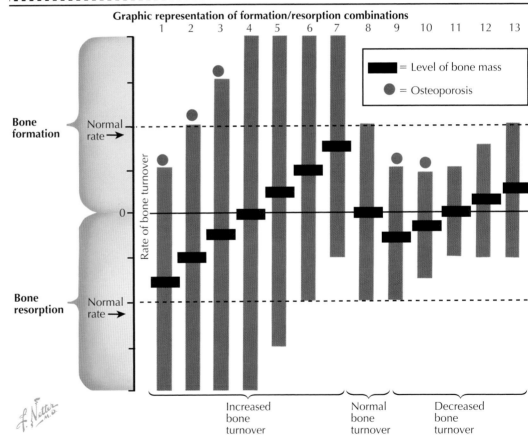

EFFECTS OF BONE FORMATION AND RESORPTION ON SKELETAL MASS

Plate 2-31   Musculoskeletal System: PART III

REGULATION OF BONE MASS
(Continued)

resorption. In this circumstance, bone mass increases with time. Such a generalized state of remodeling does not occur naturally in the adult skeleton, but it can occur when once-daily PTH injection is administered to osteoporosis patients, a treatment now referred to as intermittent PTH therapy. In a pathologic context, a localized (focal) phenomenon of increased bone formation and resorption with formation exceeding resorption occurs in the osteoblastic stage of Paget disease.

Example 6 illustrates normal bone resorption paired with an increase in the rate of bone formation, which leads to a net increase in bone mass with time. This is typical during normal growth and development, especially between late adolescence (when longitudinal growth ceases) and approximately age 35 (when peak adult bone mass is reached).

Example 7 shows the highly uncoupled state of increased bone formation and decreased bone resorption that result in a net increase in bone mass. Such a state of remodeling is seen in the adult, or autosomal dominant, form of osteopetrosis (see Section 3, Metabolic Diseases, Plate 3-43). In this disorder, the reduced rate of bone resorption is due to the relative decline in osteoclastic bone resorption; the rate of bone formation may be normal or increased. This form of uncoupling may also be induced by pharmacologic doses of fluoride administered to stimulate bone formation and stabilize bone apatite crystal and render it more resistant to breakdown.

Decreased Bone Turnover. *Example 9* shows a state of normal bone resorption with decreased bone formation, which leads to reduced bone mass and osteoporosis. This can occur after exposure to a poison or toxin that affects the osteoblasts, as with use of certain chemotherapeutic agents and chronic alcohol abuse.

In *example 10*, both bone formation and resorption are decreased but bone resorption still exceeds bone formation. This is seen when calcium and vitamin D supplementation helps to diminish age-related bone loss.

Example 13 shows a positive bone balance resulting from a normal rate of bone formation and a decreased rate of bone resorption. This occurs in women receiving replacement therapy with calcium and estrogen or calcium and calcitonin soon after menopause. These agents, administered independently or in combination, act to decrease bone resorption. The coupling process then causes bone formation rates to adjust downward accordingly (*example 12*); eventually, bone mass stabilizes at a much lower rate of bone remodeling (*example 11*). In a more extreme example, administration of bisphosphonates to patients with osteoporosis nearly eliminates bone resorption rates and, as a consequence of coupling, bone formation rates also substantially decline over treatment time.

FOUR MECHANISMS OF BONE MASS REGULATION

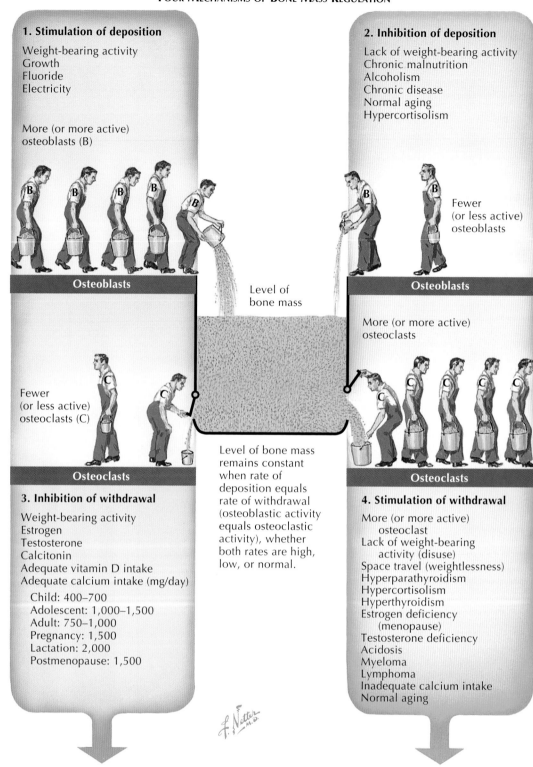

FOUR MECHANISMS OF BONE MASS REGULATION

1. Stimulation of deposition

Weight-bearing activity
Growth
Fluoride
Electricity

More (or more active) osteoblasts (B)

Osteoblasts

Fewer (or less active) osteoclasts (C)

Osteoclasts

3. Inhibition of withdrawal

Weight-bearing activity
Estrogen
Testosterone
Calcitonin
Adequate vitamin D intake
Adequate calcium intake (mg/day)

   Child: 400–700
   Adolescent: 1,000–1,500
   Adult: 750–1,000
   Pregnancy: 1,500
   Lactation: 2,000
   Postmenopause: 1,500

Net increase in bone mass

2. Inhibition of deposition

Lack of weight-bearing activity
Chronic malnutrition
Alcoholism
Chronic disease
Normal aging
Hypercortisolism

Fewer (or less active) osteoblasts

Osteoblasts

More (or more active) osteoclasts

Osteoclasts

4. Stimulation of withdrawal

More (or more active) osteoclast
Lack of weight-bearing activity (disuse)
Space travel (weightlessness)
Hyperparathyroidism
Hypercortisolism
Hyperthyroidism
Estrogen deficiency (menopause)
Testosterone deficiency
Acidosis
Myeloma
Lymphoma
Inadequate calcium intake
Normal aging

Net decrease in bone mass

Level of bone mass

Level of bone mass remains constant when rate of deposition equals rate of withdrawal (osteoblastic activity equals osteoclastic activity), whether both rates are high, low, or normal.

Plate 2-31 illustrates four basic mechanisms of bone mass regulation: (1) stimulation and (2) inhibition of bone formation, or deposition, and (3) stimulation and (4) inhibition of bone resorption, or withdrawal. However, in many cases, early changes will be checked by concomitant stimulation of the opposing bone cell population—stimulation of osteoclasts (resorption) leads to a coupled stimulation of osteoblasts (formation).

Plate 2-32

Physiology

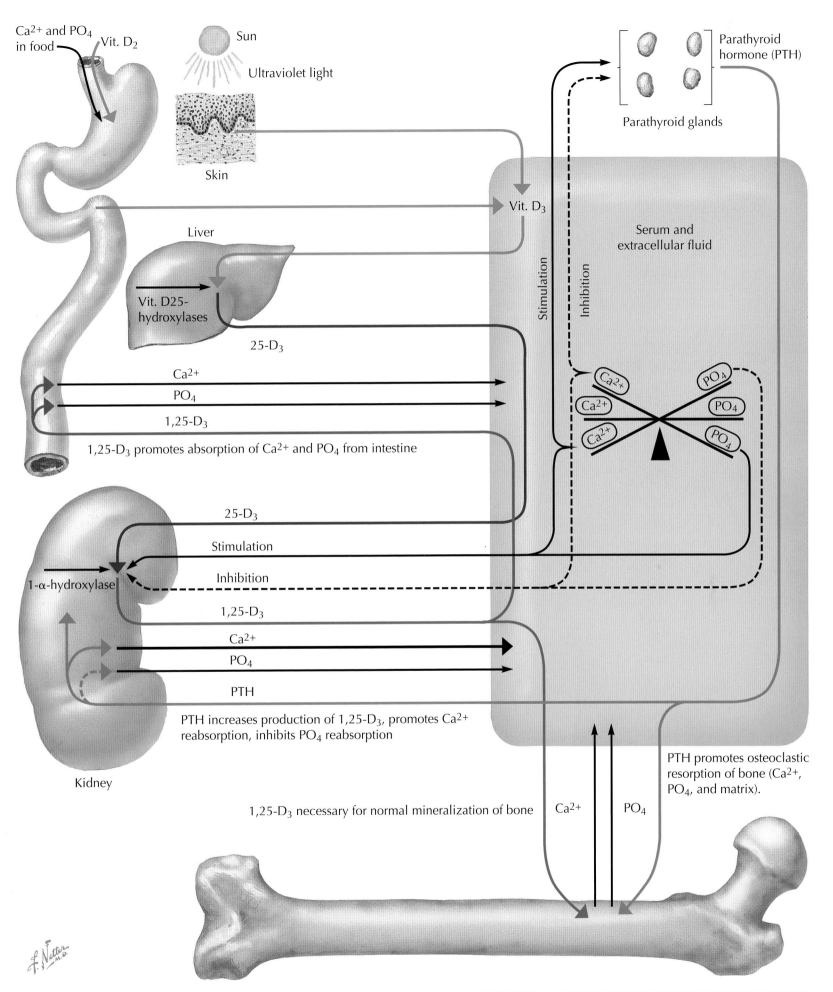

Ca^{2+} and PO_4 in food

Vit. D_2

Sun

Ultraviolet light

Skin

Parathyroid hormone (PTH)

Parathyroid glands

Vit. D_3

Serum and extracellular fluid

Liver

Vit. D25-hydroxylases

Stimulation

Inhibition

$25\text{-}D_3$

Ca^{2+}

PO_4

$1,25\text{-}D_3$

$1,25\text{-}D_3$ promotes absorption of Ca^{2+} and PO_4 from intestine

Ca^{2+}

Ca^{2+}

Ca^{2+}

PO_4

PO_4

PO_4

$25\text{-}D_3$

Stimulation

$1\text{-}\alpha\text{-hydroxylase}$

Inhibition

$1,25\text{-}D_3$

Ca^{2+}

PO_4

PTH

PTH increases production of $1,25\text{-}D_3$, promotes Ca^{2+} reabsorption, inhibits PO_4 reabsorption

Kidney

$1,25\text{-}D_3$ necessary for normal mineralization of bone

Ca^{2+}

PO_4

PTH promotes osteoclastic resorption of bone (Ca^{2+}, PO_4, and matrix).

Plate 2-32

Musculoskeletal System: PART III

NORMAL CALCIUM AND PHOSPHATE METABOLISM

Three major axioms govern the metabolism of calcium and phosphate and in large measure explain systems that are closely regulated by a complex homeostatic mechanism. These axioms are distinct, representing chemical, physiologic, and biologic facts.

1. Calcium phosphate is minimally soluble in water. In fact, at the pH of body fluids and the concentrations of calcium and phosphate ions found in extracellular fluids, the critical solubility product is approached and sometimes exceeded. Any calcium phosphate precipitation is prevented by various soluble and extracellular matrix-bound inhibitor systems that buffer the critical (and "metastable") concentrations of calcium and phosphate ions in blood and tissues, respectively.

2. The irritability, contractility, and conductivity of skeletal and smooth muscles and the irritability and conductivity of nerves are exquisitely sensitive and inversely proportional to the concentration of calcium. (The relationship between the calcium level and cardiac muscle is an equally sensitive but direct one.) The body goes to great lengths to protect these important systems from the danger of hypocalcemia or hypercalcemia.

3. Absorption of calcium across the gut lining cells, reabsorption of filtered calcium by the renal tubule, and resorption of calcium released from the apatite crystals of bone cannot take place without calcium transport systems. These systems include voltage-gated calcium-channel proteins and calcium-binding transporter proteins that transport calcium ions from the exterior to the interior of gut lining or renal tubule cells. The mechanism by which calcium-binding proteins (CBP) are synthesized and act to transport calcium from the lumen of the distal duodenum (and proximal jejunum) across the lining cells and into the extracellular fluid is principally dependent on 1,25-dihydroxyvitamin D, or 1,25$(OH)_2$D, which enhances the transcription of messenger ribonucleic acid (mRNA) for the synthesis of CBP polypeptide. PTH plays a role in this process by enhancing 25-hydroxyvitamin D–α-hydroxylase activity in the kidney, which forms 1,25$(OH)_2$D from 25-hydroxyvitamin D. In addition, PTH helps render the gut lining cells more permeable for calcium transport and helps to lower serum phosphate ion concentration by increasing its secretion by renal tubule cells in urine (a high phosphate ion concentration can interfere with calcium absorption).

1,25-Dihydroxyvitamin D's potent effects on calcium transport in gut lining cells and the release of calcium from bone is mitigated by its relatively short-acting half-life, thereby emphasizing a constant metabolic need to acquire vitamin D precursors. Provitamin D_2 (ergosterol) is ingested or provitamin D_3 (7-dehydrocholesterol) is synthesized from cholesterol by the liver, and both are stored in the skin. Sunlight at wavelengths of approximately 315 nm (ultraviolet range) activates the provitamins into vitamin D_2 (calciferol) or vitamin D_3 (cholecalciferol), respectively, which

are then transported to the liver. Here, they are acted on by a vitamin D, 25-hydroxylase (vitamin D, 25-OH$_{ase}$) to form 25-hydroxyvitamin D, or 25(OH)D. (Because both D_2 and D_3 are treated identically and act in similar manners, the numerical designator has been omitted.) The 25(OH)D then travels to the renal tubule and, in response to lowered calcium, high PTH, and low phosphate levels in serum, is transformed by 25-hydroxyvitamin D–α-hydroxylase, or 25(OH)D-1α-OH$_{ase}$, into the highly potent metabolite 1,25$(OH)_2$D. If a surplus of either calcium or phosphate is present (indicated by a high serum concentration of calcium or phosphate, or both, or a low PTH level), an alternate pathway is selected in which the 25$(OH)_2$D is acted on by 25(OH)D-24-OH$_{ase}$ and the far less potent 24,25$(OH)_2$D is synthesized.

In a balanced diet, calcium and phosphate are ingested in adequate amounts. However, adequate calcium can be difficult to obtain in many reasonable diets and has led to fortifying food products with supplementary calcium. On the other hand, phosphate is present in almost all foods and dietary deficiencies are uncommon. Accessory factors promoting absorption of calcium from the gut include an acid pH, a low serum phosphate concentration (to avoid exceeding the critical solubility product mentioned in the first axiom above), and the absence of chelators such as phytate, oxalate, or excessive free fatty acids. Transport across the gut lining cells is controlled principally by the interaction of PTH, which renders the cells more permeable to luminal calcium, and 1,25$(OH)_2$D, which activates the transport polypeptide CBP.

Reabsorption of filtered calcium from the proximal tubule obeys the same rules. A diminished PTH level or decreased synthesis of 1,25$(OH)_2$D leads to decreased tubular reabsorption of calcium, whereas a high level of PTH and an increased level of 1,25$(OH)_2$D enhance reabsorption. Although both PTH and 1,25$(OH)_2$D are apparently able to cause resorption of bone, the vitamin D metabolite is at least partly responsible for the normal mineralization of bone.

The mechanism of phosphate absorption is less selective than that of calcium absorption but also appears to be at least partly dependent on the vitamin D metabolites. Because dietary intake of phosphate varies widely and absorption is almost unrestricted, the first axiom might suggest that humans stand poised on the brink of metastatic calcification and ossification because of a high, uncontrollable intake of phosphate. In fact, the renal excretory mechanisms exert a fine-tuned control over phosphate ion levels. In addition, tubular reabsorption of phosphate is exquisitely and inversely responsive to the concentration of PTH. Thus, PTH, which acts to *increase* tubular reabsorption of calcium, *diminishes* tubular reabsorption of phosphate, thus avoiding the potential disaster associated with exceeding the critical solubility product.

PTH plays a critical role in regulating levels of calcium and phosphate in serum and extracellular fluid. If the normal calcium concentration is not maintained, the diminished level signals the parathyroid glands to produce more PTH. The release of PTH, which is almost entirely dependent on the calcium level, has six separate functions, five of which are designed to correct the calcium deficit in serum and extracellular fluid. The five functions of PTH are as follows:

1. Increasing the synthesis of 1,25$(OH)_2$D in the kidney

2. Acting at the level of the gut lining cell (with vitamin D) to increase absorption of calcium

3. Acting at the level of the renal tubule (with vitamin D) to increase tubular reabsorption of filtered calcium

4. Acting at the level of bone (with vitamin D) to increase the population of activated osteoclasts, which destroy not only the hydroxyapatite crystals but also segments of organic bone matrix, thus releasing both calcium and phosphate ions

5. After releasing phosphate ions from bone (see 4), lowering the tubular reabsorption of phosphate to reduce the potential danger of violating the critical solubility product

A brief mention of two other homeostatic systems should be included in this discussion, namely, the body's response system to hypercalcemia and hyperphosphatemia.

The standard physiologic mechanism that controls hypercalcemia (see first and second axioms above) is twofold: (1) "Turnoff" of the vitamin D/PTH/calcium-sparing system, resulting in limited production of 1,25$(OH)_2$D, greatly diminished PTH elaboration, diminished gut absorption of calcium, diminished resorption of bone, and greatly diminished tubular reabsorption of calcium. (2) Increased elaboration of calcitonin, a hormone of low molecular weight secreted by the parafollicular cells (C cells) of the thyroid gland, which acts to lower the serum calcium concentration. This is achieved principally by diminishing the osteoclast population and activity and, to some extent, by reducing gastrointestinal absorption. However, it should be clearly noted that although the second mechanism may be well developed in avian species and although administration of exogenous, non-species-specific calcitonin may have a profound effect on the skeleton, the natural mechanism in humans appears to be too limited to protect the body from hypercalcemia.

Hyperphosphatemia, or increased concentration of serum phosphate, may lead to metastatic calcification, particularly in renal failure, since the critical solubility product can be exceeded even if calcium levels are normal. An increase in phosphate ions, however, appears to effectively impair the vitamin D/PTH/calcium-sparing system. Thus, with increase of phosphate levels in serum and extracellular fluid, synthesis of 1,25$(OH)_2$D markedly declines. Also, gastrointestinal absorption and tubular reabsorption of calcium, and even bone breakdown, are initially reduced, thus diminishing the concentration of calcium. (If these mechanisms continue for a long period of time, however, they will induce a secondary hyperparathyroidism in response to the lowered serum calcium level.)

The system of calcium and phosphate metabolism is complex, and the variables are multiple. The fundamental axioms and the interactions of the various hormonal and mineral materials discussed here are important in understanding the principles that govern and control the homeostatic mechanisms and the alterations that lead to the rachitic syndrome (see Plates 2-28 and 2-29, and Section 3, Metabolic Diseases, Plates 3-13 to 3-23).

Plate 2-33

Physiology

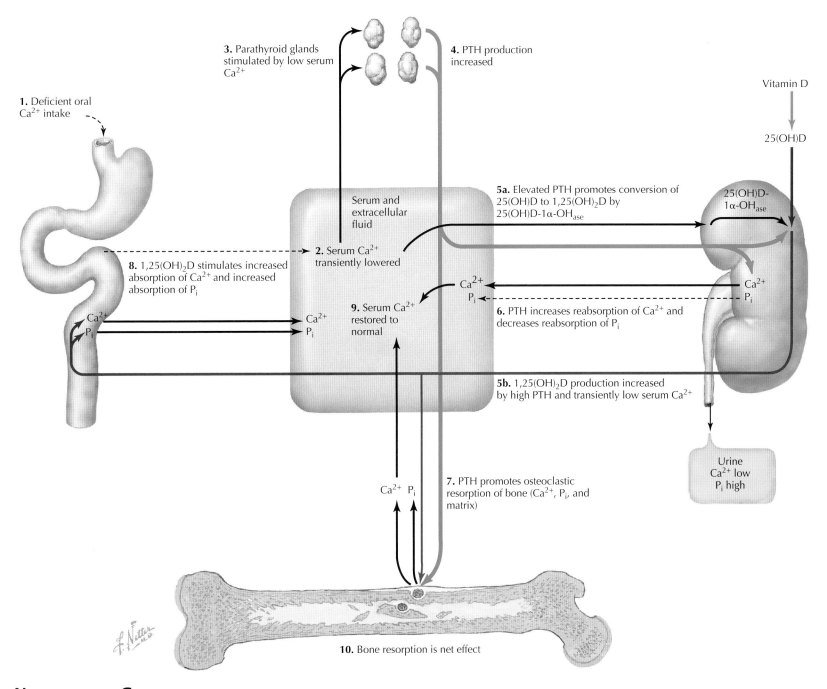

1. Deficient oral Ca²⁺ intake

3. Parathyroid glands stimulated by low serum Ca²⁺

4. PTH production increased

Vitamin D

25(OH)D

Serum and extracellular fluid

5a. Elevated PTH promotes conversion of 25(OH)D to 1,25(OH)₂D by 25(OH)D-1α-OH_ase

25(OH)D-1α-OH_ase

2. Serum Ca²⁺ transiently lowered

8. 1,25(OH)₂D stimulates increased absorption of Ca²⁺ and increased absorption of P_i

Ca²⁺
P_i

Ca²⁺
P_i

9. Serum Ca²⁺ restored to normal

Ca²⁺
P_i

Ca²⁺
P_i

6. PTH increases reabsorption of Ca²⁺ and decreases reabsorption of P_i

5b. 1,25(OH)₂D production increased by high PTH and transiently low serum Ca²⁺

Urine Ca²⁺ low P_i high

Ca²⁺ P_i

7. PTH promotes osteoclastic resorption of bone (Ca²⁺, P_i, and matrix)

10. Bone resorption is net effect

NUTRITIONAL CALCIUM DEFICIENCY

Calcium deficiency poses a constant threat to all life forms. Although 99% of the body's total calcium is stored in bone in the form of imperfect hydroxyapatite crystals, it is the 1% remaining in the extracellular fluid (including serum) that the body monitors vigilantly and controls assiduously. Many functions critical to life such as cell proliferation, differentiation, secretion, coagulation, excitation, and contraction require a stable and steep gradient of calcium across cell membranes. That gradient is dependent on the concentration of calcium in the extracellular fluid.

An intricate physiologic mechanism has evolved to prevent dangerous hypocalcemia: a reduction in calcium intake stimulates calcium absorption by the gastrointestinal tract, promotes renal calcium conservation, and stimulates net bone resorption (mineral plus matrix), thus restoring the serum calcium level to normal.

Take as an example a 30-year-old woman who begins a diet with a very low calcium intake. Let us explore the mechanisms that maintain a constant calcium level in the extracellular fluid.

In response to reduced calcium intake, net absorption decreases and serum calcium levels decline transiently. As a result, secretion of PTH increases. The target organs for PTH are the bones and the kidneys. In bone, osteoclastic activity is stimulated via a complex "coupling" mechanism involving interactions with osteoblasts. PTH stimulates osteoblasts to produce Receptor for Activation of Nuclear Factor κB ligand (RANKL), which then interacts with RANK receptors on osteoclast precursor cells. This ligand-receptor interaction leads to an activation of osteoclastic activities that result in a net resorption of both bone matrix and bone mineral. In the kidney, PTH promotes the tubular reabsorption of filtered calcium and impairs the reabsorption of P_i. In addition, via the cyclic adenosine monophosphate (cyclic AMP)–mediated pathway, PTH activates the enzyme

25-hydroxyvitamin D–1α-hydroxylase, or 25(OH)D-1α-OH_ase, in the mitochondria of the proximal tubular cells, thus promoting the conversion of the 25(OH)D substrate to the potent hormonal metabolite 1,25-dihydroxyvitamin D (1,25[OH]₂D, or calcitriol). The major target organs for 1,25(OH)₂D are the bones, the duodenum, and the jejunum. The mechanism of 1,25(OH)₂D-induced bone resorption involves a stimulation of osteoclastic precursors. It promotes calcium absorption in the duodenum and jejunum by stimulating numerous events and proteins, including the production of CBP in the enterocytes. However, the kidney's ability to adapt to low calcium intake by the mechanisms described declines with age. An age-related decline in 1,25(OH)₂D production by the kidneys impairs the efficiency of gastrointestinal absorption of calcium; thus, an even greater resorption of bone is required to maintain serum calcium at normal levels. This latter mechanism is thought to play a major role in the evolution of type II, or age-related, osteoporosis.

Plate 2-34

Musculoskeletal System: PART III

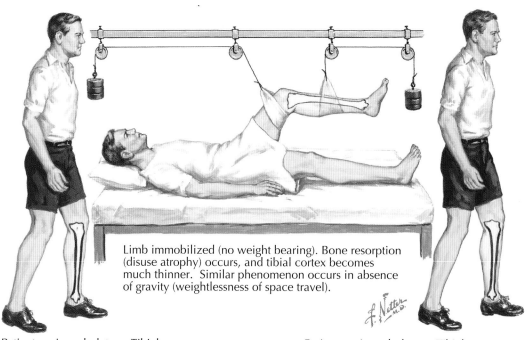

Limb immobilized (no weight bearing). Bone resorption (disuse atrophy) occurs, and tibial cortex becomes much thinner. Similar phenomenon occurs in absence of gravity (weightlessness of space travel).

Patient again ambulatory. Tibial cortex was eventually restored to near original thickness.

Patient again ambulatory. Tibial cortex was soon restored almost to original thickness.

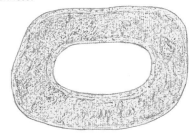 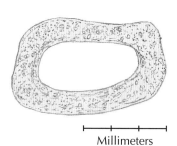

Millimeters

Cross sections of metacarpals of young adult dog (metacarpals weight bearing in dogs). Left from control limb. Right from limb immobilized 40 weeks. Right shows greatly decreased cortical thickness, reduced bone diameter (periosteal resorption), increased bone porosity, and enlarged medullary cavity. (Endosteal resorption predominates in older animals.)

EFFECTS OF DISUSE AND STRESS (WEIGHT BEARING) ON BONE MASS

Disuse osteoporosis is an important example of Wolff's law (see Plate 2-36). Normally, the tibial cortex in the midshaft region is quite thick. If the limb is immobilized, disuse osteoporosis sets in rapidly, and the cortex thins measurably. With resumption of weight bearing, the bone gradually rebuilds and the cortical mass and thickness are eventually restored, though the time for restoration is much longer than the immobilization time period. However, in some cases, the level of bone mass before immobilization may not be fully restored.

Disuse osteoporosis may be focal, involving a single bone or limb (arthritis or limb immobilization), or it may be generalized (prolonged bed rest or paralysis). With generalized immobilization, bone loss is most profound and rapid in the trabecular bone tissues of the axial skeleton and weight-bearing appendicular long bones.

Nevertheless, even with prolonged immobilization, loss of bone mass does not continue indefinitely. Results of studies carried out on dogs show that tubular bones exhibited temporal and envelope-specific patterns of change in bone mass after long-term immobilization in a cast. In these studies, a rapid initial loss of bone occurred over the first 6 weeks of immobilization. By the 12th week of immobilization, a rebound in bone

Pattern of bone loss in metacarpal 3 of dog in relation to duration of immobilization (expressed as percentage of control). Partial recovery from 8th to 12th week; then progressive bone loss to lower steady state.

mass occurred, although these levels were still below those before immobilization. Thereafter, a slower, longer-lasting bone loss continued and ended at 32 weeks of immobilization, with bone mass levels reaching a plateau at approximately 50% of original values.

In the short first phase, bone loss involved the periosteal, osteonal (haversian), and corticoendosteal envelopes. In the later, sustained-loss phase, the periosteal envelope was affected, resulting in a smaller bone with a slightly widened medullary canal and a thinner, more porous cortex. This latter trend was noted more so in relatively younger dogs (less so in older dogs) and may be in part attributed to a suppression of residual cortical bone growth in girth by immobilization of the younger dogs. Also, a similar suppression of cortical bone growth at mid-diaphysis has been reported for young rats flown in space experiencing weeks of weightlessness and mechanical disuse.

Plate 2-35

Physiology

MUSCULOSKELETAL EFFECTS OF WEIGHTLESSNESS (SPACE FLIGHT)

Gravity has played a major role in the evolution of life on Earth. The structure of living organisms and basic physiologic processes such as growth, development, and locomotion evolved in the presence of a gravitational field. Space flight has made it possible for humans to escape the pervasive influence of Earth's gravitational field and to experience the consequences of true weightlessness. Although there are several physiologic consequences to humans when exposed to long-term space flight, only those affecting bone are discussed here.

One consequence of space flight is a significant loss of bone mass (both matrix and mineral) in a weightless environment. During the early Gemini and Apollo flights, x-ray densitometry studies of the calcaneus of astronauts indicated that bone loss may be extensive and rapid even during a brief period of weightlessness. In later Apollo and Skylab space missions, a more precise technique, photon absorptiometry, was employed to assess the preflight and the postflight bone mass of the calcaneus. Findings showed a direct dose-response relationship between time spent in a weightless environment and loss of bone mass, although wide variations between astronauts were observed. These findings were corroborated by Mir space flight studies of changes in bone mass carried out on Soviet cosmonauts. Overall, for the proximal femur and spinal vertebra locations, there is an average loss of 1.0% to 1.5% bone mass and density for every month in space. In relative comparison, this level of bone loss would occur during menopausal osteoporosis over a 10- to 12-month time period.

The just-mentioned bone losses occur mostly in the weight-bearing bones of the lower limb and axial skeleton, with the greatest changes seen in the trabecular bone tissues having high-remodeling rates. After return from space, skeletal mass is gradually restored, although the recovery times on Earth are usually much longer than the actual space flight duration times. In some cases, bone mass recovery on Earth after a space mission is not completely restored, even after a prolonged recovery in Earth's gravitational field. For these cases with greatly prolonged weightlessness, full recovery is not anticipated because of irreversible loss of the surface scaffolding that is necessary for bone cell activity. Studies of metabolic balance, performed on the Skylab crew during flights lasting 28 to 84 days, revealed a striking increase in urinary calcium levels, which reached a plateau after 28 days in space. Fecal calcium levels, however, continued to increase, with no sign of leveling off even after 84 days in space. After only 10 days of weightlessness, the preflight positive calcium balance was abolished and a net negative calcium balance prevailed for the remainder of the flight. Apparently, dietary calcium sources used by the Skylab crew were not effectively absorbed during space flight. Rather, systemic calcium homeostasis was seemingly maintained in these astronauts by release of calcium from the skeleton.

Space flight's loss of total body calcium was much greater than that predicted from bed rest studies. Assuming that bone loss was continuous without a stabilizing end point during space flight, these findings led Rambaut and Johnston to calculate that a year of weightlessness might result in a loss of up to 20% of the body's total calcium reserve removed principally from trabecular bone surfaces. As occurs with immobilization, hypercalciuria is accompanied by hydroxyprolinuria, indicating that bone's organic matrix as well as

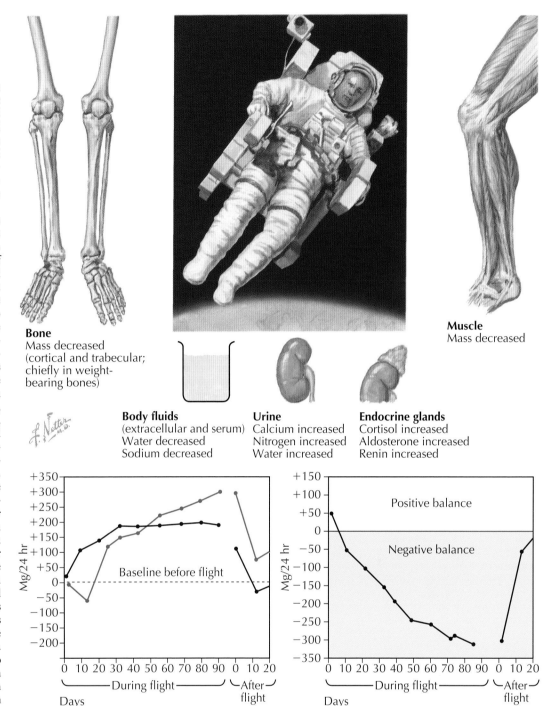

Bone
Mass decreased (cortical and trabecular; chiefly in weight-bearing bones)

Muscle
Mass decreased

Body fluids
(extracellular and serum)
Water decreased
Sodium decreased

Urine
Calcium increased
Nitrogen increased
Water increased

Endocrine glands
Cortisol increased
Aldosterone increased
Renin increased

— **Fecal calcium level** — **Urinary calcium level**

Total body calcium balance
(intake minus output)

mineral is lost. This finding was confirmed by the detection of elevated levels of collagen degradation products in the urine of Skylab astronauts. Results of studies of metabolic balance also showed a profound loss of total body nitrogen, reflecting a concomitant precipitous loss of muscle mass. Astronauts on later Skylab missions exercised vigorously, but these particular exercises did not restore or lessen their calcium loss.

Within 10 days after return to Earth, the astronauts' urinary calcium levels returned to normal but the fecal calcium content remained elevated. Thus, total body calcium balance remained negative even 20 days after the space flight.

Osteoporosis caused by weightlessness is more severe and unrelenting than any form of disuse osteoporosis here on Earth. The roles played by muscle contraction, periosteal tension, circulatory physiology, and bioelectric and piezoelectric properties of bone in weightlessness provide intriguing topics for further investigations. The study of bone physiology in the weightless environment of space is important for several reasons. First, the prolonged time in space required for interplanetary travel could result in the severe and permanently disabling complications of profound osteopenia, which would elevate the risk for fracture on reattaining weight-bearing activities under normal gravity loads. Therefore, protective countermeasures must be developed to mitigate bone loss during long space missions. Second, the weightless environment provides a natural opportunity for studying the complexities of normal bone physiology as well as a multitude of osteopenic conditions.

Plate 2-36

Musculoskeletal System: PART III

PHYSICAL FACTORS IN BONE REMODELING

In 1683, Galileo first recognized the relationship between applied load and bone morphology, noting a direct correlation between body weight and bone size. During the next 2 centuries, others observed that bone remodels, but Julius Wolff, a German anatomist, was the first to describe changes in bone mass accompanied changes in load, through the process of skeletal remodeling. In "The Law of Bone Transformation," published in 1892, Wolff explained: "Every change in the function of a bone is followed by certain definite changes in internal architecture and external conformation in accordance with mathematical laws." Stated more simply, *form follows function*. Although the mechanism by which bone cells transform mechanical or other biophysical signals into a useful biologic response is not fully understood, Wolff's observations are as valid today as they were nearly a century ago.

BONE ARCHITECTURE

The architecture of the proximal femur beautifully illustrates the general principle that the external form and shape of bone *as an organ* and the internal organization of bone *as a tissue* are well adapted to the forces placed upon them. There are dynamic internal forces as well as static and dynamic external forces on bone. The internal forces are created by muscle contraction; the external forces, by Earth's ubiquitous gravitational field and by the dynamic compressive forces of weight bearing. The upper half of Plate 2-36 depicts the bony trabeculae of the proximal femur aligned along the lines of stress according to Wolff's law. This intersecting network of trabeculae is the biologic response to the sum of internal and external physical forces on that region of the skeleton. These trabecular networks form arches that disperse and distribute loads corresponding to the principal tensile and compressive lines of force. Reduced weight bearing resulting from disuse or immobilization leads to a progressive thinning and eventual loss of these trabecular networks; those experiencing the greatest reduction in weight-bearing loads are resorbed first. A similar pattern is seen in all weight-bearing bones, including the loss of trabecular networks in the axial skeleton, especially in the vertebral bodies, which are largely composed of weight-bearing trabecular bone.

Mechanical forces also play a significant role in the external shape of bone. For example, the applied dynamic force of contraction of the gluteal muscles influences both the size and shape of the greater trochanter. If these muscles are paralyzed during skeletal development (as in certain types of poliomyelitis or in meningomyelocele), the greater trochanter does not attain its normal size and shape.

BONE ARCHITECTURE AND REMODELING IN RELATION TO STRESS

Bone architecture in relation to physical stress

Wolff's law. Bony structures orient themselves in form and mass to best resist extrinsic forces (i.e., form and mass follow function).

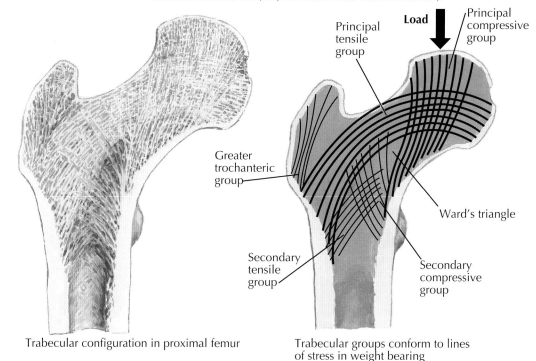

Trabecular configuration in proximal femur

Trabecular groups conform to lines of stress in weight bearing

Bone remodeling in response to stress

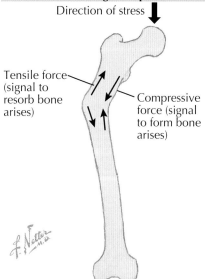

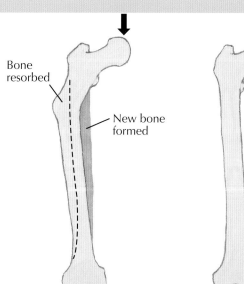

Malunion of long bone, with angulation. During weight bearing, compressive force develops on concave side of bone, and tensile force develops on convex side.

Compression signals osteoblasts to deposit bone on concave side, while tension signals osteoclasts to resorb bone on convex side.

Bone thus remodeled to a form best suited for weight bearing. Although weight bearing might be expected to increase angulation, opposite occurs.

BONE REMODELING

Wolff's law is also demonstrated by the straightening of a malunion of a long bone. With time, growth, and weight bearing, a malunion that has an angulation of as much as 30 degrees will straighten completely, at least in the infant and young child (lower half of Plate 2-36). This phenomenon would seem contrary to mechanical loading principles predicting that an

angulated structure repetitively bent should eventually fatigue and fail. However, the exact opposite happens and the bone straightens with growth.

What is the explanation of this phenomenon? Some biologic or physical signal must arise from the concave side of the bone at the site of the malunion, inducing the osteoblasts there to lay down additional bone tissue, and a corresponding signal must arise from the convex side of the malunion, stimulating the osteoclasts there

Plate 2-37

Physiology

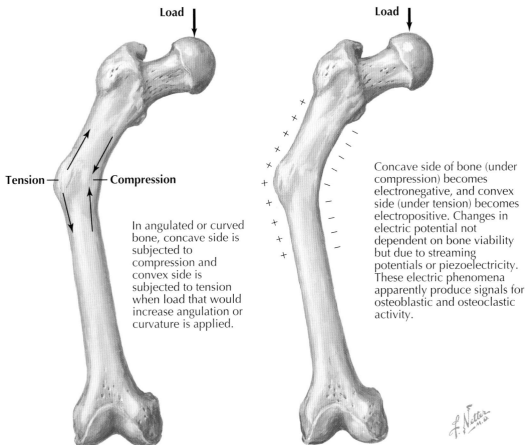

STRESS-GENERATED ELECTRIC POTENTIALS IN BONE

Strip of bone held in clamp at one end

Pressure applied to free end of flexed bone. Concave side of flexed bone (under compression) becomes electronegative, and convex side (under tension) becomes electropositive.

In angulated or curved bone, concave side is subjected to compression and convex side is subjected to tension when load that would increase angulation or curvature is applied.

Concave side of bone (under compression) becomes electronegative, and convex side (under tension) becomes electropositive. Changes in electric potential not dependent on bone viability but due to streaming potentials or piezoelectricity. These electric phenomena apparently produce signals for osteoblastic and osteoclastic activity.

PHYSICAL FACTORS IN BONE REMODELING (Continued)

to remove bone tissue. The working hypothesis to explain this phenomenon lies in bone's principal function—namely, to bear repetitive loads—whereby biophysical signals direct bone formation and resorption. Various investigations of this hypothesis identified the nature of signals in stressed bone and those in viable nonstressed bone. These studies determined that two types of electrical action potentials are present in bone: *stress-generated*, or strain-related, potentials and *bioelectric*, or standing, potentials.

STRESS-GENERATED ELECTRIC POTENTIALS IN BONE

Under stress, the concave side of the bone (the area under compression) becomes net negatively charged, or electronegative and the convex side of the bone (the area under tension) becomes net positively charged, or electropositive (see Plate 2-37). In the malunion of a long bone, the area of compression, where new bone will be formed, is electronegative and the area under tension, where bone will be removed, is electropositive. These stress/strain-generated potentials arise when the ionic fluid volume distributed in bone flows out of the compressed tissue areas and flows into the expanding tissue areas under tension. Under repetitive bending moments, this charged fluid movement flows back and forth across a fixed-charge scaffold matrix, thereby generating cyclical electrical potentials. It is conjectured that low-intensity, pulsed-ultrasonic waves externally applied to the skin in proximity of bone tissue may induce localized fluid movements that then could induce stress-generated electrical potentials at those application sites in bone.

BIOELECTRIC POTENTIALS IN BONE

Bioelectric potentials are measured from the surface of nonstressed bone (see Plate 2-38). In the intact tibia, the metaphyseal and epiphyseal regions are net electronegative, whereas the diaphyseal, or midshaft, region is relatively neutral in net charge. When a fracture occurs in the diaphysis, the entire tibial surface becomes electronegative, with a large peak of electronegativity occurring over the fracture site and persisting well after the fracture heals. A second peak of electronegativity occurs over the farthest growth plate. This latter finding is fascinating because a fractured extremity in a child frequently exhibits overgrowth not at the fracture site but in the growth plate near the end of the bone. The nature of the signal directing the growth plate to accelerate growth has never been identified, but the increased

electronegativity over the growth plate/metaphyseal area that accompanies a midshaft fracture may be involved.

To determine the source of action potentials in nonstressed bone, a series of experiments were performed on rabbit tibiae indicating that viable cells and tissues were involved. When the vascular (or nerve) supply of the leg was interrupted, the electric potential over the proximal tibia did not change even 30 minutes after

ligation (or denervation). The introduction of cytotoxic drugs (or other necrosis-inducing agents) led to a significant drop in electronegative potential to the bone, suggesting that cell viability was necessary for bioelectric potentials. In particular, localized necrosis led to a significant drop in bioelectric potential just at the nonviable site.

Potentials arising from nonstressed bone are called bioelectric potentials, meaning that they arise from

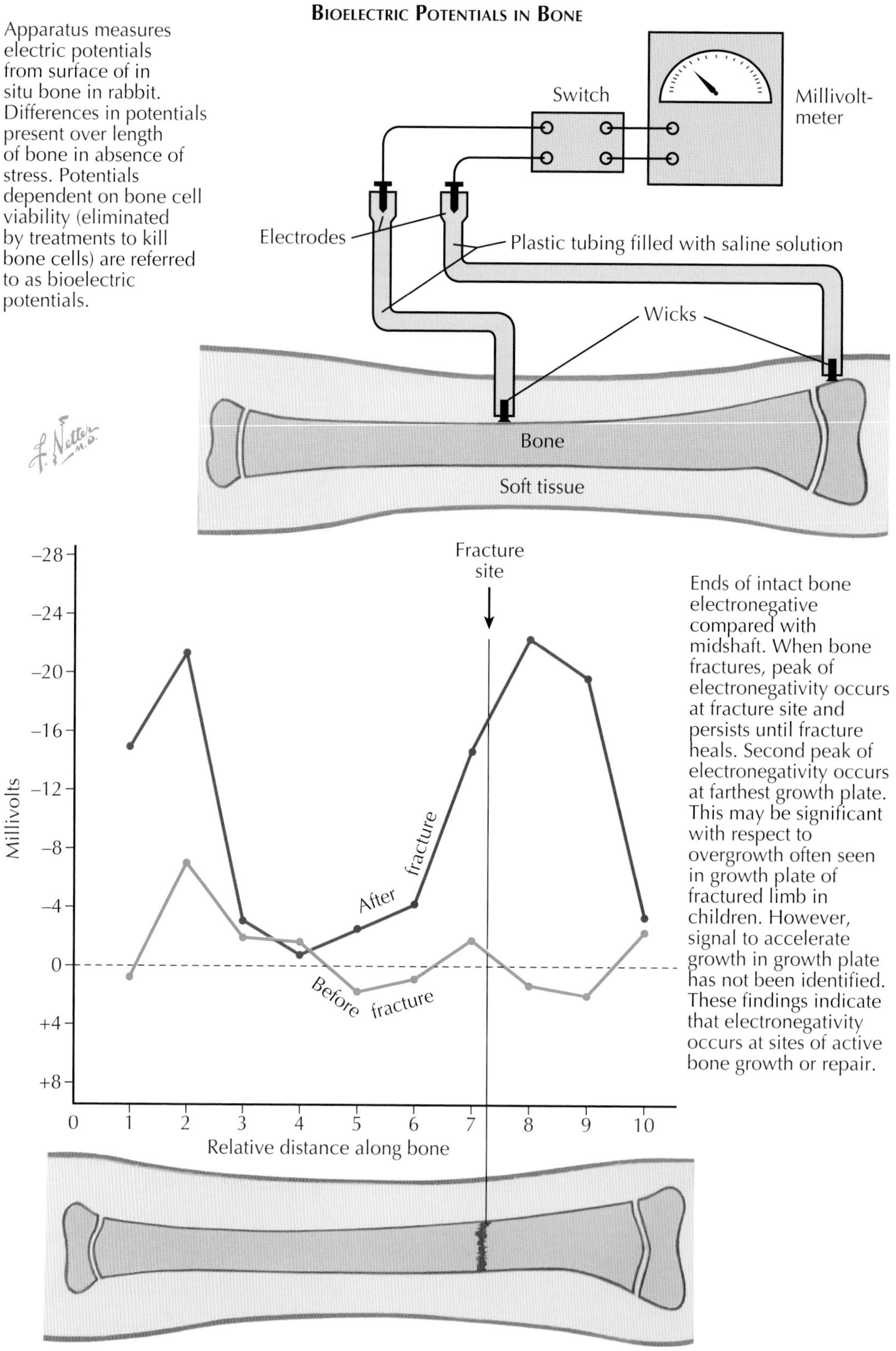

Plate 2-38

BIOELECTRIC POTENTIALS IN BONE

Apparatus measures electric potentials from surface of in situ bone in rabbit. Differences in potentials present over length of bone in absence of stress. Potentials dependent on bone cell viability (eliminated by treatments to kill bone cells) are referred to as bioelectric potentials.

PHYSICAL FACTORS IN BONE REMODELING (Continued)

living bone. Such potentials are dependent on cell viability and not on stress. Active areas of growth and repair are electronegative, and less active areas are electrically neutral or electropositive. Studies have also shown that the application of small electric currents to bone stimulates osteogenesis at the site of the negative electrode (cathode).

Various in vitro and in vivo models have identified the processes and results of electrically induced osteogenesis. Mainly in the vicinity of the cathode, electrically induced osteogenesis exhibits a dose-response over a relatively narrow, low current range. Within this proper range, electricity can induce bone formation in the absence of trauma and in areas of inactive bone formation, such as in the medullary canal of an adult animal. It has also been shown that the application of small electric currents can favorably influence fracture healing in laboratory animals, but for this to occur the cathode must be placed directly in the fracture site.

In addition, electricity can be induced in bone by means of an electric field with the electric apparatus remaining completely external to the limb; however, the amplitude and frequency of the applied current needs to be increased to effectively cross the cutaneous resistance barrier. The electric field can be inductively or capacitively coupled to the bone. In inductive coupling, a current varying over time within external wire coils produces a time-varying magnetic field, which in turn induces a time-varying direct current electric field within biological tissues contained inside the space between the wire coils. In capacitive coupling, an electric field is induced in bone by an external capacitor (two charged metal plates are placed on either side of the limb and attached to a voltage source). Several studies have shown that both inductive- and capacitive-coupled pulsed electric fields can favorably influence fracture repair in experimental animals and humans.

The mechanism by which electricity induces osteogenesis is unclear. It is known that the cathode consumes oxygen and produces hydroxyl radicals according to the equation $2H_2O + O_2 + 4e^- \rightarrow 4OH^-$. Thus, the oxygen tension (Po_2) could be lowered in the local tissue, and pH is raised in the vicinity of the cathode. Studies have also shown that low Po_2 in tissue encourages bone formation at the growth plate and within fracture calluses. Other studies have determined that the pH in the growth plate at the calcification front is

Ends of intact bone electronegative compared with midshaft. When bone fractures, peak of electronegativity occurs at fracture site and persists until fracture heals. Second peak of electronegativity occurs at farthest growth plate. This may be significant with respect to overgrowth often seen in growth plate of fractured limb in children. However, signal to accelerate growth in growth plate has not been identified. These findings indicate that electronegativity occurs at sites of active bone growth or repair.

rather high (7.70 ± 0.05), and this information is consistent with the previous concept.

These local microenvironmental changes in the vicinity of the cathode lead to cellular changes that ultimately result in osteogenesis. Both capacitive- and inductive-coupled pulsed electric fields act directly on bone and cartilage cells resulting in transient elevations in intracellular calcium ions contributed by two sources: (1) the opening of voltage-gated calcium channels allowing external calcium ions to flow into cells and (2)

those calcium ions released from endoplasmic reticulum storage depots. In addition, evidence shows that these pulsed electromagnetic treatments activate other intracellular signal transduction pathways in bone and cartilage cells, leading to the stimulation of cell proliferation and/or the production and secretion of additional extracellular matrix. These findings have enabled the application of bioelectricity in one or more of its many forms to modulate growth, maintenance, and repair of bone and cartilage.

Plate 2-39

Physiology

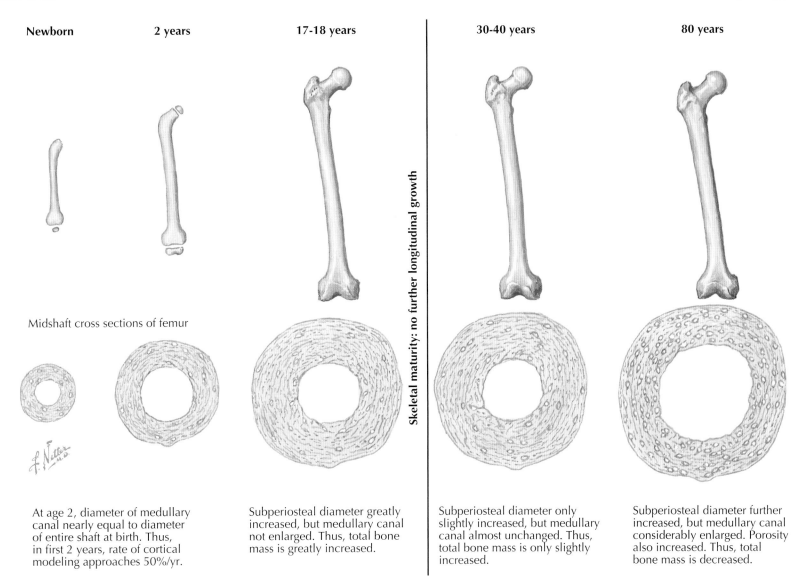

| Newborn | 2 years | 17-18 years | 30-40 years | 80 years |

Skeletal maturity: no further longitudinal growth

Midshaft cross sections of femur

At age 2, diameter of medullary canal nearly equal to diameter of entire shaft at birth. Thus, in first 2 years, rate of cortical modeling approaches 50%/yr.

Subperiosteal diameter greatly increased, but medullary canal not enlarged. Thus, total bone mass is greatly increased.

Subperiosteal diameter only slightly increased, but medullary canal almost unchanged. Thus, total bone mass is only slightly increased.

Subperiosteal diameter further increased, but medullary canal considerably enlarged. Porosity also increased. Thus, total bone mass is decreased.

AGE-RELATED CHANGES IN BONE GEOMETRY

The long bones of the appendicular skeleton grow in length by endochondral ossification and in width by a process of subperiosteal bone formation and endosteal bone resorption. Even after longitudinal growth ceases at skeletal maturity, both bone modeling and remodeling continues throughout life. Age-related changes in the geometry of long bones reflect the body's ability to rearrange its remaining skeletal assets in the most biomechanically useful way—another example of Wolff's law (see Plate 2-36).

The growth in width of a long bone is due primarily to subperiosteal formation of new bone, a process referred to as modeling, which begins before birth and continues even into the ninth and tenth decades. In all population samples studied, subperiosteal formation of new bone is greater in males than in females. The growth in width of long bones is particularly accelerated in the first 2 years of life. For example, by age 2, the diameter of the medullary canal at the mid-diaphysis of the femur is nearly equal to the diameter of the entire mid-diaphysis at birth. Thus, the rate of cortical

modeling approaches 50% per year in the first 2 years of life. The growth in width of long bones continues at a slower rate in childhood and then increases rapidly during the adolescent growth spurt. During this period of rapid longitudinal as well as latitudinal growth, as much as 300 mg of elemental calcium is incorporated into bone apatite every day.

Most traditional views of bone development imply that all growth ceases after skeletal maturity, near the beginning of the third decade. However, results of cross-sectional studies on large samples of the adult population and longitudinal studies on individuals indicate that subperiosteal bone apposition continues throughout adulthood and into old age. The greatest increase in bone width occurs in the femur, but the general process is observed in the entire skeleton, in bones as diverse as the skull, ribs, and vertebrae. Also, subperiosteal bone formation occurs in both men and women and in all population samples studied. Although the total subperiosteal area is greater in men than in women, the percentage of gain is greater in women.

In conjunction with the age-specific subperiosteal bone apposition that continues throughout life, a complex age-related activity, characterized by alternating phases of resorption and apposition in a process referred to as remodeling, occurs at the endosteal

surface. Whereas subperiosteal activity determines the width of the bone, endosteal activity determines the width of the medullary canal. The combination of the relative activities at the two surfaces over a period of time determines the thickness of the cortex, and remodeling within the individual osteons of the cortex determines intracortical porosity.

During the first few years of life, a great deal of modeling and remodeling activities takes place at both the subperiosteal and the endosteal surface of cortical bone, tremendously increasing the width of both the bone and the medullary canal. Then, for the next several years, subperiosteal bone formation continues at a slower rate, accompanied by a large decrease in endosteal resorption and a short period of endosteal apposition. These processes enlarge the diameter of the bone and reduce the width of the medullary canal. Then, from about age 6 until the middle teenage years, endosteal bone resorption resumes, with resultant enlargement of the medullary canal.

The greatest natural uncoupling of bone activity in favor of bone formation occurs during adolescence. (For a more complete discussion of coupling, see Plates 2-30 and 2-31.) The growth in bone length by endochondral bone formation at the growth plates is accompanied by a corresponding burst of subperiosteal bone

Plate 2-40

Musculoskeletal System: PART III

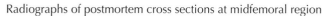
Radiographs of postmortem cross sections at midfemoral region

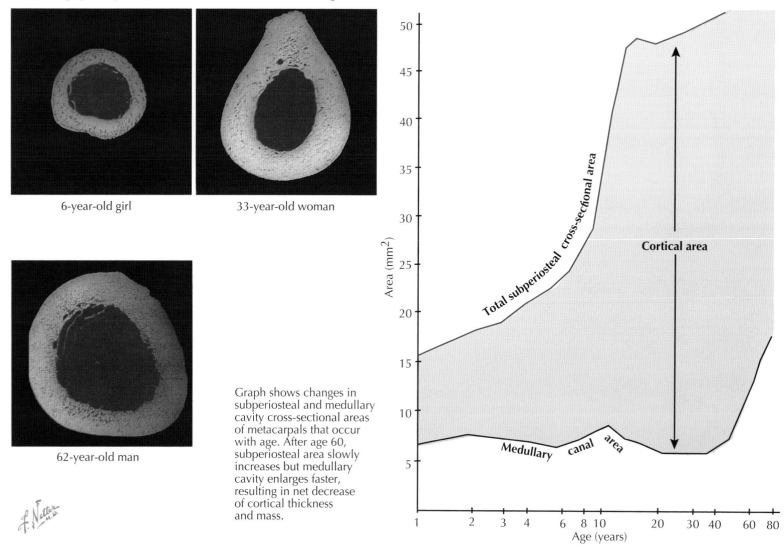

6-year-old girl

33-year-old woman

62-year-old man

Graph shows changes in subperiosteal and medullary cavity cross-sectional areas of metacarpals that occur with age. After age 60, subperiosteal area slowly increases but medullary cavity enlarges faster, resulting in net decrease of cortical thickness and mass.

AGE-RELATED CHANGES IN BONE GEOMETRY (Continued)

formation at mid-diaphysis; once again, endosteal activity is reversed, with a new wave of endosteal bone apposition taking place. These processes increase the length and width of the bone, increase the thickness of the cortex, and decrease the width of the medullary canal. The apposition of bone at the endosteal surface begins earlier in females and continues until nearly age 40 in both sexes. After age 40, the activity at the endosteal surface again reverses, with endosteal bone resorption persisting for the remainder of life. Subperiosteal bone formation continues for the rest of life as well, at a slow but steady rate.

As a result of these two activities at the bone surfaces, the width of the bone increases slightly throughout adulthood and into old age; the width of the medullary canal also increases, resulting in a wider but thinner cortex. Although these changes in bone geometry have been noted in all long bones studied, they are most striking in the femur. However, the changes in the metacarpals (the bones most extensively studied and documented) provide an excellent means of assessing the state of cortical bone modeling in the appendicular skeleton. However, changes in the cross-sectional geometry of the bone surfaces do not take into account changes in intracortical bone density.

The age-related subperiosteal expansion of long bones partially compensates mechanically for the endosteal resorption and resultant cortical thinning and increased porosity that occurs with aging. This radial

outward displacement of the cortical mass provides an increase in a bone's moment of inertia, thereby serving to protect the long bones from bending and torsional stresses. This can best be understood by envisioning a solid rod of a certain cross-sectional area. If the material in the solid rod were displaced radially from the central axis of the rod to create a hollow tube, the result would be a structure that was stronger in both bending and torsion and thus better able to resist fracture. Thus, rearranging the same amount of material into a hollow tube improves the structural properties. It is no coincidence that the long bones are hollow and that the osteon is also essentially a hollow tube with a central haversian canal. By a process of natural selection, a structure has evolved that best accommodates the local biomechanical requirements of a system whose metabolic resources are under strict systemic control.

METABOLIC DISEASES

Plate 3-1   Musculoskeletal System: PART III

Synthesis, Secretion, and Function of Parathyroid Hormone (PTH)

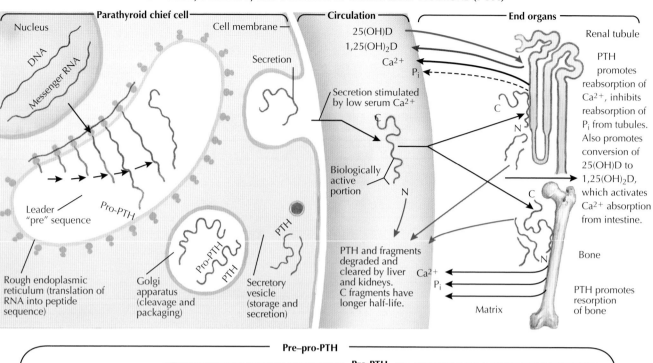

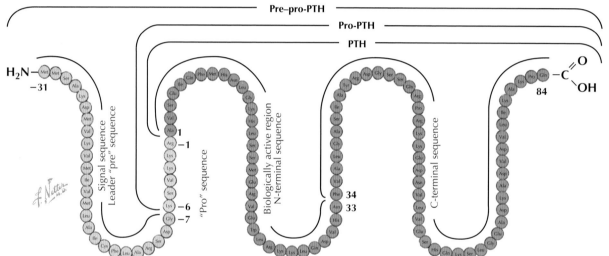

Parathyroid Hormone

The parathyroid gland regulates the calcium in the extracellular fluid by sensing small changes in calcium levels and rapidly modifying the secretion of parathyroid hormone (PTH). With a fall in the calcium level, PTH secretion is increased and, in turn, leads to increased calcium concentration and suppressed PTH secretion, thus completing a feedback loop. PTH raises the calcium level by promoting the entry of calcium from bone, renal tubule, and intestine. In bone, PTH increases resorption of formed bone, which contains calcium and phosphate. In the kidney, PTH enhances renal tubular reabsorption of calcium (which decreases urinary calcium excretion) and decreases tubular reabsorption of phosphate (which eliminates the phosphate released from bone). PTH indirectly increases calcium absorption from the gut by increasing the synthesis of the active form of 1,25-dihydroxyvitamin D, or 1,25(OH)$_2$D, from its precursor 25-hydroxyvitamin D, or 25(OH)D. This metabolite of vitamin D mediates

the gut effect of PTH by directly activating calcium absorption in the small intestine.

Compared with other secretory systems, the parathyroid cell contains minimal amounts of hormone stored in the granules. Consequently, regulation of secretion occurs at the gene level and by cell proliferation. PTH is initially synthesized as pre–pro-PTH, a large precursor peptide of 115 amino acids. During translation from its messenger ribonucleic acid (mRNA), the initial "pre" sequence directs the growing peptide across the membrane of the endoplasmic reticulum and is then cleaved before synthesis of the entire hormone is completed. The 90-amino-acid pro-PTH is then transported through membrane channels to the Golgi apparatus where the hexapeptide extension of pro-PTH is removed. PTH is stored in the secretory vesicles until secretion occurs. Once secreted it is metabolized to inactive products composed of fragments from the carboxyl (C)-terminal end. Modern-day assays for PTH recognize the intact molecule and do not measure the inactive C-terminal fragments.

The regulation of PTH secretion is more complex than previously recognized. Its secretion is controlled

not only by serum calcium and phosphorus but also by the active form of 1,25-dihydroxyvitamin D (1,25-DHVD) and by fibroblastic growth factor-23 [FGF23] and its membrane receptor Klotho.

Serum calcium and phosphorus have a post-transcriptional effect on gene PTH expression. Hypocalcemia increases mRNA levels and PTH secretion. Chronic low-calcium states also induce cell proliferation. Increased serum phosphorus has opposite effects. It decreases secretion of PTH via a regulatory step at the mRNA level where specific proteins stabilize or destabilize the concentration of PTH mRNA.

FGF23 is a regulatory protein of phosphorus. It is a skeletal protein that acts on the kidney to decrease synthesis of 1,25-DHVD and increase phosphorus excretion through binding to a renal membrane protein called Klotho. The parathyroid cell also has this Klotho receptor protein. The binding of FGF23 to parathyroid cell Klotho receptor causes an activation of specific intracellular kinases that suppress PTH gene expression and subsequent secretion of the hormone.

Plate 3-2   Metabolic Diseases

PRIMARY HYPERPARATHYROIDISM

PATHOLOGIC PHYSIOLOGY

Primary hyperparathyroidism is caused by excessive production of parathyroid hormone (PTH) by enlarged parathyroid glands (see Plate 3-2). In 85% of cases, only a single parathyroid gland is enlarged (adenoma); in 15% of cases, all four glands are enlarged (hyperplasia). These two pathologic types of hyperparathyroidism have identical clinical manifestations and can only be distinguished at surgery, although nuclear imaging may sometimes identify hyperplasia of all the glands. This technique is a localizing procedure and not a diagnostic test for hyperparathyroidism. Parathyroid carcinoma occurs in less than 1% of patients, and severe hypercalcemia is often the initial symptom. Histologic diagnosis is helpful. Clinically this problem is suggested when recurring parathyroid "adenomas" develop after repeated removal of an adenoma.

Hyperparathyroidism causes hypercalcemia as a result of increased resorption of bone, reabsorption of calcium in the renal tubule, and absorption of calcium from the gut. PTH also decreases reabsorption of phosphate in the renal tubule, and in moderate-to-severe hyperparathyroidism the serum phosphate level is reduced; in the mild form of the disease, the serum phosphate level is often normal. Another form of the disease, although less often appreciated, is the entity called normocalcemic or eucalcemic hyperparathyroidism.

CLINICAL MANIFESTATIONS

Hyperparathyroidism is a chronic indolent disorder that slowly increases serum calcium levels over many years and may be evident for decades before it produces significant clinical problems. It was considered a rare disorder until 2 decades ago, but routine screening of serum by automated techniques greatly increased recognition of increased serum calcium in many patients and the suspicion for this disorder. Most patients have mild hypercalcemia (serum calcium level < 12 mg/dL) and have few or no symptoms. The most common clinical complaint in newly diagnosed hyperparathyroidism is no complaint at all. Those patients with clinical manifestations may show a spectrum of problems such as fatigue, lethargy, constipation, nocturia, abdominal discomfort, changes in mental status of minor degree (e.g., poor concentration, forgetfulness, depression) osteoporosis, bone pain, fractures, renal colic and stones, unexplained anemia, and weight loss. With severe hypercalcemia (>12 mg/dL), confusion and coma may supervene along with anorexia, nausea, vomiting, and dehydration. It is a clinical observation that older patients tolerate high serum calcium levels poorly and may manifest these later problems more often than younger patients. In a small number of patients there is

PATHOPHYSIOLOGY OF PRIMARY HYPERPARATHYROIDISM

| Adenoma (93% of cases) | Hyperplasia (6% of cases) | Carcinoma (1% of cases) |

Variable reduction in bone density. In rare, severe cases, cysts and brown tumors form (due to osteitis fibrosa cystica) and subperiosteal resorption.

clinical or radiographic evidence of hyperparathyroid bone disease. Typical findings include serum calcium levels greater than 12 mg/dL, serum PTH levels several times higher than normal, high serum alkaline phosphatase, and diffuse bone pain.

In patients with severe hyperparathyroidism and bone disease, radiographs may show subperiosteal bone resorption (highly specific to hyperparathyroidism) around the phalanges and distal ends of the clavicles and diffuse decalcification of the skull (salt-and-pepper skull) that resembles multiple myeloma. Bone cysts (also called brown tumors), if present, are often the sites of pathologic fractures. With bone loss in the spine, the intervertebral discs herniate into the vertebral bodies, creating a "codfish" appearance on radiographs. Even if there is no radiographic evidence of bone disease, excessive, PTH-mediated bone resorption may increase the risk of osteoporosis, a situation of particular concern

Plate 3-3   Musculoskeletal System: PART III

CLINICAL MANIFESTATIONS OF PRIMARY HYPERPARATHYROIDISM

Mild, asymptomatic: Most common (serum Ca^{2+} often <12 mg/dL)	Moderate-to-severe, symptomatic: Uncommon (serum Ca^{2+} often >12 mg/dL)

PRIMARY HYPERPARATHYROIDISM
(Continued)

in postmenopausal women who display the greatest incidence of this problem and already are at high risk for primary osteoporosis. This problem is often diagnosed as osteoporosis from a low bone density test. Histologically, the bone changes are more complex than simple osteoporosis. PTH activates osteoclastic resorption of bone, which can lead to significant bone loss. There is also a compensatory increase in osteoblastic bone formation; however, resorption ultimately exceeds formation, leading to bone loss. Osteoblasts release alkaline phosphatase, and serum levels may be elevated in patients with significant bone involvement. In severe cases of hyperparathyroidism, cystic areas of skeletal erosions may appear along with areas of fibrous tissue in adjacent bone marrow (osteitis fibrosa cystica).

Nephrolithiasis (urinary calculi) occurs in approximately 10% of patients with hyperparathyroidism (see Plate 3-3). Nephrocalcinosis is rarer and is typically seen in severe hyperparathyroidism with bone involvement. PTH increases calcium reabsorption in the renal tubule, the increased renal filtration produced by elevated serum calcium levels does not compensate, and the result is hypercalciuria. In some patients, calcium precipitates in the renal tubule and forms urinary calculi, common manifestations of kidney stones.

In severe hypercalcemia, precipitates can occur in the renal interstitium and incite an inflammatory reaction (nephrocalcinosis). By the time interstitial calcium deposits are visible on radiography, renal function is already considerably reduced. Hypercalcemia also decreases the capacity to concentrate urine, which frequently leads to polyuria and dehydration (if compensatory fluid intake does not compensate for this fluid loss). Pancreatitis and peptic ulcers, although rare, may occur with hyperparathyroidism. Gastrin-secreting tumors associated with hyperparathyroidism may cause ulcers in patients with multiple endocrine neoplasia (MEN) syndromes. Prolonged or severe hypercalcemia often results in calcium deposits in the medial and lateral edges of the cornea (band keratopathy).

TREATMENT

Surgical excision of the single, enlarged parathyroid gland is the treatment of choice for patients with an adenoma. Treatment of hyperplasia is subtotal parathyroidectomy, or removal of all but one or one-half gland. However, excision of too little tissue leads to persistent hypercalcemia and removal of too much tissue causes hypoparathyroidism. Asymptomatic disease is a conundrum in clinical practice. When to intervene surgically is the topic of many guidelines published through the years.

Three familial autosomal dominant syndromes of hyperparathyroidism have been identified among patients with parathyroid hyperplasia. In two of these syndromes, MEN I and II, neoplasms occur in other endocrine glands. MEN I is characterized by pituitary

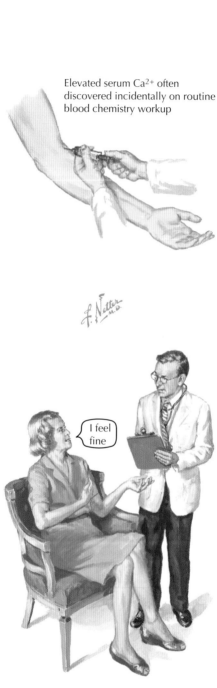

Elevated serum Ca^{2+} often discovered incidentally on routine blood chemistry workup

I feel fine

Most patients asymptomatic or have only mild systemic manifestations such as weakness, polyuria, nocturia, constipation, or hypertension

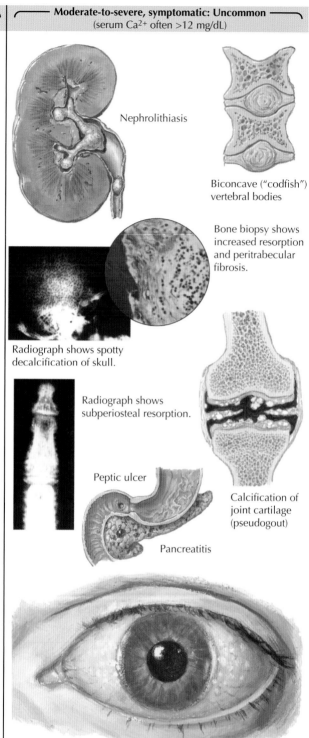

Nephrolithiasis

Biconcave ("codfish") vertebral bodies

Bone biopsy shows increased resorption and peritrabecular fibrosis.

Radiograph shows spotty decalcification of skull.

Radiograph shows subperiosteal resorption.

Peptic ulcer

Calcification of joint cartilage (pseudogout)

Pancreatitis

Conjunctival calcification; band keratopathy may be seen on slit-lamp examination.

adenomas and islet cell tumors in the pancreas, whereas MEN II is characterized by a high incidence of pheochromocytoma and medullary carcinoma of the thyroid. Patients with familial hypocalciuric hypercalcemia, the third and rarest syndrome, exhibit lifelong asymptomatic hypercalcemia that persists even after subtotal parathyroidectomy. This syndrome is distinguished from typical hyperparathyroidism by an absence of hypercalciuria and a high familial incidence

of asymptomatic hypercalcemia without other endocrinopathies. This disorder is due to abnormalities in the calcium-sensing receptors in the kidney that fail to excrete appropriate amounts of calcium, thereby raising the serum level.

Cancer of the parathyroid glands can rarely be cured by surgical excision because it has metastasized by the time it is detected. Patients with parathyroid carcinoma usually die of uncontrollable hypercalcemia.

Plate 3-4   Metabolic Diseases

DIFFERENTIAL DIAGNOSIS OF HYPERCALCEMIC STATES

The cause of hypercalcemia can often be determined on the basis of the patient's history and a careful physical examination, because most of the disorders that give rise to hypercalcemia (aside from primary hyperparathyroidism) are clinically apparent by the time the condition occurs. Tests that measure serum levels of parathyroid hormone (PTH), inorganic phosphate (P_i), and vitamin D metabolites aid in the diagnosis, but the clinical history of hypercalcemia should not be discounted as a diagnostic aid. Hyperparathyroid disease is a chronic, slowly developing disorder, and results from old laboratory tests show the existence of hypercalcemia for many years.

The serum level of PTH distinguishes primary hyperparathyroidism from other disorders causing hypercalcemia, because it is the only hypercalcemic disorder resulting from excessive production of PTH. Serum phosphate levels are inversely proportional to PTH levels because PTH promotes the urinary excretion of phosphate. Although hypophosphatemia suggests hyperparathyroidism, it may also be present in patients with cancer, because certain tumors secrete phosphaturic factors. In addition, anorexia alone will lower serum phosphorus, thereby confounding its use as a diagnostic tool for parathyroid disease. High levels of 25-hydroxyvitamin D, or 25(OH)D (also known as calcidiol) suggest an excessive intake of vitamin D. A very high concentration of this usually inactive compound can result in hypercalcemia. A high concentration of 1,25-dihy-droxyvitamin D, or 1,25(OH)₂D (also known as calcitriol) occurs only in hyperparathyroidism, granulomatous diseases, and, rarely, malignant disease.

Primary hyperparathyroidism is the most common cause of hypercalcemia; often, the hypercalcemia is the only clinical manifestation (see Plates 3-2 and 3-3). In patients with mild-to-moderate hyperparathyroidism, radiographs usually do not reveal bone disease and the serum phosphate level is often normal. Also, serum 1,25(OH)₂D levels are elevated in less than 50% of patients. Therefore, the most specific and reliable tool in the diagnosis of hyperparathyroidism is the measurement of serum PTH level.

Malignancies cause hypercalcemia by increasing bone resorption either locally through skeletal metastases (e.g., breast cancer and multiple myeloma) or by secreting hormonal factors that stimulate resorption (e.g., lung and renal cell cancer). Hypercalcemia is usually a late manifestation of hypercalcemia due to a nonparathyroid mechanism and usually occurs only after the tumor is apparent. The presence of such a tumor is therefore an important clue to the etiology of hypercalcemia. Hypercalcemia is rarely the first manifestation of occult cancer but is more typically seen in patients with widespread end-stage disease.

Sarcoidosis and, rarely, other granulomatous diseases such as tuberculosis and histoplasmosis also lead to hypercalcemia, because of an increase in the synthesis of 1,25(OH)₂D. Hyperparathyroidism is the other disease in which the level of 1,25(OH)₂D is elevated, but the PTH level is also elevated. In sarcoidosis, by contrast, the PTH level is normal or reduced and the level of the angiotensin-converting enzyme (ACE) activity is often elevated. Although this finding is not specific to sarcoidosis, the absence of high ACE activity levels makes the diagnosis very unlikely. Certain malignancies such as lymphomas cause hypercalcemia also by

increasing the synthesis of 1,25(OH)₂D. Fortunately these are rare events.

Hyperthyroidism, or thyrotoxicosis, rarely causes mild hypercalcemia. The diagnosis is based on clinical and laboratory evidence of hyperthyroidism and restoration of a normal serum calcium level with antithyroid therapy.

The *milk-alkali syndrome* is typically caused by excessive intake of both milk and absorbable alkalis such as sodium bicarbonate and calcium carbonate. Because absorbable alkalis are not often used as antacids, this

syndrome is rare; however, ingestion of large amounts of calcium (usually more than 4 g/day) can produce the syndrome. The diagnosis is made by a careful history and by observing the patient's response to withdrawal of calcium.

Immobilization due to fractures or paralysis increases calcium release from bone resulting in hypercalcemia and hypercalciuria is common. Hypercalcemia, although uncommon, may develop when the rate of bone turnover is high, as in childhood or adolescence, and in extensive Paget disease.

Condition	Serum Ca²⁺	Serum Pᵢ	Serum PTH	Serum 25(OH)D	Serum 1,25(OH)₂D	Associated findings
Primary hyperparathyroidism	↑	N or ↓	High N or ↑	N	N or ↑	80% Asymptomatic Nephrolithiasis Osteoporosis Hypercalcemic symptoms
Cancer with extensive bone metastases	↑	N or ↑	↓	N	↓ or N	History of primary tumor, destructive lesions on radiograph, bone scan
Multiple myeloma and lymphoma	↑	N or ↑	↓	N	↓ or N	Abnormal serum or urine protein electrophoresis, abnormal bone radiographs
Humoral hypercalcemia of malignancy	↑	N or ↓	↓	N	↓ or N	↑PTHrP Solid malignancy usually evident
Sarcoidosis and other granulomatous diseases	↑	N or ↑	↓	N	↑	Hilar adenopathy, interstitial lung disease, elevated angiotensin-converting enzyme
Hyperthyroidism	↑	N	↓	N	N	Symptoms of hyperthyroidism, elevated serum thyroxine
Vitamin D intoxication	↑	N or ↑	↓	Very ↑	N or ↑	History of excessive vitamin D intake
Milk-alkali syndrome	↑	N or ↑	↓	N	N or ↓	History of excessive calcium and alkali ingestion, heavy use of over-the-counter calcium-containing antacids
Total body immobilization	↑	N or ↑	↓	N	↓ or N	Multiple fractures, paralysis (children, adolescents, patients with Paget disease of bone)

Table title: DIFFERENTIAL DIAGNOSIS OF HYPERCALCEMIC STATES

Plate 3-5

Musculoskeletal System: PART III

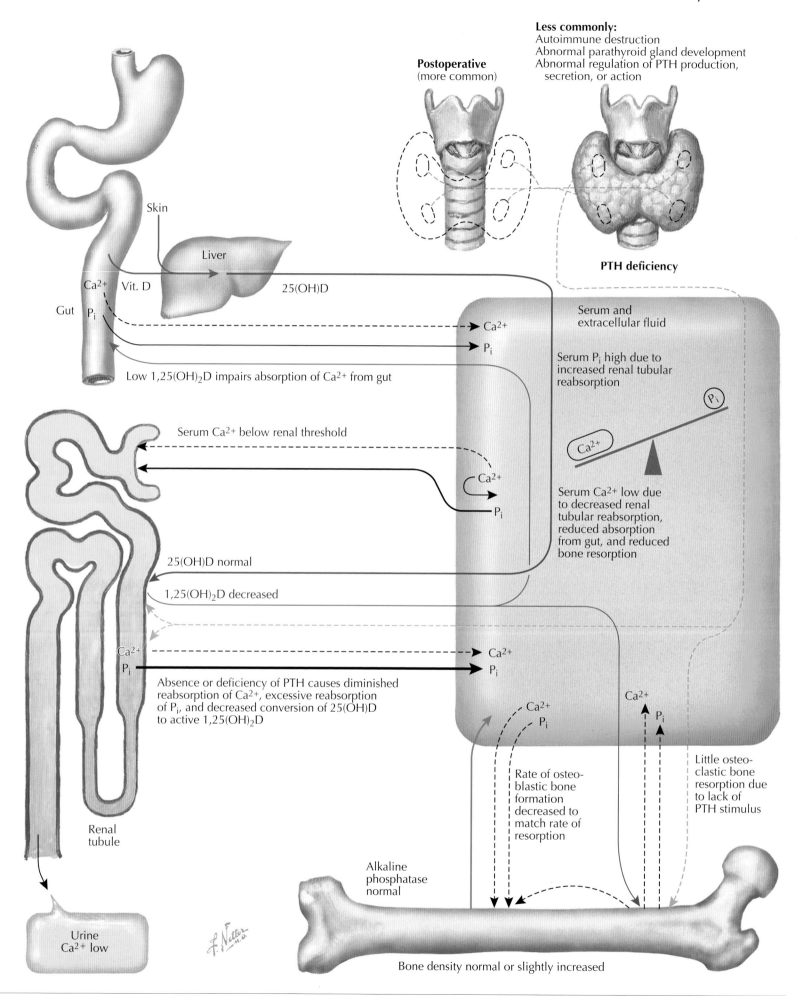

Less commonly:
Autoimmune destruction
Abnormal parathyroid gland development
Abnormal regulation of PTH production,
secretion, or action

Postoperative
(more common)

PTH deficiency

Skin

Liver

Vit. D

25(OH)D

Ca²⁺

Pᵢ

Gut

Low 1,25(OH)₂D impairs absorption of Ca²⁺ from gut

Serum and
extracellular fluid

Ca²⁺

Pᵢ

Serum Pᵢ high due to
increased renal tubular
reabsorption

Pᵢ

Ca²⁺

Serum Ca²⁺ below renal threshold

Ca²⁺

Pᵢ

Serum Ca²⁺ low due
to decreased renal
tubular reabsorption,
reduced absorption
from gut, and reduced
bone resorption

25(OH)D normal

1,25(OH)₂D decreased

Ca²⁺

Pᵢ

Ca²⁺

Pᵢ

Absence or deficiency of PTH causes diminished
reabsorption of Ca²⁺, excessive reabsorption
of Pᵢ, and decreased conversion of 25(OH)D
to active 1,25(OH)₂D

Ca²⁺

Ca²⁺

Pᵢ

Pᵢ

Little osteo-
clastic bone
resorption due
to lack of
PTH stimulus

Renal
tubule

Rate of osteo-
blastic bone
formation
decreased to
match rate of
resorption

Alkaline
phosphatase
normal

Urine
Ca²⁺ low

Bone density normal or slightly increased

Plate 3-5

Metabolic Diseases

PATHOLOGIC PHYSIOLOGY OF HYPOPARATHYROIDISM

The most common cause of hypoparathyroidism is the inadvertent removal or destruction of the parathyroid glands during thyroid or parathyroid surgery. Idiopathic hypoparathyroidism is less common and usually begins in childhood; its occurrence may be sporadic or familial. Current evidence suggests that, in many cases, the mechanism is autoimmune, and serum levels of parathyroid hormone (PTH) are low because the parathyroid glands have been destroyed by antibodies or are stimulated by antibodies that bind to the calcium-sensing receptor. Autoimmune hypoparathyroidism can occur as an isolated defect or as part of the type 1 polyendocrinopathy syndrome that affects endocrine glands as well as other tissues. In some patients with the type 1 polyendocrinopathy, a defect in cellular immunity leads to chronic mucocutaneous candidiasis (see Plate 3-6), with later development of hypoparathyroidism and Addison disease. Additional hormonal deficiencies may also arise due to destruction of other endocrine glands, including diabetes mellitus, primary hypothyroidism, and primary hypogonadism. In addition, many patients will also develop features of an ectodermal dystrophy with vitiligo and nail and dental defects. Most patients with the type 1 polyendocrinopathy syndrome have loss of function mutations in both copies of the *AIRE* gene, which encodes an autoimmune regulatory protein. Hypoparathyroidism can also be congenital and may occur as an isolated defect or as part of a complex syndrome, with the DiGeorge sequence representing the most common cause. DiGeorge sequence is a developmental field defect that affects the third and fourth branchial pouches and can arise from intrauterine exposure of the fetus to maternal alcoholism, retinoic acid, or poorly controlled diabetes mellitus. More commonly, the DiGeorge sequence is due to large deletions on chromosome 22q11 that result in the loss of multiple contiguous genes and that represent the most common chromosome deletion syndrome in humans. DiGeorge sequence is associated with facial, cardiac, thymic, and parathyroid defects that apparently occur due to the loss of a transcription factor *(TBX1)* that is required for normal development of these embryonic tissues.

Deletions within two nonoverlapping regions of 10p can lead to a phenotype similar to DiGeorge sequence, namely, the hypoparathyroidism, sensorineural deafness, and renal dysplasia (HDR) syndrome. Unlike patients with the DiGeorge sequence, individuals with HDR do not exhibit cardiac, palatal, or immunologic abnormalities. The HDR disorder is due to haploinsufficiency of the GATA binding protein-3 *(GATA3)* gene, which is located within a 200-kb critical HDR deletion

region on 10p14-10pter and encodes a C-terminal zinc-finger protein essential for DNA binding.

The hypoparathyroidism, retardation, dysmorphism (HRD) syndrome, also known as the Sanjad-Sakati (SS) syndrome, is a rare form of autosomal recessive hypoparathyroidism associated with other developmental anomalies. In addition to parathyroid dysgenesis, affected patients have severe growth and mental retardation, microcephaly, microphthalmia, small hands and feet, and abnormal teeth. This disorder is seen almost exclusively in individuals of Arab descent. The Kenny-Caffey syndrome is an allelic disorder that is characterized by hypoparathyroidism, dwarfism, medullary stenosis of the long bones, and eye abnormalities. Both disorders are due to mutations in the tubulin-specific chaperone E *(TBCE)* gene on chromosome 1q42-43.

Hypoparathyroidism may also occur as an isolated genetic condition. The leading cause of autosomal dominant hypoparathyroidism is an activating mutation of the *CASR* gene encoding the calcium-sensing receptor. Parathyroid glands are present but secrete little PTH because the activated calcium-sensing receptor behaves as if the extracellular calcium concentration is elevated. Activation of the same receptor in the distal renal tubule decreases calcium reabsorption, so urinary excretion of calcium is inappropriately high. By contrast, autosomal dominant and recessive mutations in the *GCM2* gene at 6p23-24 lead to parathyroid gland aplasia or dysplasia and cause severe isolated hypoparathyroidism in neonates.

Transient hypocalcemia and hypoparathyroidism are common in the neonatal period, presumably because of the underactivity and immaturity of the parathyroid glands and/or renal tubules. Despite hypocalcemia, serum PTH levels are low or inappropriately normal. Maternal hypercalcemia (as seen in hyperparathyroidism) may further suppress the fetal parathyroid gland and produce tetany in the neonate. In patients with alcoholism or malabsorption syndromes, hypomagnesemia leads to functional impairment of the parathyroid glands and hypocalcemia. In these patients, magnesium replacement increases serum levels of both parathyroid hormone (PTH) and calcium.

The biochemical hallmarks of hypoparathyroidism are a low serum calcium level and a high serum phosphate level, which result from a lack of PTH. Hypocalcemia occurs because less calcium is absorbed from the gut and resorbed from the skeleton and more calcium is cleared by the kidney. Absorption of calcium from the gut is reduced because synthesis of 1,25-dihydroxyvitamin D, or $1,25(OH)_2D$, which enhances absorption, is decreased in the absence of PTH. Because both PTH and $1,25(OH)_2D$ are critical activators of osteoclastic bone resorption, low levels of both hormones lead to decreased mobilization of calcium from skeletal stores. Because the renal tubular reabsorption of calcium is responsive to PTH, the threshold for calcium excretion

is reduced in subjects with hypoparathyroidism, and when the serum calcium level is therapeutically raised to normal, urinary excretion of calcium is inappropriately elevated. However, if the condition is not treated, the serum calcium concentration is usually below the renal threshold and urinary excretion of calcium is therefore low. Hyperphosphatemia in hypoparathyroidism occurs because phosphate reabsorption by the renal tubule increases when PTH levels are low.

Although acute reduction of PTH diminishes bone resorption, when PTH levels are chronically low, the rate of bone formation falls to match the rate of bone resorption. In chronic hypoparathyroidism, the net results are a reduced rate of bone turnover and a normal or slightly increased bone mass.

Most patients with idiopathic hypoparathyroidism exhibit severe hypocalcemia (serum calcium level < 7 mg/dL), but symptoms are mild when hypoparathyroidism has been chronic. On the other hand, patients with postsurgical hypoparathyroidism have variable hypocalcemia but typically have more severe clinical symptoms. Patients with the mildest form may have latent hypoparathyroidism; they can maintain normal serum calcium and phosphate levels, although physiologic or pathologic stresses, such as pregnancy or diarrhea, may cause the onset of hypocalcemia. Patients with postsurgical hypoparathyroidism often manifest moderate-to-severe hypocalcemia that is challenging to manage.

Hypoparathyroidism is treated by a combination of oral calcium supplements and vitamin D analogs; in mild cases, calcium supplementation alone is sufficient. Calcium supplements serve several important roles. First, they ensure a constant daily intake of calcium and thereby reduce day to day fluctuations in dietary calcium due to differences in food consumption. Second, they provide a ready source of gastrointestinal calcium and thereby reduce mobilization of skeletal calcium. And third, oral calcium supplements reduce absorption of dietary (and secreted) phosphorus from the intestine and thereby help maintain a normal serum phosphorus concentration. In most patients, calcium absorption from the intestine is too low, necessitating some form of supplemental vitamin D (in addition to calcium salts) to enhance absorption. Because the activation of vitamin D is impaired in these patients, large amounts of the parent compounds ergocalciferol (vitamin D_2) or cholecalciferol (vitamin D_3) are required (50,000 to 100,000 IU/day). In contrast, $1,25(OH)_2D$ (calcitriol) and dihydrotachysterol can be used at much lower doses because they do not require PTH-dependent activation by the 1α-hydroxylase enzyme in the kidney. Because the renal threshold for calcium is lower in patients with hypoparathyroidism, the total serum calcium concentration should be maintained in the low-to-normal range (8 to 9 mg/dL) to avoid hypercalciuria and nephrolithiasis.

Plate 3-6

Musculoskeletal System: PART III

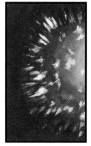

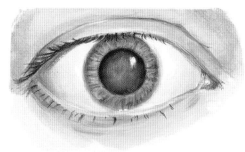

Spiculate opacities
of lens seen on
oblique slit-lamp
examination

Cataract (posterior subcapsular)

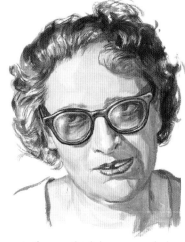

Lethargy; thick lenses needed
after cataract extraction

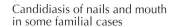

Candidiasis of nails and mouth
in some familial cases

CLINICAL MANIFESTATIONS OF CHRONIC HYPOPARATHYROIDISM

Although the manifestations of acute hypocalcemia as seen in hypoparathyroidism can be quite dramatic, the clinical signs and symptoms of chronic hypocalcemia are subtle and may be easily overlooked. For this reason, chronic hypocalcemia is often diagnosed incidentally during investigation of nonspecific symptoms, often neurocognitive, which include lassitude, irritability, depression, or even psychosis. These symptoms are due primarily to the hypocalcemia. There may also be evidence of increased neuromuscular excitability, with signs and symptoms ranging from paresthesias, described as "pins and needles" sensations around the mouth and in the hands and feet, to tetany with muscle cramps and spasms, laryngeal stridor, apnea in neonates, and seizures. The Chvostek or Trousseau sign may be elicited even in patients with asymptomatic hypocalcemia.

Despite the hypocalcemia, soft tissue calcifications may develop in patients with hypoparathyroidism when elevated serum phosphorus levels lead to an elevated (i.e., >70 mg²/dL²) calcium × phosphorus solubility product. A patient with poorly controlled, longstanding hypoparathyroidism may develop calcifications in the lens (cataracts) that opacify the lens and can impair vision. Calcifications may also develop in the basal ganglia and, if they are extensive, cause a movement disorder with features of Parkinson disease. These calcifications can be seen on standard radiographs of the skull or on computed tomography, which is a more sensitive technique.

The condition of the teeth provides a clue to the patient's age at onset of the disease. Dental hypoplasia with poor dental root formation indicates that the disease occurred before age 6. If onset was during childhood, there is crumbling of the teeth because of poor enamel structure. An increased density of the lamina dura can also be seen on dental radiographs.

In patients with hypoparathyroidism, the skeleton is usually not demineralized; in most cases, bone density is normal or slightly increased.

Hypoparathyroidism can occur as part of a familial tendency to the development of autoimmune destruction of multiple endocrine glands. The type 1 polyendocrinopathy syndrome that produces

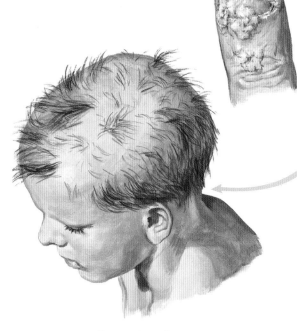

Spotty alopecia

Dental hypoplasia

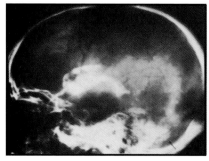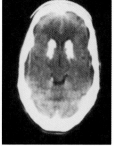

Lateral radiograph and CT scan of skull show calcification of basal ganglia.

hypoparathyroidism is due to mutations in the *AIRE* gene that encodes an immune regulatory protein (see earlier), and affected patients often manifest a defect in cell-mediated immunity and an absence of delayed cutaneous hypersensitivity reactions to *Candida*. Affected patients may have chronic *Candida* infections of the skin, especially the hands, toes, and nails, as well as infections of the oral mucosa and vagina, but systemic candidiasis is not a feature of this syndrome.

Occasionally, these lesions respond to long-term antifungal therapy. Affected patients present initially with chronic fungal infections with subsequent development of hypoparathyroidism and Addison disease. Individuals have an increased incidence of autoimmune primary hypothyroidism, diabetes mellitus, and primary hypogonadism. Alopecia, vitiligo, hepatitis, and pernicious anemia also occur with increased frequency.

Plate 3-7

Metabolic Diseases

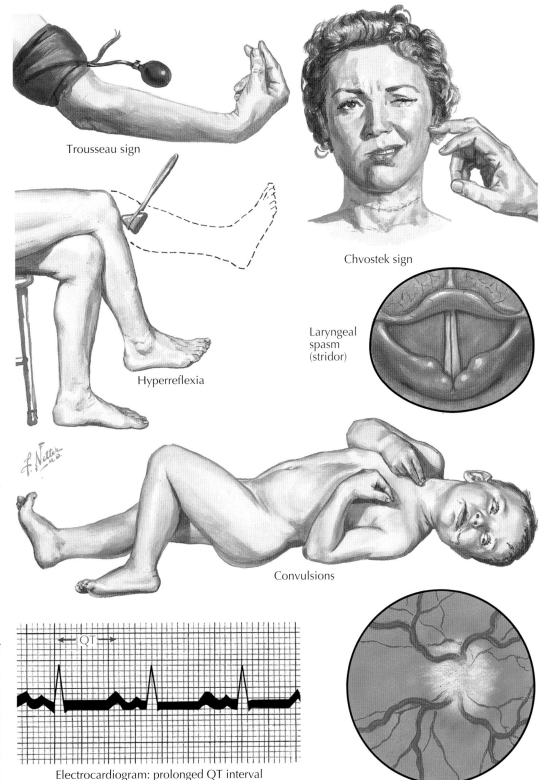

Trousseau sign

Chvostek sign

Hyperreflexia

Laryngeal spasm (stridor)

Convulsions

Electrocardiogram: prolonged QT interval

Choked disc

CLINICAL MANIFESTATIONS OF HYPOCALCEMIA

The symptoms of hypocalcemia emphasize the vital role of calcium in neuromuscular function. Hypocalcemia increases neuromuscular excitability, which can lead to tetany. The most severe form of tetany is characterized by tonic contractions of the muscles of the forearm and hand and, less commonly, by laryngospasm and seizures ranging from classic types (generalized and focal) to brief absence seizures. Often it is not clear if hypocalcemia is the direct cause of seizures or if it lowers the seizure threshold in a patient with a predisposition for epilepsy.

More typically, patients with hypocalcemia may be asymptomatic or experience milder symptoms such as muscle cramps and paresthesias. The paresthesias, described as "pins and needles" sensations in the hands, feet, and around the mouth, are episodic and often occur at times of stress, vomiting, or hyperventilation. This can be explained by the fact that metabolic or respiratory alkalosis increases the binding of serum calcium to albumin and decreases the concentration of free ionized calcium that interacts with cells.

Symptoms of hypocalcemia are also more likely to occur when the serum calcium level has fallen abruptly; chronic hypocalcemia, in contrast, can be asymptomatic with very low levels of serum calcium. Asymptomatic hypocalcemia must be differentiated from the low total serum calcium concentration (with a normal ionized calcium level) that occurs with hypoalbuminemia. The corrected total serum calcium concentration can be calculated by measuring the serum albumin level and adding 0.8 mg/dL to the total serum calcium level for each 1 g/dL reduction in the serum albumin level from 4 g/dL (corrected calcium = 0.8 × [4.0 − patient's albumin] + serum calcium).

Tetany can be elicited in patients with no overt signs of hypocalcemia by inducing the Chvostek and Trousseau signs. The Chvostek sign is produced by tapping the facial nerves at the angle of the jaw, which causes contracture of the ipsilateral facial muscles. The Trousseau sign is elicited by applying a blood pressure cuff to the upper arm and inflating it to just above the systolic blood pressure for 3 minutes. The resulting carpopedal spasm, with contractions of the fingers and inability to open the hand, is a result of increased neuromuscular irritability caused by hypocalcemia and aggravated by ischemia. This may be painful for the patient if sustained for too long but is believed to be a more specific marker of hypocalcemia than the Chvostek sign.

Other nonspecific signs and symptoms of hypocalcemia are lethargy, psychomotor depression, and impaired cognitive function with poor school performance in children. Hypocalcemia also decreases the contractility of the heart muscle, which can provoke or aggravate congestive heart failure in patients with heart disease. In these patients, heart failure can improve with administration of calcium. Hypocalcemia also leads to prolongation of the rate-corrected QT interval on an electrocardiogram. An unusual ocular manifestation of chronic hypocalcemia is papilledema, caused by increased pressure of the cerebrospinal fluid, which improves with reversal of hypocalcemia.

Plate 3-8   Musculoskeletal System: PART III

PSEUDOHYPOPARATHYROIDISM

In pseudohypoparathyroidism (PHP) type 1, tissues such as the kidney fail to respond to the action of parathyroid hormone (PTH) owing to an inability to generate the second messenger cyclic adenosine monophosphate (cyclic AMP). Signs, symptoms, and laboratory findings are those of hypoparathyroidism, with the exception of an elevated PTH level in response to hypocalcemia (see Plates 3-5 to 3-7). Both hypocalcemia and hyperphosphatemia are present, but the parathyroid glands are enlarged. PHP type 1 is divided into two major forms, type 1a and type 1b. Patients with PHP type 1a also have a characteristic physical appearance known as Albright hereditary osteodystrophy (AHO), which includes round face, subcutaneous ossifications, short stature, and brachydactyly, particularly shortening of the fourth and fifth metacarpals and metatarsals. Associated findings are mild primary hypothyroidism, growth hormone deficiency, and, occasionally, primary hypogonadism. Patients with PHP type 1b generally have only PTH resistance, although some patients have mild hypothyroidism and brachydactyly.

PTH activates its target cells by increasing the activity of adenylyl cyclase, thereby increasing cellular levels of cyclic AMP. Cyclic AMP activates a cascade of proteins that produces the physiologic effect. Patients with PHP type 1 have heterozygous mutations of the maternally derived allele that reduce expression or function of the α-subunit of the heterotrimeric G protein Gs, which couples receptors for hormones such as PTH, thyroid-stimulating hormone (TSH), and others to activation of adenylyl cyclase. Patients with PHP type 1a have mutations in the *GNAS* gene that directly affect production of Gα_s, whereas patients with PHP type 1b have mutations in or near *GNAS* that disrupt genomic imprinting and thereby reduce synthesis of Gα_s. Although PTH binds to the cell, it fails to elicit an effect because the lack of functional Gα_s "uncouples" the receptor from adenylyl cyclase. Hence, there is no production of its second messenger, cyclic AMP, and the biochemical abnormalities of hypoparathyroidism develop. Hypocalcemia occurs because of decreased calcium absorption from the intestine due to low PTH-mediated synthesis of $1,25(OH)_2D$. The serum phosphate level is high because the proximal renal tubule is resistant to PTH, and as a result the tubular reabsorption of phosphate is very high. In contrast to true hypoparathyroidism, the serum PTH level is elevated in response to hypocalcemia.

Because Gα_s couples receptors for many different hormones to adenylyl cyclase, patients with PHP type 1a have impaired responsiveness not only to PTH but also to other hormones such as TSH, growth hormone–releasing hormone (GHRH), and gonadotropins and develop obesity. By contrast, the defect in PHP type 1b tends to be less severe, and PTH resistance is the principal manifestation of the disorder. Bone is variably responsive to PTH; in most patients bone density is increased, although in some cases, osteitis fibrosa cystica occurs as a result of high PTH levels. As in hypoparathyroidism, the hypocalcemia ranges from latent to severe. Treatment of pseudohypoparathyroidism is the same as that for hypoparathyroidism, but patients rarely develop hypercalciuria because the distal renal tubule remains responsive to PTH.

Pathologic physiology and characteristic signs of pseudohypoparathyroidism

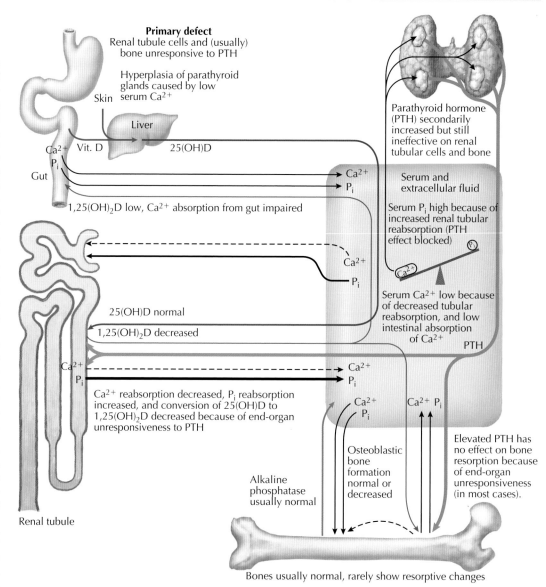

Primary defect
Renal tubule cells and (usually) bone unresponsive to PTH

Hyperplasia of parathyroid glands caused by low serum Ca^{2+}

Skin

Liver

Ca^{2+} P_i Vit. D $25(OH)D$

Gut

$1,25(OH)_2D$ low, Ca^{2+} absorption from gut impaired

Ca^{2+}
P_i

Parathyroid hormone (PTH) secondarily increased but still ineffective on renal tubular cells and bone

Serum and extracellular fluid

Serum P_i high because of increased renal tubular reabsorption (PTH effect blocked)

Ca^{2+}
P_i

Serum Ca^{2+} low because of decreased tubular reabsorption, and low intestinal absorption of Ca^{2+}

$25(OH)D$ normal

$1,25(OH)_2D$ decreased

Ca^{2+}
P_i

Ca^{2+}
P_i

Ca^{2+} reabsorption decreased, P_i reabsorption increased, and conversion of $25(OH)D$ to $1,25(OH)_2D$ decreased because of end-organ unresponsiveness to PTH

Renal tubule

Alkaline phosphatase usually normal

Osteoblastic bone formation normal or decreased

Ca^{2+}
P_i

Ca^{2+} P_i

PTH

Elevated PTH has no effect on bone resorption because of end-organ unresponsiveness (in most cases).

Bones usually normal, rarely show resorptive changes

Albright hereditary osteodystrophy

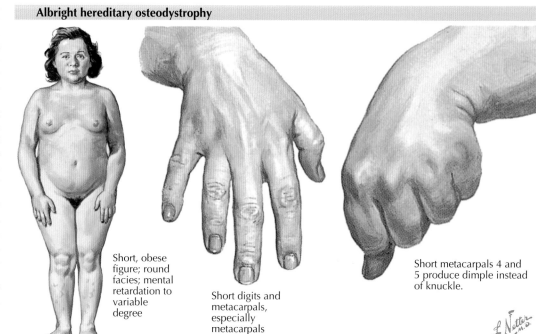

Short, obese figure; round facies; mental retardation to variable degree

Short digits and metacarpals, especially metacarpals 4 and 5

Short metacarpals 4 and 5 produce dimple instead of knuckle.

Plate 3-9

Metabolic Diseases

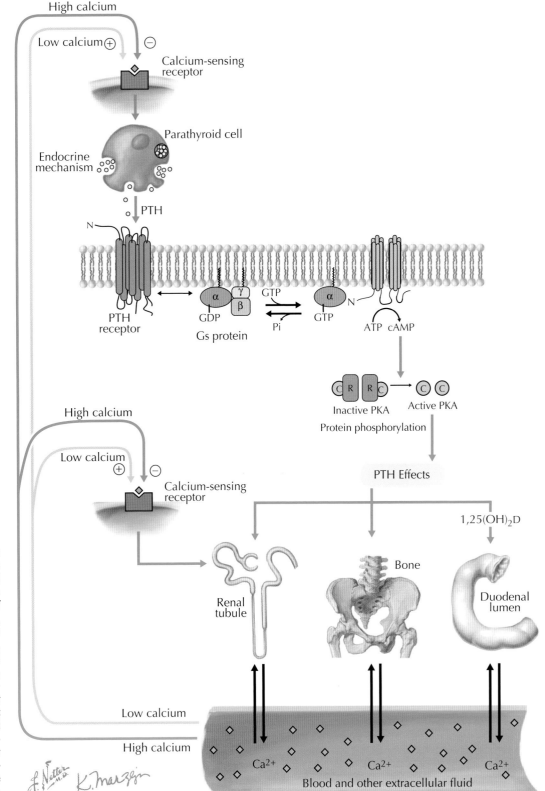

MECHANISM OF PARATHYROID HORMONE ACTIVITY ON END ORGAN

Parathyroid hormone (PTH) has two target organs: kidney and bone. In the kidney, PTH enhances the reabsorption of calcium in the distal tubule and decreases the reabsorption of phosphate in the proximal tubule. It also increases the synthesis of 1,25-dihydroxyvitamin D, or 1,25(OH)$_2$D (calcitriol), the active form of vitamin D, from its precursor 25-hydroxyvitamin D, or 25(OH)D (calcidiol). Increased secretion of 1,25(OH)$_2$D leads to increased intestinal calcium and phosphate absorption. In bone, PTH stimulates the release of minerals from hydroxyapatite. Initially, there is a rapid activation of existing osteoclasts, the large multinucleated bone cells that resorb bone. These cells resorb mineralized bone and release calcium, phosphate, and fragments of bone proteins into the circulation. After this initial phase, new osteoclasts are also recruited. There is also a compensatory increase in bone formation by osteoblasts (the process of bone remodeling is highly coordinated); however, the net effect is bone resorption.

PTH produces its effects on target cells by stimulating the synthesis of second messengers, most notably cyclic adenosine monophosphate (cyclic AMP) by the enzyme adenylate cyclase (see Plate 3-9). This intracellular second messenger activates protein kinase A, which catalyzes the phosphorylation of several cellular proteins and thereby modifies their activity.

Although all of the targets of phosphorylation have not been identified, they likely include proteins involved in the transport of calcium and phosphate, as well as proteins that regulate gene transcription. To activate

adenylyl cyclase, PTH binds to specific heptahelical receptor molecules on the surface of the cell. The first segment of PTH, containing 34 of the 84 amino acids in the hormone, is the only component required for binding and activating receptor molecules; the function, if any, of the remainder of the peptide is unknown (see Plate 3-1).

Adenylate cyclase is a separate molecule on the inner surface of the cell membrane (see Plate 3-9). However,

for adenylate cyclase to convert adenosine triphosphate (ATP) to cyclic AMP, it must interact with Gα_s, which is activated by the PTH-receptor complex. Gα_s is one component of the heterotrimeric G protein, Gs, and can bind and hydrolyze guanosine triphosphate (GTP). In the "off" state guanosine diphosphate (GDP) is bound to Gα_s, which enhances its affinity for the $\beta\gamma$ subunit. Ligand-bound receptors interact with the heterotrimeric Gs and promote release of GDP, thereby

Plate 3-10

Musculoskeletal System: PART III

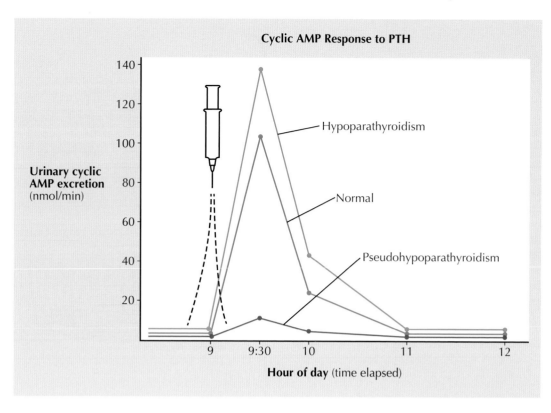

Cyclic AMP Response to PTH

Urinary cyclic AMP excretion (nmol/min)

Hypoparathyroidism

Normal

Pseudohypoparathyroidism

Hour of day (time elapsed)

MECHANISM OF PARATHYROID HORMONE ACTIVITY ON END ORGAN *(Continued)*

allowing GTP to bind to $G\alpha_s$. $G\alpha_s$-GTP dissociates from the $\beta\gamma$ subunit and in the "on" state is then able to stimulate adenylyl cyclase. After a very brief period of time the GTP is hydrolyzed to GDP, and the $G\alpha_s$-GDP molecule then reassociates with $\beta\gamma$ to end a cycle of hormone activation. As noted earlier, expression or function of $G\alpha_s$ is reduced in PHP type 1, which impairs receptor activation of adenylyl cyclase. Cyclic AMP is rapidly degraded by intracellular phosphodiesterase enzymes, although some of it also leaks out of the cell. In the kidney, cyclic AMP produced under the influence of PTH leaks out of proximal renal tubule cells and is excreted in the urine.

Normally, about half of the cyclic AMP in urine is derived from the renal action of PTH; the other half comes from circulating cyclic AMP, which is filtered through the glomerulus. Measurement of cyclic AMP excreted in the urine can be used as an index of the level of circulating PTH (see Plate 3-10); excretion of cyclic AMP is increased in hyperparathyroidism and decreased in hypoparathyroidism.

In PHP type 1, cyclic AMP is not synthesized in response to PTH, because of a deficiency of the coupling protein $G\alpha_s$. As a result, little cyclic AMP is produced in target tissues in response to PTH, and functional hypoparathyroidism develops (see Plate 3-5). This defect can be demonstrated in patients by measuring the level of cyclic AMP in urine after an injection of PTH. In normal persons and in patients with hypoparathyroidism, the rise in the excretion of cyclic AMP in urine is rapid and marked; in patients with PHP type 1, it is blunted or absent (see Plate 3-10).

The gene encoding $G\alpha_s$, *GNAS*, is a very complex transcriptional unit that derives considerable plasticity through use of alternative first exons, alternative splicing of downstream exons, antisense transcripts, and reciprocal imprinting. Four alternative exons, NESP55, XLαs, exon A/B, and exon 1, splice onto exons 2 to 13 of *GNAS*. Transcripts originating from alternative exons A/B and XLαs are expressed exclusively from the paternal allele. Exon A/B transcripts are probably nontranslated. By contrast, the XLαs protein shares C-terminal sequences with $G\alpha_s$ and functions in G-protein–coupled signal transduction. Transcripts starting with exon 1 encode $G\alpha_s$ and are expressed from both the maternal and paternal alleles in most tissues. Loss of one functional *GNAS* allele (i.e., haploinsufficiency) does not cause hormone resistance in these

tissues, because 50% of normal $G\alpha_s$ activity is sufficient to ensure normal transmembrane signal transduction. By contrast, suppression of the paternal allele occurs in cells such as renal proximal tubule cells, thyroid follicular cells, pituitary somatotrophs, and the paraventricular nucleus of the hypothalamus. Hence, mutations of the maternal *GNAS* allele results in expression of little if any $G\alpha_s$ protein in these imprinted tissues and is associated with hormone resistance. Thus, variable hormone resistance, from tissue to tissue between patients, reflects an unusual set of requirements that specifies that the tissue must exhibit imprinting of $G\alpha_s$ transcripts and the mutation must be on the maternal *GNAS* allele. By contrast, when the same *GNAS* mutation is carried on the paternal allele hormone, responsiveness is normal. Subjects with paternally inherited *GNAS* mutations have phenotypical features of AHO without hormonal resistance, a condition termed *pseudopseudohypoparathyroidism* (pseudoPHP). Subjects with pseudoPHP have a normal urinary cyclic AMP response to PTH, which distinguishes them from occasional patients with PHP type 1a who maintain normal serum calcium levels without treatment. It is not unusual to find extended families in which some members will have only AHO (pseudoPHP) whereas others will have hormone resistance as well (PHP type 1a), based on the parental origin of the identical *GNAS* mutation.

Plate 3-11

Metabolic Diseases

DIFFERENT FORMS OF PTH AND THEIR DETECTION BY WHOLE [BIOACTIVE] PTH AND I-PTH IMMUNOMETRIC ASSAYS

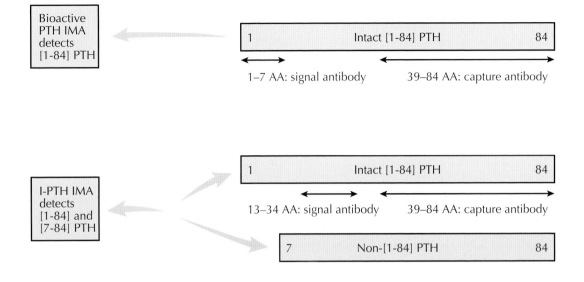

CLINICAL GUIDE TO PARATHYROID HORMONE ASSAY

The major circulating form of parathyroid hormone (PTH) in serum is an 84 amino acid [1-84] polypeptide. This form acts on type 1 PTH receptor via interaction with the first 34 amino acids. After secretion in the circulation, PTH is cleaved into C-terminal and amino (N)-terminal fragments. The N-terminal fragments contain the first 33/34 amino acids and are biologically active, just like the whole molecule, have a short half-life, and disappear rapidly from the circulation. The C-terminal fragments contain the remaining 34 to 84 amino acids (see Plate 3-11). In contrast, the half-life of the C-terminal is several times longer than that of either the N-terminal or the intact hormone; this fragment is therefore the most abundant form of PTH in serum. Because the C-terminal fragment is cleared by the kidney, renal insufficiency further causes this fragment to accumulate in the circulation.

Measurement of biologically active intact PTH is essential for accurate clinical assessment. Today most laboratories use commercially available U.S. Food and Drug Administration (FDA)–approved two sites or sandwich immunometric assays (IMAs) on different automated immunoassay platforms. These assays are designed to capture the intact molecule by using well-characterized N-terminal and C-terminal specific

monoclonal or polyclonal antibodies, one used as a capture antibody bound to solid support and the other tagged with nonisotopic ligand and used as a signal antibody. These assays improved detection of intact PTH by decreasing the detection of PTH fragments and are called intact PTH assays (I-PTH). Measurement of I-PTH provided better clinical correlation than older N-terminal or C-terminal radioimmunoassays. Most I-PTH IMAs have low detection limit and high reproducibility, facilitating the diagnosis of hypoparathyroidism and differentiating primary hyperparathyroidism from hypercalcemia of malignancy.

If primary hyperparathyroidism is the cause of hypercalcemia, the serum PTH level is usually increased; in general, the elevation is proportional to the degree of hypercalcemia. Primary hyperparathyroidism is unlikely to be the cause if the serum calcium level is substantially increased and the PTH level is in the low to normal range. The PTH assay can also determine whether hypocalcemia is due to hypoparathyroidism or due to a

nonparathyroid mechanism such as vitamin D deficiency. In patients with hypoparathyroidism, the serum PTH level is inappropriately low or even normal, despite the presence of hypocalcemia. In hypocalcemia due to nonparathyroid mechanisms, PTH secretion is stimulated (secondary hyperparathyroidism) and thus serum levels are high. In pseudohypoparathyroidism, PTH levels are high but hypocalcemia develops because of resistance to the effects of PTH (see Plate 3-12).

Although these I-PTH assays provide accurate measurement of PTH secretion and show excellent diagnostic sensitivity for primary hyperparathyroidism and of hypercalcemia of malignancy, their performance for management of secondary hyperparathyroidism in patients with renal insufficiency has been questioned owing to the presence of higher levels of a non-[1-84] PTH molecular form. This molecular form of PTH was later identified as an N-terminally truncated segment, the [7-84]PTH peptide. This molecular form accumulates in renal failure and is detected by I-PTH

Plate 3-12

Musculoskeletal System: PART III

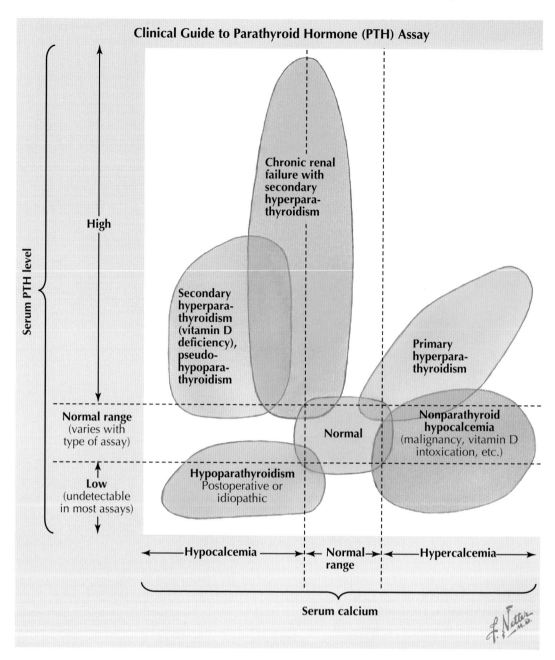

Clinical Guide to Parathyroid Hormone (PTH) Assay

CLINICAL GUIDE TO PARATHYROID HORMONE ASSAY
(Continued)

assays (see Plate 3-11). This accounts for the larger portion of I-PTH in patients with renal failure than in normal subjects and contributes to the major proportion of nonsuppressible fraction of I-PTH. This [7-84] PTH fragment is capable of binding to PTH receptor but has no biologic activity. Therefore it competes with I-PTH for receptor binding and serves as a PTH antagonist. In renal failure, a twofold increase in I-PTH is accompanied with about a sevenfold increase in [7-84]PTH fragment, leading to overestimation of I-PTH levels and of PTH-associated osseous abnormalities in uremia. After realizing this shortcoming of the I-PTH IMA assays, the efforts were made to develop the next generation of assays that employ the detection antibody that has specificity for the first four amino acids in the PTH molecule (see Plate 3-11). These assays are called "whole/total PTH assay" as well as "bioactive PTH assays." The specificity of these assays was confirmed by their inability to detect synthetic PTH fragments lacking one or more N-terminal amino acids. Although there is excellent correlation

between these two assays in normal individuals and in patients with primary hyperparathyroidism, PTH concentrations are 40% to 50% lower in patients with end-stage renal disease by "bioactive/whole PTH" assays than those obtained using the I-PTH IMA. In patients with end-stage renal disease, bioactive/whole-PTH may provide more accurate assessment of need for vitamin D and/or calcium treatment.

Primary hyperparathyroidism is often characterized as a multiglandular disease, requiring the surgical exploration and identification of all glands on both sides. One of the new applications of the I-PTH assay is the rapid measurement of intraoperative PTH. This has been suggested as a cost-effective way of predicting the necessity of other gland exploration and further neck dissection after the removal of an adenoma. PTH levels before and during surgery are measured in a timely manner by simply reducing the incubation time of I-PTH assays and hence called rapid PTH. PTH has a short half-life, and normal PTH secretion does not recover immediately after surgery. This provides a

window of time shortly after surgical removal of parathyroid adenoma (5 to 10 minutes) to monitor the decreasing levels of PTH in blood. Rapid PTH assays can accurately predict the postoperative outcome if a 50% or more drop in PTH is present and are useful in allowing selective unilateral exploration during parathyroid surgery. Therefore, the biochemical intraoperative monitoring with rapid PTH in a timely manner provides a valuable guidance to the endocrine surgeons when directing selective unilateral exploration or if there is a need to explore other parathyroid lobes during surgery.

In summary, the advent of totally automated immunometric I-PTH assays has led to improved accurate clinical discrimination of parathyroid disorders and has provided a tool to measure PTH levels in real time during surgical procedures. Also, development of bioactive I-PTH assay provides more accurate assessment of secondary hyperparathyroidism in patients with end-stage renal disease and their need for vitamin D and/or calcium treatment.

Plate 3-13

Metabolic Diseases

CHILDHOOD RICKETS

Impaired growth
Craniotabes
Frontal bossing
Dental defects
Chronic cough
Pigeon breast (tunnel chest)
Kyphosis
Rachitic rosary
Harrison groove
Flaring of ribs
Enlarged ends of long bones
Enlarged abdomen
Coxa vara
Bowleg (genu varum)

Clinical findings
(all or some present in variable degree)

Flaring of metaphyseal ends of tibia and femur. Growth plates thickened, irregular, cupped, and axially widened. Zones of provisional calcification fuzzy and indistinct. Bone cortices thinned and medullae rarefied.

Coxa vara and slipped capital femoral epiphysis. Mottled areas of lucency and density in pelvic bones.

Cartilage of epiphyseal plate in immature normal rat. Cells of middle (maturation) zone in orderly columns, with calcified cartilage between columns.

After 6 weeks of vitamin D– and phosphate-deficient diet. Large increase in axial height of maturation zone, with cells closely packed and irregularly arranged.

Radiograph of rachitic hand shows decreased bone density, irregular trabeculation, and thin cortices of metacarpals and proximal phalanges. Note increased axial width of epiphyseal line, especially in radius and ulna.

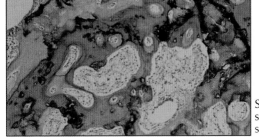

Section of rachitic bone shows sparse, thin trabeculae surrounded by much uncalcified osteoid (osteoid seams) and cavities caused by increased resorption.

RICKETS, OSTEOMALACIA, AND RENAL OSTEODYSTROPHY

Nutritional rickets, a metabolic bone disease characterized by impaired mineralization of osteoid (matrix), is reported infrequently because the basic pathophysiology is due to severe (<10 ng/mL) vitamin D deficiency, which is far less common now than in the past, since dairy products were fortified with vitamin D in the 1940s. Osteomalacia (adult rickets) has multiple causes in addition to severe vitamin D deficiency. Renal osteodystrophy compromises a group of metabolic bone diseases accompanying chronic kidney disease (CKD) and are defined by quantitative bone histomorphometry and may be associated with increase in fracture risk. Although a large number of etiologic factors may contribute to these disorders, the basic defect is a deficiency at the tissue level of calcium or phosphate, or both, which impairs the normal mineralization and growth of the skeleton in the child (rickets) or leads to impaired mineralization of osteoid in the adult (osteomalacia).

The causes of rachitic and osteomalacic syndromes are numerous and include a variety of genetic errors, nutritional abnormalities, metabolic disorders, and chronic renal diseases. Quite independent of cause, the clinical manifestations of the disorders may be remarkably similar, making it difficult for the physician to solve the often tangled puzzle of causation and introduce the appropriate treatment. However, recent discoveries relating to the disease mechanisms and the introduction of newer hormonal and drug treatments are contributing to better management and may lead to a cure.

Besides being interesting, the history of rickets and osteomalacia is important for the classification of the disorders. Both diseases were known in antiquity, but one of the clearest descriptions appeared in a 17th-century Latin text by Glisson. Investigations by Schmorl in the late 19th century established the role of sunlight in the prevention of the disease, and dietary factors were identified in the first part of the 20th century. Despite this knowledge, nutritional rickets remained a common occurrence and many children in working-class families in the temperate zones exhibited

Plate 3-14

Musculoskeletal System: PART III

RICKETS, OSTEOMALACIA, AND RENAL OSTEODYSTROPHY
(Continued)

the characteristic symptoms of short stature, rib cage deformities, and bowed extremities.

Vitamin D was discovered in the 1920s, and the use of the sterol as a food supplement made nutritional rickets rare in all but the most economically disadvantaged communities. However, within a short time, additional cases were reported, which appeared to be resistant to even massive doses of vitamin D. Scientists such as Albright, Butler, Fanconi, and others, studying the defects that led to this metabolic disorder, identified the mechanisms of calcium transport in the gut, kidneys, and bone cells, as well as the roles played by exogenous factors (the polar metabolites of vitamin D) and endogenous factors (parathyroid hormone [PTH] and phosphate). The identification and synthesis of 1,25-dihydroxyvitamin D, or $1,25(OH)_2D$, a better understanding of the handling of calcium and phosphate by the kidneys, and the discovery of the osteocyte-derived phosphaturic peptide FGF-23 (fibroblast growth factor 23) have defined mechanisms behind various forms of osteomalacia and renal bone disease.

CHILDHOOD RICKETS

Clinical Manifestations. In severe childhood rickets (see Plate 3-13), growth is impaired and height is generally below the third quartile. However, unless there is concurrent severe nutritional disturbance, weight is usually normal. Affected children are apathetic and irritable and frequently remain immobile, sitting in a Buddha-like position. The head displays a number of abnormalities, including softening and deformity of the skull (craniotabes), prominence of the frontal bones (frontal bossing), and caries and enamel defects. Examination of the thorax may reveal flaring and deformity of the ribs, funnel chest (pectus excavatum) or pigeon breast, an indentation at the insertion of the diaphragm into the lower ribs (Harrison's groove), and nodules at the costochondral junctions (rachitic rosary). Frequent manifestations are respiratory infections and a chronic cough.

Children with rickets may also have a gentle thoracic kyphosis (rachitic cat back) and a rachitic potbelly, which, together with the bowed extremities and apathetic facies, emphasize their Buddha-like appearance. Examination of the extremities also uncovers abnormalities such as symmetric enlargement of the ends of the long bones (most prominent at the elbows and wrists), bowleg (genu varum), and, less frequently, knock-knee (genu valgum). Fractures occur frequently.

Histologic Features. In patients with rickets, the histologic appearance of the epiphyseal plate is pathognomonic. Comparison of normal and rachitic epiphyseal plates in rats shows a greatly increased axial height of the epiphyseal plate (sometimes as much as 20 times), principally because of the increased number of cells in the maturation zone; the cells have lost their columnar organization and occur in profligate profusion. Both the zone of provisional calcification of the cartilage and the primary spongiosa of the metaphysis have irregular contours and lack calcific mineral deposition.

Although changes in bone structure are no less pronounced in osteomalacia, they are not specific to that

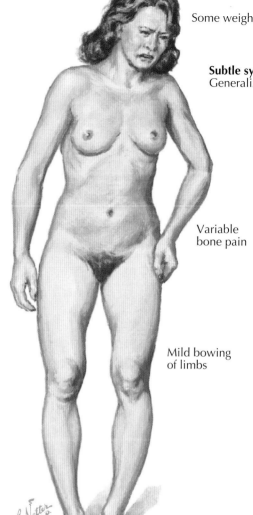

ADULT OSTEOMALACIA

Some weight loss

Subtle symptomatology (all or some present)
Generalized muscle weakness and hypotonia

Variable bone pain

Mild bowing of limbs

Osteomalacia

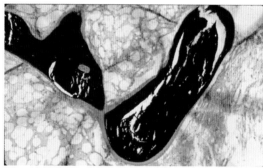

Differential diagnosis of osteomalacia
1. Nutritional vitamin D deficiency
2. Persistent hypophosphatemia (renal or GI sources)
a. Hypophosphatemic vitamin D–resistant rickets syndromes
b. Chronic malabsorption
3. Chronic metabolic acidosis
4. Oncogenic osteomalacia
5. Renal osteomalacia

Differential diagnosis of elevated bone-specific alkaline phosphatase (BSAP)
1. Paget disease
2. Metastatic cancer to bone
3. Osteomalacia
4. Hyperthyroidism
5. Hyperparathyroidism
6. Recent bone fracture
7. Chronic antiseizure medication
8. Immobilization
9. Calcineurin anti–organ rejection therapy
10. Severe (<6-7 ng/mL) 25 (OH) D deficiency
11. Treatment with PTH
12. Treatment with strontium ranelate

Radiographic findings
Radiograph shows variegated rarefaction of pelvic bones, coxa vara, deepened acetabula, and subtrochanteric pseudofracture of right femur.

disorder because similar changes may occur in several other metabolic bone disorders (most notably hyperparathyroidism and fibrous dysplasia). The cortices are thin, and the trabeculae are small and irregularly shaped, with evidence of osteoclastic resorption of bone (a mild-to-moderate secondary hyperparathyroidism is characteristic of most rachitic syndromes). The most characteristic histologic feature, however, is the presence of a wide zone of unmineralized bone, or osteoid seam, which surrounds the mineralized trabeculae. In

the section shown in Plate 3-13, the mineralized bone appears dark and the osteoid seams are pink.

Radiographic Findings. Radiographic findings reflect the histologic changes: thinned cortices and rarefied medullary bone, with indistinct and fuzzy trabecular markings. However, the radiographic hallmarks are the enormously increased axial height of the epiphyseal plate and the poor definition or absence of the zone of provisional calcification, which is normally seen as a dense, white line separating the growth plate, or physis,

Plate 3-15

Metabolic Diseases

RICKETS, OSTEOMALACIA, AND RENAL OSTEODYSTROPHY

(Continued)

from the metaphysis. Often noted are cupping and flaring of the ends of the long bones, usually because of a softening of the epiphyseal-metaphyseal region. Slipped capital femoral epiphysis at the widened and severely weakened plate is an occasional finding, particularly in patients with renal osteodystrophy (see Plate 3-22).

Unlike osteomalacia, rickets is a disease of growth. If growth slows, either for natural reasons or because the patient becomes ill with other manifestations of the disease, a phenomenon known as the paradox of rickets may occur; that is, the characteristic epiphyseal changes seen on radiography appear to improve. The radiograph of the hand in Plate 3-13 illustrates this paradox. The hand shows evidence of advanced rachitic changes in the rapidly growing distal radius and ulna, less severe manifestations in the metacarpals, even milder signs in the slowly growing proximal phalanges, and virtually no signs at all in the least active physeal regions of the middle phalanges.

ADULT OSTEOMALACIA

Clinical Manifestations. The diagnosis of adult osteomalacia (see Plate 3-14) may be difficult to establish because the changes may be considerably more subtle than those seen in childhood rickets. In early stages, the patients may be asymptomatic and the changes are biochemical—the most sensitive being an elevated serum total alkaline phosphatase. If the total alkaline phosphatase is elevated, then a bone-specific alkaline phosphatase (BSAP) should be obtained. If the BSAP is elevated, then there is a differential diagnosis of elevated BSAP (see Plate 3-14). By exclusion, osteomalacia can be strongly suspected but the gold standard is quantitative bone histomorphometry. A bone biopsy is diagnostic, and there are very specific histomorphometric criteria for the diagnosis of osteomalacia (see Plate 3-14). Once a specific diagnosis is established, then adult osteomalacia has a very narrow group of causes (see Plate 3-14). By biochemical testing, the etiology can be determined; and, by correcting the biochemical abnormalities and keeping them corrected, the symptoms of osteomalacia can be eliminated and the histomorphometry normalized.

Patients with adult and advanced osteomalacia may complain of generalized weakness, especially proximal muscle weakness, bone pain, easy fatigability, and malaise. The physical findings are minimal: tenderness of bony prominences or, in more serious cases, muscle weakness that is severe enough to cause an abductor-lurch type of gait (the gluteal, or Trendelenburg, gait). In long-standing cases, a bone deformity such as bowleg, coxa vara, or kyphosis may be common.

Radiographic signs are equally subtle, showing for the most part only a diffuse osteopenia, similar to that seen in other metabolic bone diseases such as postmenopausal or senile osteoporosis, hyperparathyroidism, hyperthyroidism, and diffuse skeletal metastatic tumors such as those seen in multiple myeloma. One distinctive feature seen in more advanced osteomalacia, present in about 25% of cases, is virtually pathognomonic of osteomalacia. Focal collections of osteoid produce localized, narrow, ribbon-like zones of

decreased density in the cortices. These zones are almost always symmetric and are located at right angles to the long axes of the bones. On radiography, they resemble partial fractures. These usually painless pseudofractures—called Looser's zones, *Umbauzonen*, or milkman syndrome—are usually seen on the concave sides of a long bone, the medial side of the femoral neck, the ischial and pubic rami, the clavicle, the ribs, and the axillary border of the scapula. They may serve as stress risers, thus leading to a true fracture (particularly in the femoral neck or in the pubis).

Primary causes

Lack of sunlight impairs endogenous vitamin D synthesis.

Sun · Ultraviolet light · Skin

Parathyroid gland hyperplasia due to low serum Ca^{2+}

Parathyroid hormone (PTH) elevated

Dietary lack of vitamin D

Marked prematurity (liver inefficient in converting vitamin D to 25[OH]D)

Anticonvulsants promote breakdown of vitamin D and 25(OH)D in liver.

Lack of bile or alimentary secretions may impair absorption of vitamin D and calcium.

High dietary intake of phosphate, phytate, oxalate, or fatty acids may impair absorption of calcium.

Gastrectomy or GI shunts may decrease absorption of calcium and vitamin D.

Antacids (aluminum salts) impair phosphate absorption.

Pregnancy

Lactation

Malabsorption, sprue (excessive loss of calcium and phosphate in stool)

Vit. D · Deficient vit. D · Vit. D

Ca^{2+} · Ca^{2+} · P_i · Al · P_i · Ca^{2+} · P_i

Ca^{2+} and P_i absorption impaired

Deposition of Ca^{2+} and P_i decreased because of low serum levels

Loss of Ca^{2+} and P_i to fetus or in milk

Serum and extracellular fluid

Ca^{2+}

Ca^{2+} low to low normal

Lack of vitamin D for activation to $1,25(OH)_2D$ by liver and kidney impairs Ca^{2+} and P_i absorption.

P_i · P_i very low

Alkaline phosphatase greatly elevated

P_i Ca^{2+} · Ca^{2+} P_i

Glomerular filtration of Ca^{2+} and P_i low because of low serum levels

Ca^{2+} · P_i · P_i

PTH inhibits P_i reabsorption, further reducing serum P_i.

Urine Ca^{2+} very low; P_i low (may be elevated initially)

Increased osteoblastic activity in response to osteoclastic destruction of bone

Elevated PTH promotes osteoclastic resorption of bone (Ca^{2+}, P_i, and matrix).

Osteoblasts · Osteoclasts

Flaring · Widened and irregular epiphyseal plate · Pseudofractures · Bowing, soft bones · Uncalcified osteoid seams · Subperiosteal resorption · Cysts and brown tumors

Rickets or osteomalacia

NUTRITIONAL-DEFICIENCY RICKETS AND OSTEOMALACIA

The classic and most clearly understood cause of nutritional-deficiency rickets and osteomalacia (see Plate 3-15) is a severe chronic deficiency of vitamin D. Deficiency of this fat-soluble sterol vitamin can be dietary, inadequate exposure to sunlight, or malabsorption. Malabsorption can be due to a variety of gastrointestinal conditions, including asymptomatic celiac disease. Because fat-soluble vitamins need to be bound to bile salts to be absorbed in the terminal ileum,

Plate 3-16

Musculoskeletal System: PART III

RICKETS, OSTEOMALACIA, AND RENAL OSTEODYSTROPHY
(Continued)

deficiency of bile salts may also lead to low vitamin D levels. Although histomorphometric changes of defective mineralization can be seen with 25(OH)D levels less than 10 ng/mL, clinical osteomalacia is usually not seen unless the serum vitamin D levels are even lower and consistently low for months before recognizable fractures or muscle weakness is seen.

Although the Institute of Medicine (IOM) nutritional dietary recommendation for the U.S. population is 800 IU/day of vitamin D, serum levels are often lower than adequate for many clinical outcomes at this intake. The widespread availability of reliable measurements of serum 25(OH)D levels has made the management of adequate vitamin D replacement a standard of care. Many professional societies recommend that the serum 25(OH)D level be kept between 30 and 50 ng/mL.

Vitamin D has receptors throughout many tissues and acts as both an endocrine as well as an autocrine/paracrine hormone. The endocrine properties have direct effects on bone and muscle tissue whereas the autocrine/paracrine pathways are involved in the immunologic system. 25(OH)D is converted into additional active metabolite 1,25(OH)$_2$D in renal tubules and monocyte cell lines. The synthesis of 1,25(OH)$_2$D is tightly regulated by serum PTH, calcium, and phosphorus such that it requires very high or very low 25(OH)D to change to serum 1,25(OH)$_2$D. This regulation is important because either high or low 1,25(OH)$_2$D can lead to either hypercalcemia or hypocalcemia. In syndromes of reduced 1,25(OH)$_2$D production, such as hypophosphatemic vitamin D–resistant rickets, oncogenic osteomalacia, or severe CKD, a secondary hyperparathyroidism develops, in part owing to hypocalcemia and in part owing to the direct effect(s) of 1,25(OH)$_2$D to regulate PTH synthesis. The biochemical abnormalities shown in Plate 3-15 lead to a syndrome that manifests all the histologic and radiographic findings of rickets and/or osteomalacia, as well as those of secondary hyperparathyroidism. In addition, the discovery of FGF-23 has led to a greater understanding of the interactions between the parathyroid gland, kidney, and bone. FGF-23, synthesized by the osteocyte, is a major regulator of renal phosphate reabsorption as well as PTH synthesis. Preliminary data suggest that FGF-23 also has effects on osteoid mineralization. FGF-23 increases early in CKD, much earlier than PTH, and is the peptide responsible for the phosphaturia and inhibition of 1,25(OH)$_2$D levels in the syndrome of oncogenic osteomalacia. The information presented in Plates 3-5 and 3-12 puts into perspective the links between bone/kidney/parathyroid glands that share common pathways in the pathophysiology of many, if not most, of the clinical conditions associated with osteomalacia.

As shown in the left half of Plate 3-15, other defects or conditions may result in a rachitic or an osteomalacic syndrome. For example, in a premature infant, the immature liver cannot adequately convert vitamin D to 25(OH)D. Chronic use of anticonvulsant medications may lead to a deficiency of 25(OH)D by interfering with the microsomal enzyme systems in the liver. Some nutritional disorders interfering with calcium absorption that may also lead to a similar syndrome are

excessive dietary ingestion of phytate (in certain coarse cereals), oxalate (in spinach), citrate or phosphate, and an increased intake of aluminum salts (usually in the form of antacids) that can cause a phosphate deficiency. Any condition in which the gut wall is damaged (e.g., tuberculosis, celiac syndromes, sarcoidosis, presence of surgical shunts) or in which rapid transit of gastrointestinal contents occurs (e.g., biliary disease, postgastrectomy syndromes) may also cause a rachitic or an

osteomalacic syndrome due to a deficiency of either calcium or vitamin D, or both.

VITAMIN D–RESISTANT RICKETS AND OSTEOMALACIA DUE TO PROXIMAL TUBULAR DEFECTS

In countries with vitamin D supplementation, genetic or acquired rachitic and osteomalacic syndromes (see

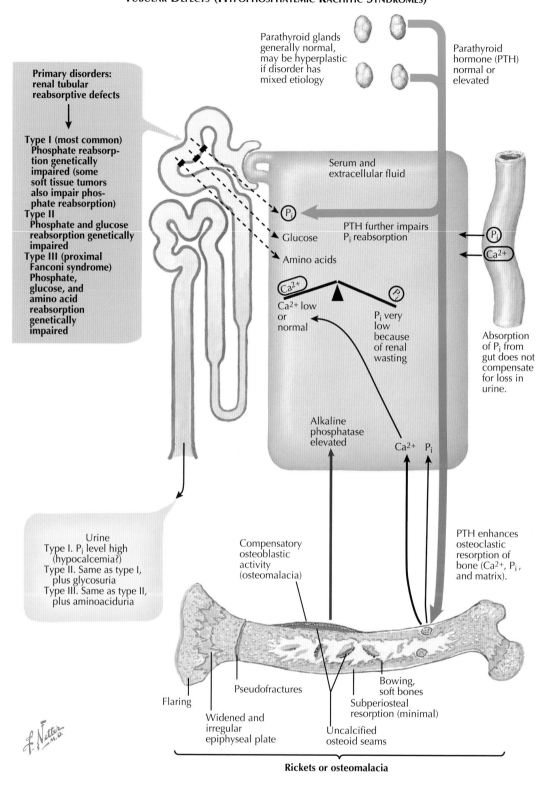

VITAMIN D–RESISTANT RICKETS AND OSTEOMALACIA DUE TO PROXIMAL RENAL TUBULAR DEFECTS (HYPOPHOSPHATEMIC RACHITIC SYNDROMES)

Parathyroid glands generally normal, may be hyperplastic if disorder has mixed etiology

Parathyroid hormone (PTH) normal or elevated

Primary disorders: renal tubular reabsorptive defects

Type I (most common) Phosphate reabsorption genetically impaired (some soft tissue tumors also impair phosphate reabsorption)
Type II Phosphate and glucose reabsorption genetically impaired
Type III (proximal Fanconi syndrome) Phosphate, glucose, and amino acid reabsorption genetically impaired

Serum and extracellular fluid

Glucose

PTH further impairs P$_i$ reabsorption

Amino acids

Ca^{2+}

Ca^{2+} low or normal

P$_i$ very low because of renal wasting

Alkaline phosphatase elevated

Ca^{2+} P$_i$

Absorption of P$_i$ from gut does not compensate for loss in urine.

Urine
Type I. P$_i$ level high (hypocalcemia?)
Type II. Same as type I, plus glycosuria
Type III. Same as type II, plus aminoaciduria

Compensatory osteoblastic activity (osteomalacia)

PTH enhances osteoclastic resorption of bone (Ca^{2+}, P$_i$, and matrix).

Flaring

Widened and irregular epiphyseal plate

Pseudofractures

Uncalcified osteoid seams

Bowing, soft bones

Subperiosteal resorption (minimal)

Rickets or osteomalacia

Plate 3-17

Metabolic Diseases

RICKETS, OSTEOMALACIA, AND RENAL OSTEODYSTROPHY
(Continued)

Plate 3-16) that are resistant to high therapeutic doses of vitamin D are now more common than those associated with vitamin D deficiencies. Almost all of these syndromes are renal in origin and are associated with a narrow or broad reabsorptive defect in the renal tubule that leads to hypophosphatemia (thus, they are also known as hypophosphatemic vitamin D–resistant rickets, or phosphate diabetes).

The most common of these disorders is type I, a sex-linked dominant genetic disorder in which the renal tubule does not reabsorb phosphate; as a result, the disease produces all the features of rickets or osteomalacia, as seen on histologic and radiographic examinations. In the purest form of the disorder there is no abnormality of calcium or vitamin D metabolism and results of serum analysis and urinalysis demonstrate profound hypophosphatemia, marked lowering of the percent tubular reabsorption of phosphate (%TRP), and an increased serum alkaline phosphatase level. Many of the syndromes are impure, however, and either show evidence of a defect in vitamin D metabolism (see Plate 3-18) or some degree of loss of calcium as fixed base (see Plates 3-17 and 3-19). Under these circumstances, the serum calcium concentration may be low or low to normal and the PTH level may be increased, which aggravates the already severely phosphate-depleted state.

Three phosphate-wasting lesions in the proximal tubule have been identified. *Type I*, first described by Albright, is seen most frequently. It is transmitted as a sex-linked dominant trait and the reabsorptive defect is confined to phosphate only. In *type II*, the defect is broader and involves both phosphate and glucose. In *type III*, the proximal Fanconi syndrome, the reabsorptive defect is for phosphate, glucose, and various amino acids.

VITAMIN D–RESISTANT RICKETS AND OSTEOMALACIA DUE TO PROXIMAL AND DISTAL RENAL TUBULAR DEFECTS

In another group of vitamin D–resistant rachitic and osteomalacic syndromes, the range of renal tubular defects is considerably broader and may interfere more severely with normal metabolism (see Plate 3-17). Reabsorption of phosphate, glucose, and amino acids in the proximal tubule is impaired, and, in addition, the functions of the distal tubule are significantly altered. Consequently, in patients with type I syndrome, known as the proximal and distal Fanconi syndrome, or the Debré-de Toni-Fanconi syndrome, the kidney's ability to reabsorb water, bicarbonate, proteins, and fixed base is to some degree impaired. This represents a severe challenge to the patient, particularly the newborn, and requires major replacement therapy.

Typically, the patient is a very ill child, often dehydrated and hypoproteinemic, with rachitic changes in the bones. The rachitic and osteomalacic patterns in these patients result from the failure of tubular reabsorption of phosphate coupled with the loss of fixed base, including calcium. This unfortunate combination results in both rachitic changes and a mild-to-moderate secondary hyperparathyroidism (which worsens the bone lesions and intensifies the hypophosphatemia).

VITAMIN D–RESISTANT RICKETS AND OSTEOMALACIA DUE TO PROXIMAL AND DISTAL RENAL TUBULAR DEFECTS

Type I. Proximal and distal Fanconi syndrome

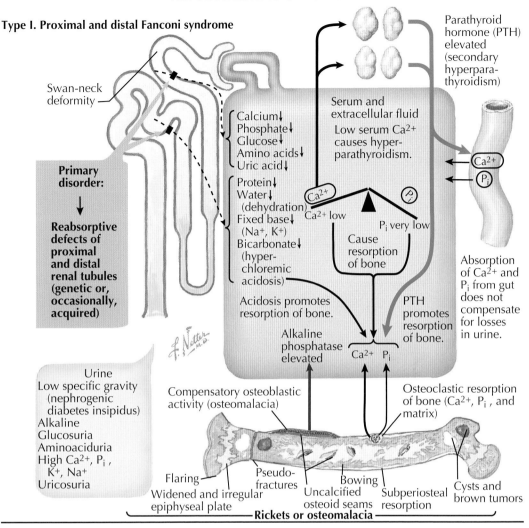

Parathyroid hormone (PTH) elevated (secondary hyperparathyroidism)

Swan-neck deformity

Serum and extracellular fluid

Low serum Ca^{2+} causes hyperparathyroidism.

Calcium↓
Phosphate↓
Glucose↓
Amino acids↓
Uric acid↓

Protein↓
Water↓ (dehydration)
Fixed base↓ (Na$^+$, K$^+$)
Bicarbonate↓ (hyperchloremic acidosis)

Ca^{2+} low   P$_i$ very low

Cause resorption of bone

Absorption of Ca^{2+} and P$_i$ from gut does not compensate for losses in urine.

Primary disorder:
↓
Reabsorptive defects of proximal and distal renal tubules (genetic or, occasionally, acquired)

Acidosis promotes resorption of bone.

PTH promotes resorption of bone.

Alkaline phosphatase elevated

Ca^{2+} P$_i$

Urine
Low specific gravity (nephrogenic diabetes insipidus)
Alkaline
Glucosuria
Aminoaciduria
High Ca^{2+}, P$_i$, K$^+$, Na$^+$
Uricosuria

Compensatory osteoblastic activity (osteomalacia)

Osteoclastic resorption of bone (Ca^{2+}, P$_i$, and matrix)

Flaring
Widened and irregular epiphyseal plate
Pseudofractures
Uncalcified osteoid seams
Bowing
Subperiosteal resorption
Cysts and brown tumors

— Rickets or osteomalacia —

Type II. Lignac-Fanconi syndrome (cystinosis)

All manifestations of type I, plus generalized disorder of cystine metabolism: deposition of cystine crystals in tissues (cornea, conjunctiva, spleen, bone marrow, liver, lymph nodes)

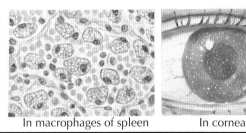

In macrophages of spleen   In cornea

Type III. Oculocerebrorenal syndrome (Lowe syndrome), rare
Most manifestations of type I, plus congenital glaucoma, cataracts, nystagmus, mental retardation, hyperexcitability, inattentiveness, muscular hypotonia, diminished or absent tendon reflexes, decreased motor power

Type IV. Superglycine syndrome, very rare
Teenage onset; many manifestations of type I, plus severe muscle weakness or atrophy, very high urinary glycine and glycylproline levels

These conditions have little relationship to vitamin D; in fact, treatment with even high doses of the sterol vitamin has little effect.

Biochemical changes in type I disease include hypocalcemia, hypophosphatemia, increased serum alkaline phosphatase level, and normal serum levels of 25(OH)D and 1,25(OH)$_2$D. The patient is likely to have signs of renal tubular acidosis (hyperchloremia, hyponatremia, and hypokalemia in association with an alkaline urine). Urinalysis reveals a low fixed specific gravity and the presence of excessive concentrations of metabolites, including calcium, sodium, and potassium ions; phosphate (as a result of a greatly lowered %TRP); uric acid; amino acids; and proteins.

Three other less common types of the severe form of vitamin D–resistant rickets and osteomalacia are often included under the proximal and distal Fanconi syndrome. (1) *Type II*, Lignac-Fanconi syndrome, is almost

Plate 3-18

Musculoskeletal System: PART III

RICKETS, OSTEOMALACIA, AND RENAL OSTEODYSTROPHY
(Continued)

identical to type I but has an additional defect in the metabolism of cystine. This defect leads to the deposition of crystals of the amino acid in the viscera, bone marrow, and eyes (the diagnosis may be made by slit-lamp examination). As a result of the deposits, cirrhosis of the liver and renal failure frequently supervene by puberty. (2) *Type III* disease is known as oculocerebrorenal, or Lowe, syndrome. Patients with this condition have many of the manifestations of type I disease but may also have a broad range of ocular and neurologic abnormalities, which include congenital glaucoma, nystagmus, mental retardation, muscular hypotonia, and weakness. (3) *Type IV*, the superglycine syndrome, is rare. It is less severe than the other types and usually has a later onset. Presenting symptoms are profound motor weakness and very high urinary concentrations of glycine and glycylproline.

VITAMIN D–DEPENDENT (PSEUDODEFICIENCY) RICKETS AND OSTEOMALACIA

This major category of vitamin D–dependent rickets is characterized by abnormalities of vitamin D metabolism (see Plate 3-18). In this group of syndromes, the error is also almost always inherited but involves either a failure of conversion of 25(OH)D to the potent 1,25(OH)$_2$D or a relative end-organ insensitivity of the gut (and, presumably under certain circumstances, the renal cell as well) to the patient's autogenous 1,25(OH)$_2$D. In both of these circumstances, orally administered vitamin D in standard or therapeutic doses does not help to increase reabsorption of calcium by the renal tubule, and hypocalcemia and rachitic manifestations develop. In response to the lowered serum calcium level, the parathyroid glands elaborate PTH, which further depletes the skeleton's calcium reserves and produces hyperphosphaturia and hypophosphatemia.

All of the findings and chemical abnormalities are similar to those seen in the classic nutritional deficiency syndrome, with the exception of the concentrations of the polar metabolites of vitamin D. In the first form of the disorder—failure of conversion of 25(OH)D to 1,25(OH)$_2$D in the kidney—serum levels of 25(OH)D may be very high (hence, the term *pseudo*) while levels of 1,25(OH)$_2$D may be low. In the latter form of the disorder—end-organ insensitivity to the action of 1,25(OH)$_2$D—the serum levels of both 25(OH)D and 1,25(OH)$_2$D are usually normal or high. Both forms are often successfully treated with administration of 1,25(OH)$_2$D.

A specific disorder that fits into the so-called pseudodeficiency is oncogenic osteomalacia. This syndrome is due to mesenchymal tumors that develop in adults for unknown cause. These tumors are often very small, subcutaneous, and, more often than not, benign. However, these tumors secrete FGF-23 and induce renal phosphate wasting and hypophosphatemia and inhibit renal production of 1,25(OH)$_2$D. Hence, the classical biochemical triad is hypophosphatemia, normal 25(OH)D, and low 1,25(OH)$_2$D. Serum levels of FGF-23 are available clinically and can help confirm the diagnosis. Although patients with oncogenic

osteomalacia can have symptomatic improvement with oral phosphorus and 1,25(OH)$_2$D replacement, the cure is finding the mesenchymal tumor responsible for producing FGF-23 and having it removed. The latter is often a diagnostic challenge because these tumors are small and may be located anywhere in the human body. The radioisotope, octreotide, is taken up by these tumors such that periodic scans, often with positron emission tomographic accentuation, are necessary to find these tumors. Removal of the tumor is a cure. Total

tumor removal will be accompanied by normalization of the BSAP, serum phosphorus, 1,25(OH)$_2$D, and FGF-23 levels and the patient will never again need oral phosphorus or 1,25(OH)$_2$D replacement.

VITAMIN D-RESISTANT RICKETS DUE TO RENAL TUBULAR ACIDOSIS

The group of diseases classified under renal tubular acidosis includes metabolic disorders of diverse and

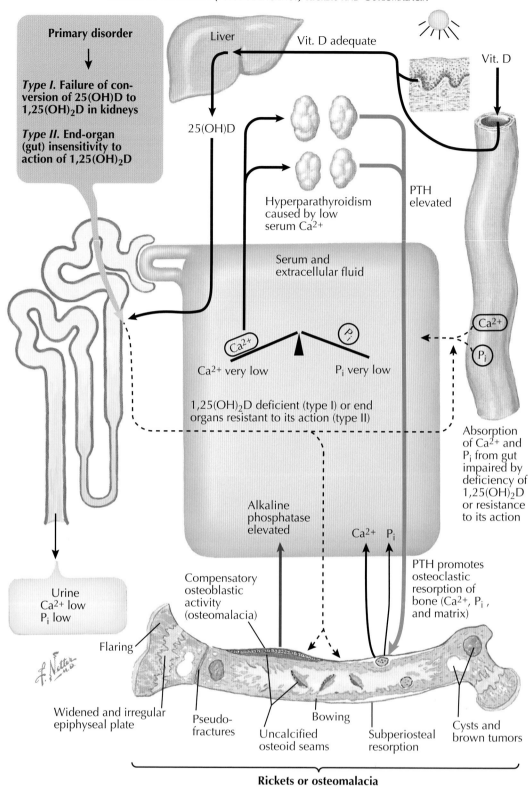

VITAMIN D–DEPENDENT (PSEUDODEFICIENCY) RICKETS AND OSTEOMALACIA

Primary disorder

Type I. Failure of conversion of 25(OH)D to 1,25(OH)$_2$D in kidneys

Type II. End-organ (gut) insensitivity to action of 1,25(OH)$_2$D

Liver

Vit. D adequate

Vit. D

25(OH)D

PTH elevated

Hyperparathyroidism caused by low serum Ca^{2+}

Serum and extracellular fluid

Ca^{2+}

P$_i$

Ca^{2+}

P$_i$

Ca^{2+} very low

P$_i$ very low

1,25(OH)$_2$D deficient (type I) or end organs resistant to its action (type II)

Absorption of Ca^{2+} and P$_i$ from gut impaired by deficiency of 1,25(OH)$_2$D or resistance to its action

Alkaline phosphatase elevated

Ca^{2+} P$_i$

PTH promotes osteoclastic resorption of bone (Ca^{2+}, P$_i$, and matrix)

Urine
Ca^{2+} low
P$_i$ low

Compensatory osteoblastic activity (osteomalacia)

Flaring

Widened and irregular epiphyseal plate

Pseudo-fractures

Uncalcified osteoid seams

Bowing

Subperiosteal resorption

Cysts and brown tumors

Rickets or osteomalacia

Plate 3-19

Metabolic Diseases

VITAMIN D–RESISTANT RICKETS AND OSTEOMALACIA DUE TO RENAL TUBULAR ACIDOSIS

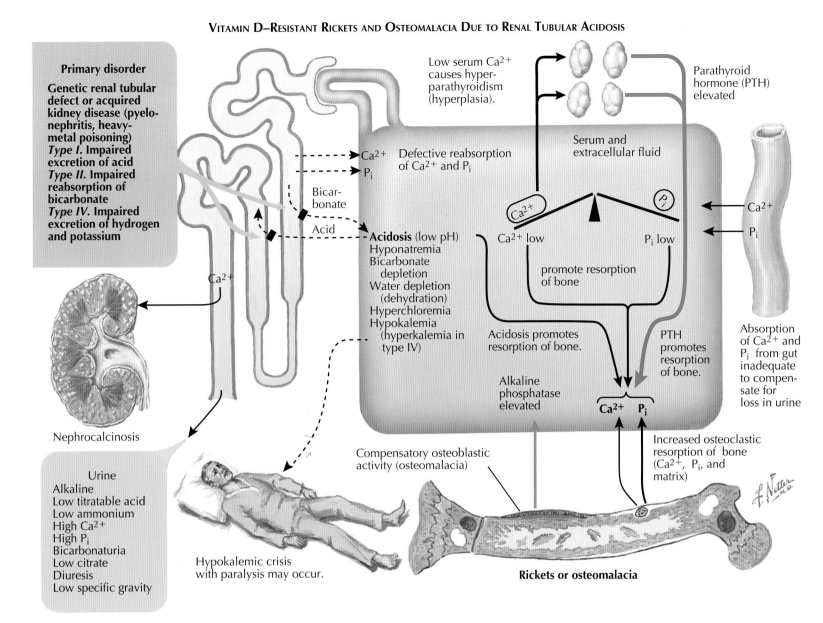

Primary disorder

Genetic renal tubular defect or acquired kidney disease (pyelonephritis, heavy-metal poisoning)
Type I. **Impaired excretion of acid**
Type II. **Impaired reabsorption of bicarbonate**
Type IV. **Impaired excretion of hydrogen and potassium**

Low serum Ca^{2+} causes hyperparathyroidism (hyperplasia).

Parathyroid hormone (PTH) elevated

Ca^{2+} Defective reabsorption of Ca^{2+} and P_i

P_i

Serum and extracellular fluid

Bicarbonate

Acid

Ca^{2+}

P_i

Ca^{2+}

Ca^{2+} low

P_i low

Ca^{2+}

P_i

Acidosis (low pH)
Hyponatremia
Bicarbonate depletion
Water depletion (dehydration)
Hyperchloremia
Hypokalemia (hyperkalemia in type IV)

promote resorption of bone

Acidosis promotes resorption of bone.

PTH promotes resorption of bone.

Absorption of Ca^{2+} and P_i from gut inadequate to compensate for loss in urine

Nephrocalcinosis

Alkaline phosphatase elevated

Ca^{2+} P_i

Compensatory osteoblastic activity (osteomalacia)

Increased osteoclastic resorption of bone (Ca^{2+}, P_i, and matrix)

Urine
Alkaline
Low titratable acid
Low ammonium
High Ca^{2+}
High P_i
Bicarbonaturia
Low citrate
Diuresis
Low specific gravity

Hypokalemic crisis with paralysis may occur.

Rickets or osteomalacia

RICKETS, OSTEOMALACIA, AND RENAL OSTEODYSTROPHY
(Continued)

multiple causes (see Plate 3-19). The basic mechanism common to them all is the kidney's inability to substitute hydrogen ions for fixed base. The diseases are now subclassified into three types. In *type I* (classic or distal), proton exchange is defective; in *type II* (proximal), the cause appears to be a failure of reabsorption of bicarbonate in the proximal tubule; and in *type IV* (generalized distal), through one of several mechanisms, the excretion of both hydrogen and potassium ions in the distal tubule is defective. (Type III is a poorly defined mixture of types I and II and is usually excluded from current classifications.)

All three syndromes are characterized by a hyperchloremic, acidosis, non–anion gap metabolic acidosis and an alkaline urine. Type II is also characterized by a lowered serum bicarbonate level, and types I and II are characterized by hypokalemia, which at times may become so severe as to be life threatening.

(Hypokalemia does not occur in type IV, which is associated with hyperkalemia.) In about 70% of patients, the urinary citrate concentration is inadequate (<50 mg/day), which, coupled with the alkaline pH and hypercalciuria, leads to some degree of nephrocalcinosis. Nephrocalcinosis is rare in proximal renal tubular acidosis because the normal urinary citrate inhibits calcium crystallization. In addition, in distal renal tubular acidosis, the urinary pH cannot be lowered less than 5.4 even with an acid load. Hence, in the rare form of incomplete distal renal tubular acidosis in which there may be nephrocalcinosis, hypercalciuria, and normal serum chloride and bicarbonate levels, an ammonium chloride challenge test may be necessary to make a diagnosis. The ammonium chloride test is conducted by giving a patient 0.1 g/kg of ammonium chloride (placed best in tomato juice to mitigate nausea) and performing urine pH by a pH meter every hour for 4 hours post load. The urine pH should drop less than 5.4 in patients with normal ability to excrete an H+ load.

Rickets or osteomalacia of variable degrees is a common manifestation of all the diverse conditions associated with renal tubular acidosis. Some of the rachitic disorders are life threatening, such as vitamin

D–resistant rickets and osteomalacia due to proximal and distal tubular defects (see Plate 3-17). Other disorders are mild and, in some cases, do not require prolonged treatment. These include the genetically determined, sometimes self-limiting, Butler-Albright syndrome and disorders associated with altered globulin states or hyperthyroidism.

The mechanisms by which renal tubular acidosis contributes to the development of rickets and osteomalacia are not completely understood. Chronic acidosis alone can deplete the bones of calcium and phosphate but is considered to be, at most, a minor mechanism. Many investigators believe that calcium, as well as sodium and potassium, is lost in the urine as fixed base due to a failure to substitute hydrogen or to reabsorb bicarbonate (in types I and II). In some of the syndromes, the %TRP appears to be diminished (either because of a primary renal defect or as a result of secondary hyperparathyroidism and the action of increased concentrations of PTH on the reabsorptive mechanism for phosphate in the renal tubule; or, if found, an elevated FGF-23). The combination of diminished serum calcium and phosphate levels results in rachitic and/or osteomalacic findings that are identical to those seen

Plate 3-20

Musculoskeletal System: PART III

RICKETS, OSTEOMALACIA, AND RENAL OSTEODYSTROPHY
(Continued)

with other syndromes yet are clearly refractory to even very large doses of vitamin D.

In patients with classic rachitic or osteomalacic changes in the epiphyseal growth plates and bones, renal tubular acidosis should be suspected as the underlying cause of the disease. Characteristic findings on biochemical analysis are hyperchloremia, hyponatremia, hypokalemia (except in type IV), hypophosphatemia, and hypocalcemia, often with a lowered serum bicarbonate level. Serum alkaline phosphatase and PTH concentrations are usually also increased. Urinalysis reveals striking findings: alkaline urine with very low concentrations of acid, ammonia, and citrate; increased levels of fixed base (including calcium); and, occasionally, a fixed low specific gravity. Patients usually fail to respond to an acid-loading test (with ammonium chloride) by acidification of the urine.

Treatment of rachitic and osteomalacic syndromes due to renal tubular acidosis should focus on the primary process rather than on the bone disease. Administration of alkali in the form of sodium bicarbonate or similar materials (e.g., polycitrate K) may be all that is required to correct the metabolic disorder, including the rachitic or osteomalacic syndrome. At times (particularly in type IV), sterol treatment may be necessary.

RENAL OSTEODYSTROPHY

Metabolic Aberrations. Chronic renal failure causes an extraordinary number of metabolic abnormalities that affect almost all of the body's homeostatic mechanisms (see Plate 3-20). There are now five stages of chronic kidney disease (CKD) defined by criteria established by the National Kidney Foundation (NKF) (see Plate 3-20). Although abnormalities in bone turnover, volume, and mineralization occur in all stages of CKD and are now defined in broader terms, *chronic kidney disease–mineral and bone disorder* (CKD-MBD), the histomorphometric abnormalities called renal osteodystrophy become manifest by quantitative bone histomorphometry in stage 4-5 CKD. In the patient with azotemia and chronic renal failure, aberrations in water distribution, electrolyte and acid-base balances, protein synthesis, nutrition, and hormonal activities produce extensive changes in bodily structure and functions. The manifestations of chronic renal failure on the body's connective tissues predominate in bone as a multifaceted syndrome. Known in the past as renal rickets, renal hyperparathyroidism, and renal osteomalacia, this

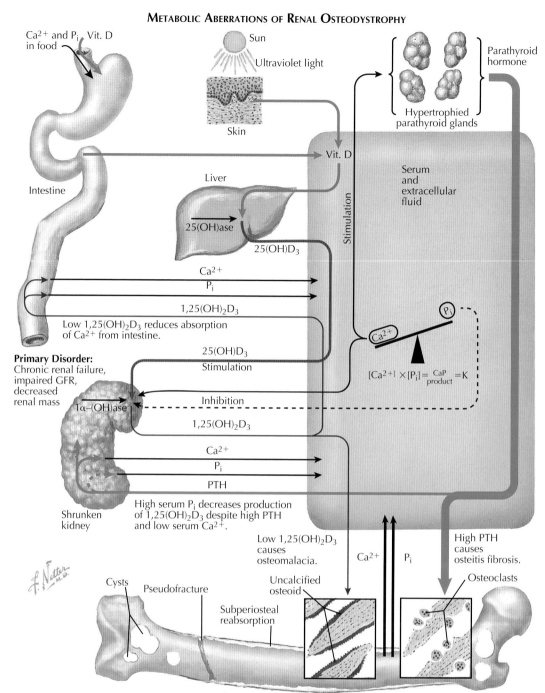

METABOLIC ABERRATIONS OF RENAL OSTEODYSTROPHY

Ca^{2+} and P$_i$ Vit. D in food

Sun

Ultraviolet light

Skin

Parathyroid hormone

Hypertrophied parathyroid glands

Vit. D

Liver

Intestine

25(OH)ase

25(OH)D$_3$

Serum and extracellular fluid

Ca^{2+}

P$_i$

1,25(OH)$_2$D$_3$

Low 1,25(OH)$_2$D$_3$ reduces absorption of Ca^{2+} from intestine.

Stimulation

25(OH)D$_3$

Primary Disorder:
Chronic renal failure, impaired GFR, decreased renal mass

Stimulation

1α-(OH)ase

Inhibition

1,25(OH)$_2$D$_3$

P$_i$

Ca^{2+}

$[Ca^{2+}] \times [P_i] = \dfrac{CaP}{product} = K$

Ca^{2+}

P$_i$

PTH

Shrunken kidney

High serum P$_i$ decreases production of 1,25(OH)$_2$D$_3$ despite high PTH and low serum Ca^{2+}.

Low 1,25(OH)$_2$D$_3$ causes osteomalacia.

Ca^{2+} P$_i$

High PTH causes osteitis fibrosis.

Cysts   Pseudofracture

Subperiosteal reabsorption

Uncalcified osteoid

Osteoclasts

National Kidney Foundation—Stages of chronic kidney disease
Stage 1: GFR < 110 mL/min with evidence of intrinsic renal damage (proteinuria, etc.)
Stage 2: GFR < 90-60 mL/min (with evidence of intrinsic renal damage)
Stage 3: GFR 60-30 mL/min (no need for evidence of intrinsic renal damage)
Stage 4: GFR 30-15 mL/min
Stage 5: < 15 mL/min or ESRD

Data from National Kidney Foundation: K/DOQI clinical practice, guidelines for chronic kidney disease: evaluation, classification and stratification. Am J Kidney Dis 2002;39(Suppl. 1):S1–266.

syndrome is now generally called renal osteodystrophy (see Plates 3-20 to 3-23).

Manifestations of renal osteodystrophy in both children and adults include a number of chronic disorders of epiphyseal cartilage and bone. Among them are rickets and osteomalacia, osteitis fibrosa cystica (secondary hyperparathyroidism), osteosclerosis, and metastatic calcification. In a child with chronic disease, slipped capital femoral epiphysis may be an additional complication. Osteoporosis, osteomyelitis, and (if corticosteroids are administered) osteonecrosis are also seen frequently in both children and adults.

The pathogenetic mechanisms for the bone changes in renal osteodystrophy are complex (see Plates 3-20 to 3-23). The underlying defect is kidney damage, which includes not only a failure of glomerular filtration that results in azotemia and hyperphosphatemia but almost always a reduced renal, and thus a reduced tubular,

Plate 3-21   Metabolic Diseases

Mechanism of development of chemical and bony changes in renal osteodystrophy

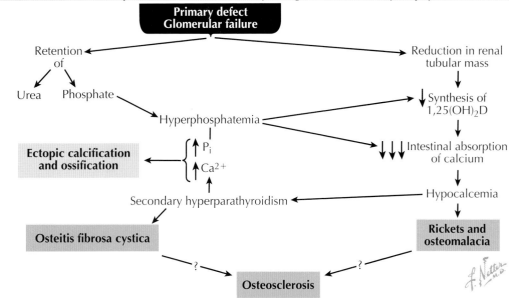

RICKETS, OSTEOMALACIA, AND RENAL OSTEODYSTROPHY
(Continued)

mass. Even when vitamin D intake is normal or increased, the high phosphate concentration and the reduction in tubular function greatly reduce the synthesis of $1,25(OH)_2D$ and lead to elevated PTH and FGF-23. Increased serum phosphate levels and the severely lowered concentration of $1,25(OH)_2D$ lead to a markedly reduced absorption of calcium from the gastrointestinal tract and profound hypocalcemia. Despite acidosis, which promotes the solubilization of calcium salts, the hypocalcemia is so severe that it not only causes all the bony and soft tissue manifestations of rickets or osteomalacia but also induces a secondary hyperparathyroidism. The excessive secretion of PTH leads to osteitis fibrosa cystica (marked osteoclastic resorption of bone and brown tumors). The resorption of bone partially restores serum calcium levels to normal. The elevated FGF-23 may contribute to the impairment of bone mineralization as well and be one of the leading mechanisms for the very low bone turnover now labeled adynamic renal bone disease.

In patients with renal osteodystrophy, the critical solubility product for calcium phosphate is in danger of being exceeded and resulting in vascular calcification. This is a consequence of both the hyperphosphatemia and the reduction in tubular mass, which results in a failure of the increased PTH and FGF-23 concentrations to induce an adequate phosphate diuresis. Because calcium salts are more soluble in an acid medium, chronic acidosis helps to prevent deposition of calcific salts. However, the level of calcium or phosphate (or both) may sometimes rise sufficiently or the pH may increase, resulting in ectopic calcification or ossification.

The biochemical alterations in renal osteodystrophy can be summarized as follows:

1. Azotemia, hyperphosphatemia, and changes in acid-base balance and electrolytes that reflect the chronic acidotic state
2. Low serum calcium level, in which case a larger percentage of the calcium is ionized because of the acidotic state but the total amount (including the nonionized calcium) is reduced not only as a result of the factors just described but because of a commonly observed decline in serum proteins.
3. Increased bone alkaline phosphatase activity due to the increased rate of new bone synthesis in hyperparathyroid and osteomalacic renal bone disease
4. Increased PTH level, which indicates the usually marked secondary hyperparathyroidism in hyperparathyroid renal bone disease. However, the

Reduced renal function and glomerular failure cause retention of urea and phosphate, leading to hyperphosphatemia, which, along with reduction in tubular mass, causes profound reduction in synthesis of $1,25(OH)_2D$. This, plus the direct effect of increased concentration of serum phosphate, reduces intestinal absorption of calcium, causing profound hypocalcemia and severe secondary hyperparathyroidism. These changes produce clinical syndromes of rickets and osteitis fibrosa cystica; 20% of patients with this combination of chemical abnormalities also have osteosclerosis. Because phosphate concentration is chronically increased, an occasional increase in serum calcium level can lead to rapid ectopic calcification and ossification in conjunctiva, skin, blood vessels, and periarticular regions.

Renal adynamic bone disease

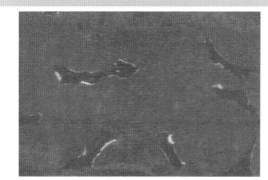

Von Kossa 40× osteopenia

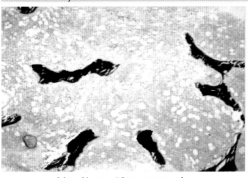

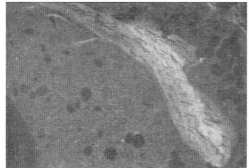

Von Kossa 40× fluorescence osteoid yellow

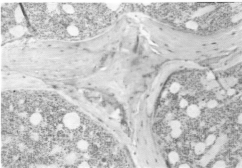

TRAP-Azure 100× no osteoclasts

Unstained fluorescence 100× no tetracycline label

serum PTH is often low for stage 4 and 5 CKD patients (<150 pg/mL) in adynamic renal bone disease.
5. Greatly diminished $1,25(OH)_2D$ levels, even with increased intake of vitamin D, and normal or high levels of $25(OH)D$
6. Increased serum FGF-23 levels

Clinical Manifestations. In the growing child with renal osteodystrophy, rachitic changes in the epiphyseal plates are virtually identical to those seen in patients with other forms of rickets (see Plates 3-15 and 3-21). However, the growth rate of children with renal osteodystrophy is often greatly reduced, with the result that radiographic manifestations of the disease may appear somewhat less severe than the chemical aberrations suggest (see the paradox of rickets). However, increased axial height of the epiphyseal plates, cupping and flaring, and diminished density in the zone of

Plate 3-22

Musculoskeletal System: PART III

BONY MANIFESTATION OF RENAL OSTEODYSTROPHY

Secondary hyperparathyroidism

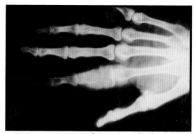

Radiograph shows
banded sclerosis of
spine and sclerosis of
upper and lower
margins of vertebrae,
with rarefaction
between. Note
compression
fracture.

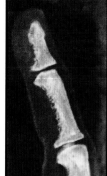

Radiograph shows spotty
decalcification of skull
("salt-and-pepper" skull).

Brown tumor of proximal phalanx

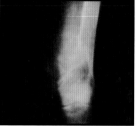

Loss of lamina dura of
teeth (*broken lines*
indicate normal contours)

Osteitis fibrosa cystica
of distal femur

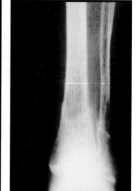

Subperiosteal
resorption of
phalanges (chiefly
on palmar aspect
of middle phalanx)

Osteitis fibrosa cystica
of tibia with brown
tumor

RICKETS, OSTEOMALACIA, AND RENAL OSTEODYSTROPHY

(Continued)

provisional calcification are characteristic radiographic findings and are indistinguishable from the changes seen in the other forms of rachitic disease. For some unknown reason, slipped capital femoral epiphysis occurs much more frequently in patients with azotemic rickets than it does in patients with vitamin D deficiency or vitamin D–resistant disease.

Radiographic examination of the bones reveals all the features of osteomalacia—thin cortices, fuzzy trabecular markings, and Looser's zones—but may also reveal striking features of osteitis fibrosa cystica, which differentiate renal osteodystrophy from the nutritional or vitamin D–resistant forms of the disease. Histologic examination is likely to show more severe degrees of osteoclastic resorption of bone, with fibrosis of the marrow and brown tumors, and large (macroscopic) regions in which resorption is so great that the cortices are enormously thinned and no medullary bone can be found. Islands of osteoblastic activity are frequently observed and account for the increased alkaline phosphatase activity in the serum and the patchy and occasionally significant increment in activity observed on radionuclide bone scans.

Radiographic examination of the skull may show irregular rarefaction of the calvaria ("salt-and-pepper" skull) and loss of the dense white line cast by the lamina dura surrounding the roots of the teeth. Cortical thinning and fuzzy trabeculae characteristic of both osteomalacia and osteitis fibrosa cystica are seen in radiographs of the long bones, with additional findings of small or large, rarefied, rounded lytic lesions characteristic of brown tumors; "disappearance" of the lateral portion of the clavicle; and subperiosteal resorption of the proximal medial tibia. The most noticeable changes are seen in the bones of the hand, with erosion of the terminal phalangeal tufts and subperiosteal resorption

Osteomalacia

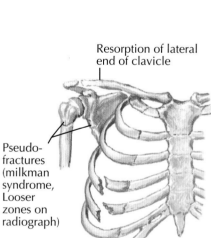

Fracture of
long bones

Resorption of lateral
end of clavicle

Pseudo-
fractures
(milkman
syndrome,
Looser
zones on
radiograph)

Fractured ribs

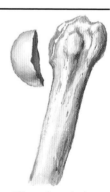

Slipped capital
femoral epiphysis

of the proximal and distal phalanges most marked on the radial sides.

For reasons not clearly understood, about 20% of the patients with the combination of chronic renal disease, osteomalacia, and osteitis fibrosa cystica also develop a type of osteosclerosis. Histologic findings reveal an increased number of trabeculae per unit volume rather than a healing of the demineralized bone of osteomalacia (osteoid seams) or an alteration in the resorptive

changes of osteitis fibrosa cystica. The disease most commonly affects the subchondral cortices of the vertebrae and the shafts of the long bones, producing a radiographic appearance of alternating light and dark shadows (banded sclerosis, or "rugger-jersey spine"). The small bones or digits of the hands and feet are rarely involved.

Renal adynamic bone disease is characterized by low bone mineral density (BMD) by either dual energy

Plate 3-23

Metabolic Diseases

VASCULAR AND SOFT TISSUE CALCIFICATION IN SECONDARY HYPERPARATHYROIDISM OF CHRONIC RENAL DISEASE

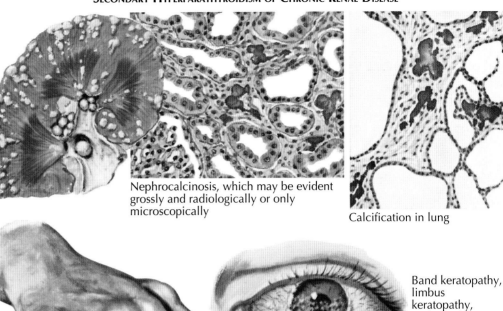

Nephrocalcinosis, which may be evident grossly and radiologically or only microscopically

Calcification in lung

Band keratopathy, limbus keratopathy, and/or calcium deposits in conjunctiva with conjunctivitis

Periarticular calcium deposits of hand

Calcium deposits in conduction system of heart, which may cause serious or fatal arrhythmias

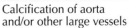

Intra- and periarticular calcium deposits of shoulder

Calcification of aorta and/or other large vessels

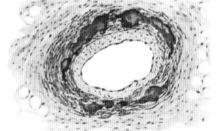

Medial calcification of coronary and/or other small arteries

RICKETS, OSTEOMALACIA, AND RENAL OSTEODYSTROPHY
(Continued)

x-ray absorptiometry (DXA) or quantitative computed tomography (QCT) or by low bone turnover on biopsy or suspected by low bone turnover markers (BSAP and PTH), hypercalcemia, and fractures. Renal adynamic bone disease may be "idiopathic," more often seen in patients with diabetes and on peritoneal dialysis, or iatrogenic from excess lowering of PTH levels by agents that inhibit PTH production (vitamin D analogs or cinacalcet). Recently, the Kidney Disease Improving Global Outcomes (KDOGO) Bone Working Group has published their guidelines on managing these more complex bone and mineral disorders.

Metastatic or ectopic calcification and ossification are seen in many sites (see Plate 3-21). The most common articular sites are the articular cartilages and menisci of the knees; the triangular ligaments of the distal radioulnar joints; the soft tissues surrounding the shoulder, elbow, knee, and ankle; and the tunica media or the tunica muscularis of the larger arterial and arteriolar vessels. In many cases, the skin and the conjunctivae (the "red eyes of renal failure") are also involved (see Plate 3-23).

Treatment. Treatment of renal osteodystrophy is complex and the recent KDIGO guidelines are the best evidence-based guides for management. The first requirement is appropriate management of the chronic renal disease, which includes procedures such as chronic dialysis and renal transplantation. Additional measures are administration of agents to mitigate hyperphosphatemia, judicious administration of vitamin D analogs to inhibit PTH production, and, if necessary, parathyroidectomy to control the sometimes autonomous (tertiary) hyperparathyroidism. Fractures that occur in CKD may or may not be related to CKD and may be osteoporosis. The differentiation between renal bone disease and osteoporosis is a challenge. Patients with stages 1 to 3 CKD can be diagnosed as other patients with

osteoporosis (e.g., by DXA). Patients with stages 4 and 5 CKD often require bone biopsy to exclude the forms of renal osteodystrophy that may also cause low bone mass or fragility fractures.

Orthopedic problems are sometimes severe, and treatment may include internal fixation of slipped capital femoral epiphysis with threaded devices, management of bowleg and knock-knee by bracing or osteotomy, and use of open or closed fixation for the

frequent fractures that occur during the course of the disease.

Rickets, osteomalacia, and renal osteodystrophy are distinct entities. They can all be diagnosed by appropriate laboratory testing. Osteomalacia and renal osteodystrophy often require quantitative bone histomorphometry to make a correct diagnosis. Once a diagnosis is made, each entity can be managed by specific interventions.

Plate 3-24

Musculoskeletal System: PART III

CLINICAL GUIDE TO VITAMIN D MEASUREMENT

Vitamin D is crucial to the bone health and overall well-being of humans. Vitamin D deficiency or insufficiency is recognized as the common cause of hyperparathyroidism with consequent bone loss and osteoporosis. Vitamin D is now recognized as a prohormone that is biologically inactive until metabolized into a secosteroid, similar to steroid hormones. Vitamin D is metabolized by hepatic 25-hydroxylase into biologically inactive 25-hydroxyvitamin D [25(OH)D; calcidiol], which by renal 1α-hydroxylase is converted into 1-25dihydroxyvitamin D [1-25(OH)₂D; calcitriol], the active vitamin D metabolite (see Plate 3-24). Furthermore, the discovery that most tissues have a vitamin D receptor and several possess the enzymatic machinery to convert the primary circulating form of 25(OH)D to the active form of 1-25(OH)₂D has suggested to its expanded role in decreasing the risk of many chronic diseases, including infectious diseases, cancers, and autoimmune diseases.

The circulating 25(OH)D concentration is the most reliable measure of overall vitamin D status, even though it is biologically inactive. 25(OH)D is measured by commercially available immunoassays, preferably by automated high throughput immunoassay analyzers. However, variability between these methods exists due to different antibodies sources, preliminary extraction or purification procedures, and/or incubation conditions. It is important that these immunoassays utilize antibodies that can react with both 25(OH)D₃ and 25(OH)D₂ equally for accurate assessment of vitamin D status. Alternatively, vitamin D is measured by direct detection methodologies that include both high-pressure liquid chromatography and LC-mass spectrometry (LC-MS). Both offer the advantage of separating and detecting both 25(OH)D₂ and D₃. LC-MS has recently been revitalized as a viable method to measure vitamin D levels. When properly performed, it provides accurate results; however, the throughput, although better than high-pressure liquid chromatography, cannot match the automated immunoassay platforms.

Vitamin D levels are inversely associated with PTH levels and directly associated with intestinal calcium absorption. Therefore, the optimal level of vitamin D is defined as 30 ng/mL, because at this level the PTH begins to level off and intestinal calcium absorption is maximal. Vitamin D levels between 15 and 29 ng/mL are considered insufficient and levels less than 15 ng/mL are considered deficient. Based on these definitions of optimal levels, vitamin D deficiency or insufficiency is highly prevalent worldwide. In contrast, vitamin D intoxication is rare and can occur by inadvertent ingestion of very high doses (>50,000 U), raising serum vitamin D levels to more than 150 ng/mL. It has been shown that doses up to 10,000 U/day for many months do not cause toxicity.

Although 25(OH)D levels reflect the overall vitamin D status, 1-25(OH)₂D levels, even though it is the active metabolite, do not necessarily correlate with vitamin D status. Serum levels of 1-25(OH)₂D do not increase in response to increased intake or exposure to sunlight and are often normal or even elevated in vitamin D insufficiency. Production of 1-25(OH)₂D is tightly regulated by 1α-hydroxylase in the kidneys and the serum level closely correlates with renal function. In end-stage renal disease, this hydroxylation step is severely reduced or negligible. Therefore, circulating concentrations of

1,25(OH)₂D are considerably lower in these patients than in healthy individuals. Inadequately low 1,25(OH)₂D levels decrease serum calcium concentrations and stimulate the production of PTH, resulting in secondary hyperparathyroidism and substantial bone loss. Therefore, the primary utility of measurement of 1,25(OH)₂D is in assessing secondary hyperparathyroidism and hypocalcemia in patients with renal dysfunction. It is also useful in evaluation of patients with hypoparathyroidism, sarcoidosis, and rickets.

Measurement of 1,25(OH)₂D is challenging because of its low circulating levels (normal range 18 to 86 pg/mL) and presence of interfering substances and cross-reactivity with other 1α-hydroxylated vitamin D

metabolites. Therefore, chemical extraction (C18 column) and purification of serum samples before assay is necessary. After extraction/purification, 1,25(OH)₂D is measured by radioreceptor or radioimmunoassay. An alternative method is LC-MS, which has been also difficult primarily owing to low levels, lack of ionizable polar groups, and its lipophilic nature. More recently using immunoextraction and concentrating the eluates before LC-MS have been shown to provide a sensitive alternative LC-MS method. Although 25(OH)D measurement serves as the indicator of nutritional vitamin D status, the 1-25(OH)₂D measurement is only indicated in assessing secondary hyperparathyroidism in patients with renal insufficiency.

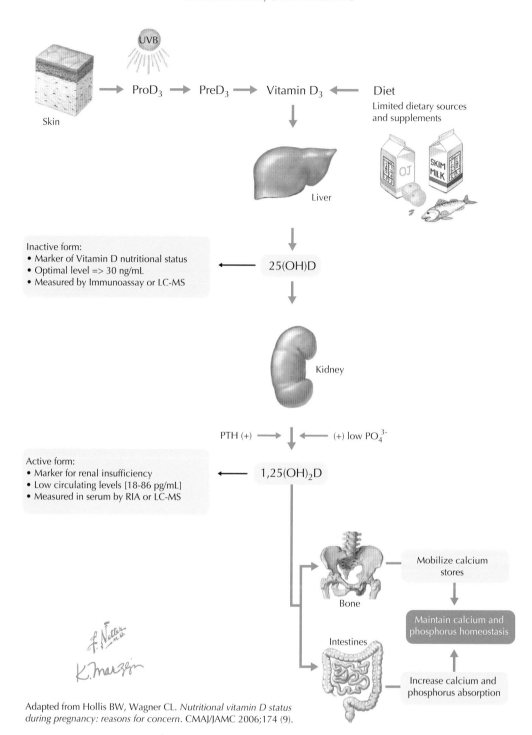

VITAMIN D METABOLISM
Endocrine Pathway (Bone Metabolism)

UVB

ProD₃ → PreD₃ → Vitamin D₃ ← Diet
Limited dietary sources and supplements

Skin

Liver

OJ   SKIM MILK

Inactive form:
• Marker of Vitamin D nutritional status
• Optimal level => 30 ng/mL
• Measured by Immunoassay or LC-MS

25(OH)D

Kidney

PTH (+) →   ← (+) low PO₄³⁻

Active form:
• Marker for renal insufficiency
• Low circulating levels [18-86 pg/mL]
• Measured in serum by RIA or LC-MS

1,25(OH)₂D

Bone — Mobilize calcium stores

Maintain calcium and phosphorus homeostasis

Intestines — Increase calcium and phosphorus absorption

Adapted from Hollis BW, Wagner CL. *Nutritional vitamin D status during pregnancy: reasons for concern.* CMAJ/JAMC 2006;174 (9).

Plate 3-25

Metabolic Diseases

HYPOPHOSPHATASIA

Hypophosphatasia (HPP) is a rare heritable metabolic bone disease characterized by a defect in bone mineralization and a deficiency of tissue-nonspecific alkaline phosphatase (TNSALP). The diagnosis is based on low serum alkaline phosphatase and genetic identification of mutations in the alkaline phosphatase gene. The gene encoding TNSALP is on chromosome 1. Over 200 mutations in the gene that cause HPP have been identified. Alkaline phosphatase (ALP) has numerous roles related to the function of inorganic phosphate and mineralization. In humans, four ALP isoenzymes exist and three are tissue specific (intestinal, placental, and germ cell). Tissue-nonspecific ALP is present in all cells but has especially high concentrations in liver, kidney, and bone.

In patients with HPP the predominant organs involved are the skeleton and teeth, which are hard tissues, even though there are high levels of TNSALP in many organs. Four of the five principal forms of HPP are based on age at diagnosis: perinatal, infantile, childhood, and adult, with earlier disease onset being more severe. The fifth form, which has dental manifestations only, is termed *odonto-HPP*. The most severe form is perinatal HPP, which presents in utero, with skeletal abnormalities at birth including extreme hypomineralization and short, deformed limbs. Life expectancy is short. Skeletal manifestations of infantile HPP present before 6 months of age and are inherited as an autosomal recessive trait. Clinical manifestations result from poor skeletal mineralization and include growth failure, rachitic deformities, hypercalcemia, and renal compromise from nephrocalcinosis. Cranial sutures appear widened but are representative of severe skull hypomineralization. Death occurs soon after initial clinical manifestations appear.

The childhood form occurs after 6 months of age and has a variable but more benign course. Premature loss of deciduous teeth, the most consistent clinical sign, is a result of hypoplasia of the cementum. Radiographs may reveal characteristic tongues, which are lucent projections from rachitic growth plates into abnormal metaphyses.

The adult form is the least severe and is clinically heterogeneous. It is inherited as an autosomal dominant trait with variable penetrance. There may be a childhood history of premature loss of deciduous teeth

or of rachitic deformity but often young adult life is relatively normal. As the patient ages, multiple recurrent, poorly healing metatarsal fractures and femoral pseudofractures are common clinical features. Patients may have pseudogout with chondrocalcinosis. Total serum alkaline phosphatase level is well below normal in patients with adult HPP. Low levels of alkaline phosphatase can be seen in pregnancy, hypothyroidism, cleidocranial dysplasia, and severe osteogenesis

imperfecta. Pyridoxal 5′-phosphate (PLP, vitamin B6) is usually elevated and is a good marker for HPP. Serum 25(OH)D, 1,25(OH)D, and PTH values are typically normal.

There is no established treatment for HPP. Bone marrow transplant has been tried in infants. Teriparatide has been used with some success in several case reports. Enzyme replacement using a bone-targeted recombinant TNSALP is undergoing clinical trials.

Elevated intracranial pressure due to craniosynostosis

Pneumonia related to chest deformity

Hypercalciuria, nephrocalcinosis, renal failure

Rachitic deformities

Infantile form
(most serious, often fatal)

Early loss of deciduous teeth

Characteristic rachitic deformities

Childhood form (less serious than infantile form)

Premature loss of teeth

Osteomalacia, pseudofractures, true fractures

Adult form
(least serious but clinically heterogeneous)

Serum and extracellular fluid

Serum P_i normal

Pyrophosphate (PP_i), Phosphoethanolamine, Phosphoserine, Phosphorylcholine, Pyridoxal 5-phosphate

Serum alkaline phosphatase activity very low or absent

Serum Ca^{2+} normal or elevated because not deposited in bone

Alkaline phosphatase, which normally promotes bone mineralization by hydrolyzing PP_i, is absent, deficient, or ineffective in hypophosphatasia.

Pyrophosphate (PP_i) inhibits bone mineralization.

Osteoblasts

Collagen Noncollagenous proteins and proteoglycans

PP_i → Ca^{2+}

Uncalcified matrix

Mineralized bone

Urine

Calcium elevated

Inorganic pyrophosphate greatly elevated

Phosphoethanolamine greatly elevated

Phosphoserine greatly elevated

Section of trabecular bone from patient with infantile hypophosphatasia shows very broad seams of uncalcified matrix (stained red) overlying thin trabeculae of mineralized bone (stained blue).
M = marrow; O = osteoblasts;
OC = osteoclasts. (Outlined panel is area shown in enlargement.)

Plate 3-26

Musculoskeletal System: PART III

Causes of Osteoporosis

Traditionally, osteoporosis has been defined based on bone density, with a T-score less than or equal to −2.5. This definition does not take into account the architectural changes in bone tissue that increase fracture risk independent of bone density. Now osteoporosis is defined as a skeletal disease characterized by low bone mass and microarchitectural deterioration of bone tissue that results in bone fragility and increased fracture risk. Fracture risk is now assessed using both bone density and clinical risk factors that predict 10-year absolute fracture risk. The FRAX tool incorporates risk factors such as age, previous fracture, family history, smoking, alcohol, and rheumatoid arthritis that increase the sensitivity for fracture prediction over and above that provided by bone density. An estimated 10 million Americans have osteoporosis, defined as a T-score of −2.5 or less, and another 34 million have low bone mass, defined as a T-score between −1.0 and −2.5.

Osteoporosis is a heterogeneous disorder that is caused by multiple pathogenetic mechanisms. The clinical manifestation of osteoporosis is fracture, and the mechanisms that lead to fracture are multifactorial and include factors that result in low peak bone mass, bone loss after menopause, and factors involved in falls (see Plate 3-26).

Age and Sex Factors. The development of osteoporosis in postmenopausal women is linked to a number of factors, the most important being estrogen deficiency. Before menopause, bone formation and resorption are balanced. At menopause, the rate of bone turnover increases with the rate of bone resorption increasing more than formation. Biochemical markers of bone resorption are increased. Estrogen plays a central role in regulating RANK ligand (RANKL), a molecule that is critical for osteoclast formation and activity. As estrogen declines, RANKL is unregulated and osteoclast activity is increased. Because men do not undergo the abrupt hormonal equivalent of menopause, they experience a slower rate of decline in bone mass and fewer fractures. Other risk factors include low peak bone mass, reduced levels of 1,25(OH)$_2$D, a calcium-deficient diet, and reduced calcium absorption from the intestine (characteristic of elderly persons).

Genetic Factors. Studies of monozygotic and dizygotic twins show a high heritability, between 60% and 80%, of bone mass. The heritability of fracture risk is less because environmental factors such as exercise, diet, and fall risk have a significant effect with aging. Genetic factors are likely to be important in the development of peak bone mass. Candidate genes for low bone mass include those responsible for receptors or proteins involved in bone biology such as lipoprotein receptor 5 *(LRP5)* and sclerostin (involved in Wnt signaling), vitamin D receptor, estrogen receptor, and type I collagen among others. Polymorphisms in candidate genes have a small effect size, indicating that osteoporosis is multifactorial with many genes involved.

Endocrine Abnormalities. Endocrine-mediated osteoporosis should be suspected in any young or middle-aged person with osteopenia. In the elderly person, endocrine-mediated osteoporosis can occur in conjunction with postmenopausal or age-related osteoporosis.

Hypogonadism causes bone loss in both men and women. In postmenopausal women estrogen deficiency plays a key role in increasing osteoclast activity and bone resorption. Other hypogonadal conditions that lead to bone loss are panhypopituitarism, Klinefelter

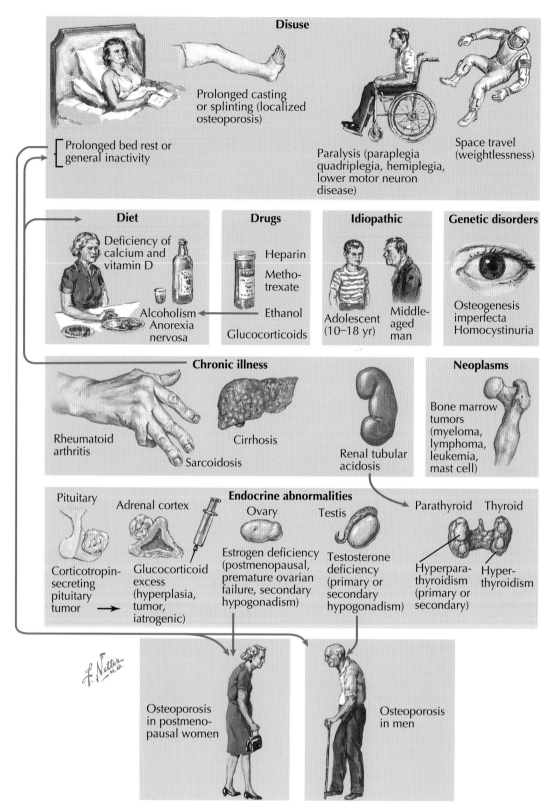

syndrome, Turner syndrome, and idiopathic hypogonadotropic hypogonadism. Medications that lower the level of estrogens, such as medroxyprogesterone (inhibits pituitary gonadotropin release) and aromatase inhibitors (inhibit enzymatic androgen conversion to estrogen), increase the rate of bone loss in women. Medications that lower the level of androgens, such as bicalutamide (binds and inhibits androgen receptors) and leuprolide (inhibits gonadotropin release

suppressing ovarian and testicular steroidogenesis) increase the rate of bone loss in men.

Thyrotoxicosis, caused by glandular hyperactivity or by excessive replacement of thyroid hormone, increases bone turnover and bone resorption. Older postmenopausal women with TSH levels below 0.1 have been shown to have a significant increase in hip, vertebral, and nonvertebral fracture risk compared with women with levels between 0.5 and 5.5.

Plate 3-27

Metabolic Diseases

CAUSES OF OSTEOPOROSIS
(Continued)

Hyperparathyroidism, either primary or secondary, increases bone turnover, causing a net increase in bone resorption. Primary hyperparathyroidism should be suspected with hypercalcemia and hypophosphatemia. The most common causes of secondary hyperparathyroidism are renal insufficiency and vitamin D deficiency. Most cases of primary hyperparathyroidism are caused by solitary adenoma. Surgical treatment is indicated in patients with symptomatic disease (gastrointestinal disease, renal stones, or neuromuscular syndromes) and in patients with asymptomatic disease who are younger than age 50, have significant hypercalcemia, urine calcium greater than or equal to 400 mg/24 hr, or a T-score less than or equal to −2.5.

Hyperadrenalism, or chronic glucocorticoid excess, whether endogenous (Cushing syndrome) or iatrogenic, leads to decreased bone mass. Glucocorticoid therapy results in a transient increase in bone resorption followed by a suppression of bone formation. Glucocorticoids decrease intestinal absorption of calcium. This stimulates the PTH–vitamin D endocrine axis to restore the serum concentration of ionized calcium by increasing bone resorption.

The combined direct and indirect effects of glucocorticoids often result in osteoporosis that is more severe in the axial than in the appendicular skeleton. Numerous guidelines have been published for the prevention and treatment of glucocorticoid-induced osteoporosis. Drugs approved for the prevention and treatment of glucocorticoid-induced osteoporosis include alendronate, risedronate, zoledronate, and teriparatide.

Nutritional. Various nutritional deficiencies can lead to osteoporosis. Adequate nutrition is critical during the accrual of peak bone mass when in a short period of time 40% of bone mass is acquired. Calcium is the principal mineral in bone. Chronic dietary deficiencies in calcium increase bone loss through PTH-mediated increase in bone remodeling. Dairy products are the major source of calcium. Total calcium intake in diet or supplements should be between 1000 and 1500 mg/day. Other food groups may affect bone health by altering acid-base balance; fruits and vegetables favor an alkaline environment, whereas meats favor an acid environment, which is buffered in bone and increases calcium loss in the urine. Dietary salt increases urine calcium excretion because sodium and calcium share transport pathways in the kidney. Adequate vitamin D is important because vitamin D deficiency decreases calcium absorption and increases PTH levels, which increases bone resorption. The major source of vitamin D is conversion of 7-dehydrocholesterol by sunlight in the skin. Very few foods contain vitamin D; fish and fish liver oils are the richest source. Vitamin D supplementation with between 400 and 1000 IU/day is recommended.

Alcoholism increases the risk for fractures. The development of osteoporosis is related to increase fall risk, poor nutrition, renal loss of calcium, and hypogonadism. In addition, ethanol decreases osteocalcin levels, a marker of osteoblast function.

Anorexia nervosa is prevalent in adolescents, affecting 0.2% to 1.0% of girls. Between 50% and 75% of patients with anorexia will have low bone mass for age. The mechanisms include amenorrhea and hypogonadism, increased levels of cortisol, and metabolic acidosis.

OSTEOPOROSIS	
World Health Organization	T-score ≥ -2.5
Consensus Development Conference	A systemic skeletal disease characterized by low bone mass and microarchitectural deterioration of bone tissue with a consequent increase in bone fragility and susceptibility to fracture
Fracture incidence, U.S.	Hip 300,000 Vertebral 700,000 Wrist 250,000 Others 300,000 _____ Total 1,550,000
Pathophysiology	Multifactorial: Bone resorption (osteoclast activity) exceeds bone formation (osteoblast activity) • Low peak bone mass, family history • Menopause and estrogen deficiency • Medications including glucocorticoids, estrogen/androgen deprivation therapy • Nutrition including low body weight, eating disorders • Calcium and vitamin D deficiency • Sedentary lifestyle • Smoking

The most effective treatment is correction of the eating disorder and resumption of menses.

Drug-Induced Bone Loss. Long-term glucocorticoid therapy is the most common cause of drug-induced osteoporosis. Use of the anticoagulant heparin may lead to osteopenia. Androgen deprivation and estrogen deprivation therapies (GnRH analogs and aromatase inhibitors) reduced bone mass by inducing hypogonadism. Anticonvulsants such as phenytoin and phenobarbital reduce vitamin D levels by increasing vitamin D metabolism. Serotonin reuptake inhibitors have been reported to increase fractures (serotonin has a role in bone metabolism) as have proton pump inhibitors, which may inhibit calcium absorption.

Disuse Osteoporosis. Weight-bearing exercise stimulates bone formation. Osteocytes have a mechanotransduction role and translate mechanical loading to cellular signals that stimulate osteoblast activity. After

Plate 3-28

Musculoskeletal System: PART III

CAUSES OF OSTEOPOROSIS
(Continued)

immobilization, bone density decreases rapidly. No-gravity environments such as spaceflight result in a loss of 1% to 2% of bone mass every month, a rate 10 times normal. Disuse osteopenia is common in degenerative lower motor neuron disease and in paraplegia and quadriplegia resulting from spinal cord injury.

Disease-Related Bone Loss. Chronic inflammatory diseases are associated with increase bone loss because of the effects of inflammatory cytokines such as tumor necrosis factor, which increase bone turnover and resorption. Rheumatoid arthritis patients have elevated levels of inflammatory cytokines such as interleukin-17 that increase osteoclast activity and cause periarticular osteopenia and bone erosions.

Multiple myeloma, the most common primary malignant bone tumor in adults, may be associated with profound generalized axial and appendicular osteopenia. Myeloma cells produce potent osteoclast-activating factors that stimulate bone resorption. A particularly lytic form of multiple myeloma is associated with secretion of Dkk-1, an inhibitor of Wnt signaling. Multiple myeloma should be suspected in any person older than age 50 who has symptomatic osteopenia, anemia, proteinuria, and a sedimentation rate greater than 100 mm/hr. Serum protein electrophoresis helps establish the diagnosis, but if the results are inconclusive, urinary immunoelectrophoresis should be performed. Approximately 1% of myelomas are nonsecretory, and bone marrow biopsy is required in all patients. Leukemia, lymphoma, and systemic mastocytosis may also be associated with osteoporosis.

CLINICAL MANIFESTATIONS AND PROGRESSIVE SPINAL DEFORMITY

A long latent period often precedes the clinical symptoms or complications of osteoporosis (see Plates 3-28 and 3-29). Skeletal resources are depleted, often for decades, before the bone mass is so compromised that the skeletal framework can no longer withstand *everyday* mechanical stresses.

The entire skeleton is susceptible to age-related and postmenopausal bone loss, but trabecular bone remodeling is greater in regions such as the thoracic and lumbar vertebral bodies, ribs, proximal femur and humerus, and distal radius. The most prevalent complications are vertebral compression fractures.

VERTEBRAL COMPRESSION FRACTURES

Approximately two thirds of all vertebral fractures are asymptomatic. An important clue to occult vertebral fractures is height loss. A loss of height from peak height of more than 1.5 inches is associated with an increased risk of vertebral fractures. One third of patients with vertebral compression fracture have acute back pain, which is often precipitated by routine activities—standing, bending, lifting—that under normal circumstances would not be stressful enough to cause a fracture.

The onset of pain is sudden. Spinal movement is severely restricted. The pain intensifies with sitting or standing and is exacerbated by coughing, sneezing, and straining to move the bowels. Bed rest in the fully recumbent position provides relief.

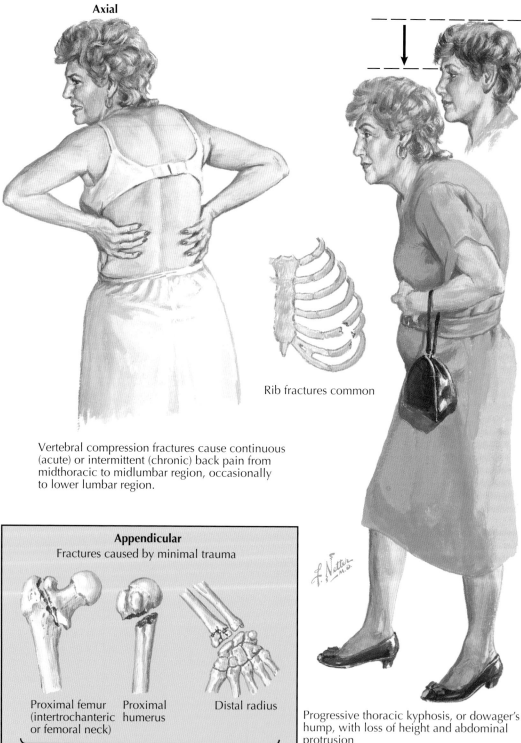

CLINICAL MANIFESTATIONS OF OSTEOPOROSIS

Axial

Rib fractures common

Vertebral compression fractures cause continuous (acute) or intermittent (chronic) back pain from midthoracic to midlumbar region, occasionally to lower lumbar region.

Appendicular
Fractures caused by minimal trauma

Proximal femur (intertrochanteric or femoral neck)   Proximal humerus   Distal radius

Most common types

Progressive thoracic kyphosis, or dowager's hump, with loss of height and abdominal protrusion

Radiculopathies may occur with thoracic or upper lumbar compression fractures and cause pain that radiates anteriorly along the costal margin of the affected nerve root.

Approximately 30% of patients continue to be plagued with chronic, dull, aching, postural pain in the midthoracic and upper lumbar regions. As each episode of segmental vertebral collapse causes progressive kyphosis, the patient's height may decrease. Both kyphosis and decreased height are reliable clinical signs of the late stage of the disease. With severe osteoporosis and multiple compression fractures, the lower ribs may rest on the iliac crest (see Plate 3-29).

Progressive vertebral compression fractures cause a decreased size of the thoracic and abdominal cavities and result in hypoventilation. Early satiety as well as abdominal protrusion secondary to severe lumbar vertebral collapse may occur.

Plate 3-29

Metabolic Diseases

CAUSES OF OSTEOPOROSIS
(Continued)

APPENDICULAR FRACTURES

Although the most common clinical symptom of osteoporosis is back pain due to vertebral fractures, fractures in the appendicular skeleton may be the first evidence of the disease. The most frequent appendicular injuries are fractures of the proximal femur (hip) sustained after a sideways fall or a fracture of the distal radius after a fall on the outstretched hand. The incidence of fractures of the proximal femur increases with age and shows a bimodal peak. Intracapsular fractures of the femur occur most often between ages 65 and 75, whereas the incidence of intertrochanteric fractures peaks about 10 years later.

WORKUP IN SYMPTOMATIC DISEASE

Causes of symptomatic bone loss must be systematically excluded. The patient's history may suggest bone loss secondary to hyperthyroidism, primary hyperparathyroidism, chronic glucocorticoid excess (hyperadrenalism or hypercorticism), myeloma, or osteomalacia. Therefore, a thorough history is essential in making the differential diagnosis and should include the following:

1. *History of Acute Illness.* Onset and duration of symptoms; location and radiation of pain; exacerbating and remitting factors; relationship of pain to posture, activity, time of day
2. *Review of Related Symptoms.* Malaise; recent weight loss or weight gain; loss of height; hot flashes; changes in visual fields; purpura or acne; amenorrhea; hypertension; goiter or neck swelling; change in voice, skin texture, or hair consistency; sensitivity to temperature change; palpitations; epigastric pain or burning, change in bowel habits, diarrhea, loose or bulky foul-smelling stools; dysuria, flank pain, fever, renal colic, nephrolithiasis; joint pain or swelling; generalized bone pain or muscle weakness; psychiatric problems
3. *Medical and Personal History.* Menstrual history, pregnancy, lactation, oophorectomy; thyroidectomy; pituitary surgery; ulcer or bowel surgery; surgery for cancer, spinal disorders (e.g., scoliosis), or bone or joint fractures
   Medications: Anticonvulsants; tranquilizers; antimetabolites; vitamins and minerals; nutritional supplements; contraceptives; thyroid hormone replacement; glucocorticoids
   Dietary history: Daily intake of dairy products, protein, alcohol; any discomfort with ingestion of dairy products; abuse of laxatives
   Activity level: Daily weight-bearing activity; work history (physical or sedentary); exercise; sports; activity limitations; prolonged immobilization; exposure to sunlight
4. *Family History.* Osteoporosis; bone or joint disorders; other growth disturbances; fractures; blue sclerae; deafness; scoliosis; childhood dental problems; joint laxity
5. *Radiographs.* Anteroposterior and standing lateral radiographs of the thoracic and lumbar spine should be considered along with bone density analysis (see Plate 3-31).

Routine laboratory tests include a complete blood cell count and leukocyte differential; determination of

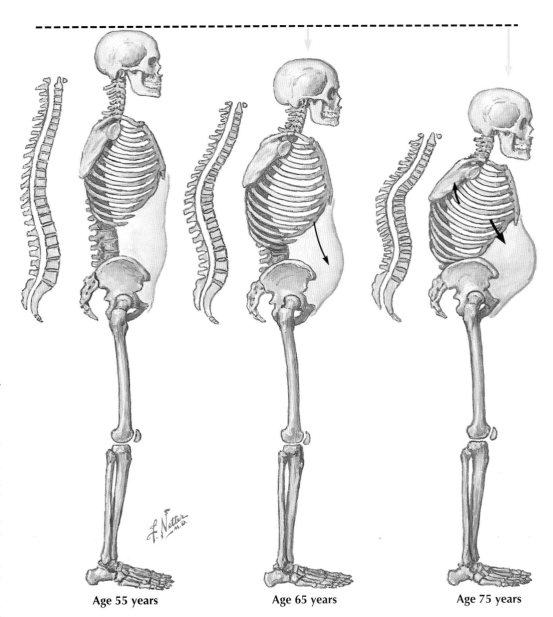

PROGRESSIVE SPINAL DEFORMITY IN OSTEOPOROSIS

Age 55 years   **Age 65 years**   **Age 75 years**

Compression fractures of thoracic vertebrae lead to loss of height and progressive thoracic kyphosis (dowager's hump). Lower ribs eventually rest on iliac crests, and downward pressure on viscera causes abdominal distention.

the erythrocyte sedimentation rate; 24-hour urinalysis for calcium; and evaluation of serum calcium, phosphate, alkaline phosphatase, blood urea nitrogen, and creatinine levels. Concentration of 25(OH)D accurately reflects the total body stores of vitamin D. In uncomplicated postmenopausal osteoporosis, results of routine laboratory tests are normal. Even in severe postmenopausal disease, serum calcium, phosphate, and alkaline phosphatase levels are usually within the normal range.

If bone loss secondary to conditions other than age-related and postmenopausal osteoporosis is suspected, additional tests are performed as necessary. For patients with suspected primary or iatrogenic hyperthyroidism, thyroid hormone and TSH levels should be obtained. Serum or urine protein electrophoresis is required when multiple myeloma is suspected. In patients with hypercalcemia, PTH levels should be measured.

Osteomalacia must be considered in the differential diagnosis of osteopenia (see Plates 3-13 and 3-14). Osteomalacia should be suspected in a patient with myopathy, bone pain and tenderness, and symmetric long bone fractures. Because abnormalities of vitamin D absorption and metabolism often play a role in the pathogenesis, serum levels of 25(OH)D and 1,25(OH)₂D should also be ascertained. A fluorescent microscopic examination of undecalcified trabecular bone tissue obtained by a transiliac bone biopsy after double-tetracycline labeling is occasionally needed (see Plate 3-33). Noninvasive diagnostic techniques to monitor the progression of bone loss and the response to treatment include quantitative assessments of bone mineral content (see Plate 3-32). The technetium-99m methylene diphosphonate bone scan or magnetic resonance imaging (MRI) is useful in documenting new fractures.

Plate 3-30

Musculoskeletal System: PART III

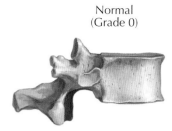

Normal
(Grade 0)

RADIOLOGY OF OSTEOPENIA

Radiology of osteopenia, the identifiable demineralization of bone on an image, utilizes many technologies including radiographs, computed tomography (CT)/ quantitative computed tomography (QCT), MRI, quantitative ultrasonography (QUS), and dual-energy x-ray absorptiometry (DXA). Each technique has a role in identifying osteopenia and in identifying fractures that allows the clinical diagnosis of osteoporosis. The only radiologic technique that allows the diagnosis of osteoporosis using World Health Organization (WHO) criteria without the presence of a fracture is DXA. The other techniques can be utilized to either determine fracture risk, loss of trabeculae (architectural integrity) or cortical bone, and the presence of a fracture.

Radiography

The identification of osteopenia on a radiograph requires a significant, 30% or greater, loss of bone mineral. There are two general types of bone loss, and the differentiation between them determines whether osteopenia/osteoporosis is in the differential. Regional bone loss may be seen in post-traumatic events, such as fracture, transient osteopenia, and reflex sympathetic dystrophy. Generalized osteopenia is either involutional or senile. Osteopenia is also seen with other metabolic disease such as osteomalacia, hyperparathyroidism, hyperthyroidism, drug-induced bone loss, and osteogenesis imperfecta.

Bone loss is manifested on radiographs differently depending on the disease process and the ratio of cortical to trabecular bone. Trabecular bone is remodeled four to eight times faster than cortical bone, and in osteopenia/osteoporosis the vertebral (especially thoracic) bodies are the first bones to demonstrate demineralization. The appearance of a picture frame vertebral body, density of intervertebral disc equal to or greater than the vertebral body, and prominent vertical trabeculae all are radiographic signs of bone loss. Vertical trabeculae become prominent when secondary and tertiary trabeculae are resorbed with resultant hypertrophy of the vertical primary trabeculae. Osteopenia can be identified in any bone. When cortical bone loss is present, the osteopenia is more severe.

A radiologic technique known as the second metacarpal index can be used to determine cortical bone loss. The width of the midpoint of the second metacarpal is measured, and the width of the combined cortex is determined at the same level. If cortical combined thickness is less than 50% of the width of the diaphysis, then the bone is osteopenic.

Film-based radiographs are being replaced by digital images. Because of window and leveling capabilities that digital imaging workstations provide, it is possible to make normally mineralized bone look osteopenic.

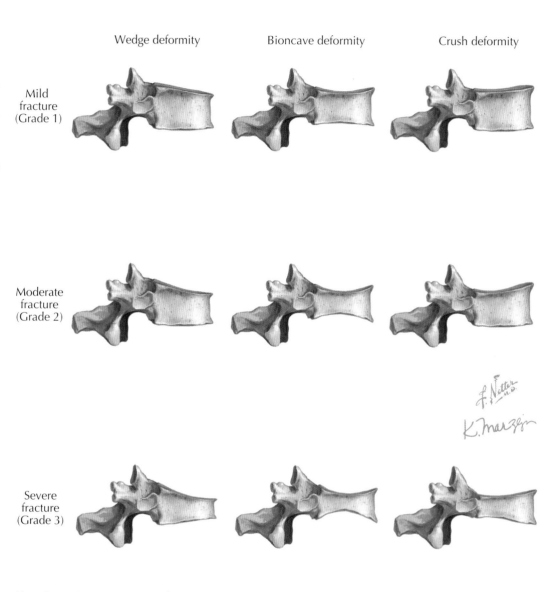

| | Wedge deformity | Bioncave deformity | Crush deformity |

Mild fracture (Grade 1)

Moderate fracture (Grade 2)

Severe fracture (Grade 3)

From Genant HK, Wu CY, van Kuijk C, Nevitt MC. *Vertebral fracture assessment using a semiquantitative technique.* J Bone Miner Res 1993;8:1137-1148.

Therefore, use of more reliable objective criteria than visual appearance of bone should be used to confirm demineralization.

Low-impact fractures that can be attributed to osteopenia are a significant finding and allow the diagnosis of osteoporosis without quantitative assessment of bone mass. The presence of a vertebral fracture on a radiographic image is termed *prevalent* if noted on the first film and *incident* if a new finding on subsequent radiographs. Vertebral fractures are classified as mild, 20% to 25% loss of height; moderate, 25% to 40% loss of height; or severe, greater than 40% loss of height. Height loss can be anterior, concave, or crush. Other traditionally associated fractures are the radius and the hip (see Plate 3-31). Fragility fractures are defined as a fall from standing height of the individual or less. Insufficiency fractures of the sacral ala, pubic ring, and ribs may also be seen in osteopenic patients. Fractures may be occult and require additional imaging for detection.

Plate 3-31

Metabolic Diseases

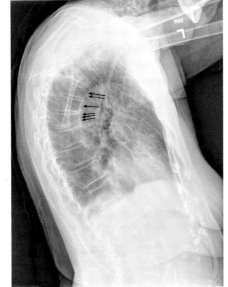
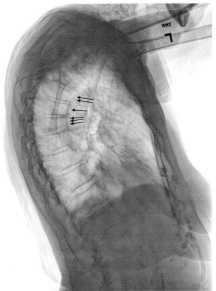

Vertebral compression fractures. One arrow, mild fracture; two arrows, moderate fracture; three arrows, severe fracture; conventional windowing (left) and inverted gray scale (right) can be useful to enhance the bone edge.

RADIOLOGY OF OSTEOPENIA
(Continued)

Dual-Energy X-ray Absorptiometry (DXA)

Quantitative techniques are used for assessment of BMD of the vertebral body: hip, radius, and calcaneus (see Plate 3-32). DXA is the only quantitative method to diagnosis osteoporosis using WHO criteria. The DXA scanner can determine bone density by generating two x-rays of different energies to determine mineral content. Additionally, DXA can be used for total body composition analysis and thoracolumbar fracture identification (see Plate 3-32). DXA results are expressed as T- and Z-scores. The T-score compares the patient's BMD to a young normal database determining the number of standard deviations from estimated peak bone mass, ages 20 to 30. The Z-score compares the patient's BMD to an aged-matched similar demographic reference database.

BMD determined by DXA is an areal measurement. The density in grams is divided by the area scanned to determine g/cm². Meticulous detail is necessary to ensure follow-up scans measure the same area and same size region of interest, ensuring that real change has occurred in patients being observed or treated. Changes in measured area can falsely alter the BMD. Guidelines for use of DXA are found in many sources; however, the most commonly used are those of the International Society for Clinical Densitometry, National Osteoporosis Foundation, and Medicare Guidelines.

Quantitative Computed Tomography (QCT)

QCT utilizes software and a phantom with existing CT scanners. The two general techniques employed are single slice and spiral CT acquisition. With either technique BMD is volumetric; a volume is measured with BMD resulting in density as g/cm³.

A phantom is scanned with the patient or before the patient being scanned. The phantom contains several different hydroxyapatite densities along with fat and soft tissue equivalents. A regression curve from phantom data is generated so the density of the patient can be determined using Hounsfield units from the scanner compared with the curve. Each manufacturer of QCT software develops its own normative database to determine the T-score of the patient compared with young normal data. The T-score using QCT is always lower than that seen with DXA because the QCT generally measures density of trabeculae. The WHO definition of osteoporosis (T-score < −2.5) is based on DXA not QCT. QCT can also measure cortical bone alone or

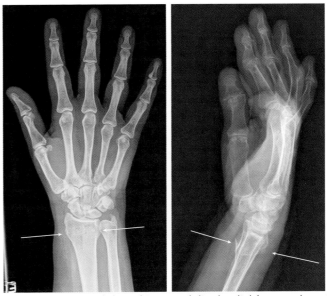

Impacted distal radial fracture PA view (left) and impacted distal radial fracture, lateral view (right)

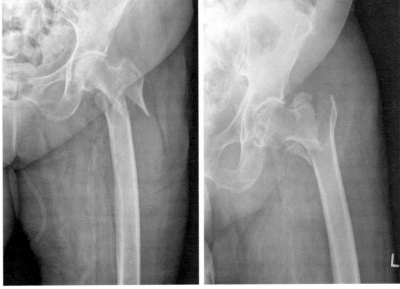

Two-part intertrochanteric fracture (left) and four-part intertrochanteric fracture (right)

Plate 3-32

Musculoskeletal System: PART III

RADIOLOGY OF OSTEOPENIA
(Continued)

cortical and trabecular bone together. Follow-up studies require meticulous detail to ensure precise results. QCT has been used to measure vertebral body, distal radius, and hip density.

CT can identify fractures and is used to determine occult fracture in patients who cannot undergo an MRI. Fractures can also be identified incidental to another study. A star in the sky appearance in a vertebral body indicates secondary and tertiary trabecular resorption and primary trabecular hypertrophy and is consistent with demineralization. Using reconstruction algorithms, trabecular volume and thickness can be determined demonstrating bone loss and structure changes. This technique has been used in the spine, distal radius, hip, and calcaneus, as well as other bones. In addition, CT as well as fluoroscopy guidance has been used in vertebroplasty and kyphoplasty.

Quantitative Ultrasonography (QUS)

QUS, unlike diagnostic ultrasonography, uses a transmitting and receiving transducer. Frequencies are higher than used for diagnostic ultrasonography. The measurement reflects structure and mineral content by determining ultrasound attenuation and speed of sound. The measurement is reported as a T-score.

The most common site of measuring bone is the calcaneus followed by the distal radius. Many other bones have been assessed without benefit of reference databases. This technology can be used to assess fracture risk but cannot be used to observe patients for density changes or treatment efficacy.

Magnetic Resonance Imaging (MRI)

Magnetic resonance imaging is used clinically to identify occult fractures that are not visualized on plain radiographs. MRI demonstrates bone marrow edema and the fracture line whether it may be partial or complete. MRI uses different sequences that result in identifiable signal characteristics dependent on radiofrequency and length of time the radiofrequency is on and off. Magnetic gradients allow the computer to reconstruct anatomy based on small differences in precession frequency of protons in the gradients. The energy that changes the position and frequency of the proton precession in the gradients applied is released by the protons returning to their normal alignment in the main magnetic field. The energy is detected by a receiving antenna, and the signal is reconstructed into an image.

Clinically, MRI is used to differentiate between osteoporotic and pathologic vertebral fractures and identify occult osteoporotic fractures of other bones, most commonly nondisplaced fractures of the hip.

MRI research, using signal intensity and spatial density, can be used to determine trabecular volume, density, and connectivity. Structural models can be reconstructed for three-dimensional rendering of trabeculae. Unfortunately, the calculation of these volumes and densities with structural models have yet to be useful for fracture prediction in individuals even though they relate to bone strength.

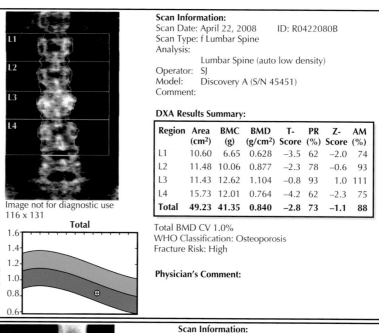

Scan Information:
Scan Date: April 22, 2008   ID: R0422080B
Scan Type: f Lumbar Spine
Analysis:
            Lumbar Spine (auto low density)
Operator: SJ
Model: Discovery A (S/N 45451)
Comment:

DXA Results Summary:

Region	Area (cm²)	BMC (g)	BMD (g/cm²)	T-Score	PR (%)	Z-Score	AM (%)
L1	10.60	6.65	0.628	–3.5	62	–2.0	74
L2	11.48	10.06	0.877	–2.3	78	–0.6	93
L3	11.43	12.62	1.104	–0.8	93	1.0	111
L4	15.73	12.01	0.764	–4.2	62	–2.3	75
Total	**49.23**	**41.35**	**0.840**	**–2.8**	**73**	**–1.1**	**88**

Image not for diagnostic use
116 x 131

Total BMD CV 1.0%
WHO Classification: Osteoporosis
Fracture Risk: High

Physician's Comment:

(graph labeled "Total", BMD axis 0.6 to 1.6)

AP spine DXA. The T-score is consistent with a DXA diagnosis of osteoporosis in this patient. Note the L3 vertebral body density is significantly higher than the other vertebral bodies because of degenerative changes. In practice this vertebral body would not be included in the BMD analysis.

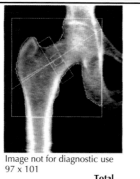

Scan Information:
Scan Date: April 22, 2008   ID: R0422080A
Scan Type: f Right Hip
Analysis:
            Right Hip
Operator: SJ
Model: Discovery A (S/N 45451)
Comment:

DXA Results Summary:

Region	Area (cm²)	BMC (g)	BMD (g/cm²)	T-Score	PR (%)	Z-Score	AM (%)
Neck	5.07	3.49	0.688	–1.9	72	–0.7	87
Troch	11.62	7.54	0.648	–0.9	85	–0.1	99
Inter	15.20	16.33	1.075	–0.8	88	0.1	101
Total	**31.90**	**27.36**	**0.858**	**–1.1**	**83**	**–0.2**	**96**
Ward's	1.17	0.66	0.562	–1.9	67	–0.0	100

Image not for diagnostic use
97 x 101

Total BMD CV 1.0%
WHO Classification: Osteopenia
Fracture Risk: Increased

Physician's Comment:

(graph labeled "Total", BMD axis 0.2 to 1.6, Age axis 20 25 30 35 40 45 50 55 60 65 70 75 80 85)

Right hip DXA. The lowest T-score is consistent with a diagnosis of osteopenia in this patient.

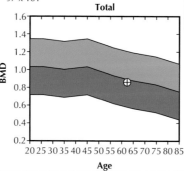

Region [1]	Avg. Ht. [2] (cm)	Z-Score	M/P Ratio [2] (%)	Z-Score	A/P Ratio [2] (%)	Z-Score
T8	1.63	–0.3	95	0.7	92	0.3
→T9	1.26	–3.4	67	–3.9	66	–4.1
L1	2.31	0.2	96	0.4	92	–0.5
L2	2.41	0.3	96	0.5	98	–0.2
L3	2.38	–0.1	101	0.9	114	2.0
L4	2.36	–0.2	96	0.4	102	–0.5

→Severe Wedge

T8
T9 Severe Wedge
L1
L2
L3
L4

Comments:

Image for vertebral deformation assessment only
Printed: 2/21/2008 3:30:11 PM (11.40)76:3.00:22.24:54.0 0.00:18.72
1.20x1.05 25.4:%Fat=13.2%
0.00:0.00 0.00:0.00
Filename: 1rgetj6g08.dfm
Scan Mode: Standard 83.0 µGy

1 -Reference based on L2, L3, and L4
2 -The precision (±1SD) is 1 mm for heights and 0.05 for ratios

Plate 3-33   Metabolic Diseases

TRANSILIAC BONE BIOPSY

The use of undecalcified histologic sections of bone (see Plate 3-33) has facilitated the diagnosis of metabolic bone diseases. Because metabolic bone diseases are generalized skeletal disorders, a small sample of bone is representative of the entire disease process. The iliac crest region is a readily accessible biopsy site and has been shown to reflect changes that may be occurring at more clinically relevant sites, such as the spine or the long bones. Commercially available trocars ranging from 5 to 8 mm in diameter are used to remove a core, or cylinder, of bone from the anterior portion of the iliac crest. Optimum biopsy samples contain both cortices and intervening cancellous bone in a single, unfragmented cylinder. The sample is taken transcutaneously, under local anesthesia.

Histologic Analysis of Undecalcified Bone. Because the differentiation between the two major metabolic bone diseases, osteoporosis and osteomalacia, is based in part on the quantity and quality of bone mineral, the ability to distinguish between calcified and uncalcified bone matrix (osteoid) is critical. The traditional procedures for processing bone for histology requires decalcification to facilitate sectioning. To preserve the distinction between mineralized bone and osteoid, tissue can be processed without decalcification, embedded in plastic, sectioned on a heavy-duty microtome, and stained with a trichrome connective tissue stain to produce thin histologic sections suitable for microscopic examination.

Osteomalacia is the consequence of insufficient mineralization, so undecalcified sections show an increase in the proportion of unmineralized bone compared with normal bone. The overall bone volume (density) may be normal but is often decreased. The overall amount of osteoid can also be increased in metabolic states characterized by increased bone turnover in general. Differentiation between these states is based on the determination of mineralization rates, using tetracycline as an in vivo bone marker.

Dynamic Tetracycline Labeling. Tetracycline antibiotics are autofluorescent and bind to immature bone mineral. These properties can be used to quantify the rate of bone mineralization, an index that can help determine if the increased osteoid in a biopsy is due to a mineralization defect (osteomalacia) or increased bone remodeling in general. One dose of a tetracycline based on the rate of bone mineralization is administered for 3 days, followed by a second 3-day dose about 14 days later. The bone biopsy is obtained 3 to 4 days after the last dose of tetracycline, and tetracycline fluorescence is evaluated on unstained, nondecalcified tissue sections by ultraviolet light. The first course of tetracycline appears as a discrete fluorescent band within the mineralized bone. The second, more recently administered course of tetracycline is located at the current mineralization front.

The mean distance between the midpoints of the tetracycline labels is measured, and this divided by the number of days between the two courses of tetracycline indicates the mineral appositional rate, which normally ranges from 0.4 to 0.9 μm/day (mean = 0.65 μm/day). This represents the amount of new bone synthesized and mineralized over the tetracycline-free interval.

When the mineral appositional rate increases, the distance between the labels grows wider. In contrast, with a reduced mineralization rate, the parallel bands become narrow and may fuse to produce single labels.

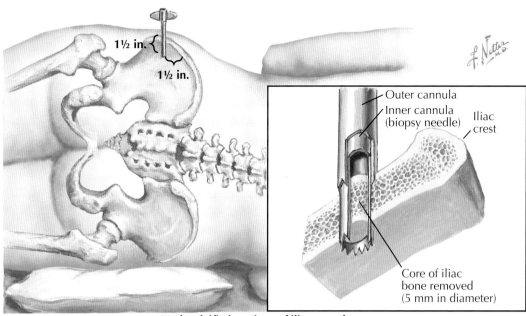

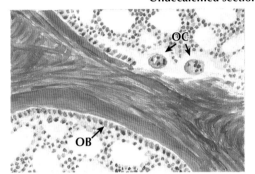

Red-staining osteoid seams (hypomineralized matrix) lined with osteoblasts (OB). Osteoclasts (OC) are in resorption bays (Masson's trichrome).

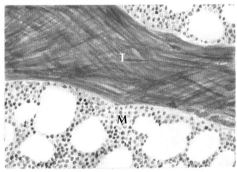

Section shows few osteoid seams, osteoblasts, or osteoclasts, indicating little bone formation or resorption.

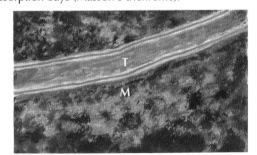

Yellow lines (tetracycline deposition at mineralization front), seen on fluorescent microscopy after 2 courses of tetracycline, indicate normal mineralization.

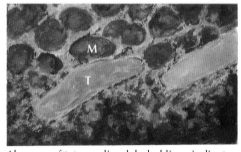

Absence of tetracycline-labeled lines indicates lack of bone formation.
T, trabecular bone; M, marrow

Abnormal patterns of fluorescent label deposition are the hallmark of osteomalacia. The amount of tetracycline fluorescence is proportional to the amount of immature amorphous calcium phosphate deposits in the mineralizing foci of the osteoid seam. If osteoid seams are deficient in mineral, the osteoid is incapable of binding tetracycline, leading to an absence of fluorescence. The mineralization front activity (percentage of osteoid seams bearing *normal* tetracycline labels) is therefore reduced.

Bone Histomorphometry. This technique is the quantitative analysis of undecalcified bone, in which the parameters of skeletal remodeling are expressed in terms of volumes, surfaces, and cell numbers. To obtain these data from a two-dimensional section, the principles of stereology are used to reconstruct the third dimension. This statistical principle states that if

measurements are made at random, the ratio of areas is equal to the ratio of volumes. Although qualitative features of a bone biopsy can usually distinguish conditions of increased bone remodeling such as hyperparathyroidism from osteomalacia, histomorphometry can be helpful in individual cases as well as when following populations of patients as part of a prospective study.

Adynamic Bone. Some patients with osteoporosis, and on long-term therapy with antiresorptive agents, as well as some patients with chronic renal failure in whom PTH has been suppressed develop bone with a reduced rate of remodeling, a condition called "adynamic bone." Patients with adynamic bone may be at increased risk of fracture. Undecalcified biopsies in patients with adynamic bone show features of low remodeling, including minimal osteoid, few osteoclasts, and low bone formation and mineralization rates.

Plate 3-34

Musculoskeletal System: PART III

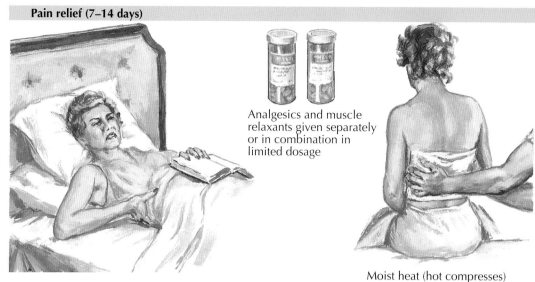

Pain relief (7–14 days)

Analgesics and muscle relaxants given separately or in combination in limited dosage

Moist heat (hot compresses)

Bed rest only as long as necessary

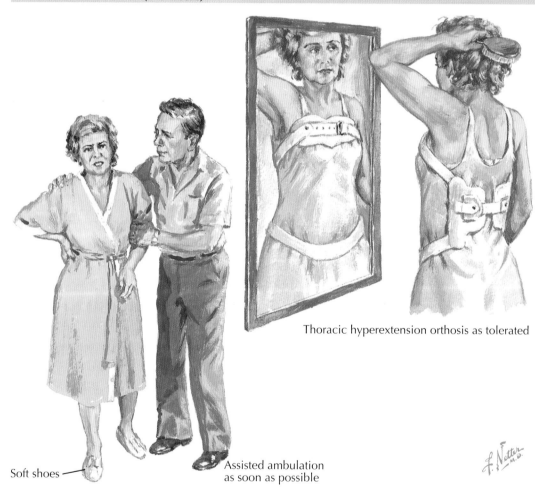

Gradual mobilization (2–5 weeks)

Thoracic hyperextension orthosis as tolerated

Soft shoes

Assisted ambulation as soon as possible

TREATMENT OF COMPLICATIONS OF SPINAL OSTEOPOROSIS

MANAGEMENT OF VERTEBRAL FRACTURES

Acute pain after a vertebral fracture usually resolves in 4 to 6 weeks. Simple and narcotic analgesics, muscle relaxants, short periods of bed rest, and physical therapy are useful. Spinal orthotics such as Jewitt and Cash orthoses are three-point (sternum, pubic symphysis, lumbar spine) hyperextension contact braces used to reduce kyphosis and relieve pain. Postural training may help to decrease kyphosis, move the center of gravity backward, and encourage the use of back extensor muscles. Patients should be shown how to avoid unnecessary spinal compressive forces in lifting and bending. They should take great precautions to prevent falls. After 6 to 8 weeks, most patients are relatively pain free and can resume normal activity.

Operative Management

Two percutaneous treatment options for painful vertebral compression fractures—vertebroplasty and kyphoplasty—involve the injection of polymethyl methacrylate (PMMA) into a compressed vertebral body. Studies show that the procedures may restore vertebral height especially if performed within 6 to 12 weeks of the fracture and relieve pain. Kyphoplasty employs a balloon tamp to create a cavity into which the PMMA is injected. Compared with vertebroplasty, which does not utilize a balloon, kyphoplasty allows for greater fill of the vertebral body and height restoration with lower risk of PMMA extravasation. The mechanism of pain relief is not proven, but micromotion of fractured vertebral bodies may be a source of pain and is reduced after the procedure. Complications include PMMA extravasation (up to 30% with vertebroplasty and 10% with kyphoplasty), which can result in neurologic sequelae, embolization to the vertebral venous plexus and to distant sites, and possibly adjacent vertebral fractures. These procedures appear to be most effective if performed soon after fracture. One study that compared vertebroplasty and kyphoplasty showed little difference between the two procedures and recommended vertebroplasty based on the higher cost of kyphoplasty.

Plate 3-35   Metabolic Diseases

TREATMENT OF OSTEOPOROSIS

Recommendations for Treatment

In 2008, the WHO opened the online fracture risk assessment calculator (FRAX) (World Health Organization fracture risk assessment tool, http://www.shef.ac.uk/FRAX/) and the National Osteoporosis Foundation (NOF) released new guidelines for the prevention and treatment of osteoporosis in the United States. Previous guidelines were based on previous fracture, T-score, and risk factors but did not apply to men, lacked weighting of risk factors, did not account for the effect of age on fracture risk, and expressed fracture risk as "relative risk" and not "absolute risk." More than 50% of all fractures occur in individuals who have low bone mineral density (BMD) (osteopenia = T-score between −1.0 to −2.5), not osteoporosis. Risk factors plus BMD allows selection of higher-risk patients needing treatment.

The 2008 NOF guidelines are based on the FRAX calculator, which expresses fracture risk as a 10-year probability of fracture. Treatment is recommended if bone density T-score is less than −2.5 at the hip or spine, if the patient has had a hip or vertebral fracture, or with a T-score between −1.0 and −2.5 at hip or spine if there is a 10-year fracture risk of 3% or more for a hip fracture or 20% or more for a major osteoporosis-related fracture (humerus, forearm, hip, or clinical vertebral fracture). The WHO FRAX tool allows individual assessment for race in the United States and calculates fracture risk based on sex, height, previous fragility fracture as an adult, family history of a parent with a hip fracture, glucocorticoid use, rheumatoid arthritis, secondary osteoporosis, and alcohol use. The NOF guidelines and FRAX are applicable to previously untreated postmenopausal women and men older than age 50.

EVALUATION FOR SECONDARY OSTEOPOROSIS

Evaluation of patients requires attention to possible secondary causes for low bone mass. Individuals with low bone mass may have diseases or take medications that may increase the risk of osteoporosis. Laboratory investigations in patients with low bone mass reveal that up to 50% may have underlying disorders such as vitamin D deficiency or hypercalciuria. Laboratory tests to identify common causes of secondary osteoporosis include a complete blood cell count and differential, erythrocyte sedimentation rate, routine chemistry profile, 25-hydroxyvitamin D level, thyroid stimulating hormone, parathyroid hormone, and 24-hour urine for measurement of calcium excretion. Correction of the underlying cause may impact BMD and fracture risk.

NONPHARMACOLOGIC THERAPY

Patient and Physician Education. Education strategies coupled with appropriate follow-up and reinforcement can increase compliance. Education on fall risk, exercise programs, dietary advice including adequate calcium and vitamin D intake, and other life style modifications are an important first step. Propensity to fall should be undertaken, with modification of such risk factors through effective intervention when possible.

Exercise. Exercise induces skeletal mechanotransduction that increases bone strength by creating small gains in bone mass. Exercise in children appears to be

Antiresorptive	Bisphosphonates

Estrogen
 	
• WHI—Vertebral and hip fracture reduction
• DVTs, breast cancer, heart disease
 	
Estrogen agonist antagonist (SERM)(raloxifene)
 	
• Only vertebral fracture reduction
• DVTs
• Decreases breast cancer risk
 	
Bisphosphonates
 	
• Vertebral, nonvertebral, hip fracture reduction
• Oral
• Intravenous
• Osteonecrosis of the jaw, atypical femur fracture (both rare)
 	
Calcitonin
 	
• Only vertebral fracture reduction
• Weak, fracture reduction in doubt
 	
Denosumab
 	
• Vertebral, nonvertebral, hip fracture reduction
• Antibody to RANK ligand
• SC injection q6m
• Increased infection risk
	Oral
	
	• Fosamax
	  • Generic cheaper
	
	• Actonel
	  • Weekly and monthly
	
	• Boniva
	  • Monthly
	  • Registration trial did not demonstrate nonvertebral fracture effect
	
	Intravenous
	
	• Reclast
	  • Yearly, reduction in hip, nonvertebral, vertebral infusion center—20 min
	  • Atrial fibrillation
	
	• Boniva
	  • 3 months. Given as a push, no infusion pump
	
	• Pamidronate
	  • 3 months, rarely used

Indications for therapy in postmenopausal women and men over age 50

1. After hip or spine fracture
2. BMD T-score in spine or proximal femur ≤−2.5
3. BMD between −1 and −2.5 and one of the following:
    a. 10-year risk of major fracture of 20% or more*
    b. 10-year risk of hip fracture of 3% or more*
 	
* Calculated by FRAX® algorithm
Based on the 2008 Guidelines from the National Osteoporosis Foundation

most effective prior to attainment of peak bone mass especially combined with calcium intake. Moderate, regular weight-bearing exercise is essential for skeletal health, both for effects on bone strength and fall prevention.

Smoking, Alcohol, and Caffeine. Smoking is toxic to bone cells, and smokers have lower hip BMD and increased fracture risk. In postmenopausal women, bone density has been shown to be inversely correlated to pack-years of smoking and rates of bone loss were greater in smokers. Serum vitamin D levels were lower in smokers, and estradiol levels were lower in patients on estrogen replacement therapy. The Nurses' Health Study found that fracture risk fell after 10 years of abstinence from smoking. Excess alcohol, three or more drinks per day, is associated with lower bone mass and increased fall propensity. Excessive caffeine may decrease intestinal calcium absorption, lower dietary calcium intake, and induce hypercalciuria.

Calcium and Vitamin D. Prepubertal twins randomized to calcium supplements have been shown to have greater gains in BMD over a 3-year period than placebo patients. Calcium alone is not sufficient to prevent early postmenopausal bone loss but may slow the rate of loss. In the U.S. NHANES III survey, higher calcium intake

was associated with higher BMD in women. In men and women, BMD was shown to be higher with increasing 25(OH)D levels and vitamin D was the dominant predictor of BMD relative to calcium intake.

Vitamin D promotes calcium absorption from the gut, retention in the body, and incorporation into bone. Dietary sources of vitamin D are limited to certain fish products. Most of our vitamin D comes from dermal synthesis after ultraviolet light exposure. Doses of 800 to 1000 IU/day and in some instances larger doses may be needed. Severe vitamin D deficiency may cause osteomalacia and is associated with secondary hyperparathyroidism, decreased intestinal calcium absorption, and calcium loss from the skeleton to maintain serum calcium. Gains in BMD may be seen in individuals with correction of severe deficiency within several months. Patients supplemented with vitamin D have improved muscle function and fall risk.

Individuals with osteoporosis randomized to calcium and vitamin D significantly reduced the risk of vertebral, nonvertebral, and hip fractures. Oral vitamin D has been shown to reduce nonvertebral fractures by at least 20%.

Fall Prevention. Almost one third of persons aged 70 years and older will sustain a fall each year, with

Plate 3-36

Musculoskeletal System: PART III

TREATMENT OF OSTEOPOROSIS
(Continued)

higher numbers reported in women, older individuals, and nursing home residents. Falls are a major source of morbidity and increased mortality, and about 5% result in a fracture. Studies show fall risk is related to a history of falls, medications, or conditions that may predispose to falls including cognitive, visual or auditory impairments, decreased muscle strength, increased body sway, and poor balance. Such conditions are more prevalent in older individuals, and falls increase as the number of risk factors rises.

Modifiable risk factors that should be corrected include poor vision, hearing or cognition, and myopathies. Diseases including alcoholism, neuromuscular disorders, and dementia should be treated, and medications such as sedatives and hypnotics in elderly patients should be avoided. A multidisciplinary team approach to fall prevention can be effective. Adjustments to flooring and lighting, footwear, showers, bathtubs, and staircases, and avoidance of restraints should also be emphasized.

Hip Pads and Other Assistive Devices. Hip protectors have been shown to prevent hip fractures in compliant subjects at significant risk of falling. An observational study in nursing homes using hip protectors showed a 60% reduction in hip fractures. Assistive devices such as canes, walkers, and other gait stabilizers are useful.

PHARMACOLOGIC INTERVENTIONS
Antiresorptive Medications

Hormone Replacement Therapy. In postmenopausal women, bone turnover increases, the rate of bone resorption exceeds the rate of bone formation, and bone density decreases. In the Women's Health Initiative (WHI) trial of women unselected for osteoporosis on estrogen plus progesterone, there was a reduction of all fractures by 24% and a reduction of hip fractures by 33% compared with placebo. In the WHI trial of unopposed estrogen in postmenopausal women with a prior hysterectomy, the patients taking unopposed estrogen demonstrated a reduction in hip fracture of 39% and of vertebral fracture by 38%. Unopposed estrogen therapy is associated with an increased risk of endometrial cancer, and combined estrogen-progesterone hormone therapy is associated with increased risk of breast cancer.

Estrogen Agonist-Antagonists. Estrogen agonist-antagonists possess tissue specificity and bind to estrogen receptors. Depending on the target organ, these compounds may demonstrate estrogen antagonist or agonist effects. These agents inhibit bone resorption through mechanisms similar to estrogens without stimulating breast or uterine tissue. Raloxifene decreases bone turnover and increases bone density and has been shown to reduce vertebral fracture by 30% in subjects with a prevalent fracture and by 55% in subjects without a prevalent fracture. Raloxifene does not reduce the risk of nonvertebral fracture. Women receiving raloxifene have a higher risk of venous thromboembolism, leg cramps, and hot flashes. After 8 years of therapy with raloxifene the risk of invasive breast cancer was reduced by 66%.

Calcitonin. Calcitonin, a naturally occurring 32-amino acid polypeptide hormone, is secreted in response to high plasma calcium levels. Salmon calcitonin, administered both parenterally or as a nasal spray,

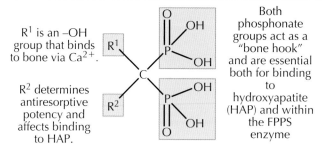

Functional domains of bisphosphonate chemical structure

R^1 is an –OH group that binds to bone via Ca^{2+}.

R^2 determines antiresorptive potency and affects binding to HAP.

Both phosphonate groups act as a "bone hook" and are essential both for binding to hydroxyapatite (HAP) and within the FPPS enzyme

Key Points
- The P–C–P moiety is common to all. The P–C–P backbone is sometime referred to as the "bone hook" and is essential for binding to calcium in hydroxyapatite.
- The R^1 group is important for binding to hydroxyapatite. R^1 is a hydroxyl (–OH) group for nearly all bisphosphonates currently used in osteoporosis.
- The R^2 group is what differentiates the actions of the bisphosphonates. The R^2 group is critically involved in both FPPS enzyme inhibition and additional mineral binding effects. The R^2 group is different for each BP and contributes to the unique chemical and pharmacologic properties of each drug.

Background
- Phosphonate: or phosphonic acid, an organic compound containing one or more $C–PO(OH)_2$ or $C–PO(OR)_2$ (with R=alkyl, aryl) groups (the phosphorous is bound to carbon)
- Phosphate: an inorganic salt of phosphoric acid, H_3PO_4 (phosphorus is not bound to carbon)
- Phosphorus: the chemical element that has the symbol P and atomic number 15
- Pyrophosphate: the anion, the salts, and the esters of pyrophosphoric acid, $H_4P_2O_7$

From Russell RGG. *Bisphosphonates: from bench to bedside. Annals of the New York Academy of Sciences.* 2006;1068:367-401.

Inhibition of FPP synthase

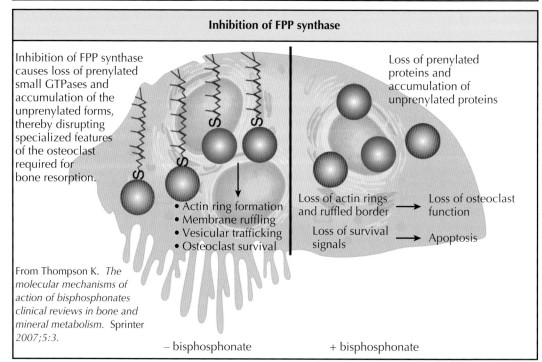

Inhibition of FPP synthase causes loss of prenylated small GTPases and accumulation of the unprenylated forms, thereby disrupting specialized features of the osteoclast required for bone resorption.

- Actin ring formation
- Membrane ruffling
- Vesicular trafficking
- Osteoclast survival

Loss of prenylated proteins and accumulation of unprenylated proteins

Loss of actin rings and ruffled border → Loss of osteoclast function

Loss of survival signals → Apoptosis

From Thompson K. *The molecular mechanisms of action of bisphosphonates clinical reviews in bone and mineral metabolism.* Sprinter 2007;5:3.

– bisphosphonate   + bisphosphonate

is used as therapy for the treatment of postmenopausal osteoporosis. Nasal calcitonin, 200 IU/day, reduced vertebral compression fractures by 33%; no reduction in hip fracture or other nonvertebral fractures was seen. Calcitonin may have analgesic effects on bone pain in patients with osteoporosis.

Bisphosphonates

Introduction and Mechanism of Action. Bisphosphonates are synthetic analogs of pyrophosphate. They suppress osteoclast-mediated bone resorption. They bind avidly to bone, a property that is primarily related to the R1 side chain (an OH group for nitrogen-containing bisphosphonates) that functions as a "bone hook." The R2 side chain determines the compound's potency and contains the nitrogen group common to all potent bisphosphonate compounds. The nitrogen-containing bisphosphonates (alendronate, risedronate, ibandronate, pamidronate, and zoledronate) interfere with the mevalonate pathway by inhibiting the enzyme farnesyl pyrophosphate. This prevents protein prenylation, the attachment of a lipid

Plate 3-36

Metabolic Diseases

TREATMENT OF OSTEOPOROSIS
(Continued)

anchor in the membrane, which inhibits osteoclast recruitment and differentiation, formation of the ruffled border, and acid production and induces apoptosis.

Pharmacologic Properties. Bisphosphonates are poorly absorbed; less than 0.7% is absorbed into the bloodstream. Food and liquids (except plain water) inhibit the absorption within the first 120 minutes after dosing. Approximately 50% of the dose is retained in the skeleton, and the remainder is excreted in the urine. Patients with impaired renal function, creatinine clearance less than 30 mL/min, retain a greater amount of the dose in the skeleton.

Bisphosphonates decrease fracture risk in patients at high risk for fracture, including those with prevalent vertebral fractures and/or low BMD.

1. **Alendronate.** Alendronate was approved for prevention and treatment of osteoporosis in 1995. In postmenopausal women with low BMD (femoral neck T-score < −1.6) and prevalent vertebral fracture (Fracture Intervention Trial Vertebral Fracture Arm (FIT 1) treated for 3 years, alendronate reduced vertebral, hip, and wrist fractures by 50% and multiple vertebral fractures by 89%; all nonvertebral fractures were reduced by 19%.

2. **Risedronate.** Risedronate was approved for prevention and treatment of osteoporosis in 2000. In clinical trials in postmenopausal women with previous fractures treated for 3 years, vertebral fractures were reduced by 41% and 49% and nonvertebral fractures were reduced by 33% and 39%, respectively (VERT-NA and VERT-MN). Multiple vertebral fractures also were reduced by 77% and 96%, respectively. A trial with hip fracture as a primary end point showed a reduction in hip fracture of 30% ($P = .02$).

3. **Ibandronate.** Ibandronate was approved for the prevention and treatment of osteoporosis in 2003. After 3 years, new morphometric vertebral fractures were reduced by 62%. Nonvertebral fractures were not reduced. The drug is also approved for use as an intravenous medication given every 3 months.

4. **Zoledronate.** Intravenous zoledronate was approved for the prevention and treatment of osteoporosis in 2007 and is given as a once-yearly intravenous infusion. After 3 years, new morphometric fractures were reduced by 70%, nonvertebral fractures by 25%, and hip fractures by 41%. All-cause mortality was reduced by 28% in a post–hip fracture population.

Side Effects with Bisphosphonates. Gastrointestinal side effects include nausea, esophageal erosions, and stricture. Patients with esophageal motility disorders and esophageal stricture are at greater risk for toxicity.

Intravenous administration of bisphosphonate associated with an influenza-like illness may be seen for 24 to 48 hours after infusion and is characterized by fever, myalgia, arthralgia, and nausea. Some patients have severe bone pain with bisphosphonates. Osteonecrosis of the jaw with bisphosphonates was first reported in 2003, usually in cancer patients treated with high doses of intravenous bisphosphonates. The incidence of this disorder with oral bisphosphonates is about 1 per 100,000 patients treated. Before bisphosphonate therapy, if teeth need to be pulled, a delay in treatment initiation is appropriate. Atypical fractures occurring in the femur shaft have been reported in patients on long-term bisphosphonate therapy.

Denosumab

Receptor activation for nuclear factor-kB ligand (RANKL), a member of the tumor necrosis factor (TNF) family, is a mediator of bone remodeling. RANKL binds to RANK, a receptor on osteoclast membranes, and induces differentiation, activation, and survival of osteoclasts. A regulator of RANK-RANKL is the soluble cytokine osteoprotegerin (OPG). OPG is a naturally occurring member of the TNF receptor family that functions as a decoy receptor by competing for binding to RANK.

Denosumab is a fully human monoclonal IgG2 antibody that binds selectively to RANKL. It was approved for the treatment of postmenopausal women at high risk for fracture in 2010. Patients given denosumab as a subcutaneous injection every 6 months had a 68% reduction in spine fractures, a 40% reduction in hip fractures, and a 20% reduction in nonvertebral fractures. Denosumab differs from the bisphosphonates:

bone turnover markers decline rapidly, as soon as 12 hours after an injection, and have a more rapid recovery after discontinuation, and there is no accumulation in bone as with bisphosphonates. Cellulitis was reported in the trial.

Parathyroid Hormone

Anabolic therapy with teriparatide (rhPTH 1-34) was approved in the United States in 2002 and is available in the European Union, as is rhPTH 1-84 ([1-34]PTH and [1-84]PTH).

Teriparatide is indicated for postmenopausal women and men who are at high risk for fracture. Recombinant hPTH (1-34) treatment in postmenopausal women for 19 months increased BMD by 9.7% in the lumbar spine and reduced vertebral fractures by 65% and nonvertebral fractures by 53%. A comparison of BMD response of teriparatide and alendronate at 18 months showed an areal BMD (DXA) increase of 10.3% with teriparatide and 5.5% with alendronate. Volumetric density (QCT) increased 19.0% with teriparatide and 3.8% with alendronate.

PTH and alendronate were compared as single agents or in combination. Alendronate with PTH blunted the BMD increase of PTH. The effects of teriparatide after 18 to 36 months of therapy with either raloxifene or alendronate showed patients previously treated with raloxifene had a greater increase in lumbar spine BMD in response to teriparatide than patients previously treated with alendronate (10.2% vs. 4.1%, respectively). A study comparing previous risedronate and alendronate on PTH response showed that previous alendronate therapy blunted both bone density and bone marker response to PTH significantly more than prior risedronate. After 12 months of therapy with teriparatide, subjects who received prior risedronate showed a 76% greater increase in QCT of trabecular bone at the spine compared with those who previously received alendronate.

Side Effects. Adverse effects from the use of rhPTH (1-34) include dizziness and leg cramps. Mild hypercalcemia is common (11%), but treatment was discontinued only very rarely. In a toxicology study, rats treated with high doses for long duration developed osteosarcoma. There has been no signal of an increased risk of osteosarcoma in humans treated with teriparatide.

Plate 3-37

Musculoskeletal System: PART III

OSTEOGENESIS IMPERFECTA

Osteogenesis imperfecta (OI), also referred to as "brittle bone disease," comprises a family of heritable disorders of connective tissue that are related to defects of type I collagen. The latter is a heterotrimeric protein composed of two $\alpha1(I)$ polypeptide collagen chains and one $\alpha2(I)$ polypeptide collagen chain, each of which undergoes extensive molecular processing before secretion from cells and the formation of mature, cross-linked collagen fibrils in the connective tissue extracellular matrix. Most cases involve mutations of either the *COL1A1* or *COL1A2* genes that code for the two polypeptide chains of type I collagen. However, in view of the numerous processing steps that are required to make mature collagens it is not surprising that recent research revealed mutations in noncollagen genes that are important in post-translational modifications, folding, or intracellular transport of the COL1A1 and COL1A2 polypeptides.

Overall, OI occurs with a prevalence of approximately 1 in 15,000 to 20,000 births. Cases due to mutations of the *CO1A1* or *COL1A2* genes occur in an autosomal dominant manner; more than 1,500 mutations of *COL1A1* and *COL1A2* are described that cause an abnormality of the quantity or structure of type I collagen. In contrast, OI that is caused by absent or defective function of a type I collagen modifying or chaperone protein occurs on an autosomal recessive basis. In view of the heterogeneity of genetic causes of OI and the diversity of mutations of those loci, it is not unexpected, therefore, that there is marked phenotypic heterogeneity of the various forms of OI. Clinical features that are common to all forms of OI include low bone mass, decreased bone strength, and increased bone fragility.

Historically, an influential early classification of the OIs was developed in the 1970s by Silence and colleagues. Current classifications include the Silence types I to IV, updated by current molecular understanding, as well as additional types that are defined on the basis of the underlying defect of the collagen modifying or chaperone gene or by histology. Type I OI comprises about 50% of cases, is due to null mutations of *COL1A1* that are autosomal dominant, and is characterized by normal stature, blue sclerae, and a propensity for fractures (see Plate 3-37). Fractures commonly occur once an affected individual begins to walk (and falls); the frequency of fractures decreases after puberty and then increases again in the fifth decade of life. The number of fractures experienced varies considerably, and fractures usually heal without deformity after appropriate management. Some persons have joint hypermobility that may progress to osteoarthritis. Other physical findings include progressive hearing deficit in about 50% of adults with OI type I. Dentinogenesis imperfecta is uncommon in this form of OI.

OI type II is the perinatal lethal form of OI, although some fetuses die in utero. Affected infants are short and underweight for gestational age and have short and bowed or deformed long bones that have sustained fractures in utero. The calvaria of an affected child is relatively large and undermineralized with a very large anterior fontanel and the sclerae are blue or gray. Most affected infants die in the first week of life, usually from pulmonary insufficiency or pneumonia related to a small thorax and rib fractures. The skeletal abnormalities of OI type II are evident by prenatal ultrasonography. Autosomal dominant mutations of either *COL1A1* or *COL1A2* cause OI type II. Because of the lethal

OSTEOGENESIS IMPERFECTA TYPE I

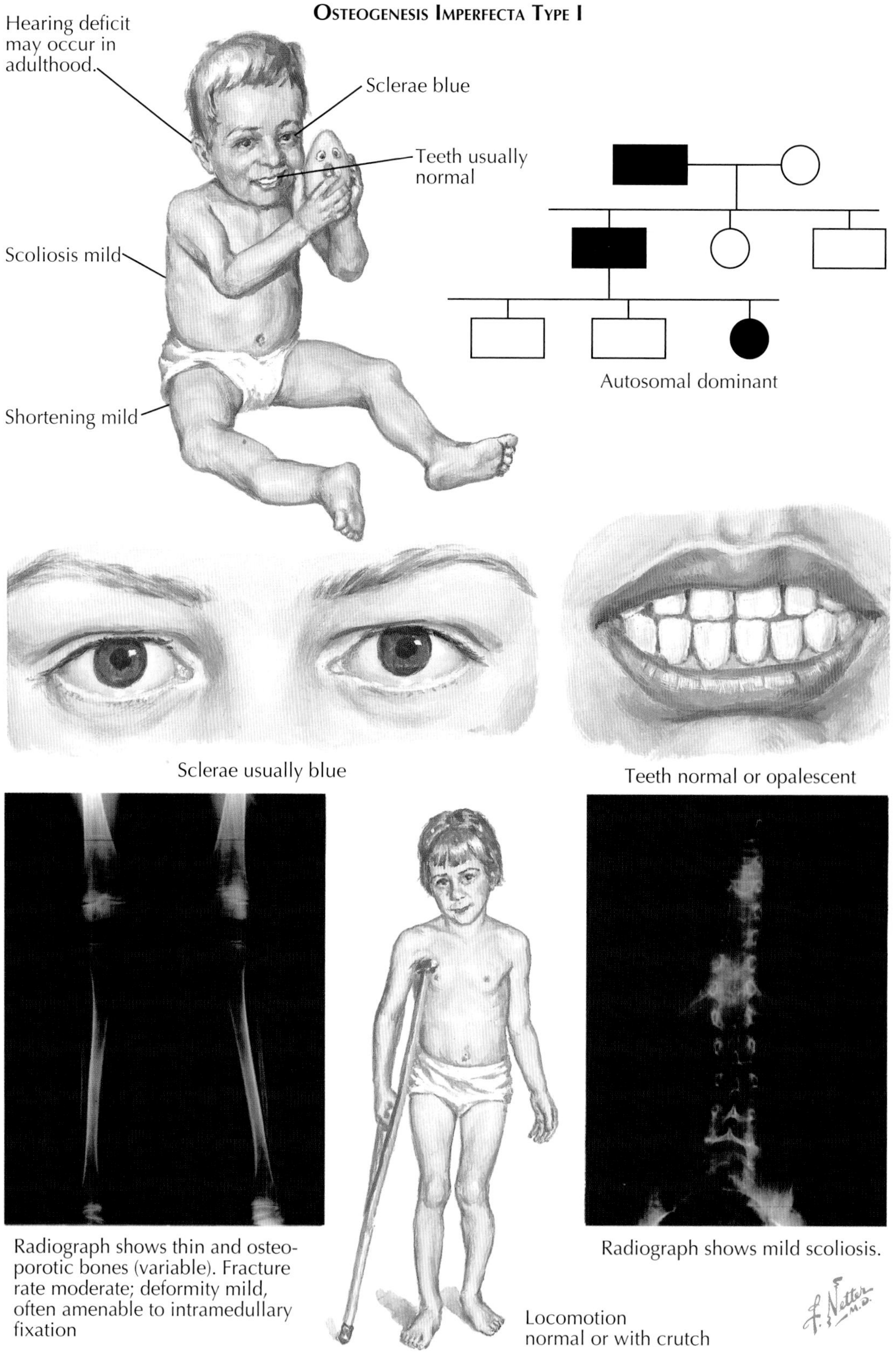

Hearing deficit may occur in adulthood.

Sclerae blue

Teeth usually normal

Scoliosis mild

Shortening mild

Autosomal dominant

Sclerae usually blue

Teeth normal or opalescent

Radiograph shows thin and osteoporotic bones (variable). Fracture rate moderate; deformity mild, often amenable to intramedullary fixation

Locomotion normal or with crutch

Radiograph shows mild scoliosis.

nature of this type of OI, most affected neonates have de novo mutations, although germline mosaicism has been reported.

OI type III, often termed the *progressive deforming* type of OI, is the most severe nonlethal form of OI; survival into adulthood can occur with this form. Affected individuals often have fractures at birth and may experience hundreds of fractures during life, even in the absence of apparent trauma. Physical findings include markedly short stature with vertebral compressions and scoliosis. Most affected individuals

are nonambulatory. Individuals with OI type III often have triangular facies, frontal bossing, blue or gray sclerae, and dentinogenesis imperfecta; hearing loss is also common and usually begins in the teenage years. Many have platybasia or basilar invagination, which is usually asymptomatic; when symptomatic, it can cause brainstem compression, obstructive hydrocephalus, or syringomyelia. Intellectual function is normal unless there has been cerebral hemorrhage that resulted in cognitive dysfunction. Life expectancy may be reduced due to severe kyphoscoliosis and abnormal chest shape

Plate 3-38

Metabolic Diseases

OSTEOGENESIS IMPERFECTA
(Continued)

that, in turn, causes restrictive lung disease and right-sided heart failure. Radiologic findings include the presence of multiple fractures, long bone deformities, thin ribs, and osteopenia.

OI type IV, a moderately severe OI, is characterized by phenotypic variability that overlaps that of types I and III. Affected individuals are usually ambulatory, and stature is variable. Dentinogenesis imperfecta is common, as is adult-onset hearing loss; sclerae are normal or have a grayish hue. Life expectancy is normal. The radiographic findings are typically intermediate between those of OI types II and III. Like OI types II and III, OI type IV is due to autosomal dominant mutations of *COL1A1* or *COL1A2*.

Few cases of OI due to mutations in genes coding for proteins that modify or chaperone newly synthesized intracellular type I collagen are described to date. Thus far, most affected individuals have had severe or lethal forms, with marked short stature and multiple fractures. At least six different genes are responsible for these types of OI, all of which are inherited on an autosomal recessive basis.

The diagnosis of any form of OI requires detailed clinical and family histories in addition to a careful physical examination based on knowledge of the common and defining features of OI. Radiologic assessment is essential and should be done by a radiologist knowledgeable in syndromic conditions. Although biochemical assessment of skin fibroblast collagens was the first confirmatory test for OI, it is now possible to sequence *COL1A1* and *COL1A2* genes as an initial diagnostic tool. Analysis of radiolabeled fibroblast collagens still has diagnostic value in selected clinical contexts.

Management of OI focuses on therapies to minimize fractures and deformities, minimize disability, and promote overall health. Orthopedic management is the mainstay of treatment, along with physical therapy and exercise. In infants, the use of soft bandages is generally adequate for the management of fractures; in children and adolescents, more rigid splints or braces are needed. Significant deformities and recurrent fractures require fixation of the long bones with intramedullary rods. Where significant longitudinal bone growth is anticipated, use of extensible rods is desirable. Physical activity should be encouraged, and immobilization should be kept to a minimum. Scoliosis can be a severe problem in OI, necessitating early and continued attention to the spine. Because braces are usually ineffective, spinal fusion may be needed to avoid severe curvature. Basilar invagination occurs with high frequency in severe OI and when present is usually slowly progressive. It requires surveillance by cranial CT or MRI; surgical intervention, when undertaken, should be done at a center experienced in the procedures used. Proper positioning on the operating room table is an important consideration when general anesthesia is needed.

Hearing loss, when present, is usually a relatively late onset complication and is of a conductive nature, although there is sometimes also a sensorineural basis. Hearing aids can be helpful and, when inadequate, stapedectomy can be a useful option. Cochlear implantation can be helpful for some individuals with significant sensorineural hearing loss. Dentinogenesis imperfecta may require restorative coverage; other dental abnormalities may include malocclusion and abnormalities of

tooth eruption. Dental treatment should be done by dentists with expertise in dentinogenesis imperfecta.

Pharmacologic therapy for OI is evolving. Bisphosphonates are now widely administered to children with OI. Positive effects on bone histology are reported, but it is not yet clear if there is a decrease of long bone fractures and there are few data thus far indicating improved strength, motor function, or decreased pain. Treatment with recombinant growth hormone can produce significant increases in linear growth and may also result in improvement of bone histology and

vertebral DXA. There is ongoing research regarding many other therapies.

The psychosocial dimensions of living with a multiple-handicapping condition are important. OI support groups can be extremely helpful for affected persons and their families. In addition, genetic counseling regarding reproductive recurrence risk issues and reproductive options should be discussed, if desired. Overall, both the diagnosis and the coordinated care of the child or adult with OI require a multidisciplinary effort by persons with expertise in OI.

OSTEOGENESIS IMPERFECTA TYPE III

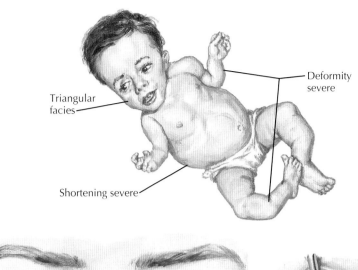

Triangular facies

Deformity severe

Shortening severe

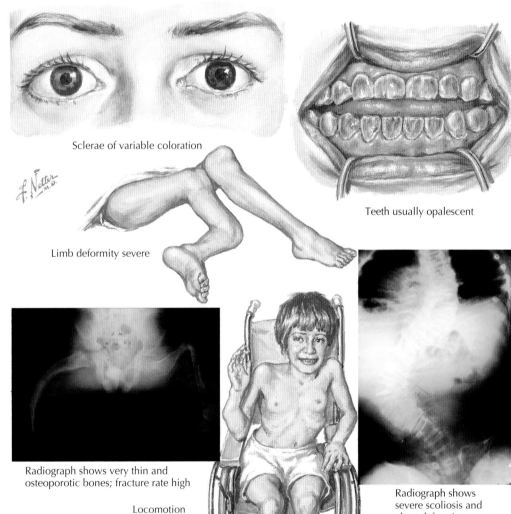

Sclerae of variable coloration

Teeth usually opalescent

Limb deformity severe

Radiograph shows very thin and osteoporotic bones; fracture rate high

Locomotion severely limited

Radiograph shows severe scoliosis and chest deformity.

Plate 3-39

Musculoskeletal System: PART III

MARFAN SYNDROME

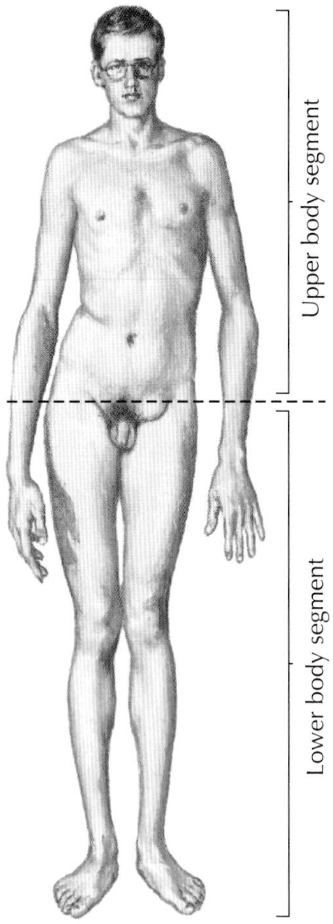

Marfan syndrome (MFS), first described by Antoine-Bernard Marfan in 1896, is a heritable and clinically variable disorder of connective tissue. Cardinal manifestations involve the cardiovascular, skeletal, and ocular systems, and its main features include disproportionate long bone overgrowth, ectopia lentis, and aortic root aneurysm (see Plate 3-39).

The prevalence of MFS is about 1 : 5,000 to 1 : 10,000 persons, with no enrichment in particular ethnic or racial groups or by gender. It is caused by mutations in the fibrillin-1 gene, *FBN1*, and is inherited in an autosomal dominant manner. Recent research indicates that at least part of the pathophysiologic basis of MFS is due to excessive activation of and signaling by transforming growth factor-β that occurs as a result of mutated fibrillin-1.

In 1986, an international group of experts developed clinical criteria for the diagnosis of Marfan syndrome. In 1991, mutations in *FBN1* were identified as the basis for MFS; and, in 1996, new diagnostic criteria, the Ghent nosology, were developed. Those criteria included both major and minor defining criteria, with major manifestations including ectopia lentis, aortic root dilatation/dissection, dural ectasia, or a combination of 4 or more of eight skeletal features. The diagnosis of MFS required major involvement of at least two organ systems and minor involvement of a third, but if an individual had an *FBN1* mutation associated with MFS or a first-degree relative with an unequivocal diagnosis, the diagnosis could then be made in the context of one major and one minor manifestation. These criteria proved extremely useful but had some limitations and, in 2010, the revised Ghent nosology for the diagnosis of MFS was developed. With these newer criteria, a diagnosis of MFS can be established for a proband not having a family history of MFS in four ways: if there is ectopia lentis and an *FBN1* mutation that has been previously associated with aortic enlargement or if there is aortic root enlargement (Z-score ≥ 2, standardized for age and body size) and either ectopia lentis, a pathogenic *FBN1* mutation, or a systemic score ≥ 7, with the latter referring to a score based on the combined presence of various physical findings that occur more commonly in persons with MFS. For individuals who have a family history of an unequivocal diagnosis of MFS, a diagnosis can be established if there is ectopia lentis, a systemic score > 7, or aortic root enlargement (with Z-score ≥ 2 for those ≥ 20 years or ≥ 3 for those < 20 years).

These diagnostic criteria highlight key clinical findings in MFS, but there is considerable additional clinical involvement that can commonly occur. Involvement of the eyes is highly variable. Myopia is the most common ocular feature, and often progresses rapidly during childhood. Ectopia lentis of varying degree occurs in about 60% of persons with MFS. Persons with MFS are also at increased risk to develop retinal detachment, glaucoma, and cataracts.

Skeletal manifestations are similarly diverse. Long bone overgrowth and joint laxity are hallmark features with limbs that are disproportionately long relative to the trunk. Scoliosis is common and, sometimes, progressive and severe. Chest wall abnormalities such as pectus excavatum or pectus carinatum are also common but usually not of major clinical significance. Other relatively common skeletal findings include pes planus, an acetabulum that can be excessively deep and

susceptible to an accelerated degenerative process, and a high and narrow palate with crowded dentition.

Abnormalities of the cardiovascular system are the major cause of significant morbidity and early mortality if MFS is untreated or treated late in its natural history. These include dilatation of the aorta at the level of the sinuses of Valsalva, predisposition for aortic dissection and rupture, mitral valve prolapse with or without regurgitation, and tricuspid valve prolapse. Each of these findings can be progressive. The risk of aortic dissection becomes significant as its diameter reaches 5 cm; secondary aortic regurgitation can develop as an aortic aneurysm enlarges. Secondary left ventricular dilatation and heart failure can occur with advanced mitral valvular dysfunction. These clinical concerns can

be minimized or prevented if diagnosis and appropriate care are provided early in the natural history of MFS.

There are numerous other clinical findings that occur with greater frequency in individuals with MFS. These include striae, inguinal hernias, lung bullae that can predispose to pneumothorax, and characteristic facial features. Stretching of the dural sac in the lumbosacral region—dural ectasia—occurs more frequently in MFS and can cause bone erosion and nerve entrapment and consequent low back and leg pain and, sometimes, additional symptoms.

The age at onset of the cardiovascular, skeletal, and ocular findings varies considerably; some features can be apparent at birth. Similarly, the pace of symptom development is variable, with a small minority of

Tall body habitus with disproportionately long extremities relative to the trunk (dolichostenomelia), scoliosis, chest wall abnormality (pectus excavation or carinatum), joint laxity, long digits (arachnodactyly), pes planus, and inguinal hernias

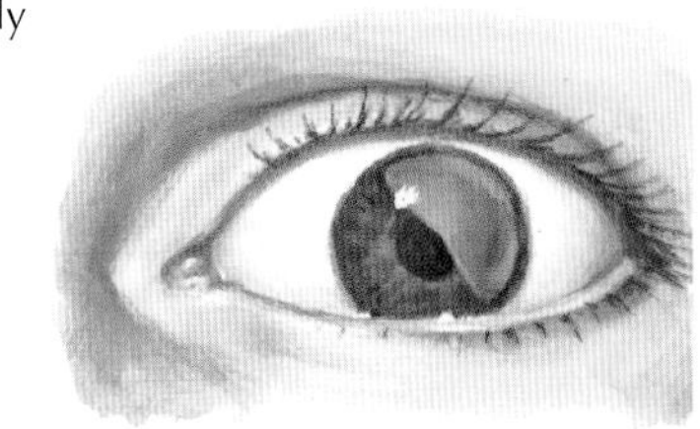

Upper body segment

Lower body segment

Ectopia lentis and myopia are common. Increased risk of retinal detachment, cataracts, and glaucoma

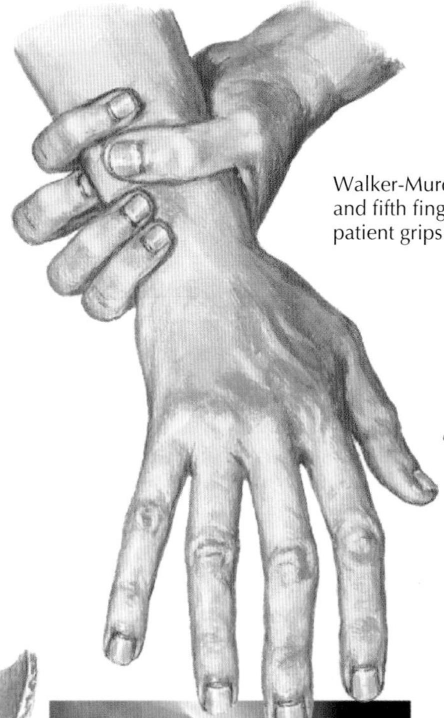

Walker-Murdoch sign. Thumb and fifth finger overlap when patient grips the wrist

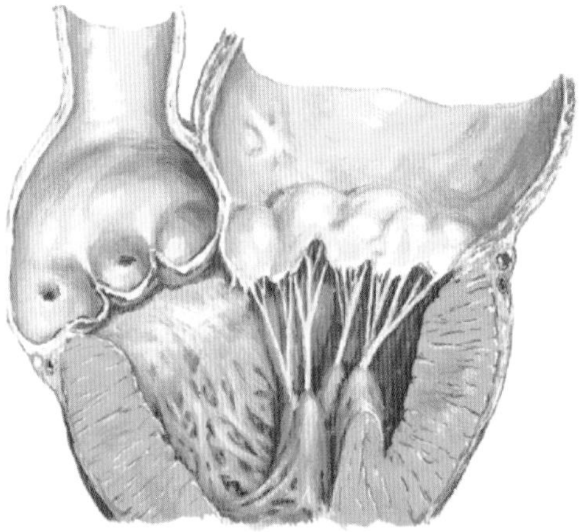

Increased risk if untreated for dilatation of aortic root due to cystic medial necrosis and for mitral valve prolapse with regurgitation

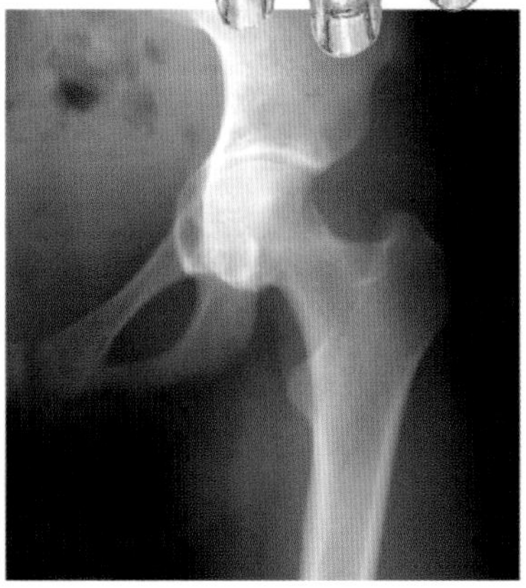

Radiograph shows acetabular protrusion (unilateral or bilateral).

Plate 3-40

Metabolic Diseases

MARFAN SYNDROME (Continued)

individuals having forms of MFS that are of early onset and that are rapidly progressive.

The diagnosis of MFS requires a careful clinical and family history, as well as a comprehensive physical examination. Knowledge of the many syndromic conditions that have phenotypical overlap with aspects of MFS is essential. In addition to use of the revised Ghent criteria, mutation analysis of *FBN1* is clinically available and has a high, but not 100%, diagnostic sensitivity. Several reasonable explanations for this incomplete diagnostic sensitivity include limitations of the diagnostic assays, genetic locus heterogeneity and, sometimes, incorrect clinical diagnosis. A majority of cases are inherited from an affected parent but about 25% of cases appear to be due to de novo mutations. However, not all individuals with mutations of the *FBN1* gene have MFS; several distinct disorders as well as individuals with "private syndromes" that are allelic to MFS are described.

The clinical management for persons with MFS requires multidisciplinary care. Evaluations by multiple specialists are recommended once a diagnosis is made, including detailed evaluations by an ophthalmologist, cardiologist, orthopedist, and medical geneticist, all of whom should have expertise in MFS. Specific testing that is recommended at that time includes slit-lamp ophthalmologic examination, intraocular pressure assessment, echocardiography, and selected radiographic tests such as evaluation of the entire aorta by magnetic resonance angiography or computed tomography and radiography of the spine.

There is a considerable literature on the medical and surgical management of the commonly occurring findings in MFS, as well as recommendations for surveillance of each at-risk organ system. Discussion of treatment of the common complications is beyond the scope of this review, but several clinical management issues merit comment.

The cardiovascular complications of untreated MFS can be severe and can lead to premature death. Normalization or near-normalization of lifespan and a marked reduction of cardiopulmonary-associated morbidity can be achieved if there is early attention to the medical and, if needed, surgical management of cardiovascular manifestations. Pharmacologic treatment with β-adrenergic blockade can prevent or decrease the progression of aortic dilatation by reducing the force of ventricular ejection, and there are specific recommendations regarding appropriate dosing. Specific criteria for when surgical repair of the aorta is indicated are also described. Surgical repair or replacement of the mitral valve is needed when there is refractory congestive heart failure due to mitral valvular disease.

There can be a significant acceleration of cardiovascular pathology in pregnant women with MFS, including a risk for rapid aortic root dilatation and dissection or rupture if the aortic root diameter exceeds 4 cm. Pregnancy should be considered only after appropriate counseling. Women with MFS who become pregnant must be carefully followed by a high-risk obstetrician

from the onset of pregnancy through delivery and the postpartum period. Beta-adrenergic blockers can be continued during a pregnancy, but certain other medications such as angiotensin-converting enzyme inhibitors or angiotensin receptor blockers should be discontinued before pregnancy because of potential teratogenic effects.

There are still other important issues in the lifelong clinical care for persons with MFS. Orthopedic surveillance is important; many individuals have chronic joint pain, and a subset of persons with MFS have significant scoliosis that requires surgical stabilization of the spine. Individuals with cardiac valvular pathology require antibiotic prophylaxis for bacterial endocarditis. There are also various situations that should be avoided, such

as contact and competitive sports and activities that will cause undue trauma to joints. Exposure to stimulants of the cardiovascular system and LASIK eye surgery should also be avoided.

Because MFS is an autosomal dominant condition, there may be others in the kindred who may be at risk to have this condition. Genetic counseling should accompany the diagnostic process. Medical genetics professionals can provide information not only about the diagnosis, natural history, and reproductive issues relating to MFS but also about relevant registries, clinical trials, and support groups. The latter, in turn, can provide important information, support, and, sometimes, access to resources for those affected with this condition and their families.

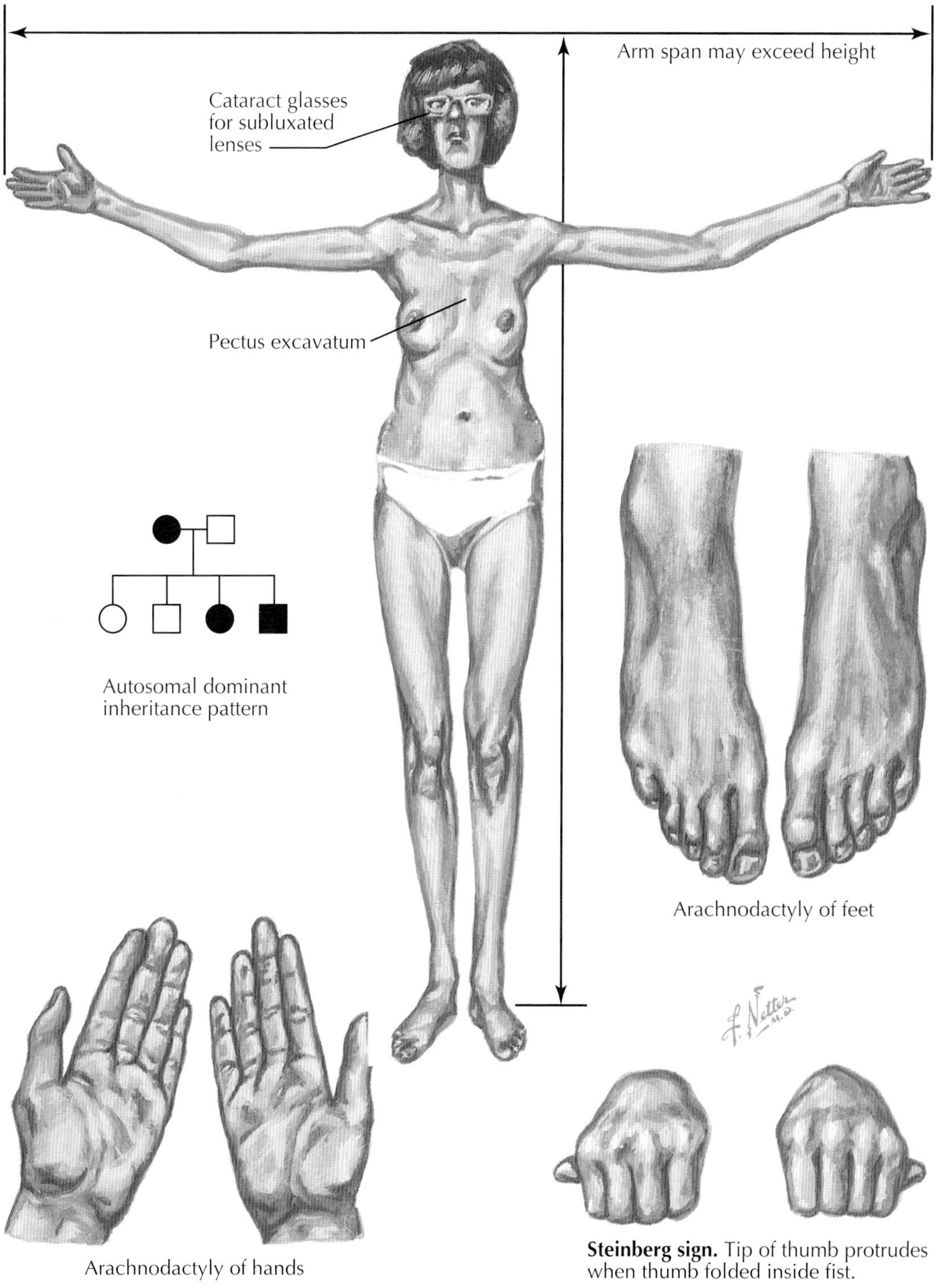

Arm span may exceed height

Cataract glasses for subluxated lenses

Pectus excavatum

Autosomal dominant inheritance pattern

Arachnodactyly of feet

Arachnodactyly of hands

Steinberg sign. Tip of thumb protrudes when thumb folded inside fist.

Plate 3-41

Musculoskeletal System: PART III

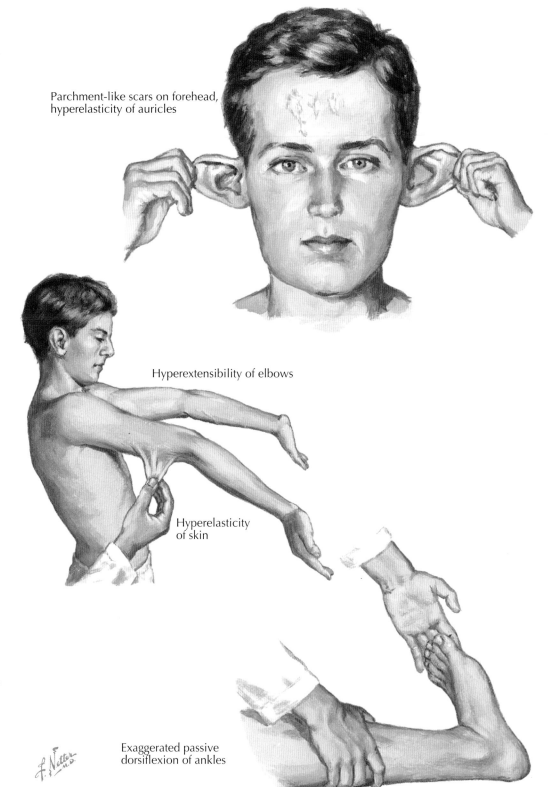

Parchment-like scars on forehead, hyperelasticity of auricles

Hyperextensibility of elbows

Hyperelasticity of skin

Exaggerated passive dorsiflexion of ankles

EHLERS-DANLOS SYNDROMES

The Ehlers-Danlos syndromes (EDS) comprise a genetically heterogeneous family of disorders that predominantly involve soft connective tissues. Hypermobility of joints, skin hyperextensibility, delayed wound healing, easy bruising, and increased fragility of soft connective tissues are common findings, but the severity of these features varies dramatically; specific clinical findings are relatively distinctive for different types of EDS (see Plate 3-41).

The birth prevalence of the EDS is about 1 in 5000 births, although this is likely an underestimate, particularly of milder forms. One commonly used classification recognizes six EDS types based on clinical features, modes of inheritance, and biochemical and molecular genetic findings. It is apparent, however, that many patients have clinical findings that overlap between recognized types and cases without a defined genetic etiology are not uncommon. Reconsideration of the nosology is needed and will require elucidation of as yet undescribed genetic etiologies. Nevertheless, in those forms of EDS with a defined etiology, the unifying features appear to be abnormalities in the expression or structure of the fibrillar collagens types I, III, and V. This is sometimes due to mutations in the genes of these collagens and in other instances due to mutations in genes coding for proteins involved in the post-translational modification or regulation of these fibrillar collagens.

The currently recognized major types of EDS include the following: classic type, hypermobility type, vascular type, kyphoscoliosis type, arthrochalasia type, and dermatosparaxis form. Classic EDS is characterized by hyperextensible, fragile, and soft skin, delayed wound healing with formation of atrophic scars, easy bruising, and generalized joint hypermobility. Hypermobility EDS is characterized by generalized joint hypermobility with frequent subluxations and dislocations and mild skin involvement. Vascular EDS is notable for characteristic facies, excessive bruising, thin and translucent skin, and a markedly increased risk of arterial, intestinal, and uterine fragility or rupture. Kyphoscoliotic EDS is notable for severe congenital hypotonia and kyphoscoliosis, generalized joint laxity, and risk of rupture of the globe. Arthrochalasia EDS is characterized by

congenital hip dislocation, severe generalized joint hypermobility with recurrent subluxations, skin hyperextensibility, and atrophic scars. The dermatosparaxis form of EDS is notable for characteristic facies, severe skin fragility, sagging and redundant skin, excessive bruising, growth retardation, frequent umbilical hernias, and delayed closure of the anterior fontanel.

Classic, hypermobility, vascular, and arthrochalasia types of EDS are associated with autosomal dominant inheritance; kyphoscoliosis and dermatosparaxis types

are inherited in an autosomal recessive manner. Heterozygous mutations in the COL5A1 and COL5A2 genes are noted in about 50% of persons with classic EDS and result in haploinsufficiency of type V procollagen. The most common subtype of EDS, the hypermobility type, is, in most instances, etiologically undefined, although heterozygous mutations of the TNX-B gene, coding for the extracellular matrix protein tenascin-X, have been reported. Vascular EDS is due to heterozygous mutations of the COL3A1 gene that result

Plate 3-42

Metabolic Diseases

Laparotomy scar from
previous GI rupture

Hyperextensibility of
thumb and fingers

Bruisability

EHLERS-DANLOS SYNDROMES
(Continued)

in deposition of a structurally abnormal type III collagen or in a diminished amount of normal type III collagen. Arthrochalasia EDS is associated with a loss of a procollagen-*N*-proteinase cleavage site on either proα1(I) or proα2(I) polypeptides due to heterozygous deletions of exon 6 of *COL1A1* or *COL1A2* genes, respectively. Kyphoscoliotic EDS is due to a deficiency of lysyl hydroxylase-I activity, an enzyme needed for collagen crosslinking, and which is due to homozygous mutations of the *PLOD1* gene. Finally, deficient activity of procollagen-*N*-proteinase due to mutations in the *ADAMTS-2* gene prevent the physiologic cleavage of the N-terminal of type I collagen and result in the dermatosparaxis type of EDS.

The diagnosis of any form of EDS requires a thorough assessment of an individual's clinical and family history and a comprehensive physical examination informed by familiarity with EDS and disorders in its differential diagnosis. Mutation analysis of candidate genes is the mainstay of diagnostic testing for most forms of EDS, although biochemical analyses of biosynthetically labeled fibroblast collagens I and III, measurement of selected enzymes involved in collagen post-translational modifications, and determination of urinary deoxypyridinoline and pyridoline can be helpful in specific contexts.

Management of EDS disorders is directed at preventative care and supportive therapy. In general, individuals with EDS should not participate in contact sports or heavy exercise. Non–weight-bearing exercise is encouraged, and physical therapy is recommended for persons with motor delays or significant hypotonia. Persons with marked skin fragility should cover particularly at-risk areas with protective pads. Individuals with mitral valve prolapse and regurgitation require antibiotic prophylaxis for bacterial endocarditis. Cardiovascular surveillance with echocardiograms is indicated for persons with any type of EDS for which cardiovascular involvement is common, as well as for persons with clinical signs or symptoms suggestive of cardiac

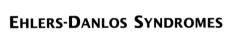

Genu recurvatum

pathology, although explicit guidelines are not yet available. Persons with vascular types of EDS require numerous precautions, including avoidance of contact sports and isometric exercise, avoidance of anticoagulant medications and antiplatelet agents, and avoidance of arteriography and other vascular procedures unless necessary. Because of vascular and skin fragility, surgeries should be done with extreme caution. Careful follow-up is recommended throughout pregnancy and postpartum, especially for pregnant women with

vascular type EDS who should be considered as high-risk patients. Psychosocial support for patients and their families is important and patient support groups are available and can be beneficial. Genetic counseling should be provided for pertinent family members who seek information about EDS, including information regarding reproductive risk and prenatal diagnosis. Overall, care for persons with EDS is best done by a multidisciplinary team with expertise in genetic connective tissue disorders.

Plate 3-43

Musculoskeletal System: PART III

OSTEOPETROSIS (ALBERS-SCHÖNBERG DISEASE)

First described by Albers-Schönberg, osteopetrosis is a family of closely related bone disorders characterized by defective osteoclast function and impaired bone resorption. Clinical features in osteopetrosis are heterogeneous, ranging from asymptomatic to fatal in infancy. Clinical classification is difficult due to extreme variability in clinical presentations and complications. Three distinct types of osteopetrosis are seen in humans, autosomal dominant (adult, benign, Albers-Schonberg disease) with few symptoms, autosomal recessive (infantile, malignant) often fatal during childhood, and X-linked inheritance patterns. The most frequent form is autosomal dominant. In this form of the disorder, disability is usually minimal and life expectancy is usually normal. The diagnosis is usually made when radiographs taken for another purpose reveal the dense, radiopaque bones that are characteristic of osteopetrosis (see Plate 3-43). Although most patients are asymptomatic, the risk of fractures is increased because there is a predominance of calcified cartilage rather than of calcified bone.

The most severe form of osteopetrosis is the congenital malignant form, which is inherited as an autosomal recessive disorder. Children usually present with recurrent infections and episodes of hypocalcemia, small medullary cavities that lead to and pancytopenia. Neurologic manifestations including retinal and brain degeneration are present. Death usually occurs in infancy or early childhood, and most patients die of the complications of anemia, bleeding, or infection.

Autosomal dominant osteopetrosis is milder, although 60% to 80% of patients have clinical manifestations. Onset is usually in adolescence. Radiographs of the spine show a "sandwich vertebra" that is diagnostic. A bone-in-bone appearance is often seen at the iliac wings. Fractures occur in about 80% of patients, with the femur most commonly involved. Hearing and visual loss occur in less than 5% of patients.

The hallmark of congenital malignant osteopetrosis is the complete failure of normal osteoclast activity. Defective osteoclastic bone resorption in the presence of normal osteoblastic bone formation results in an extreme excess of mineralized bone that encroaches on the intramedullary spaces. This leads to excessive extramedullary hematopoiesis with severe hepatosplenomegaly and a resultant anemia, thrombocytopenia, and white blood cell abnormalities. Osteoclastic dysfunction, together with loss of the medullary cavities and thickened bones, leads to encroachment on the cranial nerve foramina and neurologic complications, including optic atrophy, blindness, deafness, and any of the cranial nerve palsies. Cerebral atrophy and hydrocephalus have also been reported.

Most of the genes involved with human osteopetrosis are associated with the control of osteoclast intra- and extracellular pH. Genes the control pH include (1) the enzyme carbonic anhydrase (CAII), which catalyzes the hydration of CO_2 to H_2CO_3 and provides a source of hydrogen ions; (2) the α3 subunit of the vacuolar H^+-ATPase of the ruffled border; (3) the ruffled border Cl^- (ClCN7); (4) the ostm1 protein (OSTM1) association with Cl^- transport; and (5) plehkm1 protein (PLEHKM1) involved in vesicle trafficking and acidification. This impairment of acidification results in osteoclast inability to resorb both organic and inorganic matrix. Most patients with osteopetrosis have a normal

or increased number of osteoclasts that display no major morphologic defects but are unable to form a ruffled border, which is required for bone resorption. A few patients with osteopetrosis lack osteoclasts and likely have a defect in osteoclastogenic signaling, which in some patients is a result of mutations of the RANKL gene.

Osteoclasts are required during growth for modeling bones and enlarging the medullary cavity, in remodeling to replace woven with lamellar bone, and to remove damaged bone. The abnormalities in the medullary cavity result in hematologic manifestations. Optic and auditory nerve entrapment cause visual and auditory

defects. Persistence of calcified cartilage because of decreased resorption and inability to resorb and repair microdamage results in an abnormal skeleton that is prone to fracture.

Stem cell transplants are used to treat severe osteopetrosis. The age of transplantation is critical in determining outcome; transplantation before age 6 months is associated with better preservation of vision. Prenatal diagnosis and stem cell infusion before birth may present the best approach for a rescue in humans. Nonskeletal manifestations such as retinal atrophy and neurodegeneration may not be corrected with stem cell transplants in all genetic types of osteopetrosis.

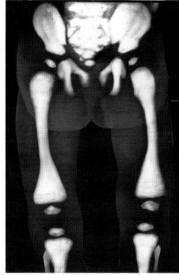

Radiograph shows marked increase in bone density, with medullary cavities obliterated.

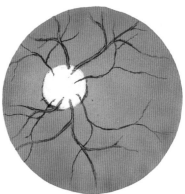

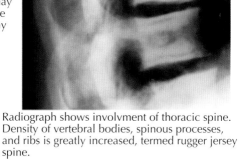

Liver and spleen greatly enlarged because of extramedullary hematopoiesis

Optic atrophy with blindness due to compression of nerve by bony encroachment of foramen. Deafness may also be caused by similar mechanism.

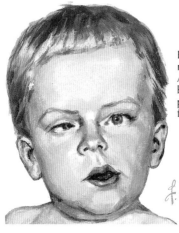

Facial and abducens nerve palsy may occur. Any cranial nerve may be compressed while passing through bony foramina.

Radiograph shows involvment of thoracic spine. Density of vertebral bodies, spinous processes, and ribs is greatly increased, termed rugger jersey spine.

Plate 3-44

Metabolic Diseases

PAGET DISEASE OF BONE

Paget disease of bone, or osteitis deformans, the second most common metabolic bone disease in the United States, was first described by Sir James Paget in 1876. It is a disorder that occurs in 2% to 7% of the population older than age 55 in North America and Western Europe. The disease occurs more frequently in men, and the incidence increases to approximately 10% by the ninth decade. It is uncommon before age 40, and its prevalence is estimated as affecting 1 million people older than age 65 in the United States. The highest prevalence of the disease is in the United Kingdom and in countries with large populations of British ancestry such as Australia, New Zealand, France, Germany, and the United States. The disease has been observed to occur in familial clusters, with 15% to 40% of patients with Paget disease reporting a positive family history.

Paget disease of bone is a localized skeletal disorder that is characterized by an increased number of osteoclasts that are large in size and contain multiple nuclei. These osteoclasts exhibit excessive activity and cause accelerated bone resorption that is tightly coupled to the recruitment of osteoblasts to the resorbed area. The result is excessive formation of disorganized osteoid tissue that is mechanically weaker, resulting in bone that is prone to deformity and fracture.

The clinical complications of the disease include bone pain, skeletal deformity, hearing loss, osteoarthritis, neurologic complications, and fractures. The skeletal sites most likely to be affected are the skull, spine, upper extremity, lower extremity, and pelvis.

Although oral bisphosphonates had been the most widely prescribed agents for the treatment of Paget disease, their use was limited by complicated dosing regimens and gastrointestinal complications. Fortunately, the advent of intravenous bisphosphonate therapy has revolutionized the treatment of this disease and has provided many patients with long-term remissions.

ETIOLOGY

The etiology of Paget disease remains unknown. Familial cases display an autosomal dominant pattern of inheritance with variable penetrance. Studies of familial patch disease have identified several susceptibility loci, including 2q36, 5q31, 5q35, 10p13, 18q21-22, and 18q23, whereas some recent investigations have focused on the sequestosome gene (SQSTSM1) on chromosome 5. However, nongenetic factors may also be involved. In 1974, some investigators demonstrated nuclear and cytoplasmic inclusion bodies in the osteoclasts of some patients with Paget disease that seemed to resemble viral particles. Electron microscopy confirmed the presence of pagetic osteoclasts with nuclear and cytoplasmic virus-like inclusion bodies resembling paramyxovirus nuclear capsids. However, this viral hypothesis remains controversial because multiple studies failed to demonstrate the presence of viruses in bone marrow cells or pagetic osteoclasts.

CLINICAL MANIFESTATIONS

Most patients with Paget disease do not initially present with clinical symptoms, and the diagnosis is frequently made as an incidental finding on radiographs or laboratory tests. Paget disease can affect one bone (monostotic) or multiple bones (polyostotic). The skeletal sites

Manifestations of advanced, diffuse Paget disease of bone (may occur singly or in combination)

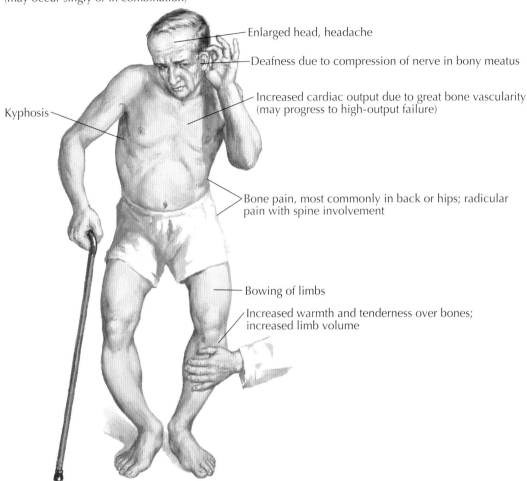

- Enlarged head, headache
- Deafness due to compression of nerve in bony meatus
- Increased cardiac output due to great bone vascularity (may progress to high-output failure)
- Kyphosis
- Bone pain, most commonly in back or hips; radicular pain with spine involvement
- Bowing of limbs
- Increased warmth and tenderness over bones; increased limb volume

Mild cases often asymptomatic (may be discovered incidentally on radiographs taken for other reasons)

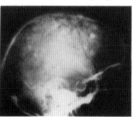

Lateral radiograph shows patchy density of skull, with areas of osteopenia (osteoporosis circumscripta cranii)

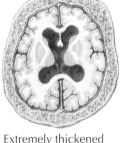

Extremely thickened skull bones, which may encroach on nerve foramina or brainstem and cause hydrocephalus (shown) by compressing cerebral aqueduct

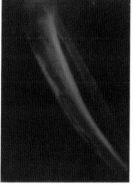

Characteristic radiographic findings in tibia include thickening, bowing, and coarse trabeculation, with advancing radiolucent wedge.

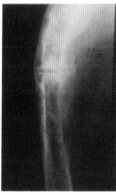

Healing chalk-stick fracture

most commonly affected are the pelvis (70%), femur (55%), lumbar spine (55%), skull (42%), and tibia (32%).

The skeletal deformities that can result include bowing of the long bones, increased skull size, dilated skull veins, hearing loss, and increased skin temperature over the affected long bones. Osteoarthritis with resultant pain of the knee or hip that occurs adjacent to the pagetic bone is commonly reported by patients with

Paget disease. The pain is frequently described as deep and aching and persists during the night, which may help differentiate it from other forms of osteoarthritis. Femur and tibia pain may be exacerbated by weight-bearing activity.

Involvement of the skull may be associated with headaches, tinnitus, vertigo, and dilated scalp veins. When the jaw is involved with Paget disease, dental complications can include loosening of the teeth or

Plate 3-45

Musculoskeletal System: PART III

PAGET DISEASE OF BONE
(Continued)

swollen gums. Spinal involvement may result in vertebral enlargement or compression fractures as well as kyphosis. Because of the disorganized osteoid tissue in Paget disease, the bone is prone to fracture after only minimal trauma. Long bones may be associated with transverse rather thin spiral fractures.

Hearing loss is a common complication of Paget disease and may be accompanied by tinnitus or vertigo in 20% of the patients. When the middle ear is involved, otosclerosis can result. Although neurologic complications are less common, they may result from pagetic bone impinging on intracranial or spinal tissue, and compression of nerves in the lumbar region may result in spinal stenosis or paraplegia. Involvement of the orbit may compress the optic nerve or interfere with function of the extraocular muscles.

When patients with Paget disease are immobilized, such as for surgery, hypercalcemia may result. Other conditions that have been associated with hypercalcemia in patients with Paget disease include fractures, hyperparathyroidism, hyperthyroidism, or unrelated carcinoma with skeletal metastases. Paget sarcoma is a rare complication occurring in fewer than 1% of cases and rarely before 70 years of age. Severe night pain in the area of previous pagetic involvement in an elderly patient as well as radiographic evidence of bone destruction should merit further evaluation for sarcoma.

DIAGNOSIS

Paget disease is diagnosed based on radiographic and biochemical findings. If radiographic findings are not diagnostic, further evaluation with computed tomography or MRI may be employed, but bone biopsy is rarely necessary for the diagnoses.

Radiologic appearance of Paget disease is characteristic and frequently diagnostic. In the early stages the disease is characterized by osteolytic lesions that appear as areas of bone loss in the skull or long bones. When the disease is left untreated, progression from the osteolytic phase to the combined lytic/sclerotic phase is demonstrated by cortical thickening, accentuated trabecular markings, and loss of corticomedullary distinction. The bone may appear abnormal in structure and is sometimes described as having a "cotton wool" appearance.

The key to the diagnosis of Paget disease is any elevated biochemical markers of bone turnover. These markers are helpful both in monitoring the disease progression as well as assessing response to therapy. The total serum alkaline phosphatase level is elevated in Paget disease, and other causes of elevated alkaline phosphatase including liver disease should be ruled out. The bone-specific alkaline phosphatase is elevated in up to 85% of patients with untreated Paget disease, and the levels may be related to the extensive skeletal involvement. Some patients with monostotic disease may exhibit normal serum alkaline phosphatase levels.

TREATMENT

The therapeutic goal in patients with Paget disease is to relieve symptoms such as bone pain and to prevent neurologic complications. In addition, medical treatment may be indicated for patients in whom surgery is planned in a region of pagetic bone in order to reduce

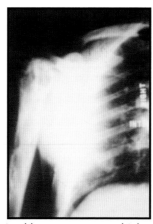
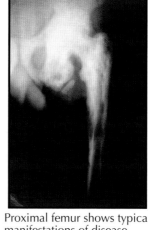
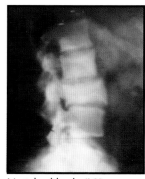

Vertebral body (L3) appears enlarged, with increased density.

Proximal humerus appears thickened and coarsely trabeculated, with patchy rarefaction.

Proximal femur shows typical manifestations of disease.

Above radiographs taken from same patient. Findings correspond to areas of increased isotope uptake in bone scan (right).

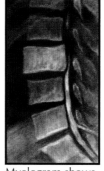
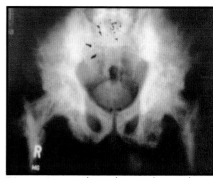

Myelogram shows obstruction of vertebral canal in L3.

Disease is seen throughout pelvis and proximal femurs, with involvment of hip joints.

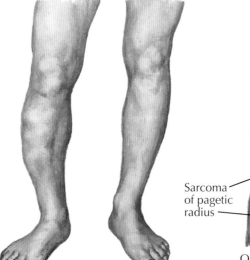

Disease may be monostotic, affecting only single bone or vertebra. Involvement of right tibia is evidenced by increased limb volume and bowing. Fibula is not involved.

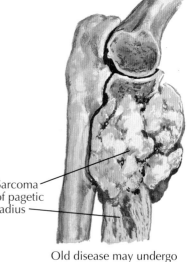

Sarcoma of pagetic radius

Old disease may undergo sarcomatous degeneration (<1% of symptomatic cases).

blood flow to the area. Treatment with antiresorptive agents can be considered for asymptomatic patients to reduce the likelihood of disease progression in the future risk of skeletal deformity, neurologic complications, hearing loss, or secondary osteoarthritis.

Nonsteroidal anti-inflammatory medications may be used to manage the pain associated with Paget disease. Because antiresorptive therapy is efficacious, surgical treatment should be limited to the management of fractures, deformity, and secondary osteoarthritis.

Antiresorptive Therapy

The goal of Paget disease therapy with antiresorptive treatment is to decrease the rate of bone turnover at the pagetic site. Therapeutic efficacy can be assessed by following the biochemical markers of bone resorption in formation.

Bisphosphonates remain the cornerstone for the treatment of Paget disease and have been demonstrated to be both efficacious and to have, in general, an acceptable safety profile.

Plate 3-46

Metabolic Diseases

PAGET DISEASE OF BONE
(Continued)

After either oral or intravenous administration, bisphosphonates bind to mineralized bone, and their antiresorptive strength is determined by the avidity of bone binding and the potency of their ability to inhibit osteoclast function. Earlier treatments with oral bisphosphonates including risedronate, etidronate, alendronate, and tiludronate are associated with several disadvantages, including complex dosing regimens over the course of several months, poor gastrointestinal absorption requiring fasting, and the potential for gastrointestinal side effects.

Although intravenous pamidronate has been available and efficacious, the requirement for a prolonged intravenous infusion over 4 hours for 3 consecutive days inhibits its use.

Zoledronic acid, a nitrogen-containing bisphosphonate, is a potent inhibitor of farnesyl pyrophosphate synthetase and induces osteoclast apoptosis. Zoledronic acid is given by intravenous infusion as a single 5-mg dose over a 15-minute period. Data indicate that a single 5-mg infusion of zoledronic acid results in remission in most patients with Paget disease for at least 24 months and possibly up to $6\frac{1}{2}$ years without further treatment. A transient acute phase reaction that is manifest as myalgias and fever may occur with any intravenous bisphosphonate infusion, although the symptoms rarely last more than 2 or 3 days and can be treated with acetaminophen or a nonsteroidal anti-inflammatory medication.

Therapeutic efficacy of bisphosphonate therapy in Paget disease can be defined as normalization of the serum alkaline phosphatase levels or a 75% reduction from baseline levels of alkaline phosphatase. Six months after the zoledronic acid infusion, 96% patient had reached the primary end point as compared with 74.3% of patients who were treated with oral risedronate. The pain score on the SF-36 improved in patients with zoledronic acid and risedronate treatment but was significantly greater with zoledronic acid compared with risedronate. The biochemical markers of bone turnover showed greater reductions with zoledronic acid then with risedronate in these comparative studies. In the first 3 days after infusion, 53.7% of patients receiving zoledronic acid reported adverse events compared with 25% of those receiving risedronate. The symptoms included flulike illness, myalgias, fever, fatigue, headaches, nausea, or bone pain, but after 3 days the rate of adverse events was comparable. Hypocalcemia can occur in patients after intravenous bisphosphonate treatment for Paget disease but seldom requires treatment. Patients should receive adequate calcium and vitamin D supplementation during the 2 weeks after zoledronic acid infusion. Zoledronic acid did not adversely affect renal function in patients with Paget disease if given over 15 to 20 minutes, but it should not be administered in patients with renal insufficiency with a glomerular filtration rate less than 35 mL/min. Studies are underway to assess the potential efficacy in Paget disease of denosumab, a monoclonal antibody that inhibits osteoclastogenesis by binding to RANKL. Denosumab is administered subcutaneously every 6 months.

PATHOPHYSIOLOGY AND TREATMENT OF PAGET DISEASE OF BONE

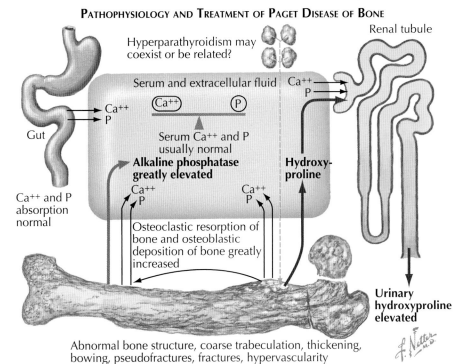

Abnormal bone structure, coarse trabeculation, thickening, bowing, pseudofractures, fractures, hypervascularity

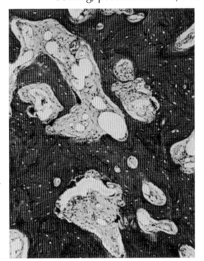

Section of bone shows intense osteoclastic and osteoblastic activity and mosaic of lamellar bone

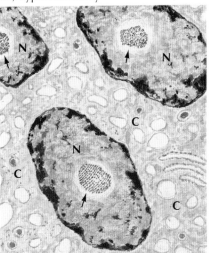

Electron-microscopic view of multinucleated osteoclast with nuclear inclusions that may be viruses (arrows). N = nuclei; C = cytoplasm

Therapeutic Agent	Zoledronic acid	Risedronate
Mode of Action	Both prevent osteoclast function by inhibiting the enzyme farnesyl pyrophosphate synthase, preventing formation of a ruffled border and hydrogen excretion and causing apoptosis	
Percentage of Patients with Response (6 months) (normalize alkaline phosphatase or >75% reduction)	96%	74%
Bone Turnover Markers	Significantly greater reduction and more rapid decline with zoledronic acid	
Quality of Life (SF36)	Significantly greater improvements in physical functioning, general health, emotional role, physical component summary with zoledronic acid	
Biochemical Relapse Rate (6.5 years)	0.7%	20%
Partial Relapse Rate (alkaline phosphatase 50% increase vs. 6 month value and 1.25 times upper limit of normal)	11%	55%

Plate 3-47

Musculoskeletal System: PART III

FIBRODYSPLASIA OSSIFICANS PROGRESSIVA

Heterotopic ossification is a pathologic condition that leads to bone formation in nonskeletal tissues. Fibrodysplasia ossificans progressive (FOP) is a rare heritable disorder, occurring with a frequency of 1 in 2 million individuals, in which bone is formed in connective tissues such as skeletal muscle, tendons, ligaments, and fascia. It is characterized by congenital skeletal malformation of the great toes, with episodes of painful soft tissue swelling that lead to severe progressive ossification of the soft tissues usually beginning in late childhood.

The gene mutation for patients with classic FOP is located on chromosome 2q23-24, a locus that includes the activin A type I receptor gene. Bone morphogenetic proteins (BMPs) are extracellular ligands that exert their effects by binding serine/threonine kinase BMP receptors that include activin A receptor, type I (ACVR1). Patients have heterozygous single nucleotide substitution (guanine to adenine at position 617), which results in a change of amino acid 206 from arginine to histidine. BMP signaling is responsible for induction of pathways that lead to endochondral bone formation. Fibrodysplasia ossificans progressiva may be inherited as an autosomal dominant disorder with full penetrance (no skipped generations) but variable expressivity (variable phenotypic expression of the gene in affected members of the same family) and no sexual or ethnic predilection. However, most cases arise as a spontaneous mutation.

Characteristic skeletal malformations of the feet include reduction defects (absent phalanges) in the toes, most commonly in the great toe. Congenital bunions are also common, and their presence suggests the possibility of the disorder long before heterotopic ossification begins. The limbs may be short, but this deformity is less prevalent than the toe anomalies. The congenital skeletal abnormalities cause few problems, and the affected child remains asymptomatic until heterotopic bone formation begins. This generally occurs by age 10 (the average age at onset is 4 years) with a series of firm, painful, asymmetric soft tissue lumps in the muscles of the neck and back. These lumps, which vary in size and shape, usually appear spontaneously but may be precipitated by trauma as minor as an intramuscular injection. The severity of FOP differs among patients, but most become immobilized and wheelchair bound by the third decade. Axial involvement precedes appendicular involvement; in the limbs, proximal ossification occurs before distal ossification. The muscles of mastication are often affected, but visceral smooth muscles, sphincters, diaphragm, larynx, tongue, extraocular muscles, and the heart are clinically uninvolved. There may be a conductive hearing loss, but ocular problems do not occur. Systemic signs of disease, such as fever and malaise, are usually absent. Flares may be spontaneous or precipitated by minor trauma such as intramuscular injections.

As heterotopic ossification develops in the soft tissues throughout the body, extra-articular ankylosis of the joints occurs, beginning proximally and axially, then progressing distally throughout the appendicular skeleton. Although longitudinal growth is normal, it may be masked by deformities caused by bony ankylosis of the spine and limbs. Paradoxically, osteoporosis resulting from immobilization may occur as the disease progresses, most notably about ankylosed joints. Fractures of the osteoporotic bone or the heterotopic new bone occur occasionally.

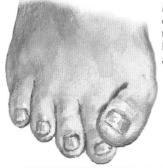

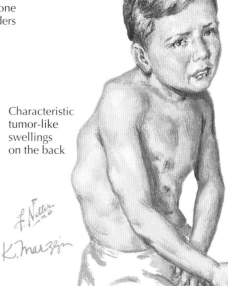

Malformed great toe, a characteristic feature that helps distinguish FOP from other bone and muscle disorders

Characteristic tumor-like swellings on the back

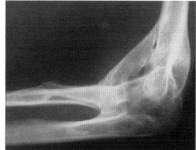

Mutation of the immune response causes fibrous tissue to ossify, as seen here in the elbow.

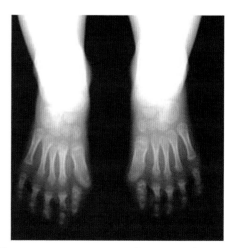

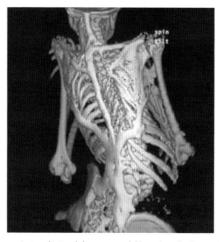

Characteristic clinical features of fibrodysplasia ossificans progressive (FOP). Left, Extensive heterotopic bone formation typical of FOP is seen on three-dimensional reconstructed computed tomography scan of the back of a 12-year-old child. Right, Anteroposterior radiograph of the feet of a 3-year-old child shows symmetrical great toe malformations. *From Shore EM, Xu G, Feldman GJ, Fenstermacher D, et al. A current mutationin the BMP type I receptor ACVR1 causes inherited and sporadic fibrodysplasia ossificans progressiva. Nature Genet 2006;38:525–527.*

Although clinical and radiographic findings are dramatic, laboratory studies of serum calcium, phosphate, and alkaline phosphatase, a complete blood cell count, and the erythrocyte sedimentation rate are normal.

Before clinical involvement, the muscles are histologically normal. Spontaneous edema of the interfascicular muscles occurs first, followed by proliferation of perivascular fibroblastic connective tissue. Involved muscle fibers degenerate rapidly and are replaced by a process of either intramembranous or endochondral ossification. Finally, formation of mature heterotopic lamellar bone that is indistinguishable from normal bone takes place. The disease process is true ossification, not calcification.

The mechanism by which the abnormal gene causes such protean regulatory defects is not known. Protein modeling of the glycine-serine domain of ACVR1 suggests that constitutive activation of ACVR1 with increased BMP signaling is the cause of the ectopic chondrogenesis and osteogenesis.

The diagnosis of FOP is based on clinical and radiographic findings. Primary malformations include the great toe almost always. Osteochondromas are common. Fusion of vertebral bodies occur. Femoral necks may be short but broad. Bone scans shows modeling and remodeling of the heterotopic bone. There is no increase in risk for fractures. There is no effective treatment, although administration of diphosphonates and glucocorticoids has been advocated. However, this treatment merely delays the mineralization of bone rather than impairing the production of heterotopic osteoid. Surgery may help a joint to fuse in a more functional position. Even in the late stages of the disease, patients should be considered severely disabled rather than ill. Genetic counseling should be provided to families in which the disease occurs.

CONGENITAL AND DEVELOPMENTAL DISORDERS

Plate 4-1

Musculoskeletal System: PART III

ACHONDROPLASIA – CLINICAL MANIFESTATIONS

Patients of various ages with body disproportion (short limbs, relatively long trunk, large head) and limited flexion of elbows and hips

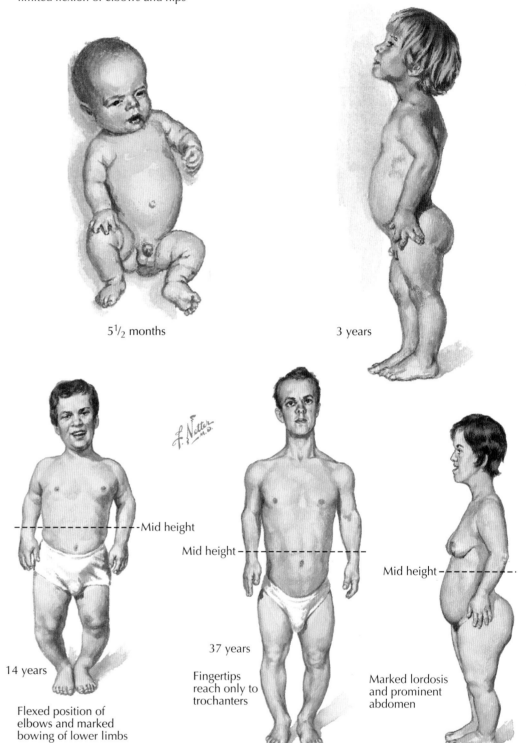

5½ months

3 years

14 years

Flexed position of elbows and marked bowing of lower limbs

Mid height

Mid height

37 years

Fingertips reach only to trochanters

Mid height

Marked lordosis and prominent abdomen

DWARFISM—OVERVIEW AND ACHONDROPLASIA

CLASSIFICATION

Although hereditary disorders of the skeleton are relatively rare, they attract a great deal of interest. Many of these disorders are associated with short stature, or dwarfism. Dwarfism can be either proportionate or disproportionate. Symmetric shortness of the trunk and limbs is common with proportionate dwarfism. Disproportionate dwarfism, in which either the trunk or limbs are more affected than the other, is common with skeletal dysplasias such as Kniest syndrome, spondyloepiphyseal dysplasia, achondroplasia, and so on.

Skeletal dysplasias, or chondrodystrophies, are a heterogeneous group of disorders resulting in short-limb or short-trunk types of disproportionate short stature. In the types of dwarfism that primarily affect the limbs, the shortening may predominate in the proximal segments (rhizomelia), the middle segments (mesomelia), or the distal segments (acromelia). The term *dwarf* has traditionally been applied to persons of disproportionate short stature, whereas the term *midget* referred to those of proportionate short stature.

Disproportionate dwarfism is caused by a hereditary intrinsic skeletal dysplasia, whereas proportionate dwarfism results from chromosomal, endocrine, nutritional, or nonosseous abnormalities. Over the past several years, we have gained further understanding regarding the mode of inheritance, the genetic defect, and the fundamental biochemical and/or molecular fault that causes the dysplasia. Many cases of dwarfism are the result of a rare genetic event, the spontaneous mutation. Unaffected parents of a child with a mutation are essentially at no risk of having another affected child, and unaffected siblings are not at risk of having children with the disorder. Affected parents may pass the trait on to their children, depending on the mode of inheritance—autosomal dominant, autosomal recessive, or X-linked.

Genetic counseling must be based on an accurate diagnosis and on familiarity with the natural history,

range of manifestations, severity, and associated findings of the specific disorder.

DIAGNOSIS

Prenatal Testing. Prenatal diagnosis of certain skeletal dysplasias without biochemical markers can be established by radiography (less commonly used), ultrasonography (most widely used), fetoscopy, amniography,

three-dimensional ultrasonography, fetal magnetic resonance imaging (MRI), and intrauterine computed tomography (CT). Knowledge of the natural history of intrauterine growth in dwarfing conditions is incomplete. Ossification of the fetal skeleton is not well established until 16 weeks, and it is not known when limb-length discrepancy becomes apparent in the fetus. Serial sonograms are necessary to recognize the decreased growth rate of the femur or to monitor the

Plate 4-2

Congenital and Developmental Disorders

ACHONDROPLASIA – CLINICAL MANIFESTATIONS (CONTINUED)

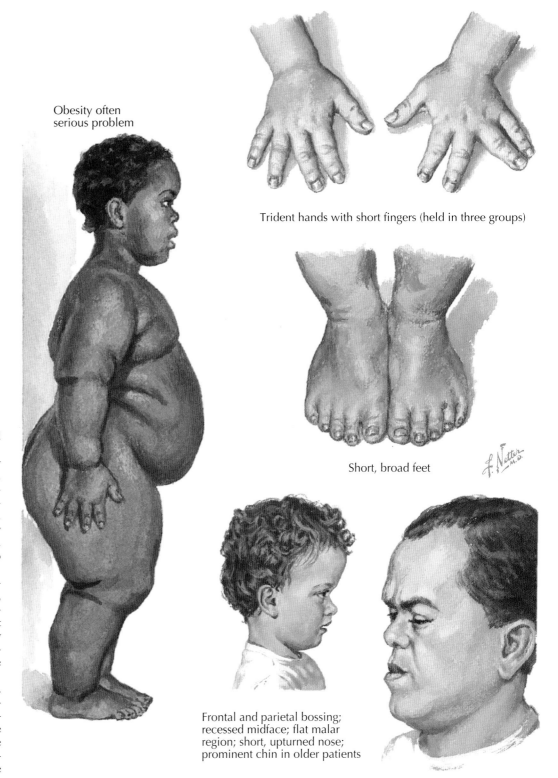

Obesity often serious problem

Trident hands with short fingers (held in three groups)

Short, broad feet

Frontal and parietal bossing; recessed midface; flat malar region; short, upturned nose; prominent chin in older patients

DWARFISM—OVERVIEW AND ACHONDROPLASIA (Continued)

fetal biparietal diameter, polydactyly, clubfoot, and other skeletal abnormalities.

History. A thorough family history is a particularly important factor in reaching the correct diagnosis. Because disorders with clinically indistinguishable features may have different patterns of inheritance, evaluation of other family members can be very helpful. Genetic testing can also be helpful because clinically some disorders can appear similar to one another. Genetic testing can help to define the disorder and also help with expectations for future generations.

Physical Examination. Measurements of head circumference, height, weight, and arm span are taken, and body proportions are evaluated. A careful examination should be done for nonosseous signs such as cleft palate, cataracts, or congenital heart disease that may contribute to the diagnosis. Ophthalmologic examination and evaluation of speech and hearing may also be needed.

Intelligence is normal in nearly all types of dwarfism. Exceptions include, but are not limited to, hypochondroplasia (see Plate 4-5), the rare Dyggve-Melchior-Clausen dysplasia (see Plate 4-16), pycnodysostosis (see Plate 4-13), and Hurler and Hunter syndromes (see Plate 4-18). The need for specific intellectual evaluation or treatment is dictated by the diagnosis and the patient's past performance.

Radiographic Findings. Radiographs must be taken of the entire skeleton (skeletal survey) because diagnosis of most bone dysplasias cannot be made on the basis of one or two radiographs of selected body parts. It is particularly important to look for atlantoaxial instability of the cervical spine. Abnormal vertebral movements occur in many bone dysplasias and, unless detected, may lead to acute compressive myelopathy. Because the radiographic characteristics of many dysplasias change with time, review of earlier radiographs is often necessary (e.g., in the epiphyseal dysplasias, the growth plates

fuse with age and all evidence of disturbed epiphyseal development is obliterated).

Laboratory Tests. Initial symptoms or the preliminary diagnosis may suggest the need for specific laboratory tests. For example, if Schmid-type metaphyseal chondrodysplasia (see Plate 4-3) is suggested, a complete blood analysis is needed to differentiate this disorder from vitamin D–resistant rickets; and if the mucopolysaccharidoses, a group of biomechanical

storage disorders, are suggested, testing for specific enzymes is required.

ACHONDROPLASIA

Achondroplasia, which occurs in about 1 in 40,000 persons, is the most common and best-known type of disproportionate short-limb dwarfism (see Plates 4-1 to 4-3). It is transmitted by a single autosomal dominant

Plate 4-3

Musculoskeletal System: PART III

DWARFISM—OVERVIEW AND ACHONDROPLASIA (Continued)

gene. Infants with homozygous achondroplasia generally do not survive for more than a few weeks or months. About 80% of cases result from a spontaneous mutation. The mutation occurs in the fibroblast growth factor receptor 3 (FGFR-3), which affects endochondral bone formation specifically in the proliferative zone of the physis. Achondroplasia is a quantitative, not qualitative, cartilage defect. The parents are usually average size, and no other family member is affected. Statistical evidence suggests that elevated paternal age (>37 years) may be linked to this type of mutation.

Clinical Manifestations. The characteristic signs of achondroplasia—disproportionate short stature, a comparatively long trunk, and rhizomelic shortening of the limbs—are evident at birth (see Plates 4-1 and 4-2). The head is both relatively and absolutely large with a prominent, or bulging, forehead (frontal bossing); parietal bossing and flattening of the occiput may also be evident. In infancy, the head increases rapidly in size and hydrocephalus can occur. It can be recognized early by using established norms for head size in patients with achondroplasia, and appropriate treatment can be instituted.

Midfacial hypoplasia of variable degree is manifested by a flat or depressed nasal bridge, narrow nasal passages, and malar hypoplasia (see Plate 4-2). The nose has a fleshy tip and upturned nostrils. These features result from restricted development of the chondrocranium and the middle third of the face.

Recurrent and chronic middle ear infections (otitis media) are common in infancy and early childhood and, if untreated, may lead to significant hearing loss. Generally, these infections become less frequent by the time the patient is 8 to 10 years of age.

A relative protrusion of the jaw is often mislabeled as prognathism. Dental development is normal, but underdevelopment of the maxilla may cause dental crowding and malocclusion. About 70% of patients have tongue thrust or other speech defects that seem to be related to the dysplastic bone structure. These problems usually subside spontaneously by school age.

The root portions of the limbs are shorter than the middle or distal segments. Soft tissues may appear excessive with redundant, partially encircling folds and grooves on the limbs. Because the long bones are shortened, the muscle mass looks bunched up, creating the appearance of great strength.

Initially, the legs appear straight but with ambulation may develop a varus position, resulting in bowleg (genu varum) with or without back knee (genu recurvatum).

The hands and feet may appear large in relation to the limbs, but the digits are short, broad, and stubby (brachydactyly). The so-called trident hand (see Plate 4-2) is common but becomes less apparent in late childhood and adulthood. The fingertips may reach only to the level of the trochanters or even the iliac crests. Elbow extension is restricted (30 to 45 degrees), but this has little functional significance. In some instances, this may be due to radial head subluxation.

Although the trunk is relatively long, deformities contribute to the overall height reduction. The chest tends to be flat and broad and the abdomen and buttocks protuberant. Excessive lumbar lordosis and a

ACHONDROPLASIA – CLINICAL MANIFESTATIONS OF SPINE

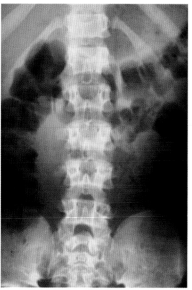

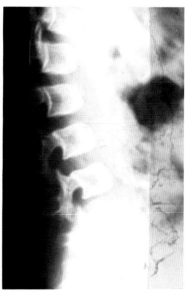

Anteroposterior radiograph shows progressive decrease in interpedicular distance (in caudad direction) in lumbar region, with resultant transverse narrowing of vertebral canal.

Lateral radiograph shows scalloped posterior borders of lumbar vertebrae and short pedicles, causing sagittal spinal stenosis.

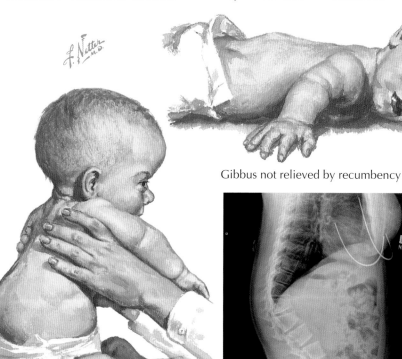

Gibbus not relieved by recumbency

Infant with severe thoracolumbar kyphosis that usually reverses to characteristic lordosis at weight-bearing age. If it does not, true gibbus with cord compression may result. Neurologic signs and vertebral wedging are indications for surgery.

Gibbus with wedging of the thoracolumbar junction

Venogram shows areas of ischemia; supply of blood to lumbar spinal cord impaired.

tilted pelvis cause a waddling gait, and fixed flexion contractures of the hip appear early.

In a sitting position, infants commonly exhibit thoracolumbar kyphosis (see Plate 4-1). A hump, or gibbus, seen in some infants, may be associated with anterior wedging of the first or second lumbar vertebra. The kyphosis is related to a variety of factors, including ligamentous laxity, hypotonia, and immature strength and motor skills. Although it requires monitoring,

the kyphosis usually disappears when the child begins to walk.

Neurologic complications are common. Respiratory abnormalities suggest stenosis of the foramen magnum and compression of the normal-sized medulla oblongata and/or cervical spinal cord. This quite frequent complication results in hypoventilation or apnea, paralysis of voluntary respiration, and compressive myelopathy at the level of the foramen magnum (see Plate 4-4).

Plate 4-4

Congenital and Developmental Disorders

DWARFISM—OVERVIEW AND ACHONDROPLASIA (Continued)

(Therefore, hyperextension of the neck and sudden, whiplash-like movement should be avoided.) Sudden infant death syndrome has also been reported. Somatosensory evoked potential (SSEP) and polysomnography coupled with CT and MRI can provide valuable information to help avert both short-term and long-term complications.

Stenosis of the lumbar spine, prolapse of intervertebral discs, osteophytes, and deformed vertebral bodies may compress the spinal cord and/or nerve roots, frequently causing neurologic manifestations. Pressure on blood vessels impairs the regional blood supply, producing focal areas of ischemia. The pedicles tend to be short and the interpedicular distance tends to decrease (instead of the normal increase) caudally in the spine.

In the teenage period, slowly progressive symptoms such as paresthesias, weakness, pain, and paraplegia develop and may be aggravated by obesity and prolonged standing or walking. Initially, the patient can quickly relieve these symptoms by flexing the spine and hips forward, squatting, or assuming a non–weight-bearing position. As the condition progresses, pain develops and may be localized to the low back or, more commonly, may radiate into the buttocks, posterior thigh, and calf. Muscle weakness and foot drop may also develop. Although these symptoms are more common in the legs, the arms may also be affected.

Patients with symptomatic spinal stenosis require a physical examination with attention to sensory levels, and a careful neurologic history should also be obtained. Specific tests such as somatosensory evoked responses, CT, MRI, and myelography all have a diagnostic function.

Growth rate is normal in the first year of life and then drops to about the third percentile, where it remains for the first decade; it may increase during puberty. Obesity is a common problem. Adult height ranges from 42 to 56 inches.

Children with achondroplasia should not be evaluated against normal developmental milestones but rather against standards developed for children with the condition. Motor skills are often delayed because of the physical difficulties posed by short limbs and hypotonia (which tends to abate by age 2); cognitive skills are usually attained at the expected ages.

Radiographic Findings. The characteristic features are present at birth and change little throughout life. Although virtually all bones of the body are affected, the abnormal configuration of the skull, lumbar spine, and pelvis are hallmarks of the disease. Typical are a shortened skull base, large cranium with prominent frontal and occipital areas, and superimposition of the spheno-occipital synchondrosis over the mastoid. The angle of the base of the skull is 85 to 120 degrees (110 to 145 degrees is normal), and the foramen magnum is small.

The radial heads may be partially or completely dislocated and dysplastic. The phalanges in the hands are short, broad, and conic. The femoral necks are short and the long bones relatively thick and short. Distinctive rectangular or oval radiolucencies in the proximal humerus and femur that are apparent in infancy disappear by age 2. The inverted-V–shaped

ACHONDROPLASIA – DIAGNOSTIC TESTING

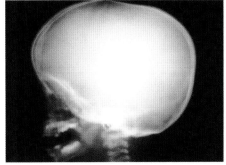

Lateral radiograph of large head shows frontal bossing, flattened occiput, open anterior fontanel, recessed midface, and occipitalization of C1.

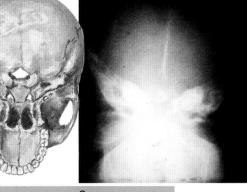

CT scan shows large ventricles but normal thickness of cortical mantle and normal CSF pressure (false hydrocephalus).

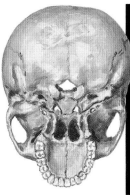

Towne projection radiograph shows constriction of foramen magnum.

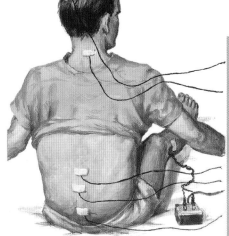

Somatosensory evoked potentials (SSEP) determine delay in neurotransmission and its location on stimulation of personal nerve (evidence of cord compression). Ulnar or radial nerve may be similarly tested.

Alignment of lower limb. (A) Good alignment, plumb line centered on hip, knee, and ankle joints; (B) hip and knee aligned but ankle inside plumb line; (C) knee outside and ankle inside plumb line. Malalignment plus pain on walking may indicate need for surgical correction.

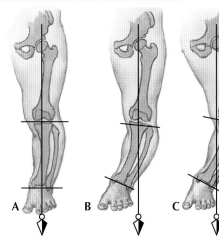

(chevron) growth plate of the distal femur is characteristic. The fibulas tend to be longer than the tibias, especially at the knees.

A diagnostic feature is a decrease of the interpedicular distance in a caudal direction, primarily in the lumbar spine (in the normal spine, the interpedicular distance increases in the caudal direction). Spinal stenosis, most evident in the lumbosacral region, is more pronounced in adulthood. Lateral radiographs reveal

posterior scalloping of the vertebral bodies. Dorsolumbar kyphosis, commonly seen in infancy, disappears with ambulation and is replaced by an exaggerated lumbar lordosis. As the lordosis increases, the plane of the sacrum becomes more horizontal. The pelvis is short and broad with relatively wide, nonflaring iliac wings, small and deep greater sciatic notches, and horizontal superior margins of the acetabulum (champagne glass shape).

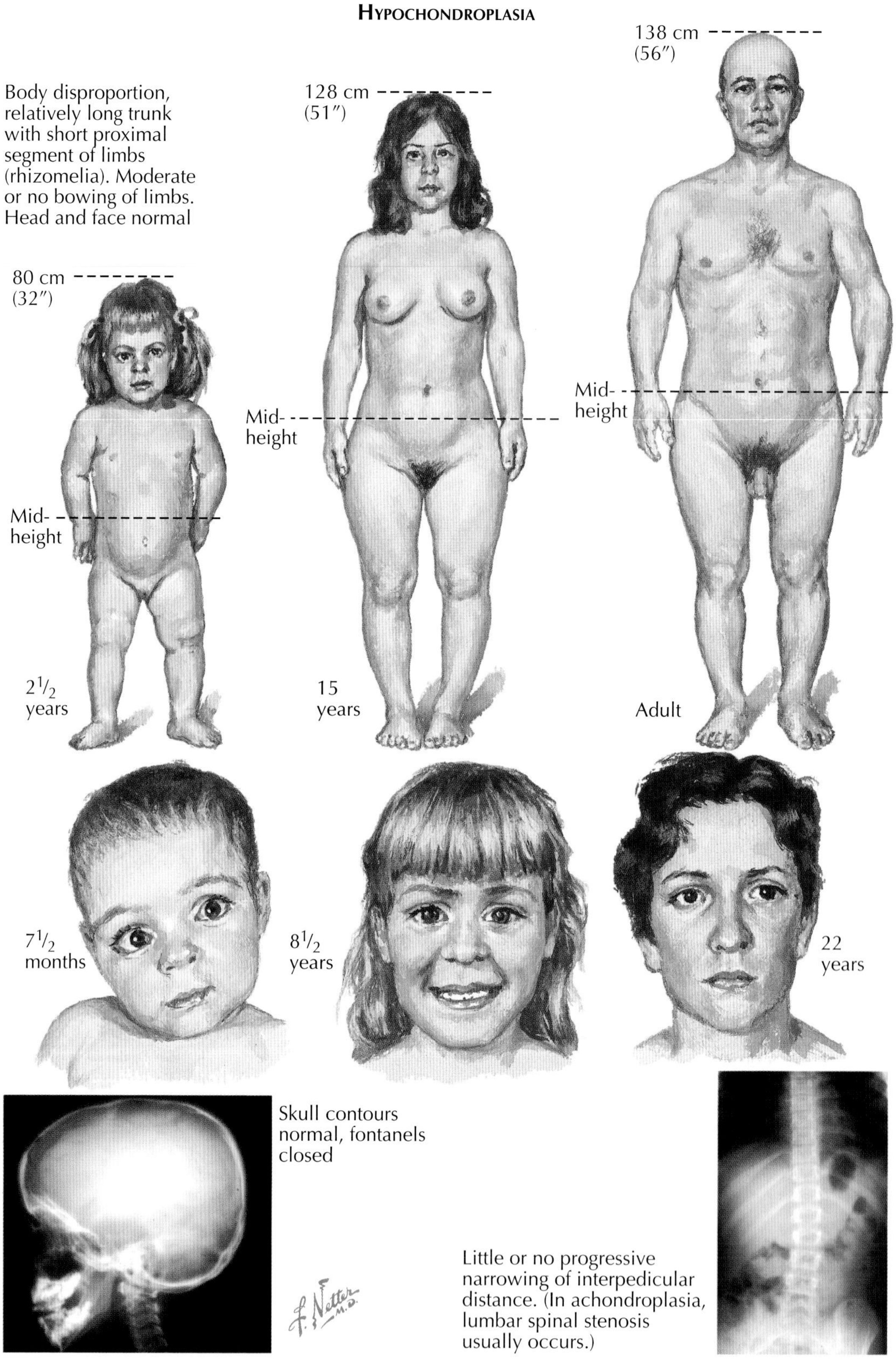

Plate 4-5

HYPOCHONDROPLASIA

Body disproportion, relatively long trunk with short proximal segment of limbs (rhizomelia). Moderate or no bowing of limbs. Head and face normal

138 cm (56")

128 cm (51")

80 cm (32")

Mid-height

Mid-height

Mid-height

2½ years

15 years

Adult

7½ months

8½ years

22 years

Skull contours normal, fontanels closed

Little or no progressive narrowing of interpedicular distance. (In achondroplasia, lumbar spinal stenosis usually occurs.)

DWARFISM— HYPOCHONDROPLASIA

For many years, hypochondroplasia was considered a mild or atypical form of achondroplasia, and many cases are probably overlooked or misdiagnosed because the height reduction and body disproportion are often relatively mild.

Hypochondroplasia is inherited as an autosomal dominant trait, but most cases appear to be sporadic, presumably the result of a spontaneous mutation affecting FGFR-3, resulting in a milder dysplasia than achondroplasia. For unknown reasons, about 10% of patients are mentally retarded.

Clinical Manifestations. Birth weight and length may be low normal, and the short stature may not be recognized until the patient is 2 or 3 years of age. The typical appearance is a thick, stocky physique with a relatively long trunk and disproportionately short limbs, making the upper body segment longer than the lower body segment.

Head circumference is normal, although the forehead may be slightly prominent. The face is also normal with no midfacial hypoplasia or depression of the nasal bridge.

The limbs are short and stocky. Mild bowleg is common, but alignment tends to improve with age. Ligamentous laxity is usually mild, and range of motion in the elbow, especially extension and supination, is often limited. The hands are broad with short fingers but no trident formation.

The trunk commonly shows mildly exaggerated lumbar lordosis with a sacral tilt and a slightly protuberant abdomen. Aching knees, elbows, and ankles and low back pain are common in adulthood. Adult height ranges from 52 to 59 inches.

Neurologic complications, particularly compressive myelopathy or radiculopathy, are much less frequent than in achondroplasia.

Radiographic Findings. Characteristic findings permit differentiation from achondroplasia. The skull is essentially normal, except for a mild bossing of the forehead. Generalized shortening of the long bones with mild metaphyseal flaring is most notable at the knees. In children, the growth plates of the distal femurs may show a shallow, V-shaped indentation, but this is not as pronounced as the chevron-shaped notch seen in achondroplasia. The femoral necks are short and broad. The pelvis may be basically normal or mildly dysplastic (e.g., the greater sciatic notches are reduced in width and the ilia are square and shortened). In the lumbar spine, interpedicular distances lack the normal caudal widening, but these alterations are not as profound as in achondroplasia. The height of the vertebral bodies is normal, and the dorsal borders are only mildly scalloped.

Plate 4-6

Congenital and Developmental Disorders

DIASTROPHIC DWARFISM

Like so many other bone dysplasias, diastrophic dwarfism, or dysplasia, was originally mistaken for a variant of achondroplasia with clubfoot or arthrogryposis multiplex congenita. The disorder is transmitted as an autosomal recessive trait affecting chromosome 5 and the diastrophic dysplasia sulfate transporter (DTDST), leading to a deficiency of the sulfate transport protein. The undersulfation of proteoglycans in the collagen matrix impairs the response of cells to fibroblast growth factor and limits endochondral growth. A lethal variant is characterized by a lower birth weight than in the classic form, radiographic evidence of overlapping joints, dislocation of the cervical spine, and congenital heart disease.

Clinical Manifestations. Clinical findings vary widely. Formerly, patients with similar but less severe signs were thought to have a variant form or a different condition. The differences, more apparent than real, were due to variable phenotypic expression.

A unique group of malformations is evident at birth, with additional characteristics appearing later. In the newborn period, the head appears normal, but many patients develop a characteristic facial appearance with a narrow root and broad midportion of the nose, long and broad lip philtrum, and square jaw. The prominent area around the mouth, coupled with the other characteristic facial features, gave rise to the now obsolete term *cherub dwarf.* The face is long and full with a high, broad forehead. Capillary hemangiomas are common in the midforehead but fade or disappear with age. Abnormalities of the palate are seen in 50% of patients and include complete, partial, or submucous clefts, bifid uvula, or double uvula with a median longitudinal ridge. These palatal abnormalities—and possibly laryngeal defects—produce the characteristic soft rasping or hoarse voice.

In 80% of patients, the ears swell in the first few days or weeks after birth, giving the appearance of acute inflammation. The swelling subsides spontaneously in 4 to 6 weeks, resulting in a cauliflower ear. Calcification and ossification occur later. Hearing is not affected by the small size of the external auditory canals but can be impaired by deformity of the middle ear ossicles.

Reduced height is primarily due to rhizomelic shortening of the limbs and is further augmented by flexion contractures of the joints, especially the hips and knees. Adult height ranges from 34 to 48 inches.

Partial and complete joint dislocation is also common, particularly in the shoulders, elbows, hips, and patellae. The dysplastic hip changes, coxa vara, and hip dislocation combine to produce a grossly abnormal gait.

Hand malformation is a hallmark of diastrophic dwarfism. The hypermobile thumb and deformed first metacarpal create an abducted hitchhiker position. The fingers are short and broad with ulnar deviation; there is limitation of movement due to ankyloses of the proximal interphalangeal joints (symphalangism). Severe progressive clubfoot is another characteristic.

The trunk is deformed by excessive lumbar lordosis that develops early in life. Scoliosis, which may also

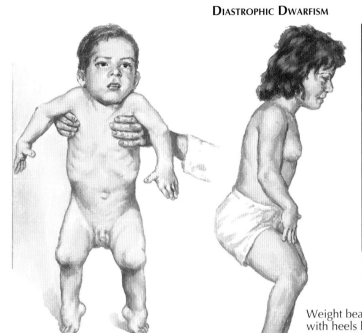

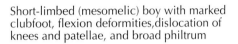

Short-limbed (mesomelic) boy with marked clubfoot, flexion deformities, dislocation of knees and patellae, and broad philtrum

Weight bearing on balls of feet and toes with heels high off floor, compensatory knee and hip flexion, lordosis, and forward position of head

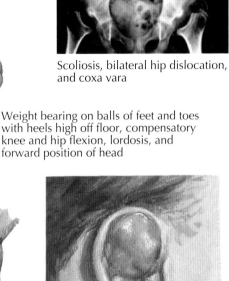

Scoliosis, bilateral hip dislocation, and coxa vara

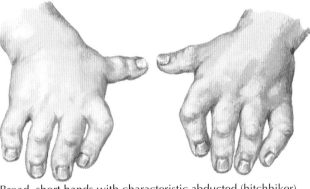

Broad, short hands with characteristic abducted (hitchhiker) thumbs and ankylosed proximal interphalangeal joints

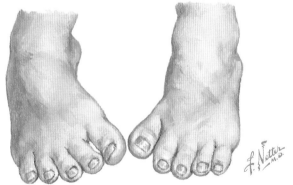

Marked clubfoot resistant to correction

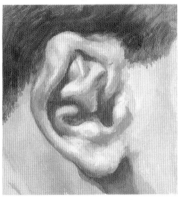

Acute inflammatory swelling of auricle in infancy

Progression to typical cauliflower deformity

begin in infancy, becomes more severe with weight bearing and leads to trunk deformity and barrel chest. Kyphosis of a variable degree accompanies the scoliosis, and the resultant deformity further reduces height. Spinal changes, especially cervical kyphosis, may cause catastrophic neurologic problems.

Radiographic Findings. Characteristic signs are short, broad, long bones with flared metaphyses. Development of the epiphyses is delayed and irregular, and stippling has been observed. The epiphyses of the proximal femurs, absent at birth, are flat and distorted when ossification does occur. The epiphyses of the proximal tibias tend to be triangular and larger than those of the distal femurs. Other findings include cervical kyphosis and dysplasia; thoracolumbar kyphoscoliosis; partial or complete dislocation of the hips; precocious ossification of the costal cartilage; small, oval, or triangular first metacarpals; irregular deformity of the metacarpals, metatarsals, and phalanges; and clubfoot.

Plate 4-7

Musculoskeletal System: PART III

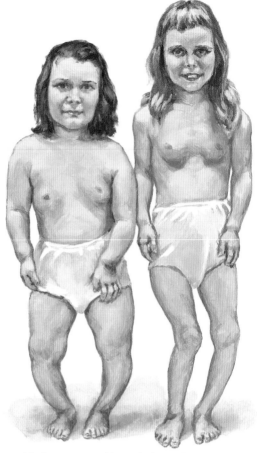

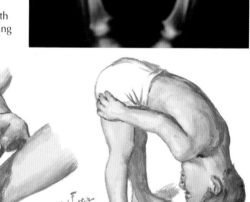

Squared-off, tonguelike projections on anterior borders of lumbar vertebrae due to defects in growth plates. This radiographic sign often disappears as growth plates mature.

Sisters with short upper and lower limbs. Girl on left has bilateral bowing of lower limbs; girl on right shows genu valgum on one side and genu varum on the other side, causing pelvic obliquity that may lead to scoliosis.

Dwarfism— Pseudoachondroplasia

For many years, pseudoachondroplasia was confused with achondroplasia (see Plates 4-1 to 4-4) and Morquio syndrome (see Plate 4-18). Pseudoachondroplasia is most often inherited as an autosomal dominant trait affecting chromosome 19 and the cartilage oligomeric matrix protein (COMP), but a rare autosomal recessive form has also been proposed. Hyaline cartilage, fibrocartilage, and growth plate cartilage are affected. Proteoglycan abnormalities have been identified and are probably related to the core protein or enzymes responsible for the formation of the glycosaminoglycan chains in cartilage.

Clinical Manifestations. Growth retardation is usually not apparent until the child is 1 year old and often not until age 2 or 3. A delay in walking or an abnormal gait is often the first clinical clue. By this time, body measurements clearly reveal the disproportionate short stature. As the growth rate slows, the typical habitus of long trunk, exaggerated lumbar lordosis, prominent abdomen, and rhizomelic shortening of the limbs develops.

Head size and face are normal. By early childhood, the patient has a waddling gait. Malalignment of the knees develops, including bowleg, knock-knee, or windswept deformities (bowleg on one limb, knock-knee on the other). Flexion contractures develop in the hips and knees, with joint pain and precocious osteoarthritis. The hands and feet are short and stubby with considerable ligamentous laxity, particularly at the wrists and fingers. Cervical instability may also be identified. Incomplete elbow extension is typical and is

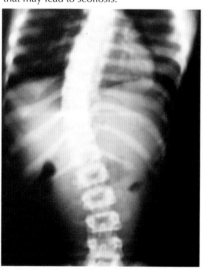

Scoliosis with some irregularity of vertebral growth plates

Wide, trumpet-like tibial metaphyses and irregular epiphyses with defecit, causing tibia vara

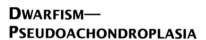

Wrist and finger hyperextension due to ligamentous laxity. Because of body disproportion, head can touch floor easily.

related to the dysplastic bone changes rather than to soft tissue problems. Adult height ranges from 32 to 51 inches.

Radiographic Findings. The skull and facial bones are normal. The long bones in the hand appear short and stubby, and the carpals are dysplastic, with late ossification. In childhood, the small, irregular epiphyses of the femoral heads may become severely deformed and fragment by early adulthood. The ilia tend to be large and straight sided, whereas the pubic and ischial

bones are short and broad; the greater sciatic notches are smaller than normal.

Spinal changes in childhood include moderate flattening of the vertebral bodies (platyspondyly) with biconvex deformity and irregularity of the superior and inferior growth plates, producing a tonguelike projection apparent on the lateral view. By adolescence, most of these characteristic vertebral changes disappear and only mild platyspondyly persists. Scoliosis and excessive lumbar lordosis may also be evident.

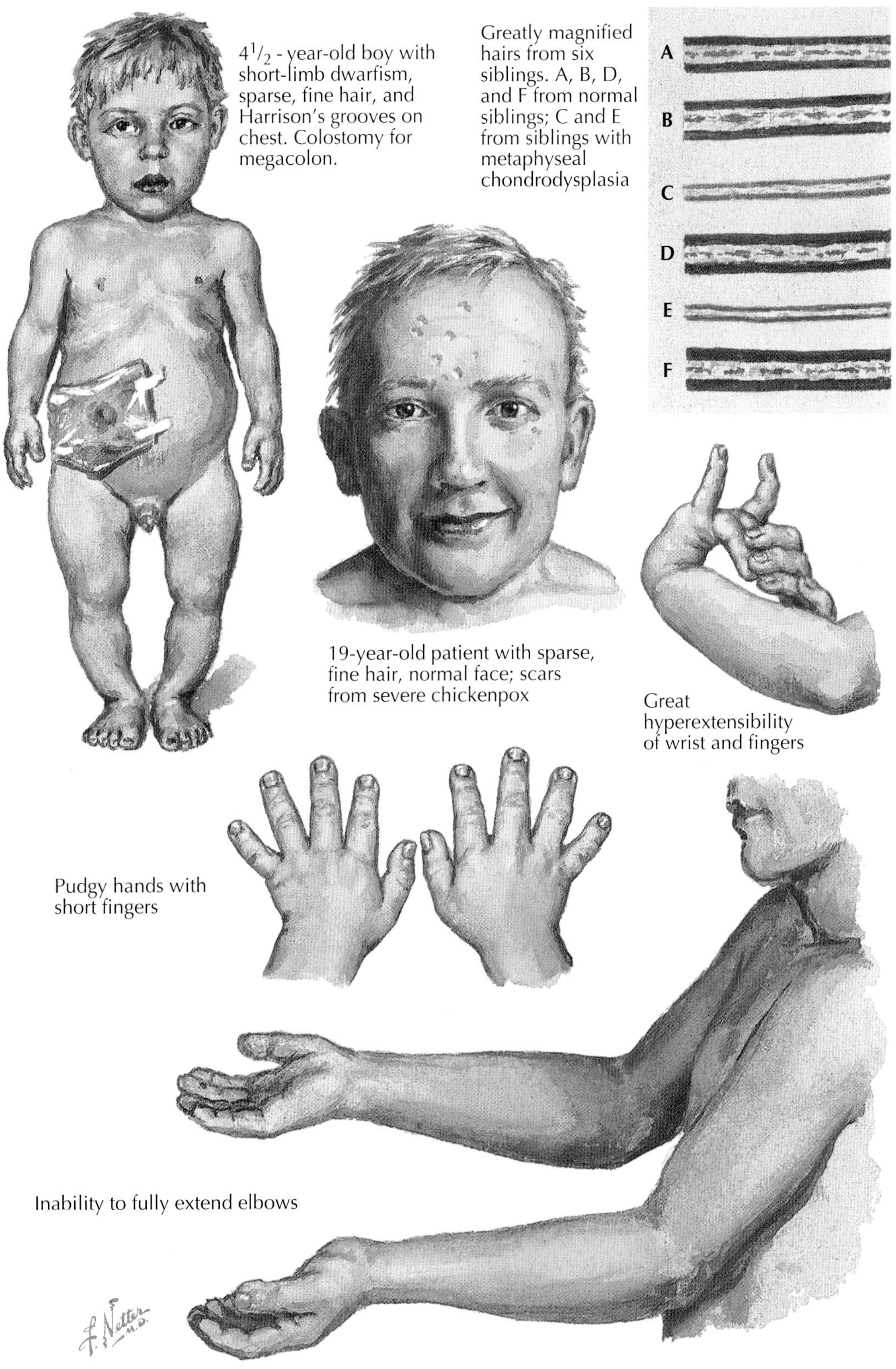

Plate 4-8

Congenital and Developmental Disorders

$4^{1}/_{2}$-year-old boy with short-limb dwarfism, sparse, fine hair, and Harrison's grooves on chest. Colostomy for megacolon.

Greatly magnified hairs from six siblings. A, B, D, and F from normal siblings; C and E from siblings with metaphyseal chondrodysplasia

19-year-old patient with sparse, fine hair, normal face; scars from severe chickenpox

Great hyperextensibility of wrist and fingers

Pudgy hands with short fingers

Inability to fully extend elbows

DWARFISM—METAPHYSEAL CHONDRODYSPLASIA, MCKUSICK TYPE

Commonly known as cartilage-hair hypoplasia, this disorder belongs to a group of intrinsic bone dysplasias characterized by significant changes in the metaphyses of the long bones and hair of small diameter. It is transmitted as an autosomal recessive trait and is relatively common in Finland and among the Old Order Amish in Pennsylvania. The genetic defect is in the ribonuclease of mitochondrial RNA-processing gene (RMPR) located in chromosome 9. At times this is due to uniparental disomy, in which the child inherits two copies of a chromosome from one parent.

Clinical Manifestations. At birth, weight is normal but body length is reduced. The configuration of the head and face is normal. The elbows do not extend fully. The excessive length of the distal fibulas in relation to the short tibias results in ankle deformity, and unilateral bowleg or knock-knee may develop in childhood. The hands and feet are short and pudgy; the foreshortened nails are normal in width and grow normally. Ligamentous laxity of the fingers and toes permits extraordinary hypermobility in the joints. Atlantoaxial instability and odontoid hypoplasia are common. A prominent sternum and mild flaring of the lower ribs with Harrison's grooves are also typical. In many patients, a distinctive feature is the sparse, fine, light-colored hair, which grows slowly and breaks easily. Cross-sectional microscopic examination reveals a reduced, somewhat elliptic hair shaft of small diameter that frequently lacks a pigment core. Body hair is similarly affected. However, in some patients, the hair is nearly normal.

About 10% of patients with the McKusick-type metaphyseal chondrodysplasia manifest intestinal malabsorption and Hirschsprung disease. They may be unusually susceptible to chickenpox. Neutropenia, persistent lymphopenia, normal serum immunoglobulins, and diminished delayed skin hypersensitivity may also be present. Adult height ranges from 41 to 57 inches.

Radiographic Findings. Radiographic abnormalities do not become evident until the patient is 9 to 12 months old. Although changes are seen primarily in the limbs and ribs and around the knees (where they are most severe), subtle changes occur in other bones such as the vertebrae and pelvic bones. The metaphyses are widened and irregular with sclerosis and cystic alterations. Other findings include cupping of the ribs and ankle deformity.

Histologic Findings. Microscopic examination of the metaphysis shows normal ossification but a hypoplastic cartilage. Chondrocytes are decreased in number, and columnization is disorganized. The cartilaginous cores on which bone mineral can deposit appear to be inadequate.

Plate 4-9

Musculoskeletal System: PART III

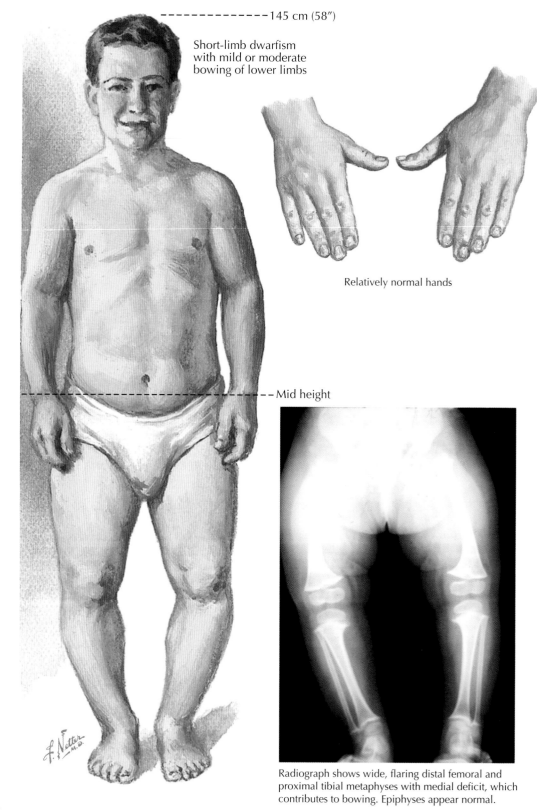

145 cm (58")

Short-limb dwarfism
with mild or moderate
bowing of lower limbs

Relatively normal hands

Mid height

Radiograph shows wide, flaring distal femoral and
proximal tibial metaphyses with medial deficit, which
contributes to bowing. Epiphyses appear normal.

DWARFISM—METAPHYSEAL CHONDRODYSPLASIA, SCHMID TYPE

In 1949, Schmid described a form of metaphyseal chondrodysplasia that has been known by many names, including metaphyseal dysostosis and familial bone disease resembling rickets. The Schmid-type metaphyseal chondrodysplasia is transmitted as an autosomal dominant trait affecting chromosome 6 and type X collagen with variable expressivity; females are usually less severely affected. Sporadic cases may be linked to advanced paternal age.

Clinical Manifestations. The moderately short stature of the short-limb type is evident by 18 to 24 months of age. The head and face are not affected. The wrists are prominent or enlarged, and often the fingers do not extend fully. Bowleg, commonly the first sign, becomes obvious shortly after the child begins to walk; if severe, the bowing produces a waddling gait and contributes to the height reduction. Poor alignment of the lower limbs can lead to symptomatic osteoarthritis in the hips and knees. Flaring of the lower rib cage signals trunk involvement, and the general habitus is stocky or chubby. Adult height is 51 to 63 inches.

Radiographic Findings. Metaphyseal abnormalities vary from mild scalloping to gross irregularities in the ankles, knees, wrists, shoulders, and hips. Although metaphyseal lesions appear to heal with bed rest, they recur once weight bearing is resumed. The epiphyseal lines are wide, and epiphyseal ossification centers appear normal.

Coxa vara and bowleg are common, and the long bones and femoral necks are short. The acetabular portions of the ilia tend to be broad, and the acetabular roof, which is normally vertical, is horizontal. Long bones in the hand and foot are mildly to moderately shortened, but metaphyseal changes are minor or absent.

Differential Diagnosis. This type of metaphyseal chondrodysplasia has frequently been confused with vitamin D–resistant rickets. Clinical and radiographic findings are quite similar. However, vitamin D–resistant rickets has an X-linked dominant inheritance, whereas the Schmid-type metaphyseal chondrodysplasia is transmitted as an autosomal dominant trait. Unlike vitamin D–resistant rickets, there are no characteristic biochemical changes (serum calcium, phosphate, and alkaline phosphatase levels are normal) and no beneficial response to administration of vitamin D.

Plate 4-10

Congenital and Developmental Disorders

DWARFISM—CHONDRODYSPLASIA PUNCTATA

CONRADI-HÜNERMANN TYPE

Chondrodysplasia punctata has been known by a bewildering array of names including chondrodystrophia calcificans congenita, Conradi-Hünermann disease, and dysplasia epiphysealis punctata. Although it is commonly considered a discrete entity characterized by radiographic evidence of punctate epiphyseal and extra-epiphyseal calcifications (stippling) in childhood, this form of intrinsic bone dysplasia actually has nonosseous manifestations. To complicate the diagnosis further, epiphyseal stippling is seen in a number of unrelated disorders, including cerebrohepatorenal syndrome, generalized gangliosidosis, cretinism, Smith-Lemli-Opitz syndrome, Down syndrome (trisomy 21), and anencephaly.

In genetic counseling, it is important to distinguish this autosomal dominant type from the clinically similar X-linked dominant type, which is fatal in hemizygous males. Severely affected infants are either stillborn or die soon after birth. Prognosis for survival is relatively good for those less severely affected. The Conradi-Hünermann type is X-linked recessive affecting Xp22 and the arylsulfatase E (ARSE) gene.

Clinical Manifestations. The major signs are usually evident at birth: a head of average circumference with a distinctive flat facies, mildly flattened nasal bridge, relatively short neck, and asymmetric shortening of the limbs. By early childhood, the characteristic facies largely disappears but the limb asymmetry may need surgical correction. Congenital cataracts are seen in about 18% of cases. Scoliosis is common after age 1; joint contractures occur later. The skin is often dry, scaly, and atrophic. The ichthyosiform skin changes and alopecia usually persist into adulthood. Adult height is 51 to 63 inches.

Radiographic Findings. Early signs consist of punctate calcifications in the vertebral column and the epiphyses of the long bones and the carpal, tarsal, and pelvic bones, usually in asymmetric distribution. The metaphyses are intact, but the epiphyses frequently become dysplastic (flattened, small, or irregularly shaped).

RHIZOMELIC TYPE

Rhizomelic-type chondrodysplasia punctata has an autosomal recessive inheritance and is more severe than the Conradi-Hünermann or X-linked dominant type. The *PEX7* gene is affected, which encodes the protein peroxin 7. Recurrent infections usually cause death in the first year of life. Survivors have a high incidence of profound psychomotor retardation and other neurologic abnormalities, such as spastic quadriparesis.

Clinical Manifestations. The features of rhizomelic-type chondrodysplasia punctata are the same as those of the Conradi-Hünermann type, but the rhizomelic shortening of the limbs is more severe and congenital cataracts are extremely common. Microcephaly, contractures, and postnatal failure to thrive are also typical.

Radiographic Findings. The epiphyseal and extra-epiphyseal calcifications are usually severe, with a symmetric distribution sparing the vertebral column. Lateral radiographs reveal vertical coronal clefts of the vertebral bodies. In the humerus and/or femur, severe shortening, splaying, and metaphyseal cupping are characteristic.

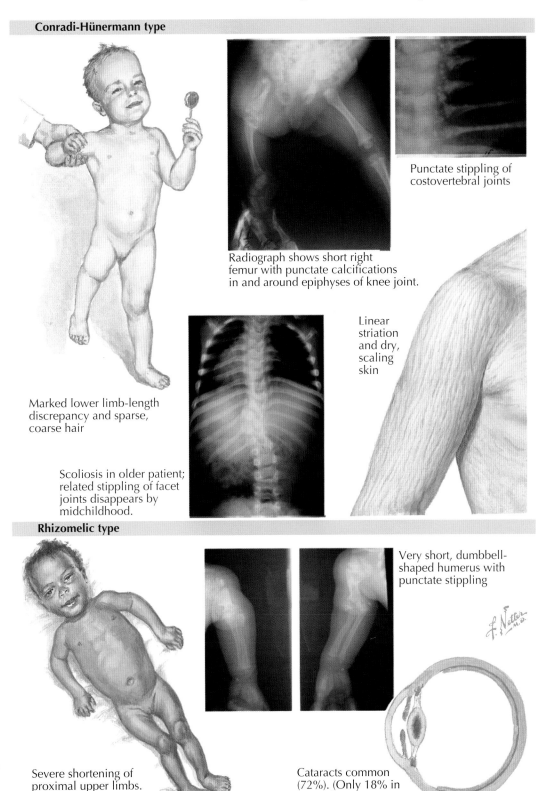

Conradi-Hünermann type

Marked lower limb-length discrepancy and sparse, coarse hair

Radiograph shows short right femur with punctate calcifications in and around epiphyses of knee joint.

Punctate stippling of costovertebral joints

Linear striation and dry, scaling skin

Scoliosis in older patient; related stippling of facet joints disappears by midchildhood.

Rhizomelic type

Severe shortening of proximal upper limbs. Femurs may also be similarly affected.

Very short, dumbbell-shaped humerus with punctate stippling

Cataracts common (72%). (Only 18% in Conradi-Hünermann type.)

X-LINKED DOMINANT TYPE

Approximately 25% of reported cases of chondrodysplasia punctata are probably transmitted as an X-linked dominant trait. This results in a mutation in the emopamil-binding protein and alters the effects on the cholesterol biosynthesis pathway. Most patients are female, and the disorder is usually fatal in males.

Clinical Manifestations. This disorder shares many features with the Conradi-Hünermann type, with hypoplasia of the distal phalanges a distinctive trait. Pathognomonic cutaneous findings in the first months of life include erythematous skin changes and striated ichthyosiform hyperkeratosis. Patterned ichthyosis, coarse and lusterless hair, and cicatricial alopecia become evident later. A variable severity, marked asymmetry of long bones, and cataracts are thought to be consistent with functional X-chromosome mosaicism in females.

Plate 4-11

Musculoskeletal System: PART III

DWARFISM— CHONDROECTODERMAL DYSPLASIA (ELLIS–VAN CREVELD SYNDROME), GREBE CHONDRODYSPLASIA, AND ACROMESOMELIC DYSPLASIA

CHONDROECTODERMAL DYSPLASIA (ELLIS-VAN CREVELD SYNDROME)

This very rare type of short-limb dwarfism has an autosomal recessive mode of inheritance with a link to chromosome 4p16.1. It is characterized by chondrodysplasia; polydactyly; ectodermal dysplasia of hair, teeth, and nails; and congenital heart defects.

Clinical Manifestations. At birth, the head and face are normal but oral and dental abnormalities are common, including natal teeth, multiple frenula that obliterate the buccolabial sulcus, and partial or pseudocleft in the midline of the upper lip. Precocious exfoliation and missing or peg-shaped teeth are evident later. Mesomelic and acromelic limb shortening is greater in the lower limbs and, with growth, knock-knee becomes serious enough to require surgical treatment. The hands are short and stubby with postaxial polydactyly, which also occurs in the feet in 10% of patients. The fingernails and toenails are hypoplastic or dysplastic. The trunk is not affected. Adult height varies from 42 to 60 inches. Congenital heart disease, typically an atrial septal defect, is seen in more than 50% of patients.

Radiographic Findings. The long bones show a progressive distal shortening with broadened metaphyses. In the hands, the capitate and hamate are fused or deformed. Delayed ossification of the lateral portions of the epiphyses and metaphyses of the proximal tibias results in knock-knee. The pelvis has short iliac crests and, in infancy, spurlike inferior projections from the medial and lateral margins of the acetabula. The configuration of the pelvis becomes normal by late childhood.

GREBE CHONDRODYSPLASIA

The rare Grebe chondrodysplasia is transmitted as an autosomal recessive trait. Mild shortness of the hands and feet may be an indicator of the carrier state (heterozygosity). Although stillbirth is frequent and neonatal mortality high, after infancy the prognosis for survival is good.

Clinical Manifestations. Marked shortening of both upper and lower limbs is apparent at birth. The legs are more affected than the arms, and length reduction of the long bones increases progressively from the proximal to the distal segments. The fingers are extremely short and toelike. In the short, valgus feet, the toes may be rudimentary, ball-like structures. Polydactyly occurs in 50% of patients. Adult height is only 39 to 41 inches.

Radiographic Findings. The skull and axial skeleton appear essentially normal. The limbs, however, show severe dysplasia or aplasia of all bony elements.

ACROMESOMELIC DYSPLASIA

Transmitted as an autosomal recessive trait, acromesomelic dysplasia results in severely restricted growth.

Clinical Manifestations. This short-limb form of dwarfism is usually apparent in the first few weeks or months of life. Head size is normal, but the frontal bones may be prominent and the midface mildly

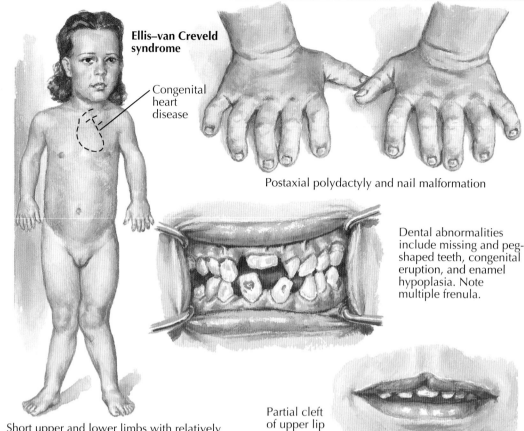

Chondroectodermal dysplasia

Ellis–van Creveld syndrome

Congenital heart disease

Postaxial polydactyly and nail malformation

Dental abnormalities include missing and peg-shaped teeth, congenital eruption, and enamel hypoplasia. Note multiple frenula.

Partial cleft of upper lip

Short upper and lower limbs with relatively long trunk, normal head circumference, and marked knock-knee (genu valgum)

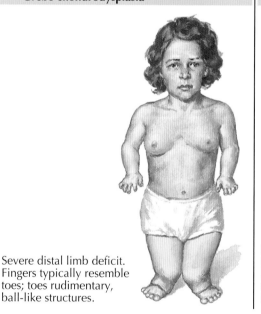

Grebe chondrodysplasia

Severe distal limb deficit. Fingers typically resemble toes; toes rudimentary, ball-like structures.

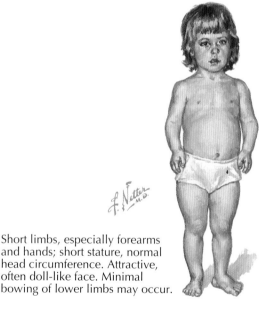

Acromesomelic dysplasia

Short limbs, especially forearms and hands; short stature, normal head circumference. Attractive, often doll-like face. Minimal bowing of lower limbs may occur.

hypoplastic and flattened. Limb shortening is greatest in the middle or distal segments. Range of motion of the elbow joints is limited by partial dislocation of the radial heads. The forearms are often bowed. Fingers, toes, and nails are very short. The thorax is small with mild anterior flaring of the lower ribs. Exaggerated lumbar lordosis makes the buttocks prominent; lower thoracic kyphosis is also common. Adult height ranges from 38 to 48 inches.

Radiographic Findings. Radiographs reveal a progressive shortening of the long bones, bowing of the radii, and often subluxation of the radial head. The epiphyses are relatively normal in infancy and become cone shaped later. The hands are unusually squat, and the phalanges appear square or sugarloaf shaped. The height of the vertebral bodies is minimally reduced, primarily in the posterior portions.

Plate 4-12

Congenital and Developmental Disorders

Dwarfism—Multiple Epiphyseal Dysplasia, Fairbank Type

Multiple epiphyseal dysplasia, Fairbank type, refers to a group of disorders with variable clinical and radiographic signs affecting the formation and maturation of the epiphyses. Usually an autosomal dominant trait, it can also be transmitted as an autosomal recessive trait. Different factors have been involved, including chromosome 19 and *COMP*, chromosome 1 and type IX collagen, and the gene encoding for matrillin-3, which is an extracellular matrix protein.

Clinical Manifestations. Multiple epiphyseal dysplasia usually remains unrecognized until the child is 5 to 10 years of age. The hands sometimes appear short and stubby, especially the thumbs. The shortening in the limbs is variable, and the trunk is normal.

Symptoms include morning stiffness, difficulty in running or climbing stairs, and a waddling gait. Joint discomfort, pain, and stiffness also develop, especially in the lower limbs. At first, symptoms tend to be episodic, transient, and fluctuating, but the waddling gait becomes more pronounced as the disorder progresses, and increased discomfort and stiffness force patients to limit their activities. Severe osteoarthritis of the hips often develops in older patients. Some affected persons, however, remain asymptomatic. Adult height ranges from 54 to 61 inches.

Radiographic Findings. Accurate diagnosis requires radiographic examination of the entire skeleton. Bilateral epiphyseal abnormalities, primarily in the hips, knees, and ankles, are the chief manifestations. The ossification centers of the epiphyses appear late, and fusion with the bone shaft is late. The epiphyses are irregular and flattened, and the ossification centers may be mottled with secondary centers, but there is no true stippling.

Mild shortening of the long bones develops, and metaphyseal irregularity is minimal. A deficiency in the lateral portion of the epiphyses of the distal tibias produces a sloping, wedge-shaped distal articular surface, which is an important diagnostic sign in adults.

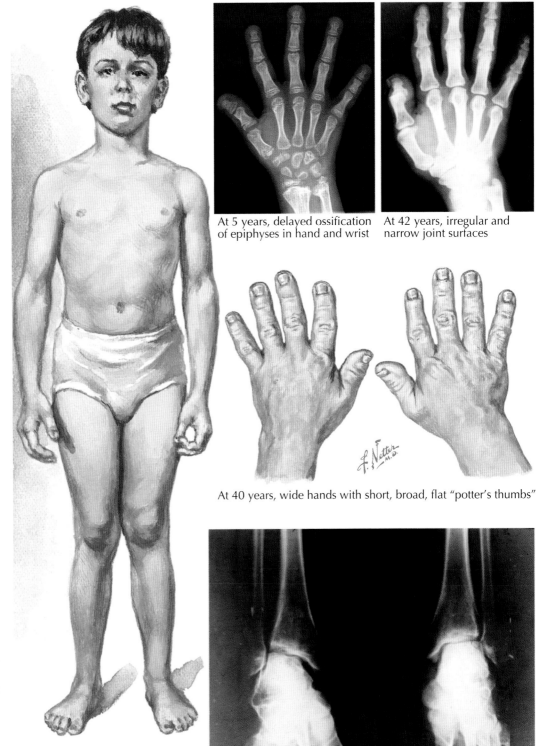

At 5 years, delayed ossification of epiphyses in hand and wrist

At 42 years, irregular and narrow joint surfaces

At 40 years, wide hands with short, broad, flat "potter's thumbs"

Relatively normal habitus, body proportions, and facies; mildly short stature. Joint stiffness may lead to progressive incapacitation.

Slanted distal articular surfaces of tibias; usually evident after epiphyseal fusion at puberty

Bipartite patella (double layer patella) is a common finding. Short, stubby phalanges and metacarpals with epiphyseal irregularities are seen. Vertebral changes are minimal and are usually manifested as Schmorl's nodules or mild anterior wedging of the vertebral bodies in the thoracolumbar area.

Differential Diagnosis. Multiple epiphyseal dysplasia is often mistakenly diagnosed as bilateral Legg-Calvé-Perthes disease. Family history, bone scans, and a radiographic survey of the entire skeleton help distinguish the two conditions. In patients with multiple epiphyseal dysplasia, the epiphyses of the femoral heads are symmetrically affected, unlike the asymmetric involvement that characterizes Legg-Calvé-Perthes disease; multiple epiphyseal dysplasia is also found in other parts of the skeleton.

Plate 4-13

Musculoskeletal System: PART III

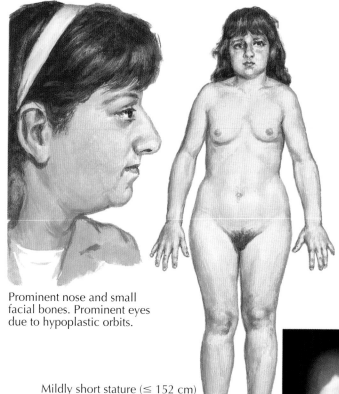

Prominent nose and small facial bones. Prominent eyes due to hypoplastic orbits.

Mildly short stature (≤ 152 cm) with relatively normal body proportion

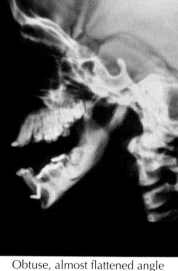

Obtuse, almost flattened angle between ramus and body of mandible

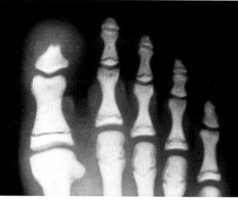

Marked shortening and tapering of distal phalanges without terminal tufts in hands and feet

DWARFISM—PYCNODYSOSTOSIS (PYKNODYSOSTOSIS)

Pycnodysostosis was once thought to be achondroplasia with cleidocranial dysostosis. Parental consanguinity has been implicated in more than 30% of cases of this autosomal recessive disease. The locus has been mapped to chromosome 1q21. Mutations lead to cathepsin K deficiency, which leads to diminished osteoclast function. Mental retardation occurs in about one sixth of patients.

Clinical Manifestations. The major signs are failure to thrive, with resultant short stature in infancy and persistence of an open anterior fontanel even into adulthood.

The head is large in relation to the body, with protrusion of the frontal and occipital bones. The major cranial sutures and anterior fontanel often remain open, giving the impression of hydrocephalus. The face is small in proportion to the cranium and is characterized by bulging or prominent eyes, parrot-like nose, receding chin, and an obtuse angle of the jaw. Dental anomalies include premature or delayed eruption of teeth, persistence of the deciduous dentition, malocclusion, and hypoplasia of the enamel. The vault of the palate is highly arched and sometimes deeply grooved. The sclerae may be blue.

Because of increased bone density, even such mild trauma as tooth extraction can cause fractures. Deformities of the long bones, often due to fractures and malunion, may exacerbate the short-limb dwarfism.

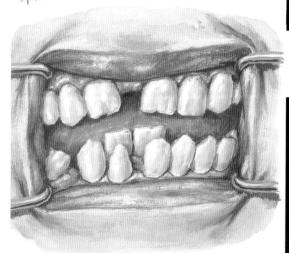

Delayed shedding of deciduous teeth results in double row of teeth, crowding, and malocclusion.

Open fontanels and wide cranial sutures are characteristic.

Arm span tends to be less than normal, and the terminal phalanges of the fingers are short and wide. Kyphosis, scoliosis, and exaggerated lumbar lordosis may develop. In some patients, the thorax is narrow and long. Adult height varies from 51 to 59 inches.

Radiographic Findings. Sclerosis is seen throughout the skeleton. The cranium is large, shortened, and brachycephalic with separation of sutures and an open anterior fontanel. Multiple sutural (wormian) bones are often present, and the facial bones, particularly the jaw,

are underdeveloped. There is variable cortical thickening of the long bones with moderate metaphyseal undermodeling, with or without evidence of fractures. In the hands and feet, partial aplasia of the tufts and distal portions of the phalanges creates a bizarre drumstick appearance on radiographs. The acromial ends of the clavicles are dysplastic and hypoplastic.

Differential Diagnosis. Pycnodysostosis is easily distinguished from cleidocranial dysostosis (see Plate 4-28) and osteopetrosis (see Plate 4-26).

Plate 4-14

Congenital and Developmental Disorders

Dwarfism—Camptomelic (Campomelic) Dysplasia

A rare form of congenital short-limb dwarfism, camptomelic dysplasia is characterized by prenatal bowing of the long bones of the lower limbs in association with anomalies of other organs. However, although bowing of the limbs is common, it is not always present or pathognomonic.

The disorder is an autosomal recessive trait, although there may be other modes of inheritance. Camptomelic dysplasia is in some cases associated with XY sex reversal. The majority of infants born with camptomelic dysplasia appear to be female, but genetic studies show that many are actually male with XY gonadal dysgenesis.

In one third of cases, hydramnios is detected during pregnancy. Stillbirth is common, and many liveborn infants die in the neonatal period or live for only several months; many develop severe respiratory distress, in part related to hypoplasia and other abnormalities of the tracheobronchial tree.

Although prognosis is guarded during the first year of life, with medical intervention, more and more children with camptomelic dysplasia survive into young adulthood.

Clinical Manifestations. At birth, infants have a low-normal weight, a relatively large and long (dolichocephalic) head, and disproportionate short length, primarily in the lower limbs.

The prominent forehead, rather flat face, depressed nasal bridge, long philtrum, small mouth, small jaw (micrognathia), and occasionally wide-set eyes and low-set ears produce a characteristic facies. Cleft palate occurs in most patients.

The arms are normal or only slightly shortened and bowed. The tibias are often bent, or boomerang shaped, with a cutaneous dimple over the apex of the bend. The femurs tend to be anterolaterally bowed, and clubfoot is common. The thorax is often small, narrow, and bell shaped. Progressive scoliosis is common. Hypotonia is an additional feature.

Stridor and laryngotracheomalacia are major hazards in infancy, leading to long-term episodes of apnea, pulmonary aspiration, cyanosis, respiratory failure, seizures, and feeding difficulties. Tracheostomy and ventilatory assistance are frequently necessary for long

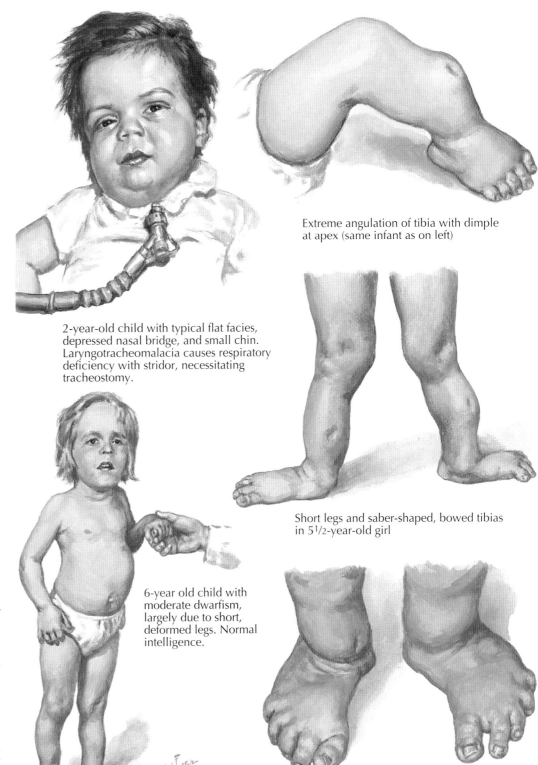

2-year-old child with typical flat facies, depressed nasal bridge, and small chin. Laryngotracheomalacia causes respiratory deficiency with stridor, necessitating tracheostomy.

Extreme angulation of tibia with dimple at apex (same infant as on left)

Short legs and saber-shaped, bowed tibias in 5½-year-old girl

6-year old child with moderate dwarfism, largely due to short, deformed legs. Normal intelligence.

Clubfoot resistant to correction; persistent metatarsus varus

periods of time. Congenital heart disease is found in nearly 25% of patients and hydronephrosis in 38%. Hemorrhagic phenomena in the central nervous system, hydrocephalus, and absence or hypoplasia of olfactory bulbs or tracts occur in 20% of patients.

Radiographic Findings. The typical findings reflect the three phenotypes: (I) classic (long-limb) type, characterized by bowed long bones with normal caliber and moderate shortening; (II) short-limb type, marked by severely shortened and bowed long bones and essentially normal neurocranium; and (III) short-limb type,

associated with premature closure of cranial sutures (craniosynostosis).

Common to all three types are a large skullcap (calvaria) in relation to facial size; a small, bell-shaped thorax with thin, wavy ribs; slender clavicles; and small scapulas. The femurs and tibias show variable degrees of bowing, and the fibulas are hypoplastic. Congenital dislocation of the hips is common. The pelvis is narrow with dysplastic pubic rami, and the ischia appear vertical or even divergent. Scoliosis or kyphoscoliosis occurs frequently.

Plate 4-15

Musculoskeletal System: PART III

DWARFISM— SPONDYLOEPIPHYSEAL DYSPLASIA TARDA AND SPONDYLOEPIPHYSEAL DYSPLASIA CONGENITA

SPONDYLOEPIPHYSEAL DYSPLASIA TARDA

This group of intrinsic bone dysplasias is characterized by progressive abnormalities of spinal and epiphyseal development. The disorders must be differentiated from spondylometaphyseal and spondyloepimetaphyseal dysplasias, which primarily involve the metaphyses instead of, or in addition to, the epiphyses.

Although most cases of spondyloepiphyseal dysplasia tarda have an X-linked recessive mode of inheritance, both autosomal dominant and autosomal recessive forms are also known. This has been mapped to the *SEDL* gene in the Xp22 chromosome affecting the protein sedlin, which plays an important role in endoplasmic reticulum/Golgi vesicular transport.

Clinical Manifestations. Growth failure does not become evident until 5 to 10 years of age. The height reduction, which is primarily due to trunk shortening, becomes quite obvious by adolescence. At this time, patients complain of pain and stiffness in the back or hips. Secondary osteoarthritis of the hip is common and may become disabling. The chest is broad or barrel shaped. Adult height ranges from 52 to 61 inches.

Radiographic Findings. The distinctive configuration of the vertebral bodies is most evident in the adult lumbar spine. Initially, the vertebral bodies are mildly flattened (platyspondyly) with a hump-shaped accumulation of bone in the posterior and central portions of the cartilage ring apophysis; the disc space appears narrowed. The thoracic cage is broad, while the pelvis is small and deep. The epiphyses of the long bones show variable dysplastic changes, and osteoarthritis of the hips is evident.

SPONDYLOEPIPHYSEAL DYSPLASIA CONGENITA

Spondyloepiphyseal dysplasia congenita is the more severe form affecting the spine and epiphyses of long bones. Most cases of spondyloepiphyseal dysplasia congenita are a result of spontaneous mutation. This type of short-trunk dwarfism is typically transmitted as an autosomal dominant trait, although cases of autosomal recessive inheritance are known. Mutations to *COL2A1* locus on chromosome 12 lead to abnormal type II collagen.

Clinical Manifestations. In the newborn, a broad or barrel chest, deep Harrison's grooves, and pigeon chest suggest the diagnosis. Flat, dishlike facies, cleft palate, and wide-set eyes are other early signs. In older children, the short neck makes the normal-sized head appear to rest directly on the shoulders. Myopia and retinal detachment or degeneration is occasionally seen.

The limbs show mild rhizomelic shortening but are long in comparison with the trunk; the hands and feet are essentially normal. Ligamentous laxity is excessive. Marked lumbar lordosis and moderate kyphoscoliosis

Spondyloepiphyseal dysplasia tarda

X-linked

Autosomal recessive

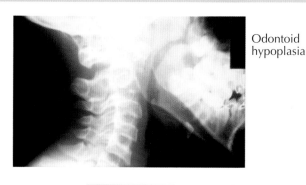

Femoral head deformity

Mid height

Mid height

Fingers reach almost to knees

Severe epiphyseal changes with pelvic tilt due to degenerative hip disease

Platyspondyly of cervical vertebrae

Spondyloepiphyseal dysplasia congenita

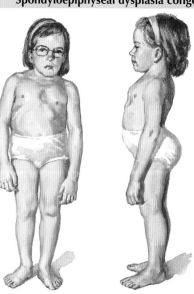

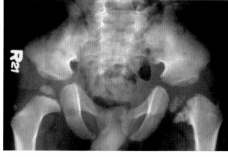

Odontoid hypoplasia

Late epiphyseal ossification, flat epiphysis of femoral head, coxa vara

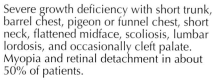

Severe growth deficiency with short trunk, barrel chest, pigeon or funnel chest, short neck, flattened midface, scoliosis, lumbar lordosis, and occasionally cleft palate. Myopia and retinal detachment in about 50% of patients.

occur in late childhood or early adulthood. Adults reach a height of only 33 to 52 inches.

Motor development is often delayed. In 50% of patients, hypotonia, ligamentous laxity, and odontoid hypoplasia result in atlantoaxial instability leading to spinal cord compression, which first manifests as overwhelming fatigue and decreased endurance.

Radiographic Findings. Retarded ossification of the pubic bones, femoral heads, and epiphyses of the knees, calcanei, and tali is the major feature in young children. Early in life, the vertebral bodies are ovoid or pear shaped but become flattened and irregular with time, resulting in kyphoscoliosis. Careful radiographic evaluation of the cervical spine is important because of the hazards associated with odontoid hypoplasia. Coxa vara is common, and rhizomelic shortening of the long bones with minimal dysplastic changes in the hands and feet may also be seen.

Plate 4-16

Congenital and Developmental Disorders

DWARFISM—SPONDYLOCOSTAL DYSOSTOSIS AND DYGGVE-MELCHIOR-CLAUSEN DYSPLASIA

Spondylocostal dysostosis

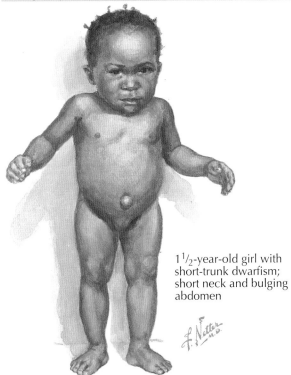

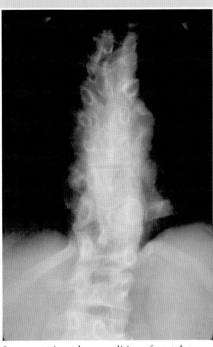

1½-year-old girl with short-trunk dwarfism; short neck and bulging abdomen

Segmentation abnormalities of vertebrae include hemivertebrae, fused vertebrae, and butterfly vertebrae. Scoliosis common.

SPONDYLOCOSTAL DYSOSTOSIS

Syndromes that comprise vertebral and thoracic abnormalities have been called by many designations, and more data are needed for a complete understanding of this group of disorders. However, evidence suggests genetic heterogeneity in spondylocostal dysostosis with at least three phenotypes: (I) autosomal recessive with high mortality in the first 2 years; (II) autosomal recessive with good prognosis for survival; and (III) autosomal dominant with mild-to-moderate clinical manifestations.

Clinical Manifestations. Posterior shortening of the thorax and thoracolumbar lordosis are the major causes of short stature. The neck is short and often nearly immobile, and the head appears to rest on the shoulders. The limbs are long in relation to the trunk. The barrel chest bulges anteriorly, the lower anterior ribs may infringe on the iliac crests, and the abdomen protrudes. Recurrent respiratory infections are common and may be related to the chest deformity, pulmonary hypoplasia, or cor pulmonale. Laryngotracheomalacia is an uncommon feature.

Radiographic Findings. Severe vertebral abnormalities—hemivertebrae, fused (block) vertebrae, absent and butterfly vertebrae—characterize this disorder. The ribs are reduced in number, and the posterior costovertebral articulations may be bizarrely approximated, producing a fanlike radiation of ribs. The posterior shortening of the spine causes anterior flaring of the chest and deformity of the rib cage. No significant abnormalities are seen in the appendicular skeleton or skull.

DYGGVE-MELCHIOR-CLAUSEN DYSPLASIA

Dyggve-Melchior-Clausen dysplasia is a rare and unusual disorder with an autosomal recessive inheritance.

Clinical Manifestations. Recognizable as early as 6 to 12 months of age, this disorder results in short-trunk dwarfism with a short neck, exaggerated lumbar lordosis, scoliosis, and prominent interphalangeal joints of the fingers with mild contractures and claw hand. Mental retardation and speech delay are common but not invariable. Adult height is about 52 inches.

Radiographic Findings. Radiographs reveal a generalized platyspondyly that usually persists into adulthood. In childhood, lateral views show anterior pointing of the vertebral bodies, with broad notches in the superior and inferior epiphyseal plates. The dens of the axis (odontoid process) may be hypoplastic. Irregular ossification of the iliac crests creates a characteristic lacelike

Dyggve-Melchior-Clausen dysplasia

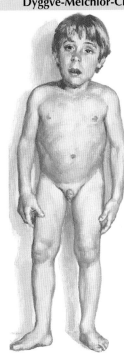

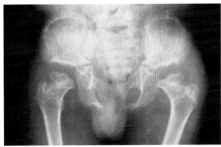

Lacelike appearance of iliac crests due to irregular ossification. Dysplastic pelvic bones and acetabula. Late appearance of femoral epiphyses.

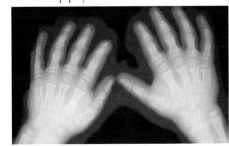

Broad and short metacarpals and phalanges; dysplastic carpals ossify late.

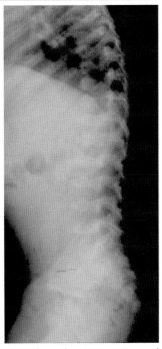

Broad notches in superior and inferior epiphyseal plates of vertebrae with anterior spurs

Boy with short-trunk dwarfism; broad chest and mental retardation

appearance on radiographs. The ilia are short and broad.

In young children, the growth plates of the proximal femurs are horizontal, with prominent spurlike projections on the medial side of the femoral necks. Ossification of the femoral epiphyses is delayed, and the long bones are short with irregular epiphyseal and metaphyseal ossification.

Differential Diagnosis. Patients with this condition bear some resemblance to persons with Morquio syndrome (see Plate 4-18). However, there is no corneal clouding and the urine contains no keratan sulfate. In fact, studies of lysosomal enzymes and histologic examination refute the hypothesis that Dyggve-Melchior-Clausen dysplasia is due to an abnormality of mucopolysaccharide metabolism.

Plate 4-17

Musculoskeletal System: PART III

KNIEST DYSPLASIA

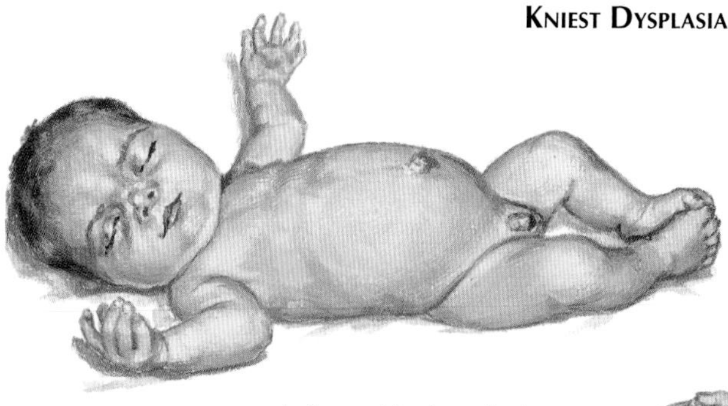

Infant with short limbs
and hypoplastic midface

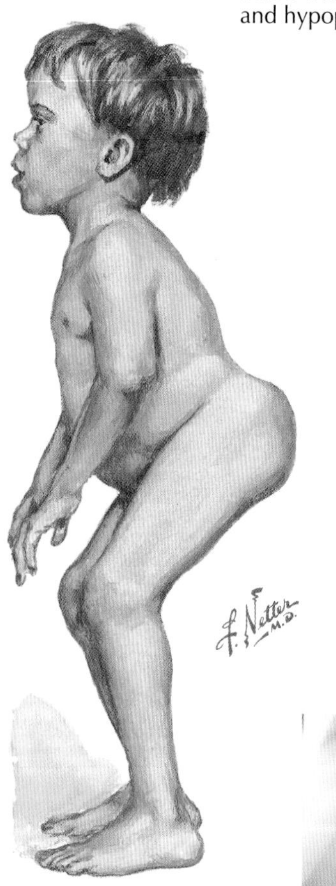

DWARFISM—KNIEST DYSPLASIA

Now considered a distinct autosomal dominant entity, Kniest dysplasia was previously thought to be a variant of metatropic dysplasia and, as a consequence, has been referred to as metatropic dwarfism, type II, and pseudometatropic dwarfism. This confusion occurred because dumbbell-shaped long bones are found in both of these skeletal disorders. Kniest dysplasia is a severe form of chondrodysplasia with significant kyphoscoliosis. Abnormal type II collagen is formed due to mutations of COL2A1.

Clinical Manifestations. The condition is usually evident at birth. Although the average birth length is $16\frac{1}{2}$ inches, adult height varies widely depending in part on the degree of contractures and kyphoscoliosis. The characteristic facies is round with midfacial flatness, a depressed and wide nasal bridge, protruding eyes in shallow orbits, and a broad mouth. Myopia occurs in 50% of patients and may become severe; retinal detachment is also common. About 50% of patients have a cleft palate without harelip. Recurrent otitis media and hearing loss, both conductive and neurosensory, are frequent.

At birth, the limbs are short in relation to the trunk but the proportions change and the trunk becomes comparatively shortened and kyphotic by early childhood. The knee and elbow joints are particularly prominent and enlarged, with limited range of motion; widespread flexion contractures develop. The fingers are relatively long and have bulbous and knobby joints. Stiffness of the metacarpophalangeal and interphalangeal joints prevents the patient from making a complete fist. Precocious osteoarthritis develops and may become incapacitating by late childhood. Lumbar lordosis is pronounced by early childhood, and kyphoscoliosis is common. Adult height ranges from 41 to 57 inches.

Radiographic Findings. Generalized platyspondyly with anterior wedging of the vertebral bodies in the lower thoracic and upper lumbar spine is a major feature. In infancy, coronal clefting may be seen in the lumbar vertebrae. The ilia are broad with hypoplastic basilar portions. Ossification of the femoral head may not be apparent until age 3 or even later. The short femoral necks are extremely broad, and in the newborn period the femurs are dumbbell shaped. The epiphyses at the knees are relatively large, and a peculiar flocculent calcification develops in the metaphyses of the long bones. The hands are affected by osteoporosis, large

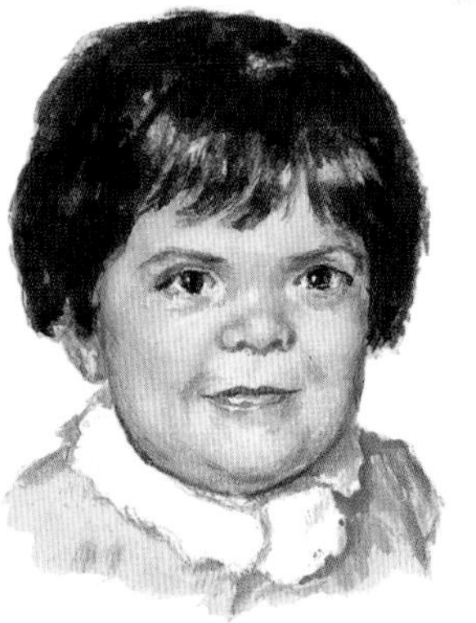

Dishlike facies with button nose, prominent eyes. Cleft palate and ear infections with hearing deficits common.

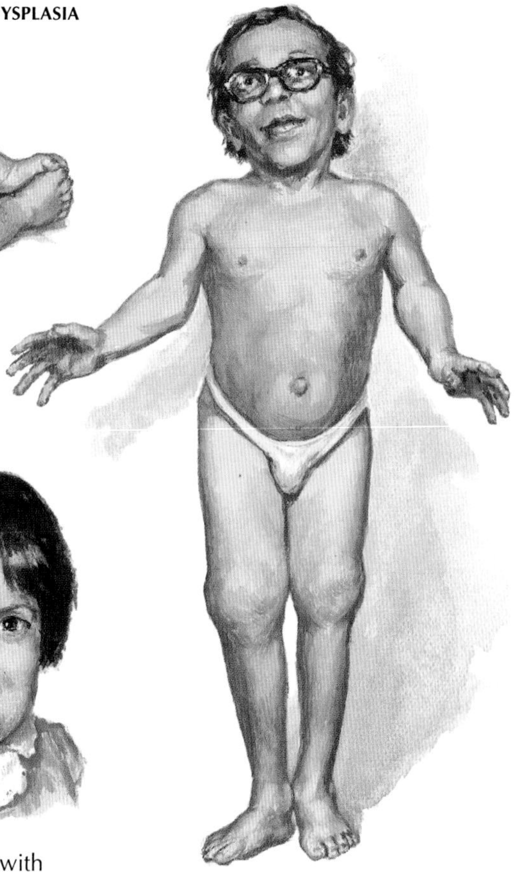

Reversal of growth pattern, short-trunk dwarfism develops with age. Knobby joints, characteristic stance, and severe myopia.

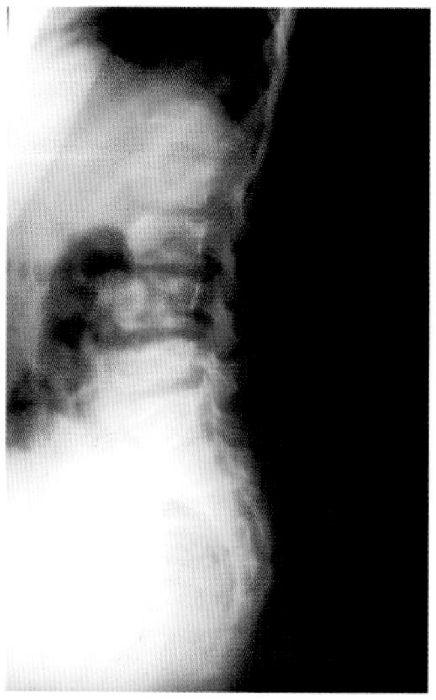

Flexion contractures and lumbar lordosis cause "about to dive" posture.

Platyspondyly, characteristic ventral spurs, and clefts in vertebrae

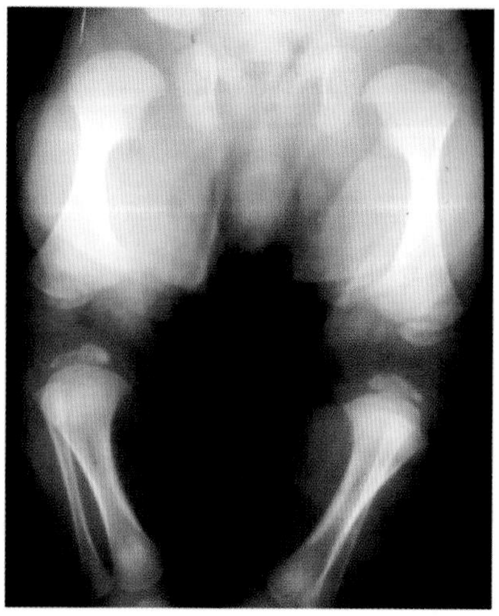

Characteristic dumbbell-shaped femurs and wide metaphyses in 1-month-old child

carpal centers, and bulbously enlarged interphalangeal joints with narrowed joint spaces.

Histologic Findings. The histopathology in Kniest dysplasia is unique. The resting cartilage contains large chondrocytes in a loosely woven matrix with numerous empty spaces (like Swiss cheese). In contrast, the growth plate is hypercellular. Electron microscopy reveals these cartilage cells to be filled with dilated cisterns of the rough endoplasmic reticulum.

Differential Diagnosis. Radiographs help to distinguish Kniest dysplasia from similar disorders; in the neonatal period, the ribs are essentially normal and there is moderately elongated platyspondyly. Metatropic dysplasia is characterized by wafer-like vertebral bodies and very short ribs. In spondyloepiphyseal dysplasia congenita (see Plate 4-15), ossification centers are not present in the neonatal period and the femurs are not dumbbell shaped.

Plate 4-18

Congenital and Developmental Disorders

DWARFISM— MUCOPOLYSACCHARIDOSES

The mucopolysaccharidoses (MPS) are a large group of biochemical storage disorders caused by lysosomal enzyme defects. More than eight major types and many subtypes have been identified, and all are hereditary and progressive.

HURLER SYNDROME

Hurler syndrome (MPS I-H) has an autosomal recessive inheritance and is caused by a deficiency in α-L-iduronidase. Elevated amounts of dermatan and heparan sulfates are identified due to the enzyme deficiency. The severity of enzyme deficiency correlates with clinical severity.

Clinical Manifestations. Affected infants are large at birth, but growth rate decreases in the early months of life. Stature is markedly restricted, and contractures develop, limiting ambulation. Facial features progressively coarsen, and the nasal bridge flattens. Corneal clouding, hepatosplenomegaly, joint stiffness, claw-hand deformity, and thoracolumbar kyphosis develop slowly. Hernias, hirsutism, macrocephaly, macroglossia, noisy respirations, and mucoid rhinorrhea are present by the second year of life.

Mental retardation is severe, with a lag in developmental milestones. Cardiac murmurs, deafness, and poor vision develop with time, and respiratory complications become more frequent. A combination of cardiac and pulmonary problems usually causes death between 6 and 12 years of age.

Radiographic Findings. Common to all the mucopolysaccharidoses are multiple skeletal changes that vary in severity. In patients with Hurler syndrome, the J-shaped sella turcica is enlarged, the skull is scaphocephalic, and the ribs are splayed. Other major findings include beaking of the lumbar vertebral bodies, kyphosis with gibbus formation in the thoracolumbar area, and abnormally short and broad long bones. Modeling of the metacarpals is poor, and their proximal ends are pointed. Broad, short phalanges contribute to claw-hand deformity.

Laboratory Findings. A high concentration of acid mucopolysaccharides, primarily dermatan sulfate and heparan sulfate, is found in the urine. There is a deficiency of lysosomal enzyme α-L-iduronidase in fibroblasts or leukocytes, and metachromatic granules may be observed in leukocytes.

HUNTER SYNDROME

Hunter syndrome (MPS II) is transmitted as an X-linked recessive trait. It is caused by a deficiency of the enzyme iduronate-2-sulfatase. Heparan sulfate is found to be in excess.

Clinical Manifestations. Clinical signs, present only in males, may not appear until age 2 or 3. The phenotypic presentations develop slowly. Two subtypes are recognizable. The severe form (MPS II-A) is marked by progressive mental retardation, and death occurs before age 15. A mild form (MPS II-B) is compatible with survival to adulthood and reproduction.

Affected persons are generally taller than those with Hurler syndrome, reaching a height of 47 to 59 inches. Coarse facies, joint stiffness and contractures, claw-hand deformity, hepatomegaly, hernias, cardiac complications, hirsutism, and deafness are major features. Usually, corneal clouding is not clinically evident,

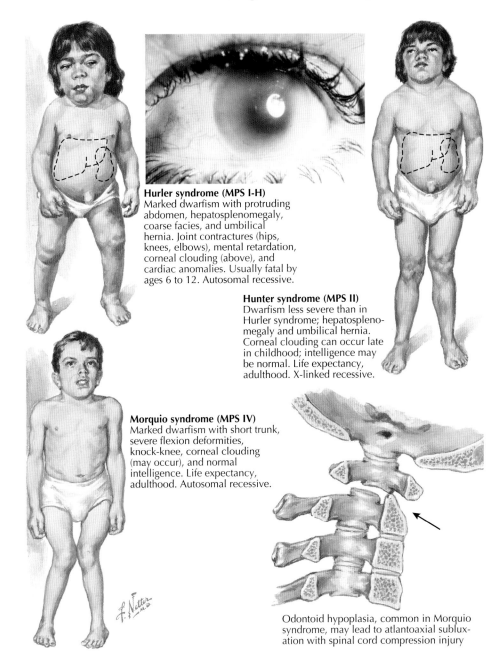

Hurler syndrome (MPS I-H)
Marked dwarfism with protruding abdomen, hepatosplenomegaly, coarse facies, and umbilical hernia. Joint contractures (hips, knees, elbows), mental retardation, corneal clouding (above), and cardiac anomalies. Usually fatal by ages 6 to 12. Autosomal recessive.

Hunter syndrome (MPS II)
Dwarfism less severe than in Hurler syndrome; hepatosplenomegaly and umbilical hernia. Corneal clouding can occur late in childhood; intelligence may be normal. Life expectancy, adulthood. X-linked recessive.

Morquio syndrome (MPS IV)
Marked dwarfism with short trunk, severe flexion deformities, knock-knee, corneal clouding (may occur), and normal intelligence. Life expectancy, adulthood. Autosomal recessive.

Odontoid hypoplasia, common in Morquio syndrome, may lead to atlantoaxial subluxation with spinal cord compression injury

although in older patients, slit lamp examination may reveal a light haze. Occasionally, a pebble-like rash is seen in regions of the scapula and upper arm.

Radiographic Findings. Findings of enlarged sella turcica, spatulate ribs, beaking of lumbar vertebrae, kyphosis, and short and broad long bones are less pronounced than those in Hurler syndrome.

Laboratory Findings. Increased levels of chondroitin sulfate B and heparan sulfate are seen in the urine. The lysosomal enzyme α-iduronidase is deficient in cultured fibroblasts.

MORQUIO SYNDROME

Morquio syndrome (MPS IV) has an autosomal recessive inheritance caused by a deficiency in the enzyme *N*-acetylgalactosamine-6-sulfate sulfatase, which is essential for the breakdown of keratan sulfate and chondroitin-6-sulfate.

Clinical Manifestations. Appearance at birth is normal, but the growth rate is usually restricted by 2 years of age and ceases by age 12. Medical attention is sought for dwarfism, awkward gait, knock-knee, bulging

sternum, flaring of the rib cage, flatfoot, prominent joints, cervical instability, or dorsal kyphosis. Corneal clouding develops between 5 and 10 years of age but is not as severe as in Hurler syndrome. The teeth are discolored and have easily fractured enamel. Ligamentous laxity can be extreme, particularly at the wrists. Severe knock-knee may interfere with ambulation.

Other complications include aortic regurgitation and atlantoaxial instability leading to spinal cord compression, which may, in turn, lead to quadriparesis. Adult height is less than in Hunter syndrome, ranging from only 32 to 47 inches.

Radiographic Findings. Flattened vertebrae with central anterior projections in the lumbar spine, odontoid aplasia or hypoplasia, delayed development of ossification centers, wide ribs, pointed proximal metacarpals, and coxa valga are the principal findings.

Laboratory Findings. The presence of keratan sulfate with normal or elevated levels of acid mucopolysaccharides in the urine is typical and is associated with a deficiency of the lysosomal enzyme *N*-acetylgalactosamine-6-sulfate sulfatase in cultured fibroblasts.

Plate 4-19

Musculoskeletal System: PART III

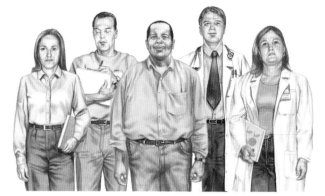

Successful treatment requires a multidisciplinary approach.

DWARFISM—PRINCIPLES OF TREATMENT OF SKELETAL DYSPLASIAS

Because of the widespread skeletal and nonosseous manifestations in many forms of dwarfism, successful treatment requires a multidisciplinary approach coordinated by the family physician. The child's growth and physical development must be monitored and compared with those of other children with the same disorder. Because eye and ear problems are fairly common in some types of dwarfism, ophthalmologic and hearing examinations should be frequent.

For genetic counseling of the family and patient faced with the choice of reproduction, it is essential to determine the specific diagnosis and mode of inheritance. It is no longer adequate to label a condition a "variant." However, in some cases the diagnosis remains unclear, and reproductive risks cannot be predicted. Psychosocial counseling may therefore be needed to promote a feeling of self-worth in the patient and social adjustment. Parents must encourage age-related—not size-related—behavior, social interaction, and independence in their affected children.

Medical Management. Patients must develop good nutritional habits early in life. Obesity is a serious problem; in a small person, even a minor weight gain is immediately apparent and may contribute to biomechanical imbalances or complications. Particularly common in persons with achondroplasia, overweight must be avoided not only to prevent hypertension and other cardiovascular diseases but also because it can precipitate or aggravate compressive myelopathy. Thus, weight loss often relieves symptoms of spinal cord ischemia. Exercise can help maintain ideal body weight, but in people with dwarfism, specific skeletal problems obviously impose some limitations, and patients should select activities that do not stress the weight-bearing joints, such as swimming and bicycling.

Custom-made shoes and orthotic devices placed in the shoe help compensate for any limb-length discrepancy, but surgery and/or a limb prosthesis may be needed in severe cases.

Surgical Treatment. Most skeletal limb deformities and malalignment problems are not amenable to conservative measures such as bracing and must eventually be corrected with surgery. Scoliosis and kyphoscoliosis are managed with bracing or spinal fusion. Symmetric extensive limb lengthening is experimental at this time and highly controversial.

Surgical decompression is the usual treatment for spinal stenosis; spinal fusion is occasionally required.

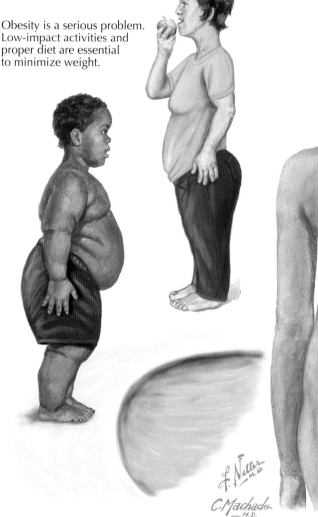

Obesity is a serious problem. Low-impact activities and proper diet are essential to minimize weight.

Custom-made orthotic devices help compensate for any limb-length discrepancy.

Scoliosis may be treated with a brace or surgical correction.

Because wide posterior laminectomy may create spinal instability, anterior vertebral body fusion followed by posterior laminectomy is often performed. Timing for surgical decompression is critical; if performed too late, it will not restore function or prevent progression. Surgery is also associated with significant morbidity.

Whenever a dwarfing condition is suspected, the cervical spine must be examined carefully for atlantoaxial instability. Radiographs should be taken with the neck in flexion, extension, and neutral position. Spinal fusion is often the treatment of choice for this hazardous complication.

Skeletal malalignment, obesity, and participation in proscribed activities may lead to or aggravate early osteoarthritis. People with dwarfism are now frequent candidates for total joint replacement, especially of the hip.

Plate 4-20

Congenital and Developmental Disorders

DIAGNOSTIC CRITERIA AND CUTANEOUS LESIONS IN NEUROFIBROMATOSIS

National Institutes of Health Neurofibromatosis Type 1 Diagnostic Criteria*

*Patient must have 2 or more of these criteria identified to be considered as having neurofibromatosis type 1 (NF1)
 	
1. More than six (6) café-au-lait spots
    a. Adult → must be ≥ 15 mm in diameter
    b. Child → must be ≥ 5 mm in diameter
2. Two (2) or more neurofibromas of any type, or one (1) plexiform neurofibroma
3. Axillary or inguinal freckling (Crowe sign)
4. Two (2) or more Lisch nodules (iris hamartomas)
5. A distinctive bone lesion, such as:
    a. Sphenoid dysplasia
    b. Anterolateral bowing of the tibia
    c. Short segmented, sharply angulated spinal deformity
    d. Cortical long bone thinning with or without pseudarthrosis
6. A first-degree relative (parent, sibling, offspring) with NF1 by the aforementioned criteria

Adapted from the NIH Consensus Development Conference statement: Neurofibromatosis. Neurofibromatosis 1988;1:172.

NEUROFIBROMATOSIS

Neurofibromatosis, first fully described by von Recklinghausen, is a disturbance in the neuroectodermal and mesodermal tissues, the supportive tissue of the nervous system. It is a multisystemic congenital and sometimes familial disorder and is progressive when it involves the central nervous and musculoskeletal systems.

Neurofibromatosis occurs in 1 in 2,500 to 4,000 persons. It is transmitted as an autosomal dominant trait with close to 100% penetrance. There is also a characteristically high rate (~50%) of spontaneous mutations, which may explain why only about 50% of patients have a family history of the disease. The gene for peripheral (von Recklinghausen) neurofibromatosis (NF1) is located on chromosome 17; the gene for central (bilateral acoustic) neurofibromatosis (NF2) has its locus on chromosome 22. This discussion is limited to von Recklinghausen neurofibromatosis.

DIAGNOSTIC CRITERIA

The diagnosis of von Recklinghausen neurofibromatosis in a child requires a high index of suspicion. If two or more of the criteria shown in Plate 4-20 are identified in a child, that individual can be considered to have NF1. By the age of 1 year, 70% will meet diagnostic criteria, with 97% fulfilling diagnostic criteria by the age of 8 years. With time, all manifestations of neurofibromatosis increase in number, size, and severity.

The most common musculoskeletal manifestations are spinal deformity, limb-length discrepancy, pseudarthrosis of the tibia, and problems such as pathologic fractures and hemihypertrophy of the foot, face, and hand. Despite multiple musculoskeletal manifestations of NF1, only approximately 10% of those affected will require orthopaedic intervention in their lifetime. Of those that require operations, many will require multiple procedures.

NF1 is characterized by the involvement of multiple organ systems outside the skeletal system. Neurologic, visual, and hearing problems are associated characteristics. In children, the incidence of several manifestations, such as sexual precocity, learning disorders, retarded sexual development, malignant hypertension secondary to diffuse renal artery changes, and mental retardation, is not statistically significant. The often-noted delay of speech and motor development may signify central nervous system involvement.

CUTANEOUS LESIONS

Café-au-lait spots—the characteristic cutaneous lesions of neurofibromatosis—are present in 90% of patients

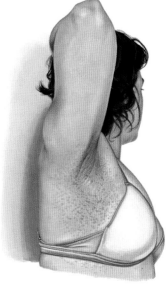

Dense axillary and inguinal freckling is rarely found in the absence of NF1.

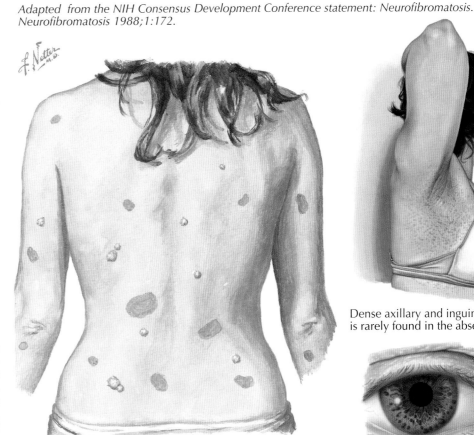

Multiple café-au-lait spots and nodules (fibroma molluscum) are most common manifestations.

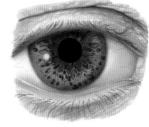

Lisch nodules are hamartomas on the iris. They are raised and frequently pigmented.

(see Plate 4-20). These spots are macular and melanotic with smooth edges, in contrast to the jagged edges seen in similar lesions of fibrous dysplasia (McCune-Albright syndrome). Café-au-lait spots in NF1 have been likened to the "coast of California," whereas lesions of fibrous dysplasia resemble the "rugged coast of Maine."

An adult with more than six café-au-lait spots with diameters of 15 mm or greater must be presumed to

have neurofibromatosis. Results of an evaluation of children younger than age 5 indicate that two or fewer café-au-lait spots occur in less than 1% of normal children and that five spots with a diameter of at least 5 mm are pathognomonic. Cutaneous neurofibroma "nodules" (fibroma molluscum), pigmented nevi, elephantiasis, and verrucous hyperplasia are other characteristic skin lesions.

Plate 4-21

Musculoskeletal System: PART III

CUTANEOUS LESIONS IN NEUROFIBROMATOSIS

NEUROFIBROMATOSIS (Continued)

Plexiform neurofibromas have a characteristic "bag of worms" proprioceptive texture, and have a 25% to 40% incidence in NF1 patients. Plexiform neurofibromas have a 10% to 24% lifetime risk for malignant transformation into malignant peripheral nerve sheath tumors (MPNST), with those patients developing MPNSTs showing a 5-year survival rate of 21%. An underlying plexiform neurofibroma is typically marked by hyperpigmented skin and can extend into underlying fascia, muscle, and bone. Severe disfigurement and pain may occur.

Over the course of their lifetime, patients with NF1 are at inherently greater risk for developing malignancy as compared with the general population. Some examples of neoplasms seen more frequently in NF1 patients include leukemia, rhabdomyosarcoma, pheochromocytoma, Wilms tumor, pancreatic endocrine tumors, and astrocytic-origin brain tumors.

BONE LESIONS

Deformity of Spine. Scoliosis is the most common bone lesion in neurofibromatosis, historically being reported in as high as 60% of NF1 patients who present to the orthopaedic surgeon. The true incidence over the general NF1 population is likely closer to 10%. Two patterns of scoliotic deformity have been identified. The deformity can vary from mild, nonprogressive forms (nondystrophic) to the less common (but more severe) form with tight, short curves (dystrophic) (see Plate 4-22). The cervical spine should also be monitored, because NF1 patients can have cervical kyphosis, rotary subluxation, and atlantoaxial instability develop.

Type I spinal deformity (dystrophic curves) are characterized by multiple abnormalities, such as foraminal enlargement, vertebral scalloping, "penciling" of ribs/transverse processes, dural ectasia (dural thinning), pedicle dysplasia, interpediculate distance widening, severe apical rotation, paravertebral soft tissue mass, and "grotesque" hairpin curves resulting in thoracic kyphoscoliosis, most commonly. This type of scoliosis tends to be progressive and to resist stabilization of the spine with the usual methods. CT and MRI are needed to rule out congenital deformity, dysplasia, and intradural pathologic processes and are necessary for preoperative planning.

The classic NF1 dystrophic curve is further divided into two subtypes: lateral curve (scoliosis) and anterior curve (kyphoscoliosis), in which the kyphotic element (>50 degrees) predominates over the scoliotic element. The kyphotic type of spinal deformity is believed to contribute more to paraplegia than the lateral deformity. Flexion of the spine causes elongation of the vertebral canal and plastic deformation of the spinal cord. Increased spinal flexion due to the kyphotic deformity increases axial tension in the spinal cord parenchyma,

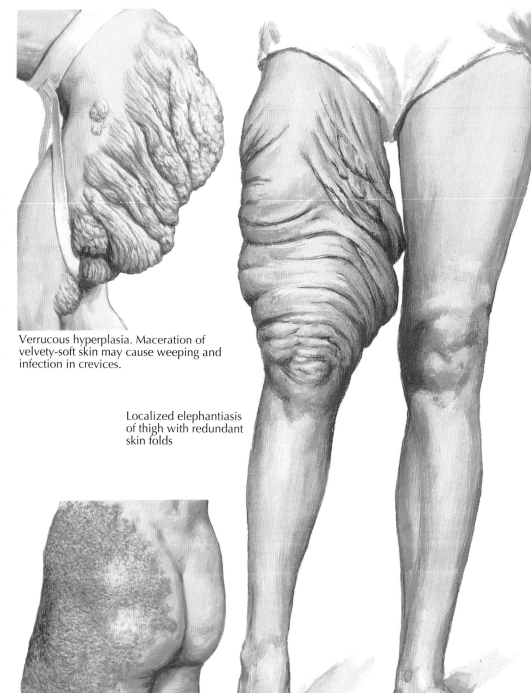

Verrucous hyperplasia. Maceration of velvety-soft skin may cause weeping and infection in crevices.

Localized elephantiasis of thigh with redundant skin folds

Nevus characteristically localized to one side of trunk and thigh

resulting in functional neurologic impairment or paraplegia. This type of deformity is not successfully treated with routine posterior spinal fusion because it tends to result in pseudarthrosis. Spinal fusion with both anterior and posterior approaches is needed to prevent progression of the deformity ("crankshaft" phenomenon) and decrease the risk of pseudarthrosis.

Type II spinal deformity appears to be indistinguishable from idiopathic scoliosis and is an incidental finding in

patients with neurofibromatosis. Follow-up studies of patients with type II deformity show less progression of the curve and better response to treatment. Despite a less severe curve pattern, careful serial examination for type II curves is essential, with as many as 65% of patients developing dystrophic changes. In contrast to idiopathic scoliosis, the incidence of pseudarthrosis in the spine tends to be higher than in NF1 scoliosis patterns.

Plate 4-22

Congenital and Developmental Disorders

SPINAL DEFORMITIES IN NEUROFIBROMATOSIS

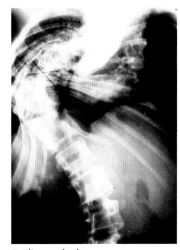

Radiograph shows severe scoliosis with characteristic short-segmented, sharply angulated curve.

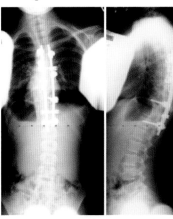

NEUROFIBROMATOSIS *(Continued)*

Operative treatment is guided by the type and severity of the curve. In general, anteroposterior surgery in anterior (predominately kyphotic) dystrophic curves progressing beyond 20 to 40 degrees is recommended. In lateral (scoliosis) dystrophic curves, early surgical intervention is also recommended, but with the advent of pedicle screws, a posterior approach alone may be sufficient to prevent deformity progression and pseudarthrosis. With type II (nondystrophic) curves, observation is indicated in curves of less than 20 degrees, bracing in curves of 20 to 40 degrees, and surgical intervention beyond 40 degrees. In very severe deformity, preoperative halo traction has been shown to reduce curve severity before fusion.

Bone Overgrowth. Disorders of bone growth are fairly common manifestations of neurofibromatosis. They are usually recognized clinically by changes in the overlying soft tissues, with some examples including hemangioma, lymphangioma, elephantiasis, and beaded plexiform neurofibroma (see Plates 4-22 and 4-23). The overgrowth in bones and soft tissue is usually unilateral, involving the limbs, head, or neck. Joseph Carey "John" Merrick, who gained fame in the 19th century as "The Elephant Man," exemplified the classic case of unilateral bone overgrowth associated with neurofibromatosis. Recently, however, Merrick's diagnosis of neurofibromatosis has been challenged, with some authors proposing that he had Proteus syndrome.

Because lesions in the limbs occasionally continue to overgrow even after skeletal maturity, epiphysiodesis to equalize limb length should be performed when the diagnosis is confirmed (see Plates 4-35 and 4-36).

Pseudarthrosis of Tibia. An anterolateral bowing deformity in neurofibromatosis may progress to multiple areas of spontaneous fracture followed by pseudarthrosis, known as congenital pseudarthrosis of the tibia (CPT) (see Plate 4-31). The tibial bowing always develops before age 2. It is often progressive and should be treated with a high degree of vigilance. In contrast, posteromedial bowing (which is not associated with neurofibromatosis) is nonprogressive and does not present severe management problems. Anteromedial tibial bowing is classically associated with congenital limb deficiency, such as fibular hemimelia. Management of a fracture associated with CPT is problematic because of its high nonunion rate.

Anterolateral bowing of the tibia in neurofibromatosis has been classified into two types according to the intactness of the medullary canal, involvement of the fibula, and risk of fracture (see Plate 4-31). *Type I* is an anterolateral bowing with increased cortical density and a sclerotic medullary canal. *Type IIA* is an anterolateral bowing with failure of tubulation (abnormal medullary canal). *Type IIB* is an anterolateral bowing associated with a cystic lesion, or prefracture. *Type IIC* includes anterolateral bowing and frank fracture with

Girl with moderate scoliosis and café-au-lait spots

Boy with kyphoscoliosis. Foreshortening of trunk secondary to kyphosis gives appearance of longer upper limbs.

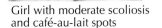

Relatively mild curve largely corrected with segmental pedicle screw and hook instrumentation

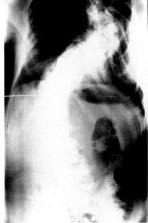

Benign-appearing scoliosis in child with neurofibromatosis

2 years later, progression of curve apparent

Spinal fusion resulted in nonunion. Exploration 3 years later revealed neurofibrosarcoma at fusion site. Section shows whorled, spindle-cell pattern of tumor (H & E stain).

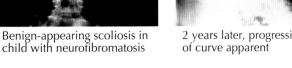

pseudarthrosis of both tibia and fibula. Overall, outcome is directly related to the presence of a fracture, location of the fracture within the tibia, and age at the time of fracture.

Type I anterolateral bowing has the best prognosis and may never progress to fracture. Management with bracing is usually unnecessary, unless the bowing starts to increase severely. Corrective osteotomy for the bowing may result in nonunion and pseudarthrosis.

Type IIA bowing may lead to fracture, and protective management with an ankle-foot orthosis (prior to walking) or a knee-ankle-foot orthosis (with weight bearing) is essential from the time of diagnosis. Whereas braces are meant to be protective, union with brace management in a fractured tibia rarely results in union. Parents should be educated on the increased likelihood for needed surgical intervention. Type IIB bowing deformity is extremely susceptible to fractures, and,

Plate 4-23   Musculoskeletal System: PART III

BONE OVERGROWTH AND EROSION IN NEUROFIBROMATOSIS

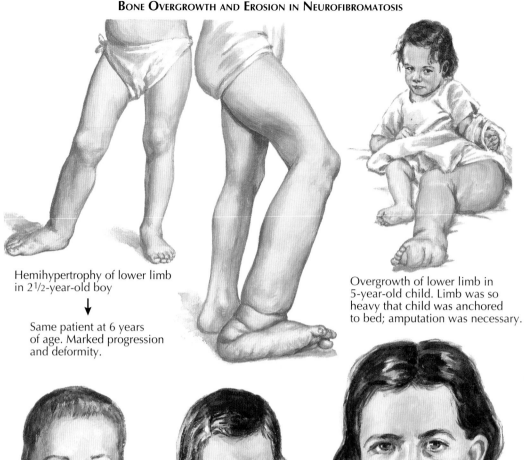

Hemihypertrophy of lower limb
in 2½-year-old boy

↓

Same patient at 6 years
of age. Marked progression
and deformity.

Overgrowth of lower limb in
5-year-old child. Limb was so
heavy that child was anchored
to bed; amputation was necessary.

NEUROFIBROMATOSIS (Continued)

therefore, risk of pseudarthrosis. Attempts to obtain osteosynthesis include various bone-grafting techniques such as massive onlay, inlay, delayed autografts, and turnaround grafts; fixation with an intramedullary rod; vascularized bone (fibular) grafts using microsurgical techniques; and electric stimulation. None of these methods has produced consistent union rates. Additionally, the risk of refracture is high. New techniques are being developed using osteoinductive materials, such as bone morphogenetic protein. This remains an off-label use, with noted variability in union rates in small sample populations. Parents should participate in deciding how many surgical procedures should be attempted before resorting to amputation.

Type IIC bowing has the worst prognosis, and amputation should be considered early in treatment. The number of operations attempted and the length of hospitalizations must be carefully considered in light of the course of the disease and the psychological and financial costs. Short-term follow-up reports of obtaining successful osteosynthesis of these pseudarthrotic lesions using the Ilizarov technique (see Plate 4-36) have not stood the test of time.

Pseudarthrosis in the context of NF1 has been reported to occur with lesser frequency in other long bone regions, such as the humerus, radius, ulna, and clavicle.

Tumors. Neurologic hamartomatous lesions in neurofibromatosis are uncommon but not rare (see Plate 4-23). A dumbbell tumor is a neurofibroma that arises in the vertebral canal and grows outward through the intervertebral (neural) foramen, its midportion being constricted by the bony foramen. Despite rare

Progression of unilateral facial deformity. Note skin pigmentation.
Infancy (left); 2½ years (center); 17 years (right).

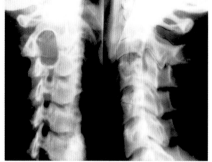

Radiographs show
enlargement of
spinal foramina
at C2–3 junction
due to erosion by
dumbbell tumor.
Excised tumor (right).

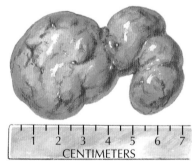

malignant transformation, retroperitoneal masses or dumbbell tumors that extend from the vertebral canal may cause mass-effect phenomena such as intestinal obstruction or neurologic compromise. Some tumors recur and overgrow into a vital area, rendering repeat excision impossible.

Bone Erosion. Erosive defects of bone in neurofibromatosis, which appear on radiographs as cysts, may be secondary to contiguous neurogenic tumors. Increased

pressure in the dural sac may give rise to dural ectasia or pseudomeningocele in the vertebral canal. Thought to be a consequence of coinciding thecal sac pulsations and elevated intrathecal pressures, expansion of a thinned dural wall can cause bony erosion, widened interpedicular distances, and narrowed pedicle canals. Likewise, dumbbell tumors of the spinal cord cause enlargement of the intervertebral foramen as they exit the vertebral canal.

Plate 4-24

Congenital and Developmental Disorders

ARTHROGRYPOSIS MULTIPLEX CONGENITA

Arthrogryposis multiplex congenita (multiple congenitally rigid joints) is a nonprogressive syndrome derived of myopathic, neuropathic, or mixed etiology that occurs in 1 in 3,000 live births. The most common form (neuropathic) is evident at birth and is believed to have at least partial etiology rooted in an intrauterine infection (probably viral), leading to developmental failure of the anterior horn cells. The resultant loss of muscle tone and function allows for fetal akinesis, which leads to thickened and fibrotic joint capsules, fibrosed tendon sheaths, and joint contractures. The autosomally inherited, nonprogressive, myogenic type of arthrogryposis is a form of congenital muscular dystrophy—the anterior horn cells, spinal cord, and nerve roots are normal with the muscle characterized by fatty infiltrates and atrophy.

Clinical Manifestations. The neonate displays multiple contractures, dislocated joints, adduction/internal rotation of the upper limbs ("waiter's tip" position), and stiff, diamond-shaped lower limbs. The deformities are usually bilateral, showing variable symmetry and involvement of the limbs. Active and passive range of motion is dramatically limited, with the joints characterized by noticeably absent skin creases. The skin is thin and smooth, and subcutaneous tissue is scanty. Muscle atrophy is striking. The bones are thin and spindly, and fractures, particularly in the lower limbs, may occur at delivery. Soft tissue webbing may also be evident.

In classic arthrogryposis, intelligence is normal. Patients display normal facies, no visceral abnormalities, retained bowel and bladder function, and intact sensation. Most remain ambulatory.

Arthrogryposis is associated with other conditions such as tuberous sclerosis, neurofibromatosis, myelodysplasia, and lumbosacral agenesis. Freeman-Sheldon syndrome, also known as "whistling face" syndrome, has many features similar to arthrogryposis but also with a characteristic puckered facial expression.

Treatment. In the newborn period, the focus of management is on treating both the deformity and the muscle weakness. Vigorous stretching is recommended to correct the rigid deformities, but care should be taken to avoid undue force because of increased fracture risk. The ultimate end goals are to allow for independent ambulation as well as independent upper extremity function in performing activities of daily living.

Deformities of Upper Limb. In the neonatal period, management of upper limb deformities comprises splinting and vigorous passive range-of-motion exercises. If the elbows are fixed in flexion, early exercises and splinting may be sufficient. More commonly, the elbows are fixed in extension and surgical release and/ or muscle transfer is necessary. Although the wrist and hand are usually severely involved, patients have adequate function. Regardless of the surgical procedure planned, the end goals should ensure bimanual hand function, with the shoulders and elbows allowing for the hands to work at tabletop level.

Deformities of Foot. The foot is nearly always involved in arthrogryposis; most common is rigid clubfoot (equinovarus). Surgical posteromedial release of the contracted structures in early infancy is necessary to allow correct positioning of the foot. Patients with severely affected feet are treated with bracing and splinting in the growth years to maintain the surgical correction. Recurrence is still common despite long-term postoperative orthotic treatment.

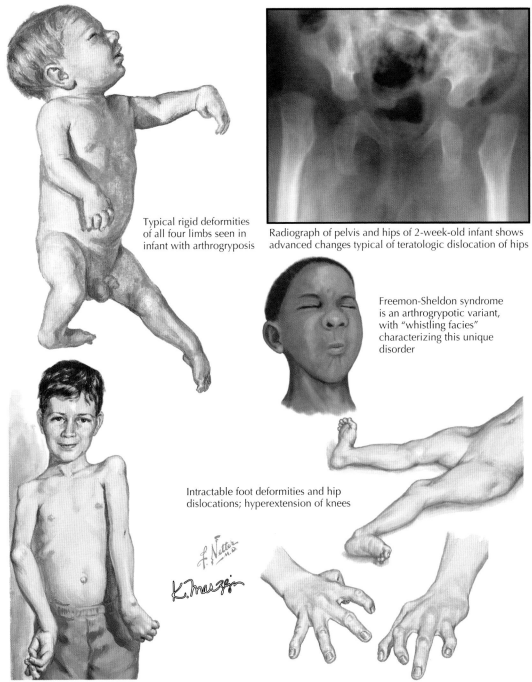

Typical rigid deformities of all four limbs seen in infant with arthrogryposis

Radiograph of pelvis and hips of 2-week-old infant shows advanced changes typical of teratologic dislocation of hips

Freemon-Sheldon syndrome is an arthrogrypotic variant, with "whistling facies" characterizing this unique disorder

Intractable foot deformities and hip dislocations; hyperextension of knees

Deformities of upper limbs in older child

Hand deformities

Deformities of Knee. The knees are commonly held in stiff extension. Although rare, flexed knee deformity is more troublesome in limiting ambulation. Early passive range-of-motion exercises, supplemented with serial casting/splinting, may be necessary to restore motion. With severe hyperextension deformity (sometimes leading to frank dislocation), surgical release or lengthening of the contracted quadriceps muscle is needed. Flexion deformity of the knee rarely responds to conservative treatment and often requires early surgical release of the posterior capsule and hamstring muscles. Perioperatively, careful wound closure and postoperative skin monitoring are essential, especially while serial casting/splinting.

Deformities of Hip. Hip involvement is characterized by two types: soft tissue contractures and dislocations.

Soft tissue contractures are evident in the neonatal period and can result in concurrent pelvic obliquity and scoliosis. Management includes early passive stretching, splinting, and surgical release. In the child with mild involvement, dislocated hips can be managed with the standard techniques used in congenital dislocation of the hip. More commonly, however, the hips are both stiff and dislocated and radiographs reveal advanced and adaptive changes similar to those seen in the older child with classic congenital dislocation of the hip. Surgery is generally performed in the first year, typically consisting of an open medial surgical reduction procedure, because closed reduction of the hips is largely unsuccessful. In the older child, surgery consists of an open anterior surgical reduction ± a femoral shortening osteotomy.

Plate 4-25

Musculoskeletal System: PART III

FIBRODYSPLASIA OSSIFICANS PROGRESSIVA AND PROGRESSIVE DIAPHYSEAL DYSPLASIA

FIBRODYSPLASIA OSSIFICANS PROGRESSIVA

Fibrodysplasia ossificans progressiva, historically referred to as myositis ossificans progressiva, is a syndrome in which the most disabling manifestation is an inflammatory-like lesion of ectopic ossification of the voluntary muscles, fascia, and tendons. The disease becomes clinically apparent during the first decade of life, and the clinician should be hyperaware of the relationship between great toe deformity (microdactyly) and fibrodysplasia ossificans progressiva in order to aid diagnosis.

The syndrome is hereditary without sex predilection. Unaffected family members may have the toe deformities without the subsequent ectopic ossification. The name of the disease indicates its histologic resemblance to the ectopic ossification found in other forms of myositis ossificans (see Section 6, Plate 6-24).

Clinical Manifestations. Congenital anomalies of the digits are initially noted at birth. Hypoplasia of the great toes is the most common manifestation, with great toe microdactyly occurring in 90% of patients. A similarly high association occurs with marked hallux valgus. Less common, microdactyly of the thumb occurs in 50% of patients.

The average age at onset is 5 years old, with characteristic localized swellings arising in the neck, back, and limbs, often accompanied by considerable tenderness, pyrexia, and occasionally draining ulcers. The ossification develops somewhat later and may cause ankylosis of the vertebral bodies and joints such as the elbow, knee, hip, and shoulder. By the midadolescent years, 95% of patients have severely restricted upper extremity range of motion. Despite the marked upper extremity involvement, the most debilitating effects are seen in the jaw muscles (inhibiting jaw motion) and chest muscles (impairing chest wall expansion and breathing). Fortunately, the tongue, diaphragm, and sphincters are not involved. Spinal involvement is common, with 65% of patients displaying scoliosis features.

Treatment. There are limited options for treatment. Clinical diagnosis is important, because surgical biopsy or excision only create robust recurrence. Supportive measures to ensure adequate nutrition and respiration may be needed, owing to the involvement of mastication and chest wall musculature. Patient falls can cause severe flareups or lifelong disability. Cervical involvement can make anesthesia management difficult. Current efforts with targeted gene therapy and bone morphogenetic protein antagonists have shown future promise. At this point, treatment measure are mainly supportive, ensuring proper nutrition, fall prevention, and pain control. Despite a marked disability, patients with fibrodysplasia ossificans progressiva can survive for many years.

PROGRESSIVE DIAPHYSEAL DYSPLASIA (ENGELMANN DISEASE)

This autosomal dominant hereditary disorder is characterized by a bilateral and symmetric cortical thickening of long bone diaphyses. The genetic pattern displays variable penetrance, with the disease becoming manifest in childhood as neuromuscular dystrophy. The child walks with legs spread apart, imparting a peculiar waddling gait. Generalized weakness and fatigability,

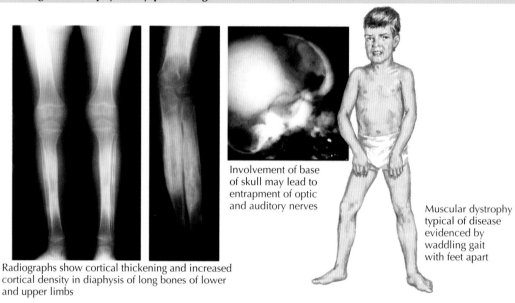

Fibrodysplasia ossificans progressiva

Left: Radiograph reveals ossification of posterolateral thoracic and arm musculature

Right: Posterior abdominal and lumbar (psoas) muscles affected

Clinical manifestations

Difficulty in opening mouth

Torticollis

Kyphosis

Bulging bony lumps

Ankylosed joints and generalized rigidity

Short first metatarsal and abnormalities of great toe

Progressive diaphyseal dysplasia (Engelmann's disease)

Involvement of base of skull may lead to entrapment of optic and auditory nerves

Muscular dystrophy typical of disease evidenced by waddling gait with feet apart

Radiographs show cortical thickening and increased cortical density in diaphysis of long bones of lower and upper limbs

along with delayed growth and sexual development, are commonly seen. Involvement of the skull in 60% of patients may lead to optic and auditory nerve entrapment.

With progression of the disease, the diameter of the diaphysis enlarges and the medullary canal becomes increasingly narrowed. The lesions spread proximally and distally toward the epiphyses. With the near obliteration of the medullary canals, hematopoiesis is diminished, resulting in secondary anemia and hepatomegaly.

Diagnostic Studies. Typical radiographic findings include (1) symmetric skeletal distribution; (2) fusiform enlargement of the diaphysis of the long bones and amorphous increase in density at the base of the skull; (3) thickening of the cortex by both periosteal and endosteal accretion of mottled bone without a recognizable trabecular pattern; (4) abrupt demarcation of the lesion; (5) progression of the lesion proximally and distally along the long axis of the bone with gradual alteration of the previously normal cortical bone; (6) relative elongation of the limb; (7) changes in soft tissue associated with underdevelopment and malnutrition; and (8) normal epiphyses and metaphyses.

Histologic examination shows that bone formation is increased on both the periosteal and endosteal surfaces. The increased osteoclastic and osteoblastic activity in the affected area destroys much of the lamellar bone and lays down large amounts of irregularly arranged trabecular bone, increasing the bone porosity.

Treatment. The only treatment for this disorder is symptomatic care. Good nutrition is essential in the treatment of secondary anemia, and blood transfusions may be needed. Anti-inflammatory medication (including corticosteroids) aids with symptomatic pain relief, with physical therapy being a staple part of treatment to increase strength and preserve joint motion. Bisphosphonates have been shown to correlate with increased bone pain in patients with progressive diaphyseal dysplasia.

Plate 4-26

Congenital and Developmental Disorders

OSTEOPETROSIS AND OSTEOPOIKILOSIS

OSTEOPETROSIS (ALBERS-SCHÖNBERG DISEASE)

Osteopetrosis ("marble bone disease") is a dysplastic process in bone characterized by a lack of osteoclastic resorption of the calcified cartilage, leading to limited remodeling of the bone in line with the mechanical stress axes and resulting in abnormal bone density and increased "brittleness" of the bone. Even the bone formed by intramembranous ossification in the skull and the periosteal surface of the long bones have this abnormal structure.

The more severe autosomal recessive form (malignant osteopetrosis, occurring in 1 in 300,000 births) is usually noted shortly after birth; death occurs in the first few years secondary to faulty hematopoiesis, in the absence of a bone transplant. The milder autosomal dominant form (tarda osteopetrosis) may not be evident until adulthood. The extent of bone involvement varies widely. The thickening of the bones at the base of the skull may cause impingement on the foramina at the base of the skull, leading to entrapment of the optic nerve (blindness) or acoustic nerves (deafness).

Pathologic fractures are a significant complication of osteopetrosis because, despite its dense appearance on radiographs, the bone is structurally weak. Normal callus formation occurs in the early stages of fracture healing but is unable to reorganize into normal trabecular bone.

Clinical Manifestations. The abnormal bone encroaches on the metaphyses and medullary canals, leaving no space for the hematopoietic marrow. This results in severe aplastic anemia, secondary enlargement of the liver and spleen, and increased susceptibility to infection (i.e., osteomyelitis). Narrowing of canals that harbor cranial nerves can rarely lead to blindness or deafness.

Radiographic Findings. The most striking characteristic is the extreme density (increased radiopacity) of the bone. On radiographs, the abnormal bone lacks an obvious trabecular pattern, cortex, or medullary canal. Occasionally, there may be transverse or longitudinal streaking. The chalklike density is caused by the persistence of irregularly shaped trabeculae of calcified cartilage surrounded by bone. Spine films show a classic "rugger jersey" appearance, with sclerotic end plates sandwiching the relatively radiolucent midportion of the vertebral bodies.

Treatment. In patients with mild-to-moderate involvement, the focus is on the management of secondary complications with good medical and surgical methods. Fractures should be treated with standard modalities. Severe secondary anemia necessitates blood transfusions, whereas bone marrow transplantation has been helpful in carefully selected patients with severe forms of the condition. Owing to the successful ability to diagnose osteopetrosis in utero, umbilical cord blood transplantation has been shown to be successful in congenital cases. In severe cases, such as threatening or impending blindness, bone marrow transplant, coupled with cranial nerve surgical decompression, has proven successful in preventing further progression. Medical treatments vary, but include corticosteroids, interferon-gamma, thyroid hormone, and erythropoietin therapies.

Osteopetrosis (Albers-Schönberg's Disease)

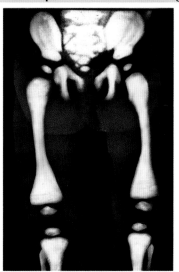

Radiograph shows marked increase in bone density with almost complete obliteration of medullary canals

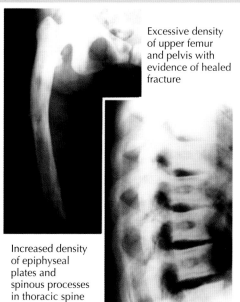

Excessive density of upper femur and pelvis with evidence of healed fracture

Increased density of epiphyseal plates and spinous processes in thoracic spine

Osteopoikilosis

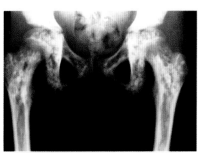

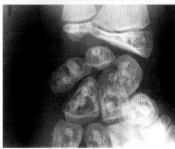

Similar dense, spotty patches in carpal bones

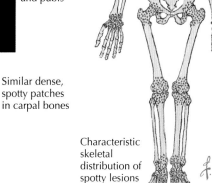

Radiograph reveals spotty patches of dense bone contrasting with radiolucent areas in proximal femur, ischium, and pubis

Characteristic skeletal distribution of spotty lesions

OSTEOPOIKILOSIS

Osteopoikilosis ("spotted bone disease") is an asymptomatic dysplasia of bone in which tiny foci of dense bone form in the spongiosa of the epiphyses and metaphyses of the long bones and the small bones of the hands and feet. Although the spine, sacrum, ribs, and sternum can be involved, occurrences in these locations are less common. The overall incidence is 0.1 per 1 million.

Dermatofibrosis lenticularis disseminata (Buschke-Ollendorf syndrome), a congenital disorder characterized by small, yellow nodular foci of subcutaneous connective tissue hyperplasia, is occasionally (~10%) associated with osteopoikilosis.

Radiographic Findings. Radiographs reveal small, rounded spots of increased density, usually less than 10 mm in diameter. The foci consist of rounded areas of normal-appearing, densely compacted bone in the spongiosa. The trabeculae in the bone surrounding the

ossification center are either decreased in number or more slender than usual. The pathologic structure of each focus is identical to that of the common hyperostotic lesion called a bone island. It is important to distinguish these lesions from metastatic bony lesions, particularly in adults. Family history may help distinguish the two.

In a closely related dysplasia called osteopathia striata, radiographs show parallel and straight-lined striations that represent slender streaks of normal bone. These striations are most common in the metaphyses of long bones and in the pelvis. The hands are rarely affected, and the clavicle is never involved. A small minority of patients may have concurrent features of osteopathia striata or melorheostosis. Existence of concurrent sclerosing conditions is known as "mixed sclerosing bone dysplasia."

Treatment. No medical or surgical treatment is indicated, because these patients are largely asymptomatic.

Plate 4-27

Musculoskeletal System: PART III

MELORHEOSTOSIS

Melorheostosis is a rare form (1 in 1 million prevalence) of "flowing" hyperostosis characterized by a linear pattern of distribution along the axis of long bones. The name—derived from the Greek words for member and flow—was suggested by the lesion's radiographic appearance, which resembles wax melting down one side of a candle. The characteristic pattern of distribution, coupled with the abnormality in other tissues of mesodermal origin overlying the bone, suggests an origin from mesodermal cells arising from somites in early embryonic development. There is no known inheritance pattern.

One or more bones of the limbs may be involved, but the spine, ribs, and skull are rarely affected. When the disease occurs along the full length of a limb, however, the hyperostotic process almost always extends to the shoulder girdle or pelvis as well. Pelvic obliquity can ensue from adduction contractures of the hips.

Clinical Manifestations. Patients report pain, stiffness, limitation of motion, and deformity. The pain, usually over the affected bones and joints, can radiate along the limb.

When the hyperostosis extends to the growth plate, growth may be altered, resulting in angular or limb length deformities. Involvement of the articular cartilage leads to osteoarthritis.

Hyperostosis affecting the full length of a limb is almost always accompanied by extensive fibromatosis, with a "ruddy wood" texture on palpation. This soft tissue manifestation lies close to the affected bones and joints (most often the hands and feet), causing contractures, muscle weakness, and limitation of joint motion. Soft tissue changes are often the first evidence of this disorder in children. Hand involvement can evolve into carpal tunnel syndrome.

Diagnostic Studies. Radiographs reveal a broad, irregular linear density along the axes of the long bones. The linear streaks may not be as evident in radiographs taken early in the disease, but they gradually increase in size and density as the child grows. In the epiphyses of the long bones and in the small bones of the hands and feet, the hyperostosis takes the form of spots and patches that resemble osteopoikilosis (see Plate 4-26).

Histologic examination reveals an excessive amount of normal-appearing bone formed by membranous ossification. Thickened, sclerotic, and somewhat

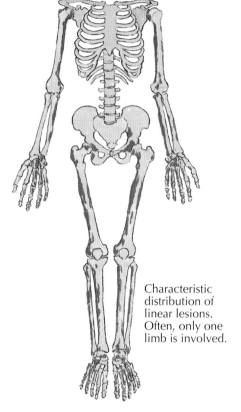

Characteristic distribution of linear lesions. Often, only one limb is involved.

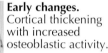

Anteroposterior (left) and lateral (right) radiographs reveal characteristic linear thickening of medial margin of ulna.

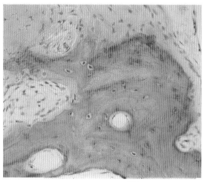

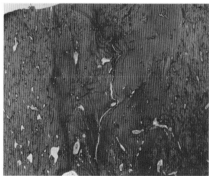

Early changes. Cortical thickening with increased osteoblastic activity.

Later changes. Dense cortical bone involving periosteal and endosteal surfaces plus intervening cortical bone.

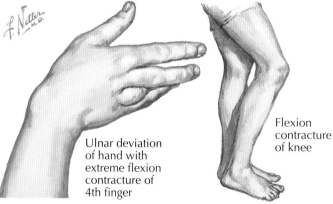

Ulnar deviation of hand with extreme flexion contracture of 4th finger

Flexion contracture of knee

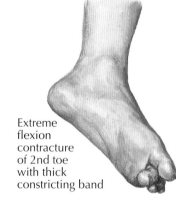

Extreme flexion contracture of 2nd toe with thick constricting band

irregular laminae surround and almost obliterate the haversian systems (osteons). Ectopic ossification may also occur near the joint or may extend into the soft tissue along the fascial planes.

Treatment. Surgical management of melorheostosis focuses on preventing or correcting deformities. To ameliorate contractures and joint stiffness, excision of the foci, fasciotomy, and capsulotomy are done. For

deformities of bone, osteotomy, epiphysiodesis (see Plate 4-35), triple arthrodesis, and, occasionally, amputations of deformed digits are performed. Myelopathy has been rarely reported in those patients with spine involvement. Unfortunately, no medical or surgical treatment can eradicate the pain of this disorder, and close partnership with a pain management team helps to improve patient comfort.

Plate 4-28

Congenital and Developmental Disorders

CONGENITAL ELEVATION OF SCAPULA, ABSENCE OF CLAVICLE, AND PSEUDARTHROSIS OF CLAVICLE

CONGENITAL ELEVATION OF SCAPULA (SPRENGEL DEFORMITY)

Sprengel deformity is a complex congenital anomaly that is associated with malposition and dysplasia of the scapula. This deformity arises from interruption of normal caudal migration and is characterized by elevation and medial rotation of the inferior scapula. In patients with this condition, the scapula is elevated and hypoplastic and the affected side of the neck is fuller and shorter than the uninvolved side, with a decrease in the cervicoscapular line and the appearance of torticollis. The involved shoulder is typically smaller and the distance from the acromion to the spine is shorter than on the normal side. A decrease in scapulocostal motion limits shoulder abduction, but motion of the scapulohumeral joint is usually normal. There is no right or left preponderance, and in one third of patients the deformity is bilateral.

Associated malformations are almost always present with a Sprengel deformity. These can include anomalies in the cervicothoracic vertebrae or the thoracic rib cage. The most common anomalies are absent or fused ribs, chest wall asymmetry, Klippel-Feil syndrome, cervical ribs, congenital scoliosis, and cervical spina bifida. When scoliosis is present, the most common curves are in the cervicothoracic or upper thoracic region. A relationship between a Sprengel deformity and diastematomyelia has also been shown. Renal anomalies occur in one third of patients. In some patients, an osseous and cartilaginous structure called an omovertebral bone originates in the upper part of the scapula and attaches to the spinous process of a cervical vertebra. This abnormal bar, occasionally in combination with contracture of the levator scapulae muscles, may further limit scapular motion. This omovertebral bone is best visualized on a lateral or oblique radiograph of the cervical spine.

If the deformity is severe enough to warrant surgical intervention, surgery provides considerable cosmetic benefit in appropriately selected patients. It restores a more natural contour to the shoulders and neck and also produces an apparent increase in neck length. The affected shoulder, however, remains smaller. Surgery is indicated for children between 3 and 8 years of age with significant deformities, both functional and cosmetic. Patients older than 8 years of age are not good candidates for scapular displacement procedures, because there is an increased risk of injury to the brachial plexus from stretching or compression by the clavicle. Removal of an omovertebral bone may increase neck and shoulder motion.

CONGENITAL ABSENCE OF CLAVICLE (CLEIDOCRANIAL DYSOSTOSIS)

A hereditary congenital disorder, absence of the clavicle is due to haploinsufficiency caused by mutations in the *CBFA1* gene, which is located on the short arm of chromosome 6. It is usually inherited in an autosomal dominant fashion, but in some cases the cause is not known. This defect results in incomplete formation of the clavicles, skull, and pubis and in some patients involves other skeletal structures as well. The entire clavicle may be absent, or simply a small segment of the middle or outer portion may be missing. The defect is bilateral in

82% of patients. Delayed closure of the cranial sutures and fontanelles and incomplete development of the pubis are frequent major manifestations. The defect in the pubis may be quite alarming and has been mistaken for erosion by a tumor.

Scoliosis and anomalies of the mandible, teeth, and small bones of the hands and feet occur in severely affected patients. The typical patient has a large head, small face, long neck, drooping shoulders, narrow chest, and short stature. In most patients, the condition is not disabling.

CONGENITAL PSEUDARTHROSIS OF CLAVICLE

A rare condition, congenital pseudarthrosis usually occurs in the middle third of the clavicle, owing to failure of union between the medial and lateral

ossification centers. The nonunion is present at birth and does not heal spontaneously. Recent studies indicate that the condition occurs most often on the right side, and the lesion may thus be due to pressure on the developing clavicle by the subclavian artery, which is normally at a higher level on the right side. The deformity may become larger and more obvious as the child grows, with a false joint developing between the enlarged ends of the clavicular fragments. The affected shoulder tends to droop forward and lower nearer the midline than the normal shoulder. The condition may be confused with a simple fracture, cleidocranial dysostosis (Plate 4-28), or neurofibromatosis (see Plates 4-20 to 4-23). The enlarged ends of the clavicular fragments are palpable, and there is a variable degree of painless motion between them. Functional problems are rare, and surgery is recommended only for patients who have pain, an unsightly lump, or shoulder weakness.

Congenital elevation of scapula (Sprengel deformity)

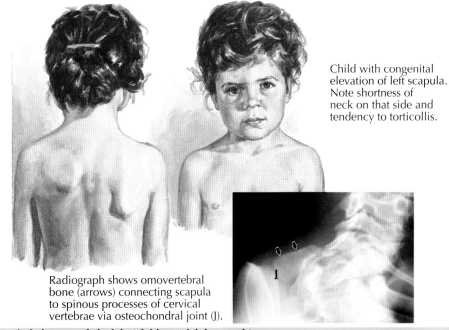

Child with congenital elevation of left scapula. Note shortness of neck on that side and tendency to torticollis.

Radiograph shows omovertebral bone (arrows) connecting scapula to spinous processes of cervical vertebrae via osteochondral joint (J).

Congenital absence of clavicle (cleidocranial dysostosis)

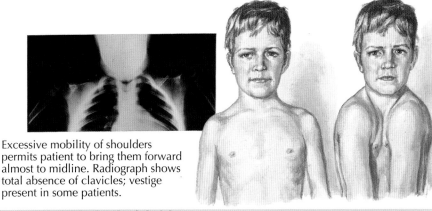

Excessive mobility of shoulders permits patient to bring them forward almost to midline. Radiograph shows total absence of clavicles; vestige present in some patients.

Congenital pseudarthrosis of clavicle

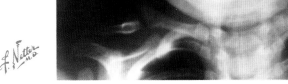

Plate 4-29

Musculoskeletal System: PART III

MADELUNG DEFORMITY

Madelung deformity of the wrist is characterized by a growth disturbance and/or an absence or underdevelopment in the volar-ulnar distal radial physis, so that it fails to contribute to the linear growth of the corresponding border of the radial diaphysis. The uninvolved radial and dorsal portions of the growth plate continue to grow. The faster growing, newly formed bone bends toward the area of slower growth, causing the articular surface of the distal radius to slant in the palmar and ulnar direction. The ulna is unaffected in Madelung deformity and remains in its usual dorsal position. This results in a volar- and ulnar-tilted distal radial articular surface, volar translation of the hand and wrist, and a dorsally prominent distal ulna. Patients experience increasing deformity and pain in the wrist with decreased range of motion. On physical examination, the hand is translated volarly to the long axis of the forearm. The ulna, being relatively unaffected, abuts the carpus and becomes prominent dorsally relative to the carpus of the hand. Range of motion is decreased, with a limitation of supination, dorsiflexion, and radial deviation. Pronation and flexion are usually normal.

Madelung deformity is bilateral in two thirds of the patients. Rarely, a reversed Madelung deformity may occur in which the articular surface of the distal radius is angulated dorsally and the distal ulna assumes a relatively palmar position.

Madelung deformity can be broken down into four etiologic groups, as follows: post-traumatic, dysplastic, chromosomal or genetic, and idiopathic or primary. The post-traumatic deformity has been found after repetitive trauma or after a single traumatic event that disrupts the growth of the distal radial ulnar-volar physis. Bone dysplasias associated with Madelung deformity include multiple hereditary osteochondromatosis, Ollier disease, achondroplasia (see Plates 4-1 to 4-3), multiple epiphysial dysplasias (see Plate 4-12), enchondromatosis, gonadal dysgenesis (Turner syndrome), and the mucopolysaccharidoses (e.g., Hurler and Morquio syndromes; see Plate 4-18). The most important dysplasia associated with Madelung deformity, however, is dyschondrosteosis.

Although Madelung deformity is considered a congenital anomaly, symptoms do not usually begin until late childhood or early adolescence (6 to 13 years of age). One third of the cases of Madelung deformity are transmitted in an autosomal dominant fashion. The condition has a variable expression and 50% penetrance. Madelung deformity is bilateral in up to two thirds of the patients, and females are affected four times as often as males. The moderately short stature of the affected person has led to some confusion as to whether Madelung deformity is an isolated deformity in the distal radius or a form of dyschondrosteosis (Léri-Weill syndrome). However, dyschondrosteosis, which is characterized by other associated skeletal deformities, particularly in the tibia, in addition to Madelung deformity at the wrist, is probably a separate entity. Furthermore, a primary chromosomal association with Madelung deformity has been observed in the patients with Turner syndrome (with and XO karyotype).

Recently, Vickers approached Madelung deformity through an anterior approach and noted for the first time the presence of a large, abnormal, anterior wrist ligament between the anterior ulnar metaphysis of the

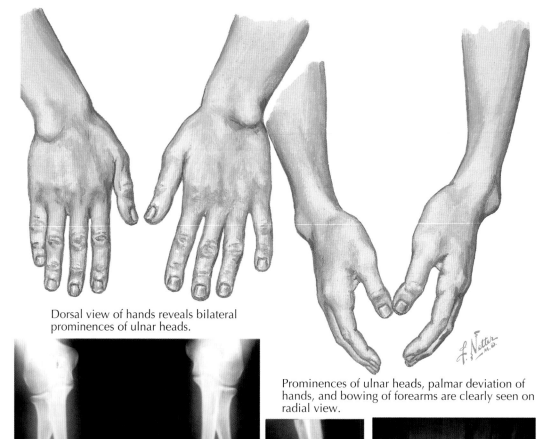

Dorsal view of hands reveals bilateral prominences of ulnar heads.

Prominences of ulnar heads, palmar deviation of hands, and bowing of forearms are clearly seen on radial view.

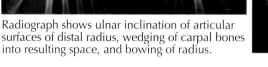

Radiograph shows ulnar inclination of articular surfaces of distal radius, wedging of carpal bones into resulting space, and bowing of radius.

Lateral radiograph demonstrates dorsal prominence of ulnar head with palmar deviation of carpal bones.

MRI showing Vickers' alignment

distal radius and the carpus (Vickers' ligament). Grossly, this ligament is a large, fibrous band about 5 to 7 mm thick. It is found under the pronator quadratus, originating well proximal to the majority of the physis, in a fossa on the ulnar side of the anterior surface of the radius. From here, it flows out onto the anterior surface of the lunate, inserting like the radiolunate ligament in the normal wrist. It may be that Vickers' ligament is a stretched out coalescence of normal structures, formed as a consequence of an abnormal growth of the radial physis beneath it. This may suggest that Vickers' ligament is a secondary rather than a primary cause of Madelung deformity. This is supported by the fact that if the ligament were present at birth, the tremendous growth of the child during the first 3 years of life should lead to Madelung deformity by the time the child is a

toddler, an age when the deformity is never seen. Regardless, releasing this ligament when reconstructing the wrists with a fully developed Madelung deformity is critical.

Treatment. Because discomfort usually resolves or remains minimal and function is excellent, surgical treatment is rarely indicated. Operative management for Madelung deformity is indicated for pain relief and cosmetic improvement. Madelung initially advised his patients to avoid forced wrist extension and to use resting splints at night to relieve the pain. Persistent pain, usually due to nerve impingement between the distal ulna and underlying carpal bones, and extreme deformity are two other reasons for operative management. Limited wrist motion is not an indication for surgery, which does little to improve it.

Plate 4-30

Congenital and Developmental Disorders

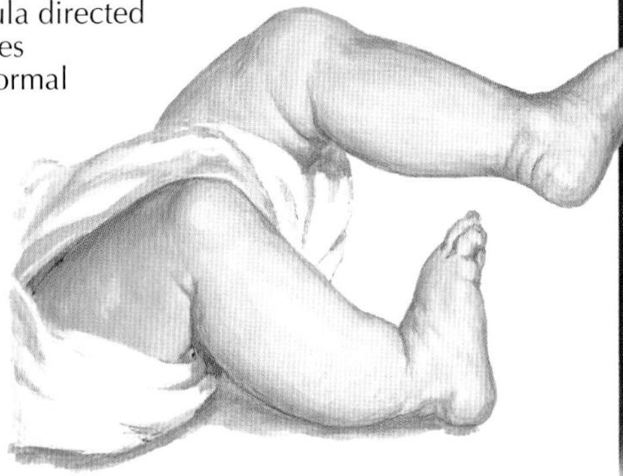

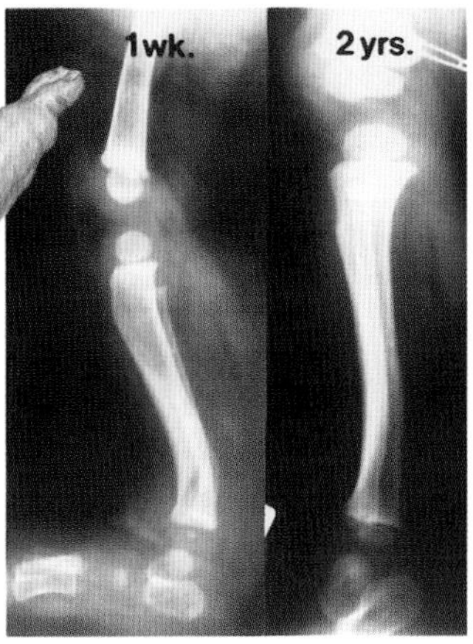

Posterior bowing. Convexity of bow in distal third of tibia and fibula directed posteriorly; usually regresses spontaneously to almost normal by 2 years of age; lower limb-length discrepancy due to growth inhibition may persist.

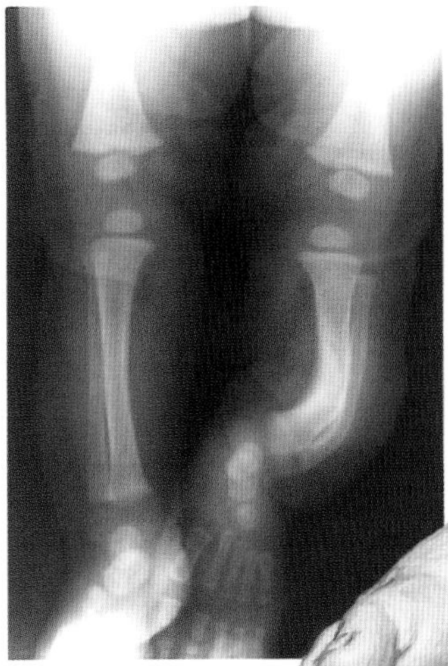

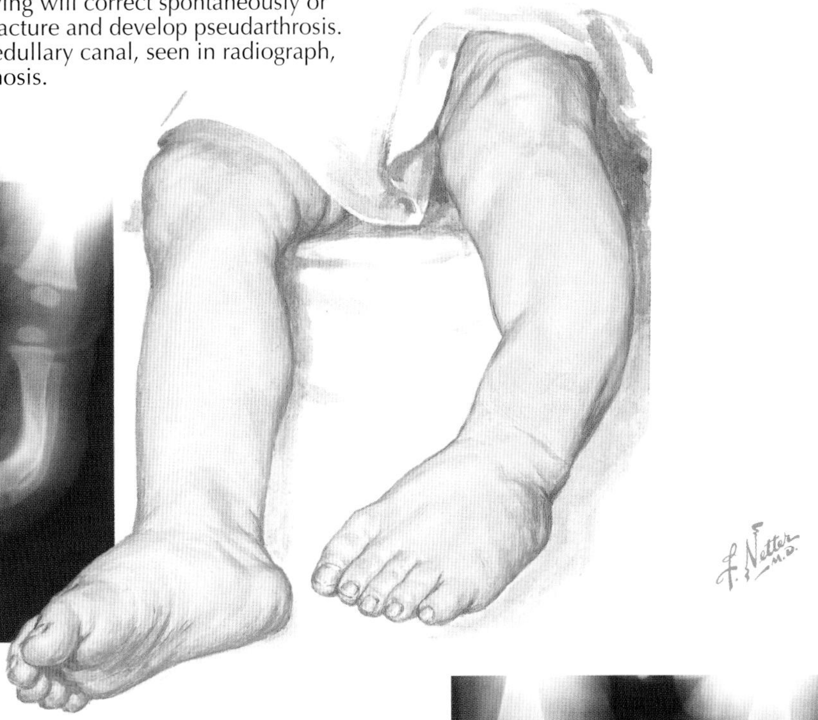

CONGENITAL BOWING OF THE TIBIA

POSTEROMEDIAL BOWING

In this condition, the posteromedial oriented apex of the tibial bow is at the junction of the lower and middle thirds of the diaphysis, typically with similar fibular bowing. The foot is in varying degrees of calcaneovalgus position and can be dorsiflexed to the shin; tightness of the anterior musculature limits plantar flexion. Although clinically the position of the foot and atrophic calf may look very impressive, the vast majority of foot deformities resolve with stretching and serial splinting, usually by 9 months of age. Etiology is thought to be secondary to intrauterine positioning and compression.

Posteromedial bowing spontaneously and markedly corrects in the first 6 months of life, with essentially normal tibial angulation noted by the age of 2 years. Surgical deformity correction is rarely needed and should not be considered until 3 to 4 years of age in those with severe residual bowing. Pseudarthrosis and increased fracture frequency are not associated with posteromedial bowing. The main orthopaedic concern tends to be limb-length discrepancy, typically ranging between 3 and 7 cm. Epiphysiodesis of the contralateral tibia is typically the mainstay treatment, but limb-lengthening procedures may also be considered in large (>5 cm) limb-length discrepancies.

ANTERIOR OR ANTEROLATERAL BOWING

Anterior or anterolateral bowing of the tibia, in association with congenital dysplasia, is highly associated with increased risk for fracture and pseudarthrosis and represents one of the most difficult and challenging treatment issues in orthopaedics. There is a high correlation of anterolateral tibial bowing and pseudarthrosis with neurofibromatosis type 1, with approximately half of all cases showing an association. Fibrous dysplasia also has a strong correlation with anterolateral bowing.

Prognosis and treatment is best guided by the presence or absence of fracture and by the age of the child at which the first fracture occurs. The bowing generally occurs in the mid-diaphysis, usually with concurrent fibular bowing. Radiographs should be carefully scrutinized for dysplastic changes in the tibia (widened medullary canal, thickened cortices, cystic or sclerotic changes, fibular pseudarthrosis, hourglass constriction) because those patients with anterolateral bowing in the setting of a nondysplastic tibia may be observed without prophylactic bracing, because the risk of fracture is markedly lower.

In the setting of dysplastic changes, the prognosis for tibial dysplasia with anterolateral bowing is very poor, with minimal chance for spontaneous fracture healing once a fracture has occurred. Prevention of fracture is a vital part of the treatment algorithm, with the mainstay of prophylactic treatment being orthotics. Bracing should be instituted as early as possible, with

Anterolateral bowing. In infancy, it may be difficult to predict whether bowing will correct spontaneously or whether bone will fracture and develop pseudarthrosis. Presence of good medullary canal, seen in radiograph, suggests better prognosis.

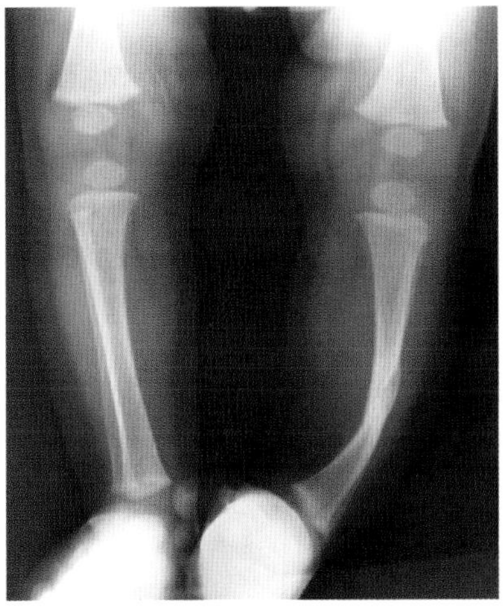

Anterior bowing. Medullary canal present but narrow with sclerotic changes; cyst apparent. Prone to spontaneous fracture and pseudarthrosis.

an ankle-foot orthosis (prior to walking) or a knee-ankle-foot orthosis (with weight bearing) being some examples. Bracing should be continued until skeletal maturity or until a fracture occurs. Once a fracture occurs, union with brace management is rarely successful.

Numerous surgical options for pseudarthrosis have been described. Intramedullary fixation is typically attempted early, although vascularized free grafts and external fixation with distraction osteogenesis are recent techniques that have been reported. New approaches are being developed using osteoinductive materials, such as bone morphogenetic protein. This remains an off-label use, with noted variability in union rates within small sample populations. Refracture, valgus malunion, and nonunion are major complications of pseudarthrosis with a high degree of prevalence, and amputation may be a final option that allows the patient to return to functional levels the quickest, utilizing new orthotic technology.

Plate 4-31   Musculoskeletal System: PART III

CONGENITAL PSEUDARTHROSIS OF THE TIBIA AND DISLOCATION OF THE KNEE

CONGENITAL PSEUDARTHROSIS OF THE TIBIA

Congenital pseudoarthrosis of the tibia (CPT) results when tibial fracture fails to heal. A dysplastic tibia (i.e., narrow, sclerotic medullary canal) with an anterolateral bow is at greatest risk of fracture. Rarely, the fracture is present at birth; 50% of fractures occur in the first year, and 25% occur in the second year. The fibula is similarly involved, with congenital fibular pseudarthrosis predisposing the patient to valgus tibial malunion. The fractured tibia and fibula fail to unite, and a pseudarthrosis forms at the fracture site.

The etiology of CPT is unclear. Approximately 55% of affected children with anterolateral bowing subsequently develop clinical findings of neurofibromatosis, although only 6% of patients with NF1 have anterolateral tibial bowing and CPT. In these patients, the lesion is thought to be the result of a neurofibroma and poor vascular ingrowth at the fracture site. Some describe the pseudarthrosis site as an "invasive fibromatosis" of abnormal collagen, and excision of this fibrous proliferation is generally stressed at the time of treatment.

Treatment. In newborns, anterolateral bowing of the tibia with concurrent dysplastic or cystic changes is an urgent problem that requires immediate treatment, because fracture and pseudarthrosis often develop soon after birth. Treatment of the newborn focuses on preventing a fracture. A custom-made plastic orthosis should be used to protect the limb until the child is ready for a standard orthosis or surgery.

Despite the most intensive conservative management, fractures occur quite frequently and extensive surgery is required to promote healing. Orthotic management is the mainstay of prophylactic treatment. Fracture prophylaxis with bone grafting of the narrowed area or cystic lesion before fracture may be considered, followed by bracing. In many children with CPT, healing does not occur and a significant number of patients ultimately need limb amputation and a prosthesis (see Plate 4-44).

CONGENITAL DISLOCATION OF THE KNEE

Congenital hyperextension and/or dislocation of the knee, although uncommon, is an orthopaedic emergency when it occurs. At birth, the knee may be simply hyperextended (genu recurvatum) or, in the severe form, completely dislocated, with the tibia displaced anterior and lateral to the femur. Dislocations are typically bilateral and associated with "syndromic" patterns, such as Larsen or Ehlers-Danlos syndromes. A mild hereditary or familial tendency has been reported, as well as an association with other "uterine packing" deformities such as torticollis (see Part II in this series, Plates 1-34 and 1-35), dislocation of the elbow (60%), ipsilateral hip dislocation (70%), and clubfoot (50%).

Dislocation of the knee is common in patients with arthrogryposis and myelodysplasia; it is related to muscle imbalance, usually fibrotic contracture of the quadriceps femoris muscle exacerbated by nonfunctional or absent hamstring muscles. In an otherwise normal child, the dislocation is believed to result from an intrauterine position (frank breech presentation), in

Congenital pseudarthrosis of tibia

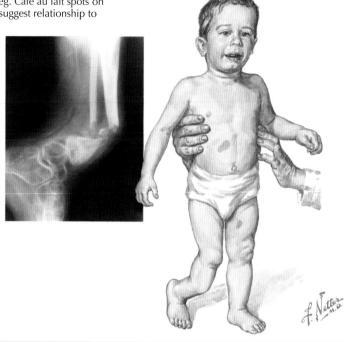

Angulation of right leg. Café au lait spots on thigh and abdomen suggest relationship to neurofibromatosis.

Congenital dislocation of knee

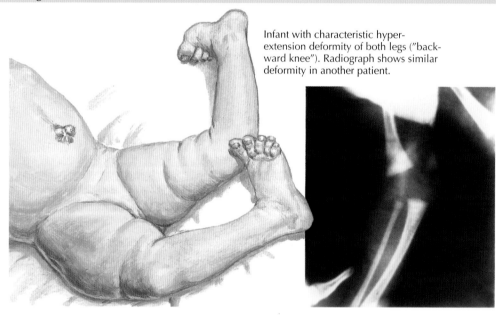

Infant with characteristic hyperextension deformity of both legs ("backward knee"). Radiograph shows similar deformity in another patient.

which the feet of the fetus are locked beneath the mandible or in the axillae.

Clinical Manifestations. The knee appears "backward" and hyperextended, with the examiner typically able to further extend the leg until it nearly touches the chest. The medial hamstring muscles are often displaced forward, anterior to the axis of the knee, thus functioning as knee extensors. The patella may be displaced laterally, and the femoral condyles are prominent posteriorly. Circulation below the knee is usually intact.

Radiographic Findings. Radiographs reveal severe genu recurvatum with malalignment of the tibia and femur, with a spectrum of findings ranging from genu recurvatum to complete anterior dislocation. Deformity of the epiphyses of the distal femur and proximal tibia can be seen in untreated older children.

Treatment. Dislocation and subluxation both require immediate treatment. Within a few hours after birth, the limb should be passively stretched to bring the knee gradually into a flexed position. In most patients, the knee can be manipulated into slight flexion (30 degrees) and splinted in this position. The splint should be changed regularly, with stretching and passive range-of-motion exercises continued until the knee can be flexed to approximately 90 degrees. A removable splint may then be used for an additional 2 to 3 months to maintain position. Recurrence is uncommon.

If gentle manipulative reduction is not possible immediately after birth, then surgical reduction and lengthening of the extensor muscles should be initiated prior to 1 year of age. Forced manipulation can lead to fracture or growth plate injury and should not be avoided.

Plate 4-32

Congenital and Developmental Disorders

LEG-LENGTH DISCREPANCY

Leg-length discrepancies include any inequality in length from the level of the pelvis to, and including, the foot. The numerous causes of the inequality include the following:

- Congenital and developmental anomalies with terminal limb deficiencies (see Plate 3-32): hemihypertrophy or hemiatrophy, Klippel-Trénaunay-Weber syndrome, Maffucci syndrome, posterior bowing of the tibia, proximal femoral focal deficiency, congenital short femur, enchondromatosis
- Paralytic disorders: poliomyelitis, encephalopathy (e.g., cerebral palsy), myelopathy (e.g., myelomeningocele)
- Infections of bone and joint that retard or arrest bone growth: osteomyelitis (may accelerate or inhibit growth), septic arthritis (may lead to avascular necrosis with partial or complete growth arrest)
- Trauma to bone and joint: injuries to the growth plate (may arrest growth); fractures of the metaphysis or diaphysis (may accelerate growth); malunion, excessive overriding, or angulation due to fracture (may result in limb shortening)
- Tumorous conditions that produce bone overgrowth: fibrous dysplasia, enchondromatosis, osteoid osteoma, hemangioma, neurofibromatosis
- Tumors that produce growth retardation: solitary enchondroma of growth plate, simple bone cyst with repeated fractures through growth plate
- Irradiation of malignant tumors of long bones that arrest growth: Ewing sarcoma, neuroblastoma

TREATMENT

The many factors to be considered in the treatment of leg-length discrepancy include (1) etiology; (2) degree of the discrepancy; (3) skeletal age; (4) progression of the discrepancy; (5) predicted adult height and predicted magnitude of the leg-length discrepancy at skeletal maturity; (6) strength and balance of the musculature of the limb, especially in neurologic disorders; (7) status of the foot and ankle (e.g., availability of muscles in the foot and ankle, presence of an equinus contracture of the short limb that allows the child to walk on tiptoe on the short side to balance the pelvis); (8) predominant site of the inequality (i.e., femur or tibia); (9) any general or extenuating health factors; and (10) the needs and desires of the patient and parents.

Evaluation

Leg-length discrepancy can be measured in several ways. A common method is to place standing blocks of measured thickness beneath the short leg to level the pelvis. Radiographic techniques, using a metal ruler on the film, include a one-exposure technique in which a single exposure is made of both entire lower limbs. The one-exposure technique may produce magnification at the ends of the lower limbs owing to the effect of parallax. A more accurate method involves three successive exposures of the hips, knees, and ankles on one long film (see Plate 4-33). Unfortunately, none of the radiographic measurement techniques accurately depicts pelvic asymmetry, differences in pelvic height, or height of the feet; therefore, it is always important to correlate the radiographic measurements with the clinical examination of pelvic obliquity.

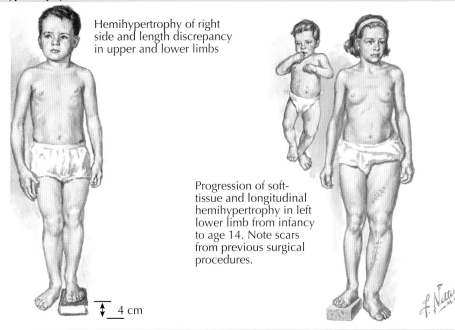

Hemihypertrophy

Hemihypertrophy of right side and length discrepancy in upper and lower limbs

Progression of soft-tissue and longitudinal hemihypertrophy in left lower limb from infancy to age 14. Note scars from previous surgical procedures.

4 cm

Maffucci syndrome

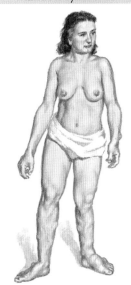

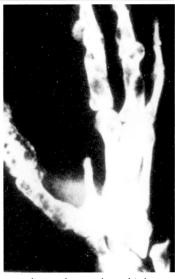

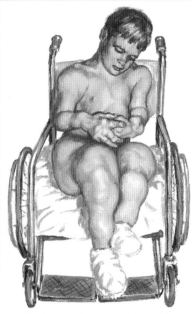

Young adult with Maffucci syndrome and hemihypertrophy of right upper and lower limbs

Radiograph reveals multiple enchondromas of metacarpals and phalanges; 2nd finger amputated

Patient with severe deformities

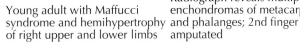

Klippel-Trénaunay-Weber syndrome

Congenital short femur

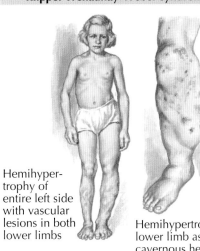

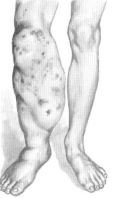

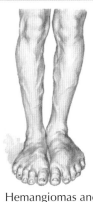

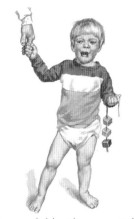

Hemihypertrophy of entire left side with vascular lesions in both lower limbs

Hemihypertrophy of right lower limb associated with cavernous hemangiomas

Hemangiomas and varicosities and hypertrophy of both feet in 9-year-old boy

Young child with congenital short left femur

Plate 4-33

Musculoskeletal System: PART III

EVALUATION OF LEG-LENGTH DISCREPANCY

LEG-LENGTH DISCREPANCY
(Continued)

Management of a leg-length discrepancy may depend more on the predicted difference at skeletal maturity than on the current degree of inequality. A final discrepancy of less than 2 cm is considered mild and usually does not require any treatment in adults. A discrepancy of 3 to 6 cm is considered moderate. The amount of growth remaining and hence the appropriate timing of an epiphysiodesis to equalize leg lengths can be calculated with the chart devised by Green and Anderson, by the arithmetic method of Menalaus, or by the Moseley straight-line graph (see Plate 4-34).

The Green and Anderson growth-remaining chart is used to estimate the effects of an epiphyseal arrest procedure on the distal femur and proximal tibia at various skeletal ages. The arithmetic method of Menalaus assumes that boys close their growth plates at an average age of 16 while girls close their growth plates at an average age of 14. Assuming 1.0 cm of growth per year from the distal femur and 0.6 cm per year from the proximal tibia, the magnitude of the final discrepancy at skeletal maturity can be predicted and therefore the appropriate timing of the epiphysiodesis determined. The Moseley straight-line graph helps determine the estimated lengths of the long and short bones at maturity, the discrepancy at maturity, and when the best equalization procedure should be performed. Although the Moseley graph is believed to be much more accurate in cases of significant growth inhibition, it is simply a logarithmic representation of the Green and Anderson chart. The child's skeletal age, which is determined by comparing the left hand to the *Greulich and Pyle Radiographic Atlas*, is used to determine the appropriate time for equalization procedures.

Regular follow-up is necessary to determine if the discrepancy is progressive and whether conservative measures (e.g., orthoses, prostheses) or surgery are the best methods of correction.

Surgical procedures for leg-length discrepancy include (1) shortening of the long side by arresting or retarding epiphyseal growth or resecting a segment of bone; (2) femoral, tibial, or transiliac lengthening of the short side; (3) combined shortening of the long side and lengthening of the short side; and (4) prosthetic fitting.

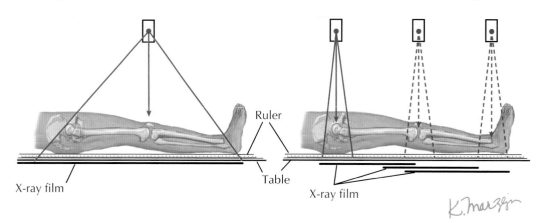

Technique for radiographic measurement by the one-exposure technique.

Technique for radiographic measurement by the three-exposure technique (scanogram).

Ruler

Table

X-ray film

X-ray film

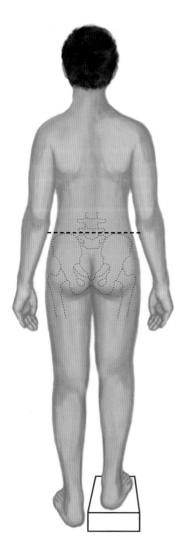

Measurement of LLD on physical examination

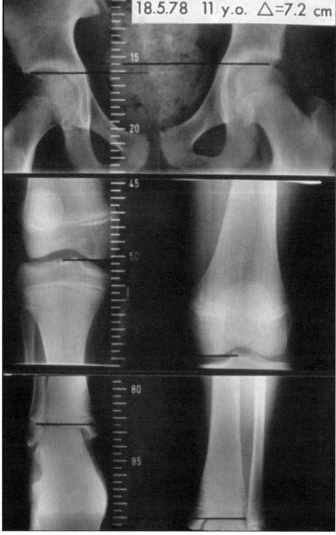

Radiographic image obtained by the three-exposure technique (scanogram).

18.5.78 11 y.o. △=7.2 cm

Plate 4-34

Congenital and Developmental Disorders

CHARTS FOR TIMING GROWTH ARREST AND DETERMINING AMOUNT OF LIMB LENGTHENING TO ACHIEVE LIMB-LENGTH EQUALITY AT MATURITY

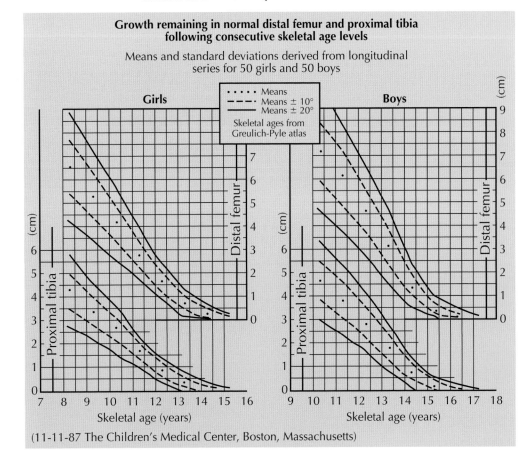

Growth remaining in normal distal femur and proximal tibia following consecutive skeletal age levels

Means and standard deviations derived from longitudinal series for 50 girls and 50 boys

(11-11-87 The Children's Medical Center, Boston, Massachusetts)

Growth-remaining chart (adapted from Green and Anderson)

LEG-LENGTH DISCREPANCY
(Continued)

Growth Arrest and Growth Retardation

Epiphysiodesis is the destruction of the growth plate by means of an open or closed surgical technique (see Plate 4-35). The open technique of Phemister involves removing a rectangular block of bone at the medial and lateral borders of the growth plate. The growth plate is then curetted from both sides under direct vision. The rectangular blocks are turned upside down and replaced.

The advent of improved clarity of intraoperative radiographic image intensification has facilitated the use of a closed technique, percutaneous epiphysiodesis. A very small incision is made over a Steinmann pin placed medially to laterally in the plane of the growth plate. A cannulated reamer is placed over the pin and used to begin removal of the growth plate, which is completed by power drilling or curettage or both. Viscous lidocaine and a radiographic contrast medium are injected into the defect, and the limb is rotated under the image intensifier to determine the adequacy of the procedure. Morbidity is quite low, and the scar is much more acceptable to patients than that of open epiphysiodesis.

Epiphyseal stapling retards, but does not stop, growth (see Plate 4-35). Unlike epiphysiodesis, the procedure must be performed on a younger patient to achieve the same growth retardation, but it should not be done before the child reaches the skeletal age of 8 years. If growth is to be resumed, the staples must be removed before growth of the epiphysis has ceased.

After the staples are removed, a rebound phenomenon, or initial growth spurt, may occur, followed by continuation of growth at the normal rate. A previously stapled epiphysis usually closes a few months prematurely, which tends to compensate for the spurt in growth. Although there are many technical problems associated with the stapling procedure, the theoretical advantages of stapling—such as the ability to control angular and length deformities—make it a worthwhile consideration.

Resection of bone from the longer limb may be performed to correct leg-length discrepancy in skeletally mature patients and may also simultaneously correct any associated angular or rotational deformities. The risk of excessive shortening is muscle weakness, which can be manifested in the femur as a knee extension lag due to decreased quadriceps strength.

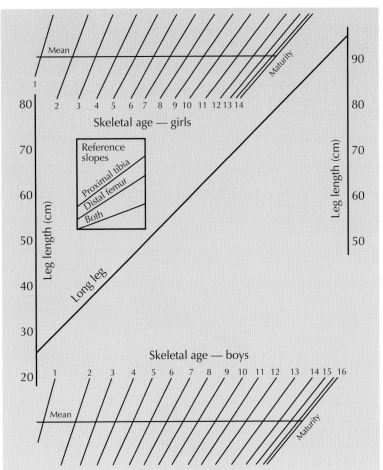

Staight-line graph for leg-length discrepancy (adapted from Moseley)

Plate 4-35

Musculoskeletal System: PART III

GROWTH ARREST

Percutaneous epiphysiodesis

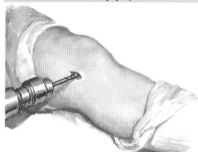
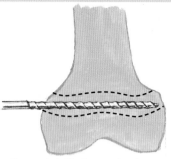
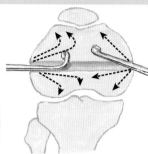

Drill introduced transversely through growth plate of distal femur along tract determined with test needle under image-intensification visualization.

Channel drilled completely through growth plate (indicated by broken lines).

Straight- and right-angled curets of various sizes used for complete removal of peripheries of growth plate (anterior view with knee and hip in flexion).

Open epiphysiodesis

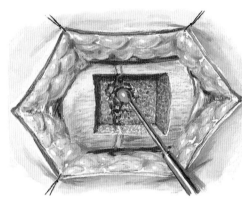
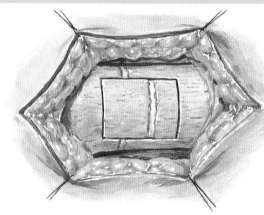

Rectangular bone plug incorporating growth plate resected from each side of distal femur. Growth plate drilled and curetted and gap filled with cancellous bone from above and below.

Bone plug reversed and impacted into its bed. Cartilaginous growth plate line on plug now more proximal.

LEG-LENGTH DISCREPANCY
(Continued)

Leg-Lengthening Procedures

Procedures for leg lengthening include (1) corticotomy and gradual distraction (distraction osteogenesis); (2) lengthening through the growth plate (chondrodiastasis); (3) osteotomy and acute distraction; (4) transiliac lengthening; and (5) lengthening and shortening in a one-stage procedure, using the bone fragment from the long side to lengthen the short side.

Lengthening is appropriate to consider in children 8 to 12 years of age who have a predicted leg-length discrepancy at maturity of 5 cm or more. The discrepancy in a skeletally immature child should be greater than can be corrected with epiphysiodesis of the long limb, which by convention has been considered to be approximately 5 cm. Muscle strength should be sufficient so that little power is lost by lengthening. However, even gradual lengthening may cause several systemic complications, including transient hypertension, anorexia and weight loss, and emotional lability. Lengthening the bone by more than 15% increases the complication rate.

The technique of limb lengthening known as distraction osteogenesis was introduced by Ilizarov in 1951 (see Plate 4-36). After subperiosteal division of the bone at the diaphysis or metaphysis (corticotomy) without disturbing the medullary canal, the bone fragments are fixed above and below with an external fixation device. The Ilizarov device incorporates metal rings that encircle the limb and attach to the bone with thin metal wires or half pins. Telescoping rods connect the rings and provide the distraction capability. The De Bastiani device, called a dynamic axial fixator, is a rigid telescoping bar that attaches to one side of the limb with screws (see Plate 4-36).

Growth retardation epiphyseal stapling

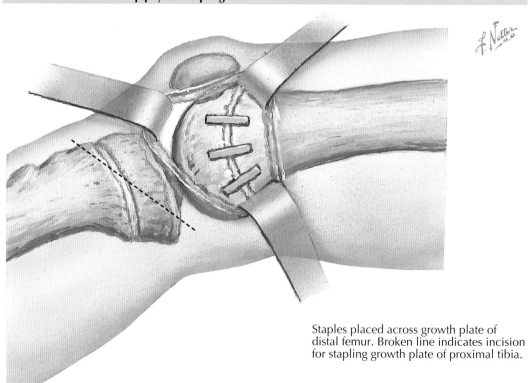

Staples placed across growth plate of distal femur. Broken line indicates incision for stapling growth plate of proximal tibia.

Plate 4-36

Congenital and Developmental Disorders

ILIZAROV AND DE BASTIANI TECHNIQUES FOR LIMB LENGTHENING

Ilizarov technique

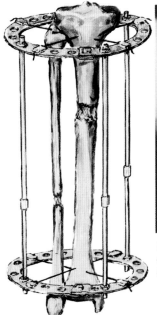

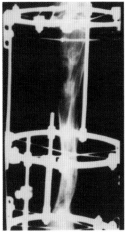

Preoperative radiograph documents short, angulated tibia.

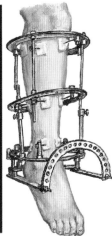

Corticotomy of tibia and fibula carried out, device in place, and distraction begun (additional corticotomy done in this patient to correct angulation).

Clinical view with device in place and wires through tibia

After percutaneous or open corticotomy, Ilizarov device secured with wires or pins passing through bone. After 7 days, device extended 0.25 mm four times a day (1 mm/day) until desired limb length attained. Cortical bone grows in to fill distraction gap.

De Bastiani technique

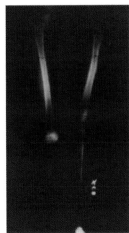

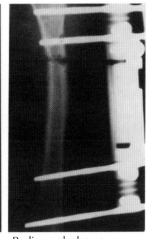

Preoperative radiograph shows unilateral congenital short femur and tibias of equal length.

Radiograph shows corticotomy of femur with dynamic axial fixator in place.

LEG-LENGTH DISCREPANCY
(Continued)

After 4 to 7 days, distraction is begun at a rate of 0.25 mm four times a day. Radiographic monitoring is critical because distraction started too early may delay formation of the regenerated bone in the distraction gap; if started too late, distraction may not be possible because of premature consolidation of the bone ends. Several variations in this technique are possible, including bone transport, in which bone is removed distally and also distracted through a proximal corticotomy to allow the intercalary fragment to fill the subsequent defect, and bifocal corticotomy, in which the bone is divided and lengthened at both proximal and distal ends, allowing overall lengthening to occur twice as rapidly.

Chondrodiastasis, or symmetric distraction of the growth plate, can be considered when the leg-length discrepancy is small. The procedure stimulates closure of the growth plate; however, its use is limited to adolescents nearing completion of growth.

Transiliac lengthening permanently corrects a static leg-length discrepancy less than 3 cm, especially when epiphysiodesis and use of a shoe lift are unacceptable. The procedure is most effective in patients with a postural imbalance in the transverse plane. The technique is similar to the Salter innominate osteotomy for congenital hip dislocation, except that the pelvic fragments are distracted and held open anteriorly and posteriorly with a quadrilateral bone graft. Unlike epiphysiodesis and epiphyseal stapling, transiliac lengthening balances the limbs directly without shortening the overall height.

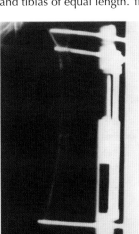

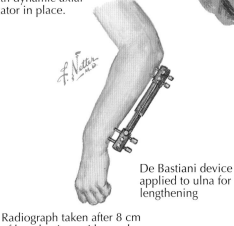

De Bastiani device applied to ulna for lengthening

Radiograph taken after 8 cm of lengthening, with new bone growth filling femoral defect. Device still in place.

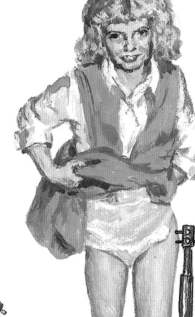

Child wears De Bastiani device.

Plate 4-37

Musculoskeletal System: PART III

CONGENITAL LIMB MALFORMATION

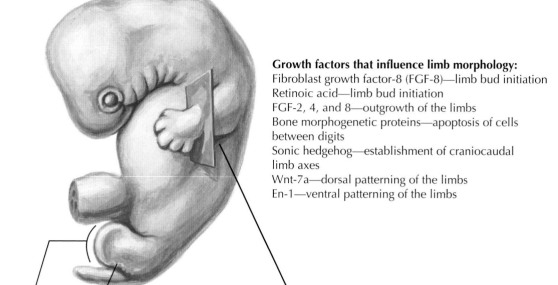

GROWTH FACTORS

Limb buds in 6-week embryo

Growth factors that influence limb morphology:
Fibroblast growth factor-8 (FGF-8)—limb bud initiation
Retinoic acid—limb bud initiation
FGF-2, 4, and 8—outgrowth of the limbs
Bone morphogenetic proteins—apoptosis of cells between digits
Sonic hedgehog—establishment of craniocaudal limb axes
Wnt-7a—dorsal patterning of the limbs
En-1—ventral patterning of the limbs

Zone of polarizing activity

Apical ectodermal ridge

Mesenchymal bone precursor

Extensor muscle

Flexor muscle

Preaxial compartment

Postaxial compartment

Ant. division nerve

Post. division nerve

Ventral compartment	Dorsal compartment
Flexor muscles	Extensor muscles
Anterior division nerves	Posterior division nerves

JOHN A. CRAIG—MD

Growth factors that promote tissue development:
Bone morphogenetic protein family—bone development
Indian hedgehog—bone development
Growth/differentiation factor 5—joint formation
Transforming growth factor-β family—myoblast proliferation
Nerve growth factor—sensory and sympathetic neurons
Insulin-like growth factor-1 (IGF-1)—general proliferation of limb mesoderm
Scatter factor (hepatic growth factor)—myotome cell migration in the limbs

ETIOLOGY AND PATHOGENESIS

Limb malformations are caused by genetic or environmental factors or a combination of both (see Plate 4-37). Limb differentiation in the human embryo occurs in a definite, sequential order. Small buds of tissue, representing the upper and lower limbs, first appear on the lateral body wall at about the 26th day. In the ensuing 4 weeks, the limb buds grow and differentiate rapidly in a proximodistal sequence (i.e., the arm and forearm appear before the hand) with the upper limbs preceding the lower limbs by 1 to 2 days.

The growth and development of the limbs are controlled by specific genes. At the tip of each limb bud is a collection of ectodermal cells called the apical ectodermal ridge (AER) that regulates limb growth in the proximodistal axis. The zone of polarizing activity (ZPA) is located at the posterior margin of the limb bud and controls the anteroposterior pattern of limb development through sonic hedgehog genes.

By the 48th day, the shape of the hand is well defined, and the skeleton is cartilaginous except for the distal phalanges, which have not yet chondrified. No further differentiation occurs after about the 50th day, and by 12 weeks the ossification centers are present in all the long bones. Later changes are essentially related only to increase in size and to the relative position and proportion of the parts.

Most limb malformations develop during the embryonic phase (approximately the 3rd to 7th weeks). During this period, teratogenic factors inhibit the rate of orderly differentiation of the part that is changing most rapidly and whose cellular components are highly sensitive at that moment. The type of deformity is determined by the stage in limb development at which the insult occurs and the location of the destructive process. The severity of the deformity reflects the degree of destruction within the limb mesenchyme.

The exact cause of limb malformations or deficiencies is rarely known. There are a few malformations associated with known genetic diseases; however, most abnormalities arise spontaneously without any identifiable genetic, environmental, or traumatic causes. The incidence of recurrence of a particular limb malformation in subsequent children is only slightly higher than that of the general population. Furthermore, although many medications and drugs are known teratogens, thalidomide is the only medication that has been widely linked to limb abnormalities.

CLASSIFICATION OF CONGENITAL LIMB DEFECTS

In the past, Greek and Latin names were used to describe common limb deficits, resulting in much semantic confusion. Despite their confusing nature, some of these terms are still commonly used to describe specific deformities. A workable classification to identify, categorize, and readily retrieve the specific diagnosis of congenital malformations had long been needed, and, in 1961, Frantz and O'Rahilly published the first attempt at such a practical classification. The method of grouping cases according to the parts that have been primarily affected by certain embryologic failures was first proposed by Swanson in 1964. Committees of the American Society for Surgery of the Hand and the International Federation of Societies for Surgery of the Hand further developed this classification, which was published in 1968 by Swanson, Barsky, and Entin. This classification, used in this discussion, has been accepted

Plate 4-38

Congenital and Developmental Disorders

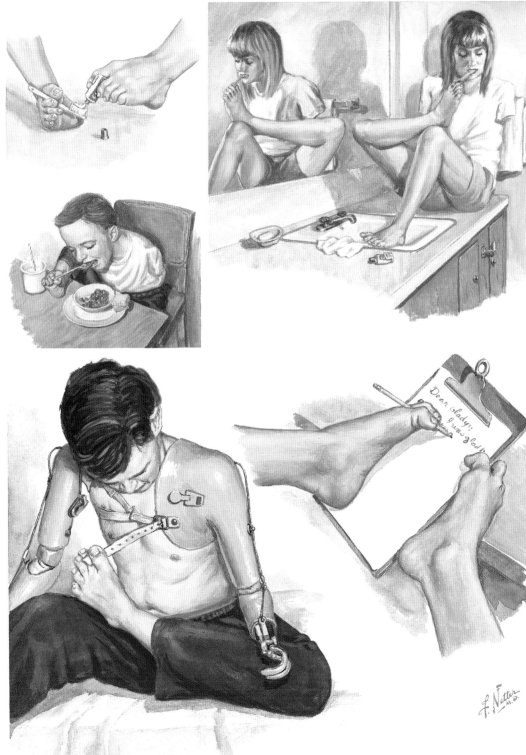

CONGENITAL LIMB MALFORMATION *(Continued)*

by both societies, as well as by the International Society of Prosthetics and Orthotics.

Although the embryologic insult to a limb usually cannot be sharply demarcated, certain similar patterns of deficit do exist. Defects may involve only the dermo-myofascial structures or all or part of both the skeletal and associated soft tissue elements of the limb. Subclassification within the major categories indicates the specific type and severity of the malformation. Deformities involving only the soft tissues are considered milder manifestations of a general deficiency pattern. The seven major categories in the classification are:

    I. Failure of Formation of Parts (Transverse and Longitudinal Arrest)
   II. Failure of Differentiation of Parts
  III. Duplication
  IV. Overgrowth
   V. Undergrowth
  VI. Congenital Constriction Band Syndrome
 VII. Generalized Skeletal Abnormalities

I. Failure of Formation of Parts: Transverse Arrest

Category I, which is subdivided into transverse arrest and longitudinal arrest, comprises congenital deficits characterized by either partial or complete failure of limb formation.

Transverse arrest deficits include all congenital amputation-type malformations and are classified by the level at which the existing portion of the limb terminates; all elements distal to that level are absent. Deficits in this group range from aphalangia (absence of a digit) to amelia (complete absence of a limb) (see Plate 4-38) and are sometimes referred to as congenital amputations, which should not be confused with intrauterine amputations. The transverse stump represents an arrest of formation in the limb anlage. It is usually well padded with soft tissue, and rudimentary digits or dimpling may be present.

Phalangeal Deficiency. One or more digits may be involved, and this defect may occur at any level of the digit. The mildest forms require no treatment. In patients with severe deficits and functional impairment, a cosmetic prosthesis or surgical reconstruction (e.g., bone lengthening, digital transposition, or transplantation) may be indicated. Phalangeal deficiencies in the foot usually require shoe correction only.

Transmetacarpal Amputation Type. This defect is relatively rare, usually unilateral, and often accompanied by a transtarsal amputation-type defect in the foot.

The hand is short and wide, and skin nubbins may be present (see Plate 4-39). Bone mass insufficiency rules out phalangization (surgical formation of a finger or thumb from a metacarpal). Children with these defects are fitted with an opposition palmar pad prosthesis secured to the distal forearm with a Velcro strap. Wrist flexion opposes the hand remnant to the prosthesis and provides a crude type of palmar prehension with sensation.

Transcarpal Amputation Type. In this rare defect, the phalanges and metacarpals are totally absent. In some patients, five skin nubbins are present. The wrist joint is normal, and the epiphyses of the distal radius and ulna appear normal on radiographs. The carpal bones are often fused to some degree. Because the limb is usually too long for a wrist disarticulation prosthesis, an opposition palmar pad prosthesis is used to provide prehension with sensation.

Plate 4-39

Musculoskeletal System: PART III

FAILURE OF FORMATION OF PARTS: TRANSVERSE ARREST
Transmetacarpal amputation type (aphalangia)

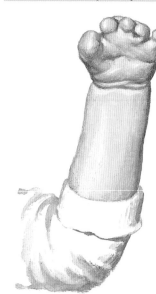

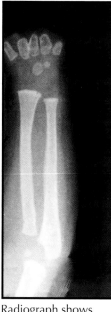

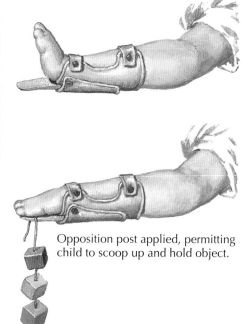

Opposition post applied, permitting child to scoop up and hold object.

Absence of all fingers. Rudimentary digits represented by skin nubbins with or without fingernails.

Radiograph shows absence of phalanges. Metacarpals present but short and osteoporotic.

CONGENITAL LIMB MALFORMATION (Continued)

Transtarsal Amputation Type. Absence of the phalanges and metatarsals, and usually the cuneiforms and cuboid, characterizes this rare deficit (see Plate 4-39). The foot is in equinus, although the tibialis anterior tendon prevents an excessive degree of deformity. Transtarsal defects are similar to Lisfranc amputations. The gastrocnemius and soleus muscles (triceps surae) are underdeveloped, and the knee tends to hyperextend. Without the forefoot, normal push-off in gait is impossible. Use of a high shoe with a reinforced steel shank and a felt foot or a foam-rubber shoe filler compensates for the defect.

Wrist Disarticulation Type. This apparently autosomal recessive trait is more common in females and is seldom bilateral. Typically, the stump is long, and skin nubbins represent failure of digit development. The epiphyses of the distal radius and ulna are present, but all skeletal elements distal to them are absent (see Plate 4-40). Pronation and supination capabilities usually exist, but a cartilaginous bar bridging the radius and ulna is occasionally present.

In patients with unilateral involvement, a forearm socket is molded to the dorsopalmar diameter of the stump to take advantage of pronation and supination capabilities. The terminal grasping device is activated by contralateral scapular abduction through a shoulder harness and cable-linkage system. With appropriate training, even young patients soon become proficient in the use of the prosthesis.

Patients with congenital bilateral absence of hands present a greater rehabilitation challenge because they lack tactile gnosis when wearing artificial limbs. The Krukenberg procedure splits the forearm stump into a prehensile forceps (see Plate 4-40). Providing the forearm stump is sufficiently long, the procedure can be used in blind patients with bilateral hand loss, in patients living in areas where prosthetic services are not available, and in any patients with bilateral hand loss. Using the simple mechanical principle of chopsticks, patients with a Krukenberg hand can function with amazing dexterity. The advantages of readily available prehension with sensation are theoretically significant; however, the Krukenberg procedure has not been shown to improve function in sighted patients. Thus, it is rarely indicated.

The goal of the procedure is to convert the forearm into a strong, active forceps with the radial ray opposing the ulnar ray. The muscles and tendons are divided between the radial and ulnar rays. The interosseous membrane is divided at the ulnar periosteal attachment, preserving the interosseous nerve and vessels. Tactile sensation should be present between the tips. Any digits present, with their associated vessels and tendons, are retained. The forceps should spread wide enough to

Transtarsal amputation type (adactyly)

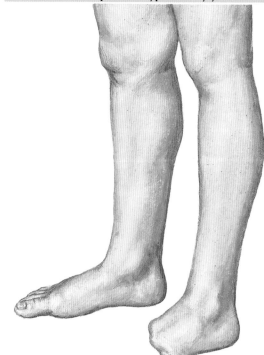

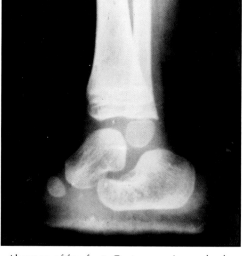

Absence of forefoot. Gastrocnemius and soleus muscles somewhat atrophied; knee tends to hyperextend. Radiograph shows complete deficit of metatarsals, phalanges, cuneiforms, and cuboid.

accommodate ordinary objects, such as a drinking glass, and should be strong enough to hold common objects securely. If the forceps is too long, it may lack strength; if it is too short, distal spread may be insufficient. The pronator teres muscle limits the proximal depth of the forceps.

Patients with a Krukenberg hand begin a training program 2 to 3 weeks after surgery. They learn how to grasp and release rapidly. Pronation and supination are strong, natural movements, but patients must learn to abduct and adduct the forceps rays for best function. Moving the radius toward or away from the relatively fixed ulna provides the principal abduction-adduction motion. In strong gripping, however, ulnar adduction is also important. The therapist plays an essential role in teaching patients to use standard implements and perform two-handed activities, using a hook on the contralateral limb.

CONGENITAL LIMB MALFORMATION (Continued)

Forearm Amputation Type. One of the most common transverse arrest deficiencies is the below-elbow defect (see Plate 4-41). Occasionally, rudimentary digits with fingernails are present at the end of the stump. The radius may also be slightly longer than the ulna. The olecranon and trochlea are usually well developed. The radial head may articulate with the capitellum or project lateroproximally beyond it. The elbow joint has lateral stability, hyperextensibility, and excellent flexion. Because of this, children are able to use their elbow for prehensile activities and often have little functional need for a prosthesis and only use one for specific purposes or occasions.

If a prosthesis is used, the length of the stump and the patient's age determine the type of prosthesis. The infant with a very short below-elbow stump is fitted with a preflexed arm. As the skeleton matures, the child can wear a preflexed socket with rigid elbow hinges. Children younger than age 10 months are fitted with a passive mitten (smooth, stuffed plastic prosthesis) or, preferably, with a hook that is not connected to a cable system. The hook is activated when the child is ready for training, which is usually near 24 months. Newer, myoelectric prosthesis can be fitted and used as the patient ages.

Elbow Disarticulation Type. The epiphysis of the distal humerus is present, but there are no bony elements distal to it. A standard elbow disarticulation prosthesis is prescribed for this type of defect. The dual-control prosthesis has a prehensile hook and an elbow lock that allows variable positioning of the forearm.

Above-Elbow Amputation Type. In this type of defect, the epiphysis of the distal humerus is absent and the standard above-elbow prosthesis is usually appropriate (see Plate 4-42). A turntable above the elbow lock allows manual rotation of the forearm piece, providing optimal function.

Shoulder Disarticulation Type. Total absence of an upper limb deprives patients of half of their prehensile power. Children with bilateral deficits present with a formidable rehabilitation challenge (see Plate 4-43). These children usually develop compensatory skills at a very early age and they frequently become very adept at using their feet for prehension (see Plate 4-38). Most patients request prostheses for the upper limbs to broaden their prehensile skills and provide a more acceptable appearance. Because motors are necessary to control the prosthetic shoulder, elbow, and terminal device, fitting these patients is extremely difficult. Fitting prostheses for lower-level amputations is much simpler.

Children with a unilateral shoulder defect should begin wearing a body-powered shoulder disarticulation

FAILURE OF FORMATION OF PARTS: TRANSVERSE ARREST (CONTINUED)

Wrist disarticulation type (acheiria)

Absence of hand. Radiograph shows radius and ulna with relatively normal distal epiphyses.

Child with Krukenberg hand on left limb. Prosthesis on right limb has terminal grasping device operated with shoulder harness.

Krukenberg hand

Biceps brachii muscle
Brachial artery and median nerve
Supinator muscle
Brachioradialis muscle
Pronator teres muscle
Flexor carpi radialis muscle
Palmaris longus muscle
Half of flexor digitorum superficialis muscle
Triceps brachii muscle
Ulnar nerve
Medial epicondyle
Brachialis muscle
Flexor carpi ulnaris muscle
Half of flexor digitorum superficialis muscle
Radial ray   Ulnar ray
Flexor aspect

Triceps brachii muscle
Olecranon of ulna
Anconeus muscle
Extensor carpi ulnaris muscle
Extensor digiti minimi muscle
Half of extensor digitorum muscle
Biceps brachii muscle
Brachioradialis muscle
Extensor carpi radialis longus muscle
Lateral epicondyle
Extensor carpi radialis brevis muscle
Half of extensor digitorum muscle
Ulnar ray   Radial ray
Extensor aspect

prosthesis during the third or fourth year. In bilateral amputations, the complexity of the harness and body movements necessary to accomplish simple tasks make the shoulder disarticulation prosthesis impractical. Therefore, patients with bilateral defects are ideal candidates for electrically powered prostheses. The prosthesis can be programmed with a feeding pattern that even a 4-year-old child can learn to use. The prosthesis on one side is programmed for use in the head and neck

area and one on the other side for use at a greater distance, such as in toilet care. However, even children who have been fitted with these devices continue to use their feet for most activities.

Ankle Disarticulation Type. This is a sporadic, nonhereditary, and usually unilateral deficit. The stump is similar to a Syme amputation. The epiphyses of the distal tibia and fibula are present and the limb is weight bearing, but because the talus and calcaneus are absent,

Plate 4-41

Musculoskeletal System: PART III

FAILURE OF FORMATION OF PARTS: TRANSVERSE ARREST (CONTINUED)

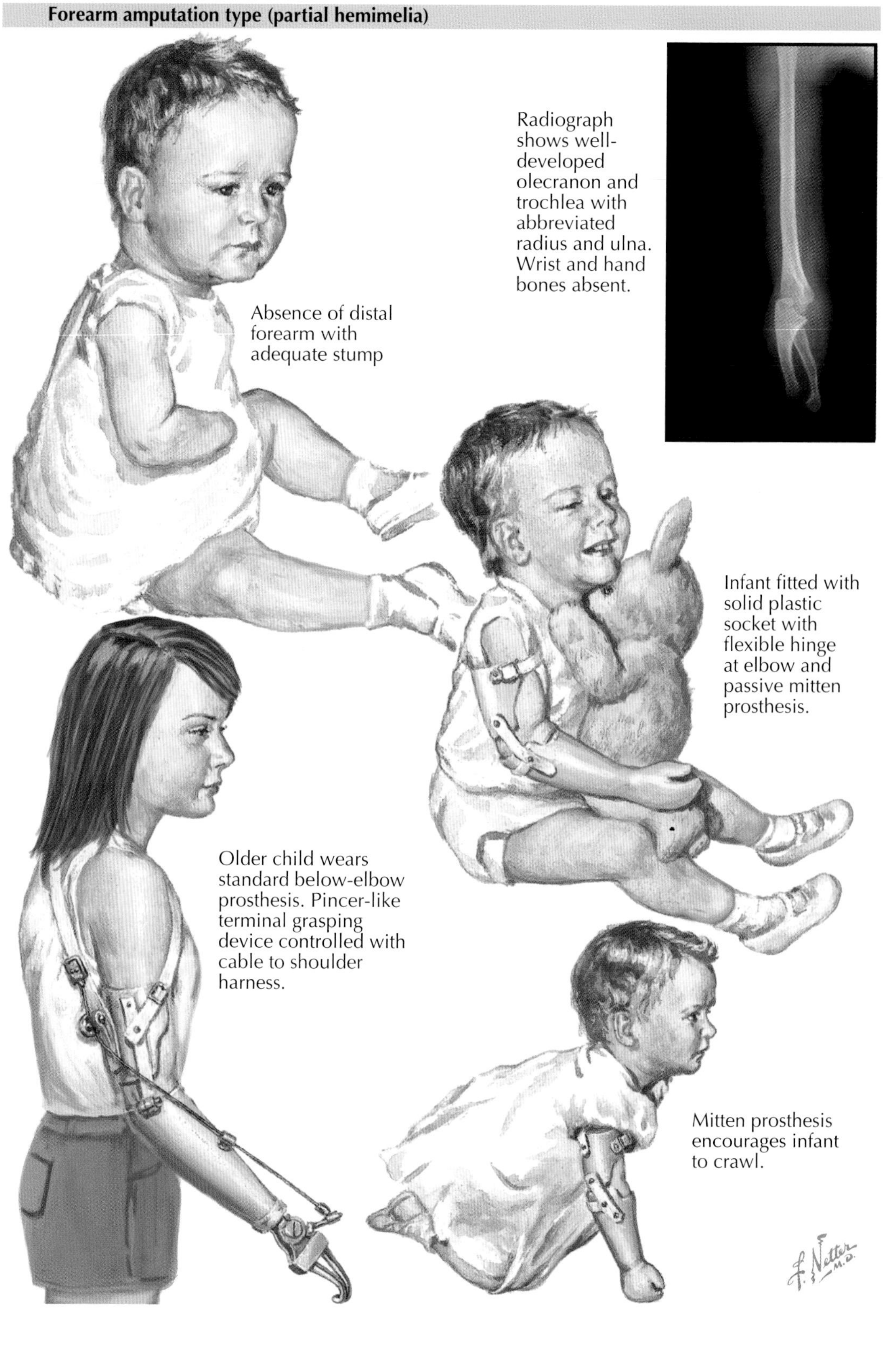

Forearm amputation type (partial hemimelia)

CONGENITAL LIMB MALFORMATION *(Continued)*

it is shorter than the normal one. Use of a standard below-knee socket with a solid ankle-cushioned heel (SACH) foot compensates for the difference in length.

Below-Knee Amputation Type. The proximal half of the tibia is usually present and the fibula is slightly shorter; distally, both bones taper to a point (see Plate 4-44). The proximal epiphyses are present; the stump is usually symmetric but may curve inward.

Children with this deformity are fitted with a below-knee prosthesis that has a plastic socket, condylar cuff, and SACH foot. In some patients, use of rigid knee joints and a leather thigh corset is necessary. The below-knee prosthesis requires little training and allows excellent function, including participation in sports.

Knee Disarticulation Type. In this deficit, the stump is symmetric without distal tapering. The entire femur, including its condyles and lower epiphysis, is present. Toddlers with unilateral defects are fitted with the simplest prosthesis so that they can learn to walk with it. The prosthesis consists of a plastic socket with two aluminum uprights that taper to a crutch tip; a SACH foot is substituted later. Initially, there is no articulated knee hinge. An over-the-shoulder harness helps to hold the prosthesis in place.

When the child is older, a knee disarticulation prosthesis is used. The knee joint is locked with an anterior strap until the child learns to stand independently in the prosthesis. When the child begins to learn thigh lifting and knee swinging, the locking strap is disengaged and later discarded. Some children can be fitted with a suction socket prosthesis as early as 5 years of age.

Above-Knee Amputation Type. In this defect, the epiphysis of the distal femur is absent (see Plate 4-44). Treatment is the same as for a knee disarticulation–type defect.

Hip Disarticulation Type. The femur is totally absent, and there is no acetabular development (see Plate 4-45). In patients with bilateral defects, pelvic contour is wide because fat accumulates over the pelvis. These patients are initially fitted with a pelvic bucket mounted on a board with casters and later with a bilateral hip disarticulation prosthesis with Canadian hip joints. Locking knee straps are used until the patient can stand alone and disengaged when training for ambulation using parallel bars begins. The upper limbs must have sufficient muscle power for these patients to lift themselves for a swing-to type of progression. Ultimately, they learn to ambulate with crutches or remain wheelchair bound.

In unilateral cases, toddlers are first fitted with the simple crutch tip prosthesis, which is later replaced with a hip disarticulation prosthesis. The prosthesis is lengthened as needed.

Absence of distal forearm with adequate stump

Radiograph shows well-developed olecranon and trochlea with abbreviated radius and ulna. Wrist and hand bones absent.

Infant fitted with solid plastic socket with flexible hinge at elbow and passive mitten prosthesis.

Older child wears standard below-elbow prosthesis. Pincer-like terminal grasping device controlled with cable to shoulder harness.

Mitten prosthesis encourages infant to crawl.

I. Failure of Formation of Parts: Longitudinal Arrest

All failures of formation of the limbs other than the transverse arrest type, are arbitrarily classified as longitudinal arrests. The deficiencies in this group reflect the separation of the preaxial (radial or tibial) and postaxial (ulnar or fibular) divisions in the limbs and include longitudinal failure of formation of all limb segments (phocomelia) or failure of either the radial, ulnar, or central components.

Radial Deficiency. Preaxial deformities in the upper limb may involve the radius and thumb, radius only, or thumb only. Malformations include deficient thenar muscles; short, floating thumb; deficient carpals, metacarpals, and radius; and classic radial clubhand. Radial deficiencies are often associated with other congenital

Plate 4-42

Congenital and Developmental Disorders

FAILURE OF FORMATION OF PARTS: TRANSVERSE ARREST (CONTINUED)
Above-elbow amputation type (hemimelia)

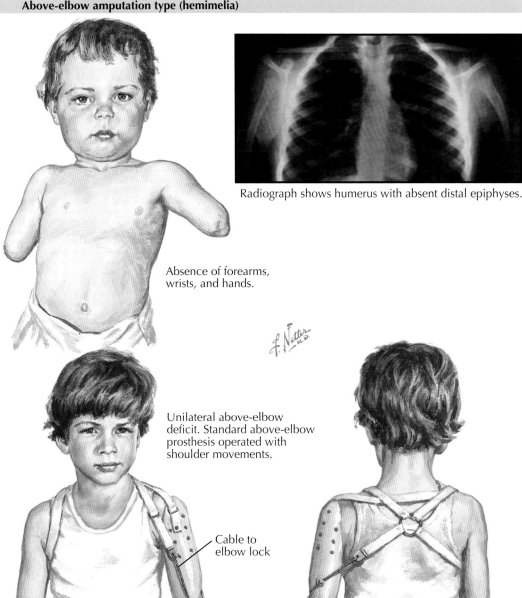

Radiograph shows humerus with absent distal epiphyses.

Absence of forearms, wrists, and hands.

Unilateral above-elbow deficit. Standard above-elbow prosthesis operated with shoulder movements.

Cable to elbow lock

Cable to terminal device

CONGENITAL LIMB MALFORMATION (Continued)

anomalies and a number of syndromes such as Holt-Oram syndrome, congenital aplastic anemia (Fanconi anemia), and thrombocytopenia-absent radius (TAR). It has also been associated with maternal use of valproic acid, thalidomide, and phenobarbital and with fetal alcohol syndrome.

In the radial clubhand the forearm is short, the hand deviates radially, and the thumb is absent (see Plate 4-46). Radiographs typically show that the radius and usually the scaphoid and trapezium are absent. The ulna is short and usually bowed, and radial deficiencies are often bilateral and rarely partial. In a partial deficiency, radiographs reveal a very short radius distal to the capitellum.

Treatment is identical for both partial and complete radial deficits. In the first few months after birth, the dislocated hand is treated with corrective plaster casts in an approach similar to that used for clubfoot. Although it is usually impossible to relocate the hand with conservative measures, serial stretching and immobilization in a cast keeps the radial soft tissue structures stretched. Aggressive stretching regimens by the parents and day and night bracing can be used to assist this correction.

Surgical centralization of the hand over the ulna improves both appearance and finger function. A careful evaluation of hand function, especially of the effects of wrist fixation on hand activity patterns, should always precede surgery. The length of the limb, elbow flexion, and the effect of the malformation on the patient's ability to reach should be noted. Flexion in the radial digits is usually inadequate, and patients tend to favor the often normal ulnar digits. In unilateral defects, wrist flexion is not essential and the advantages of surgery may outweigh the disadvantage of a fixed wrist. In bilateral defects, however, fixation of both wrists, while improving finger function, can compromise relatively good patterns of function. This is especially likely if elbow and shoulder movements are insufficient to allow functional positioning of the hands.

Surgery can be done in the patient's first or second year if great care is taken to preserve the ulnar growth plate. In the centralization procedure, the curved ulna is straightened with multiple osteotomies and the hand is centered over the ulna and held in position with an intramedullary wire extending into the metacarpal of the index, middle, or ring finger (see Plate 4-46). The ulnar growth plate will continue to grow if it is not injured and if the intramedullary wire is placed through its central portion. Pollicization of the index finger to replace the thumb on one hand is occasionally done if the defect is bilateral.

After surgery, the limb is immobilized in a plaster cast for 2 to 3 months. Day and night bracing continues for

3 more months, and continued night bracing may be necessary throughout the growing years. As the child grows, the intramedullary wire is replaced or advanced distally into the metacarpal. Despite wire fixation into the hand and bracing, recurrence of deformity is common and some hand surgeons have abandoned this procedure in favor of soft tissue reconstructions with tendon transfers.

Thumb Defects. If the thumb is absent, the index finger can be pollicized. A floating thumb can be

amputated and the index finger pollicized, or the thumb can be lengthened by metacarpal osteotomy, distraction, and bone graft. A hypoplastic thumb may be treated with metacarpal distraction and bone graft and a tendon transfer to compensate for the hypoplastic thenar muscle. Rotational osteotomy may be indicated for the nonopposed thumb.

Tibial Deficiency. Complete tibial deficiency is a serious defect; the affected leg is short, the foot is in varus position, the great toe is absent, and the knee is unstable.

Plate 4-43   Musculoskeletal System: PART III

FAILURE OF FORMATION OF PARTS: TRANSVERSE ARREST (CONTINUED)
Shoulder disarticulation type (amelia)

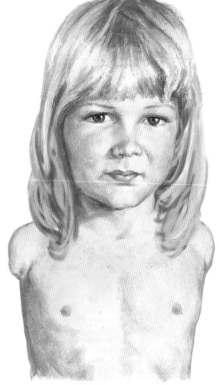

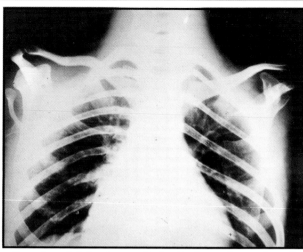

Complete deficit of upper limbs. Radiograph reveals well-formed shoulder girdle.

CONGENITAL LIMB MALFORMATION (Continued)

The tibia is absent, while the fibula is present but may be bowed. Because the fibula is completely unstable, the limb cannot bear weight. Furthermore, the patella is usually absent with no quadriceps function. Treatment with surgery and prostheses is rarely successful. The recommended treatment is knee disarticulation amputation and fitting with an end-bearing socket prosthesis.

Incomplete tibial deficiency is equally disabling. If the defect is bilateral, ambulation is impossible. Only the proximal third of the tibial shaft or only the tibial condyles are present. The tibia may be a rectangularly outlined bone with no evident epiphysis; in some cases, only a small bone cap represents the proximal epiphysis. The fibula is positioned normally or rests superiorly and posteriorly in the popliteal space. These deformities are typically managed with a Syme amputation and appropriate prosthetic management if the patient has a functioning extensor mechanism of the knee. If the patient is unable to actively extend the knee, then treatment is similar to that for a complete deficiency with a knee disarticulation and subsequent prosthesis.

Ulnar Deficiency. Longitudinal deformities of the ulnar ray (see Plate 4-47) are sporadic and nonhereditary and are among the rarest congenital anomalies of the upper limb. Ulnar ray defects are frequently associated with malformations of the radial ray (most common) or of the central rays as well. Associated deformities in the shoulder girdle, proximal humerus, or both, may also be present. (Involvement of a part proximal to the principal deformity occurs only in ulnar deficiencies, phocomelia, and Poland syndrome.) Malformations at the level of the elbow, wrist, hand, and digits vary greatly in type and severity. They include radiohumeral dislocation or synostosis, hypoplasia, partial or total absence of the ulna, curvature of the radius, ulnar deviation of the hand, fusion of carpal bones, congenital amputation at the wrist, and oligodactyly with or without syndactyly. In addition, there is a high incidence of associated anomalies in the opposite hand, lower limb, and other parts of the musculoskeletal system.

Management of ulnar ray defects is complex. Functional testing of limb position, power, and stability helps to determine the best treatment. In general, surgical treatment is reserved for the hand anomalies associated with ulnar deficiencies. Function can be improved with surgical release of syndactyly, web deepening, and thumb reconstruction or pollicization. Wrist and forearm operations are less successful. Occasionally, in partial ulnar defects with significant instability of the elbow, the ulnar remnant can be fused to the radius to provide stability.

Small child effectively uses body-powered prosthesis.

Electrically powered prosthesis on left side. Humeral section of nonfunctional right prosthesis contains rechargeable battery pack.

Fibular Deficiency. Total fibular deficiency is one of the most common long bone deficiencies and is bilateral in about 25% of patients. In patients with unilateral defects, the limb-length discrepancy is considerable. The lower part of the leg bows anteriorly, with a depressed dimple at its apex. The foot is in valgus position, because there is no ankle mortise. There are usually only three or four toes, and the distal tibial epiphysis is absent or minimal. Treatment consists of an ankle disarticulation amputation and use of an end-bearing ankle prosthesis.

Partial fibular deficiencies are quite rare. The tibia is only minimally shortened and the fibula is either shortened or its distal portion appears normal. Treatment is with a shoe lift, but surgical epiphyseal stapling to arrest growth may be necessary.

Central Ray Deficiency. Deficiencies also occur in the second, third, or fourth ray of the hand—the

Plate 4-44

Congenital and Developmental Disorders

FAILURE OF FORMATION OF PARTS: TRANSVERSE ARREST (CONTINUED)

Below-knee amputation type (partial hemimelia)

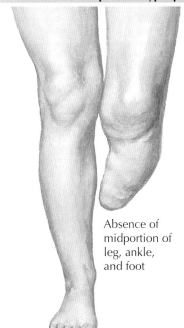

Absence of midportion of leg, ankle, and foot

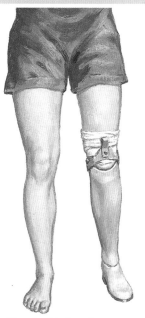

Standard below-knee prosthesis permits ambulation.

CONGENITAL LIMB MALFORMATION *(Continued)*

so-called central rays—which do not differentiate at the same time as the radial and ulnar rays.

Central ray deficiencies are further classified into typical and atypical subgroups. Typical malformations range in severity from a partial or total deficit of a phalanx, metacarpal, or carpal bone of the central rays to a monodigital hand. Atypical central ray deficiencies may be syndactylous or polydactylous. In the syndactylous type, which may be partial or complete, the elements of the third ray are fused to either the second or fourth digital ray, resembling an osseous syndactyly. The hand has a central cleft of soft tissue and the appearance of a lobster claw (see Plate 4-48). In the polydactylous deficiency, supernumerary bony elements are present in the hand, creating a cleft of soft tissue and the appearance of a lobster claw. Similar deformities may also occur in the foot.

In determining treatment for the cleft hand, existing function must be considered. The two opposing digital units are often stable, mobile, and quite functional, although not cosmetically attractive. If function (including prehension with sensation) is adequate, the appearance of the hand is of secondary importance and surgical reconstruction to improve function and appearance is not always indicated. Closure of the cleft includes reconstruction of the deep transverse metacarpal ligament. Rotational osteotomies help correct rotatory deformity of adjacent fingers. The function of a monodigital hand can be improved with rotational osteotomy, opponensplasty, use of a simple opposition post, or a combination of all three.

Intersegmental Deficiency (Phocomelia). The most profound longitudinal arrest is phocomelia (see Plate 4-49), a failure of proximodistal development. Phocomelia may be total (the hand or foot is attached directly to the trunk) or partial (the hand or foot is attached to a deficient, severely shortened limb).

The patient with *bilateral upper limb phocomelia* is unable to position the hands for feeding and toilet activities. Frequently, the problem is further compounded by associated deformities of the lower limbs that prevent good foot prehension.

The joints in phocomelia are usually unstable and hyperextensible because of ligament laxity, and muscle power is decreased. Digits may be missing or have motor deficits. As a rule, patients require a nonstandard prosthesis with external power. Many patients can use the affected limb to control the terminal device or elbow lock in a nonstandard prosthesis, which must be kept as simple as possible to be accepted by the patient.

Patients with *total upper limb phocomelia* are trained to use the lower limbs for many functions and are fitted with a shoulder disarticulation prosthesis or a

Above-knee amputation type (hemimelia)

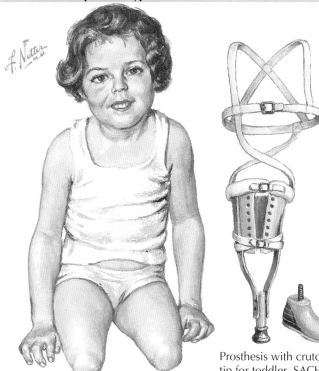

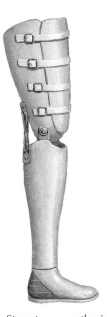

Prosthesis with crutch tip for toddler. SACH foot substituted later.

Strap-type prosthesis for older child (some children prefer suction-socket prosthesis)

myoelectric arm. In *partial phocomelia*, treatment may not be necessary, or one of the following alternatives may be indicated: clavicular transfer to replace the missing humerus, use of a nonstandard shoulder disarticulation prosthesis, hand reconstruction to improve grip or pinch, or therapy to improve function with the existing structures.

In *total lower limb phocomelia*, the foot articulates with the pelvis. Treatment in the young child is a nonstandard hip disarticulation prosthesis with a fenestration

for the foot, a Canadian hip joint held in place with shoulder straps, and a SACH foot without a knee hinge. The hinge is added when the child is older.

In *proximal lower limb phocomelia*, the ligaments are extremely lax and the tibia slides up and down in the pelvis. Motor power in the upper limb is often deficient.

In *distal lower limb phocomelia*, the foot articulates with the distal femur and is often monodigital. The pelvic joint is unstable.

Plate 4-45

Musculoskeletal System: PART III

FAILURE OF FORMATION OF PARTS: TRANSVERSE ARREST (CONTINUED)

Hip disarticulation type (amelia)

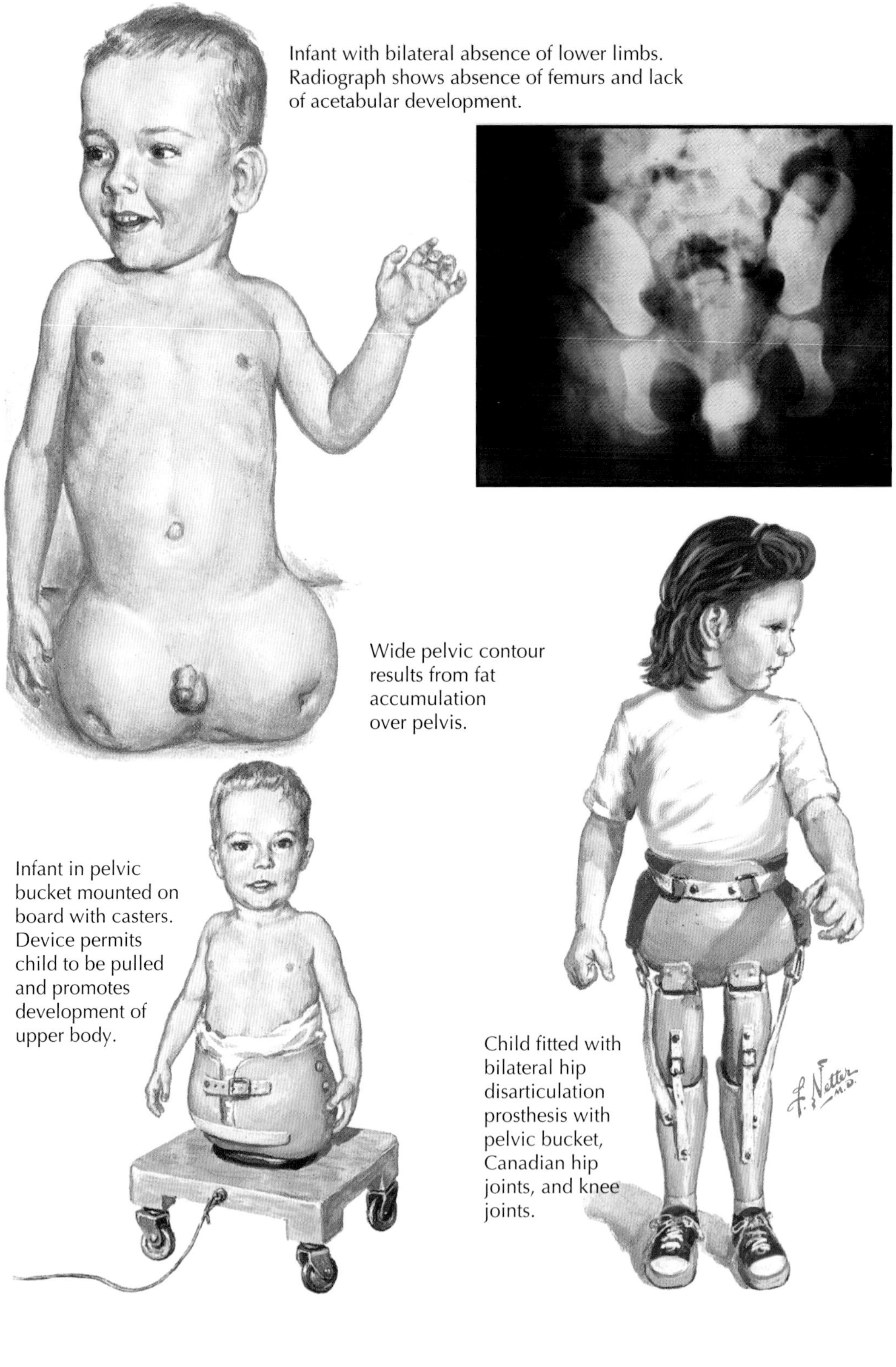

Infant with bilateral absence of lower limbs. Radiograph shows absence of femurs and lack of acetabular development.

CONGENITAL LIMB MALFORMATION *(Continued)*

II. Failure of Differentiation of Parts

Failure of differentiation (separation) of parts refers to all deficits in which the basic anatomic units are present but development is incomplete. The homogeneous anlage, or primordial, differentiates into the skeletal, dermomyofascial, and neurovascular elements found in a normal limb, but differentiation, or separation, is incomplete. Therefore, this category includes soft tissue involvement, skeletal involvement, and congenital tumors (e.g., hemangiomas, lymphomas, neuronal, connective tissue tumors, and skeletal tumors; see Section 6, Tumors of Musculoskeletal System). Upper limb defects are more disabling than those of the lower limb.

Shoulder Defects. Congenital elevation of the scapula (see Plate 4-28) and absence of the pectoral muscles are the two types of failure of differentiation in the shoulder. Skeletal involvement at this level can result in congenital humerus varus.

Elbow and Forearm Defects. Soft tissue involvement may be manifested by aberrations of the long flexor, extensor, or intrinsic muscles in the upper limb. Failure of skeletal differentiation can result in either dislocation or synostosis of the humeroradial, humeroulnar, proximal, or distal radioulnar joint. Synostosis of the proximal radioulnar joint, the most severe elbow deformity in this category, is genetically determined and often associated with synostosis elsewhere in the body. Surgical correction may be indicated if flexion/extension or pronation/supination deformities that interfere with function are present.

Wrist and Hand Defects. Failure of differentiation can occur in either the skeletal or soft tissue elements of the carpus, metacarpals, or fingers.

In *symphalangism*, an intermediary joint in the digit is missing, most commonly the proximal interphalangeal joint. This bilateral malformation most frequently involves the ring and little fingers. Symphalangism of the distal interphalangeal joint is rare and almost never seen in the thumb. The affected joint is immobile, and its flexion and extension folds are absent. Radiographs taken after closure of the epiphysis show bony ankylosis. If ankylosis is established, the deformity can be treated with implant arthroplasty or with osteotomy and fusion of the joint in a functional position.

Syndactyly, one of the two most common malformations in the hand, is often bilateral and can involve two or more digits, usually the middle and ring fingers. In some patients, only the soft tissues are fused (simple syndactyly); in other patients, the nails and bones are joined as well (complex syndactyly). Syndactyly often occurs in association with webbing of the toes (usually between the second and third toes) and is frequently

Wide pelvic contour results from fat accumulation over pelvis.

Infant in pelvic bucket mounted on board with casters. Device permits child to be pulled and promotes development of upper body.

Child fitted with bilateral hip disarticulation prosthesis with pelvic bucket, Canadian hip joints, and knee joints.

associated with other deformities in the same hand or elsewhere in the body, such as Poland syndrome, Apert syndrome, or craniofacial dysostosis. Syndactyly is occasionally hereditary, and this type affects males more often than females and is rare in African-American children. It is believed to arise during the fetal period and must be differentiated from acrosyndactyly secondary to congenital constriction band syndrome (see Plate 4-50).

If the syndactyly does not interfere with alignment of the digits, growth, or hand function, surgical repair can be postponed until the child is 2 or 3 years of age. However, syndactyly in digits of unequal length (e.g., ring and little fingers or, more commonly, the thumb and index finger) requires early surgical correction to avoid permanent deformity. In complex syndactyly, the nails of the joined digits are usually fused and the nail and bony bridge must be divided and resurfaced with a

Plate 4-46

Congenital and Developmental Disorders

FAILURE OF FORMATION OF PARTS: LONGITUDINAL ARREST

Radial deficiency (paraxial radial hemimelia)

CONGENITAL LIMB MALFORMATION (Continued)

graft. If more than two digits are affected, adjacent pairs are separated at different times to avoid compromising the blood supply. Pairs of unequal length are divided first.

Congenital Flexion Deformities. These deformities are caused by inadequate extensor tendons, flexor tendon nodules, or arthrogryposis multiplex congenita (see Plate 4-24).

Camptodactyly refers to congenital flexion contracture of the proximal interphalangeal joint of the finger (usually little finger), a condition that is often hereditary and can be bilateral. Although it usually requires no treatment, surgery may be indicated if the flexion contracture is disabling or associated with deformity of the ring finger. Moderate defects are improved by release of the flexor digitorum superficialis tendon and lengthening of the palmar skin, followed by postoperative splinting. More severe cases may require release of the palmar ligament, reconstruction of the extensor tendon, and arthroplasty or arthrodesis.

In the thumb, the absence of one or all of the extrinsic abductor or extensor pollicis tendons produces isolated postural deformities related to the missing structures. *Thumb flexion deformities* are usually bilateral and symmetric and are frequently hereditary. They must be differentiated from conditions such as trigger thumb, arthrogryposis multiplex congenita, and upper motor neuron disease (spasticity). If a thumb flexion deformity is recognized in infancy, splinting and daily manipulation can prevent soft tissue contractures. Surgery should be postponed until the child has developed more complex grasping movements, which usually occurs by 3 years of age. Surgical correction may require tendon transfers and release of skin contracture, as well as release of contracted adductor or short flexor muscles.

Trigger thumb deformity, which is characterized by flexion of both the metacarpophalangeal and interphalangeal joints, is caused by a nodule on the flexor pollicis longus tendon that interferes with tendon excursion. The condition is rare in the other digits. Surgery is indicated to release the flexor pollicis longus tendon longitudinally.

Occasionally, anomalous anchorage of the deep transverse metacarpal ligament to the first metacarpal or proximal phalanx of the thumb causes *adduction contracture of the thumb* with narrowing of the first web space. The narrowed web space and deep transverse ligament are released surgically.

Clinodactyly refers to a digit curving medially or laterally in the radioulnar plane. The deformity is due to a failure of skeletal differentiation in a phalanx and is most common in the middle phalanx; the little finger is

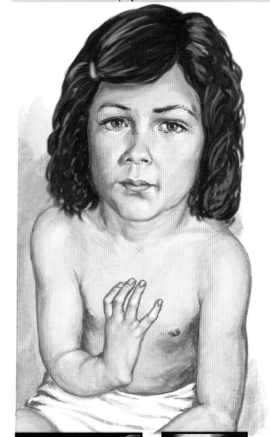

Radiograph shows double osteotomy to straighten curved ulna. Stabilized with intramedullary wire.

Partial carpal resection. Hand centralized and maintained with wire into metacarpal.

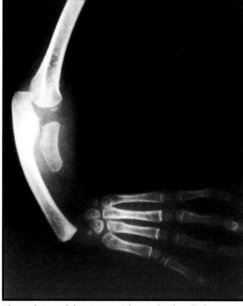

Short, bowed forearm with marked radial deviation of hand. Thumb absent. Radiograph shows partial deficit of radial ray (vestige of radius present). Scaphoid, trapezium, and metacarpal and phalanges of thumb absent.

Centralization procedure

Osteotomy of ulna

Kirschner wire

Postoperative view

most often affected. The angulation can begin at the level of the joint or the diaphysis or may result from a delta-shaped phalanx. Relatively severe deformities require surgical treatment.

Arthrogryposis Multiplex Congenita. This deformity is caused by a disseminated failure of differentiation of the soft tissue of the limbs. Isolated muscles or groups of muscles are absent, and the joints they control may become stiff and fuse spontaneously. One or all

four limbs may be affected, and usually spinal anomalies are present as well (see Plate 4-24 for a complete discussion).

III. Duplication of Parts

Duplication of parts is believed to be caused by a specific insult that causes the limb bud, or ectodermal cap, to split very early in development. Defects in the hand range from polydactyly to twinning (mirror hands) and

Plate 4-47

Musculoskeletal System: PART III

FAILURE OF FORMATION OF PARTS: LONGITUDINAL ARREST (CONTINUED)
Ulnar deficiency (paraxial ulnar hemimelia)

CONGENITAL LIMB MALFORMATION (Continued)

can involve the skin and nails, the soft tissues, or both, plus the skeletal structures. A single bone or an entire limb may be duplicated.

Polydactyly. Along with syndactyly, duplication of a digit, or polydactyly, is one of the most common malformations of the hand (see Plate 4-50), but it may also occur in the feet. Polydactyly has an autosomal dominant inheritance with variable expressivity. Unlike syndactyly, it is more prevalent in African-Americans. Duplication of the little finger is most common, followed by the thumb (see Plate 4-50). Polydactyly may be associated with a variety of syndromes, including Laurence-Moon-Biedl syndrome, Fanconi pancytopenia, and Holt-Oram syndrome..

Surgical treatment is usually performed to improve appearance. Early amputation is indicated when the polydactylous finger is a flail, poorly attached appendage. When the attachment of the extra digit is more complex, the digit to be sacrificed should be selected carefully. Bony architecture and tendon function and distribution must be considered. The marginal digit or the one that appears most normal is not necessarily the most functional one. In some patients, usable structures from the amputated digit should be preserved for transfer to the digit to be preserved. For example, if one of the two adjoining digits has greater flexor power while the other has greater extensor power, the latter is amputated and its extensor mechanism is transferred.

Duplication of the thumb can be partial or complete; partial forms include the bifid and bifurcated thumb. The thumb may be split at the interphalangeal or metacarpophalangeal joint, or the split may stem from the metacarpal diaphysis. When a polydactylous thumb is amputated, tendons should be regrouped to reinforce the power of the thumb or the part to be spared. Treatment of duplication distal to the interphalangeal joint consists of resection of a V-shaped segment of skin, nail, and bone. This principle can be adapted to the treatment of duplications proximal to the interphalangeal joint, although in children, the final correction may be delayed to avoid injury to the growth plates. When a twin digit is divided, the collateral ligaments must be reconstructed at the amputation site.

A triphalangeal thumb is another expression of thumb duplication and is often associated with serious cardiac anomalies or hematopoietic disorders. If the thumb can be positioned in opposition, treatment is optional. There may be a progressive recurvatum deformity caused by a wedge-shaped ossicle interposed between the distal and proximal phalanges; this ossicle can be removed in childhood. If the thumb cannot be

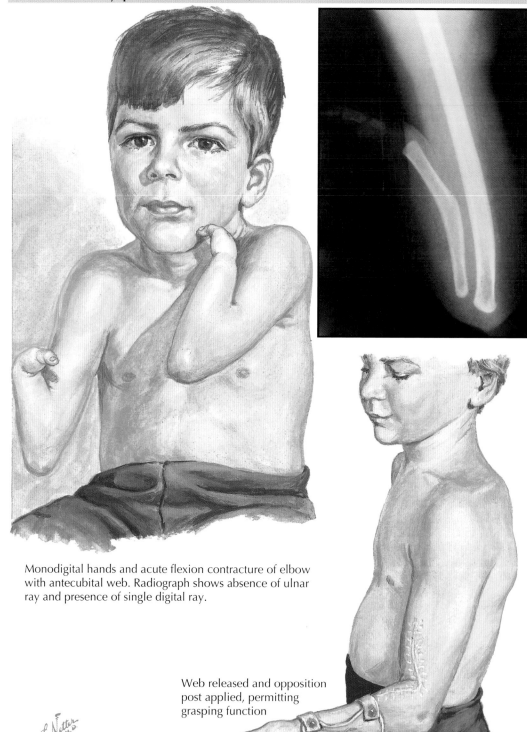

Monodigital hands and acute flexion contracture of elbow with antecubital web. Radiograph shows absence of ulnar ray and presence of single digital ray.

Web released and opposition post applied, permitting grasping function

opposed and resembles an index finger, surgical treatment may include creation of a first web space, rotational osteotomy, and tendon transfer. In complex preaxial (radial) polydactyly, the thumb is duplicated with triphalangism of one or both of the extra digits.

IV. Overgrowth

The terms *overgrowth* and *gigantism* describe conditions in which either part or all of the limb is disproportionately large. This may occur in the digit (macrodactyly),

hand, forearm, or entire limb; similar defects may occur in the lower limb. The condition is seldom bilateral and usually not hereditary.

Macrodactyly. Four types of macrodactyly have been described. In the first type, the most common type, the enlarged portion is in the distribution of a major nerve and is associated with abnormally large nerves infiltrated with large amounts of fat. It most often occurs in the distribution of the median nerve in the hand and the medial plantar nerve in the foot. The second type

Plate 4-48

Congenital and Developmental Disorders

FAILURE OF FORMATION OF PARTS: LONGITUDINAL ARREST (CONTINUED)

Central ray deficiency (lobster-claw deformity)

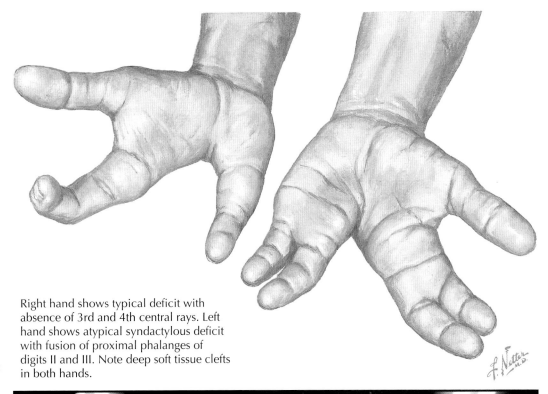

Right hand shows typical deficit with absence of 3rd and 4th central rays. Left hand shows atypical syndactylous deficit with fusion of proximal phalanges of digits II and III. Note deep soft tissue clefts in both hands.

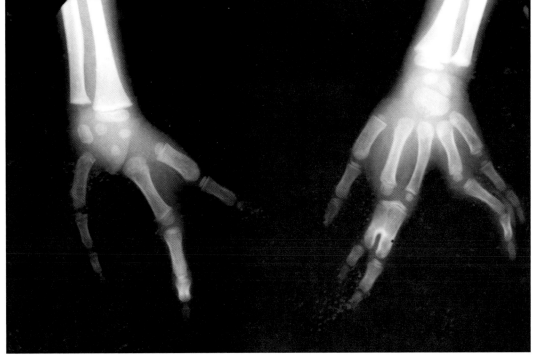

CONGENITAL LIMB MALFORMATION (Continued)

is associated with neurofibromatosis. The third type is very rare and associated with unusual hyperostosis without enchondroma. The fourth type occurs with hemihypertrophy of the ipsilateral upper and lower limb and is associated with adrenal, renal, and brain tumors.

In type I, the abnormality is usually greatest at the periphery. There are typically two clinical presentations. In the first, the child is born with an enlarged digit that grows proportionately with the child's growth. In the second, the child is born with a normal digit that enlarges in a progressive manner. Growth can be symmetric or asymmetric, resulting in increase in deformities. The thumb and the second and third fingers are most often affected.

Surgical treatment is very challenging and may include total or partial amputation or reduction in size. If the deformity is unsightly, amputation may be indicated. Although surgical reduction of an enlarged digit is possible, the procedure is difficult because of the need to preserve the neurovascular supply and joint function while reducing both the length and width of the digit. Reduction procedures can include epiphyseal arrest and progressive excision of bone and soft tissue.

V. Undergrowth

Undergrowth, or hypoplasia, denotes defective or incomplete development of the entire limb or its parts. In some classifications, the term *hypoplasia* was used to describe the condition of skeletal elements that persist after some failures of formation of parts (category I defects). However, because of their prevalence, hypoplastic defects are represented separately in the classification used here. Hypoplasia may occur in either the upper or the lower limb. In the upper limb, it may affect the arm, forearm, hand, or parts of the hand. Only the skin and nails may be involved, or the musculotendinous structures, the neurovascular structures, or both, may be affected as well.

Brachydactyly. Shortening of the digits is the most common hand malformation seen in association with syndromes and systemic disorders. It is usually transmitted as a part of an autosomal dominant phenotype with slight variation. The middle phalanges of the index through little fingers, and especially those of the index and little fingers, are most commonly affected because they develop later than the thumb. The metacarpals are involved less frequently and the deformity is rare in the distal phalanx of the thumb. Surgical lengthening of the shortened digits is usually not necessary, although

osteotomy through the anomalous or proximal phalanx can sometimes correct a deviated finger.

Brachysyndactyly. Shortening of the digits plus syndactyly could be classified in category I (failure of formation of parts) or category II (failure of differentiation of parts) because some of its features are intersegmental failure of development as well as failure of separation of parts. However, the most obvious failure, hypoplasia, explains the reason for inclusion in this category.

VI. Congenital Constriction Band Syndrome

Constriction bands are the result of focal necrosis along the course of the limb during the fetal stage of development. An area of necrosis involving the superficial tissues heals as a circular scar, creating the band. Whether constriction bands are intrinsic or extrinsic defects has not yet been fully determined. Amniotic bands have been implicated as a mechanical cause but

Plate 4-49

Musculoskeletal System: PART III

FAILURE OF FORMATION OF PARTS: LONGITUDINAL ARREST (CONTINUED)
Intersegmental deficiency (phocomelia of upper limb)

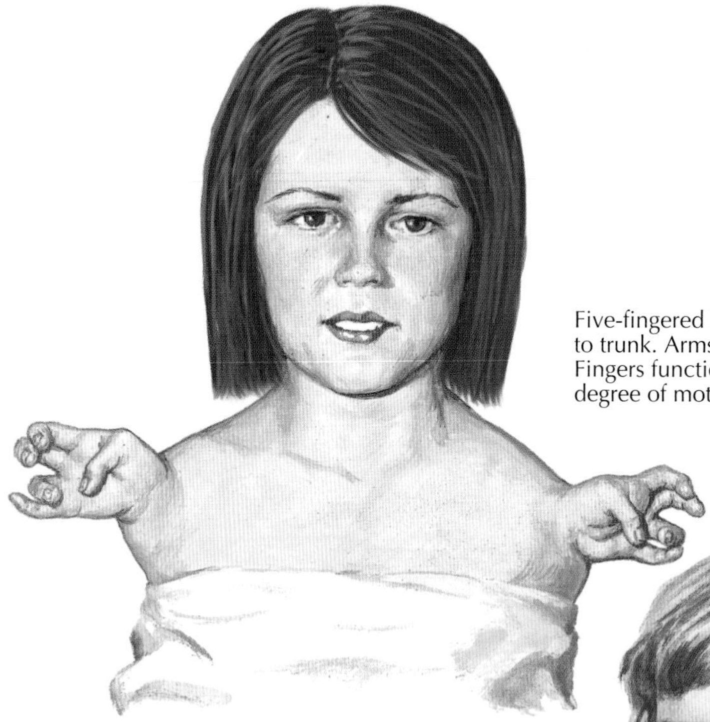

Five-fingered hands attached directly to trunk. Arms and forearms absent. Fingers functional but may have some degree of motor deficit.

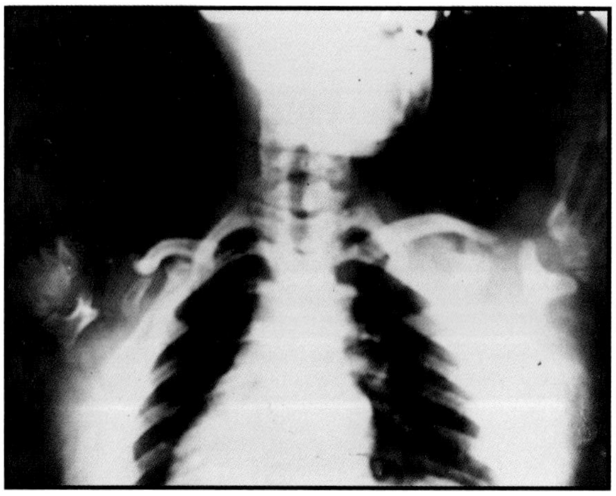

Radiograph shows absence of humerus, radius, and ulna. Rudimentary bone proximal to metacarpals cannot be identified.

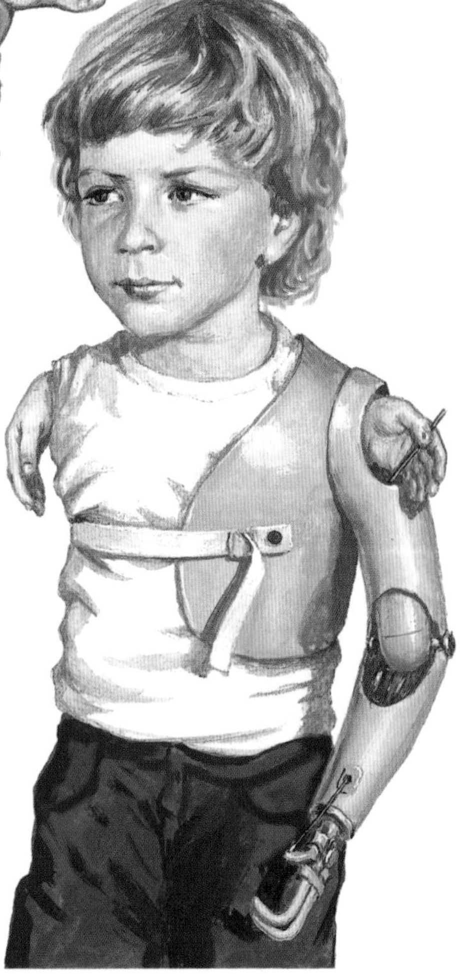

Standard shoulder disarticulation prosthesis, fenestrated at shoulder. Hand operates cable that locks and unlocks elbow and opens terminal hook device. Rubber band closes device.

CONGENITAL LIMB MALFORMATION (Continued)

may actually be secondary to a healing limb injury. The malformation is probably caused by a focal tissue defect that allows hemorrhage within the limb, with resulting tissue necrosis. The defect can be expressed as a constriction band, congenital amputation, or acrosyndactyly (see Plate 4-50). When the constriction band is severe, intrauterine gangrene may develop and a true fetal amputation occurs.

In *acrosyndactyly*, the syndactylous digits and confused arrangement of anatomic parts sometimes seen may be the result of a healed necrotic infarct that occurred during the stage of separation of parts. The tissue necrosis and the resulting fusion of parts resemble those seen in an untreated third-degree burn with bridges of scar. Unlike syndactyly, acrosyndactyly is characterized by annular grooves, transverse amputations of distal parts, and the presence of a web space or fenestration between the fused digits.

Constriction bands are more likely to involve the distal part of the limb, especially the hand and foot. The central digits are usually affected; severe acrosyndactyly is rare in the thumb. A paralytic clubfoot deformity due to compression neuropathy of the peroneal nerve caused by a deep, below-knee constriction band has been described. Deformities associated with constriction band syndrome include cleft lip and cleft palate, heart anomalies, meningocele, hemangioma, and congenital clubfoot.

Annular grooves caused by constriction bands are released by Z-plasties. If parts are missing, the surgical or prosthetic treatment depends on the level of the amputation.

VII. Generalized Skeletal Abnormalities

Hand defects may be manifestations of a generalized skeletal defect, such as dyschondroplasia, achondroplasia (see Plates 4-1 to 4-3), Marfan syndrome (with arachnodactyly), and diastrophic dwarfism (see Plate 4-6). In this category, the hand deformities are unique to each syndrome.

IMPROVING FUNCTION IN PATIENTS

Although a malformed limb may not look normal, with proper rehabilitation it can sometimes achieve almost normal function in certain prehensile patterns. Prehension requires two mobile opposing parts that either diametrically oppose each other or can be adducted parallel to each other. If these parts have normal sensation and if the proximal joints can place the hand or

foot in the desired position, functional activities can be performed with some skill.

Foot Prehension in Amelia. In children with bilateral absence of the upper limbs and functional lower limbs, a bilateral upper limb prosthesis allows prehension and is useful in social situations. However, prehension with it lacks sensory feedback and is awkward and imprecise, and foot function should be encouraged. Young children with amelia become amazingly adept at using their

feet, learning early to explore their environment by touching and manipulating objects (see Plate 4-38). In early childhood, they begin to use their feet for prehension with sensation. They develop extraordinary flexibility in the hips and legs that allows them to position their feet for functions around the head. Eventually, even small objects may be handled with precision. Some older patients learn to put on their prosthesis, take care of personal hygiene, eat, and even drive a car with their

Plate 4-50

Congenital and Developmental Disorders

Duplication of parts (polydactyly)

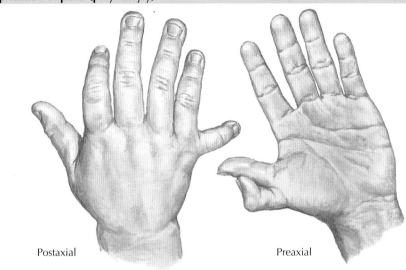

Postaxial   Preaxial

CONGENITAL LIMB MALFORMATION (Continued)

feet. Special devices extend their skills in dressing, toilet care, and other activities.

Rehabilitation in Upper Limb Defects. In patients with an upper limb defect, the capacity for prehension after treatment is determined by the type of deformity and the patient's ability to respond to training. If strong prehension with sensation can be achieved with training, no further treatment is required. Children can develop skills that will make them independent.

Surgical reconstruction is indicated if it can improve function (and possibly yield cosmetic benefit) without subjecting the patient to many operations. Surgery should be undertaken as early as possible. The goal is to obtain a good grasp-and-release mechanism, preserve good sensation, and facilitate positioning of the hand for optimal function. A very young patient should have frequent postoperative evaluations, especially during the growth period, to avoid recurrence of the deformity due to imbalance or unequal growth.

During surgery, small skin nubbins or rudimentary digits at the distal portions of the limb should be preserved, because even a small nubbin can provide excellent sensation. Amputation should be considered only if there is neurovascular insufficiency, loss of skin cover, or infection and never if there is good skin cover with sensation. Before undertaking any surgical procedure, whether an amputation or a reconstruction, the surgeon must carefully evaluate the patient's existing and potential use of the limb. For successful rehabilitation, reconstructive surgery must be individualized.

Rehabilitation in Lower Limb Defects. Children with a lower limb defect should be fitted with a prosthesis at 12 or 15 months of age, the normal age for walking. Very often, a complicated, nonstandard prosthesis must be designed for these patients. Occasionally, if function cannot be achieved with reconstructive surgery, it may be achieved with a properly performed amputation—a good example is the removal of a severely malformed foot to obtain proper fit of a prosthesis. With the prosthesis, the child will look almost normal and be almost normally active.

In the growing child, the amputation should always be through a joint, not across a long bone. Amputation through the diaphysis can result in bone overgrowth. Often, after an apparently successful amputation, the growing bone perforates distally through the stump and the ensuing infection and further overgrowth necessitate multiple surgical procedures. During a joint disarticulation, the growth plate must be preserved to ensure future growth of the stump.

Prostheses. Use of prostheses is successful in children as young as 21 months of age. They can master a voluntary opening hook and eventually become more

Overgrowth (macrodactyly)

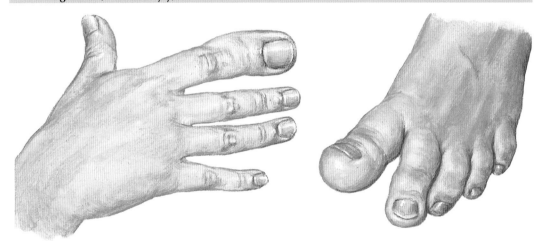

Congenital constriction band syndrome

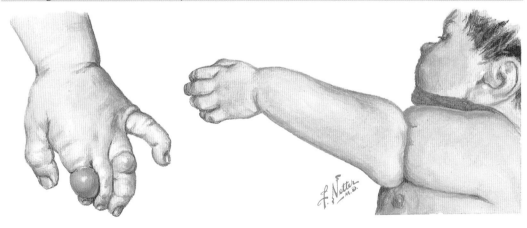

adept at using a prosthesis than adult amputees. Artificial limbs are used as long as they are tolerated by the patient, do not cause pain, and are in good working order. Children are readily accepted by playmates once the curiosity about the prosthesis is satisfied.

Children who wear upper limb prostheses are able to dress themselves and put on and take off their artificial

limbs without difficulty. The terminal hook device is a very versatile tool, and most patients prefer it to a cosmetic hand. In adolescence, a functioning cosmetic hand may be substituted.

Parents of children with limb defects should keep well informed about rehabilitation programs that include physical therapy, surgery, and prostheses.

RHEUMATIC DISEASES

Plate 5-1

Musculoskeletal System: PART III

JOINT PATHOLOGY IN RHEUMATOID ARTHRITIS

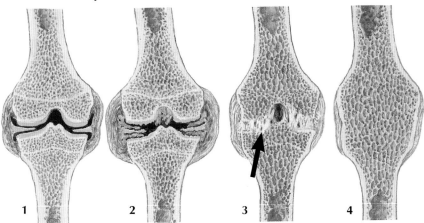

1   2   3   4

Progressive stages in joint pathology. 1. Acute inflammation of synovial membrane (synovitis) and beginning proliferative changes. 2. Progression of inflammation with pannus formation; beginning destruction of cartilage and mild osteoporosis. 3. Subsidence of inflammation; fibrous ankylosis (arrow). 4. Bony ankylosis; advanced osteoporosis.

RHEUMATIC DISEASES

The term *rheumatic disease* refers to any illness characterized by pain and stiffness in or around the joints. These diseases are divided into two main groups: disorders that involve the joints primarily (the different forms of arthritis) and disorders that, although not directly affecting the joints, involve connective tissue structures around the joints (the periarticular disorders, or nonarticular rheumatism). The many types of arthritis and nonarticular disorders differ from one another in etiology, pathogenesis, pathology, and clinical features. The focus of this section is on the more commonly encountered rheumatic conditions.

Rheumatoid arthritis and osteoarthritis (also called degenerative joint disease) are the most common forms of arthritis. Both of these chronic conditions are characterized by pain, stiffness, restricted joint motion, joint deformities, and disability, but their differences in pathogenesis, pathology, and clinical features must be distinguished because the prognosis and treatment of the two diseases differ.

RHEUMATOID ARTHRITIS

Rheumatoid arthritis is a chronic, inflammatory systemic illness with widespread involvement of connective tissue. Although rheumatoid arthritis may begin at any age, onset is usually in the fourth or fifth decade. Occurring in all parts of the world, it affects females two to three times more often than males.

The major characteristic of rheumatoid arthritis is inflammation of multiple joints (polyarthritis), usually the joints of the limbs. Although partial remissions are common, relapses and progression of active disease are common. If unchecked, the joint inflammation causes irreversible damage to the articular cartilage and bone, resulting in joint deformity and disability.

JOINT PATHOLOGY

There are one to two layers of the synovial lining cells in the synovium in normal joints, which mainly consist of two types of synovial lining cells (also called

Knee joint opened anteriorly, patella reflected downward. Thickened synovial membrane inflamed; polypoid outgrowths and numerous villi (pannus) extend over rough articular cartilages of femur and patella.

Villi (pannus)

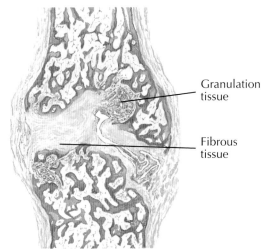

Granulation tissue

Fibrous tissue

Section of proximal interphalangeal joint. Marked destruction of both articular cartilages and subchondral bone; replacement by fibrous and granulation tissue, which has obliterated most of joint space and invaded bone.

Section of synovial membrane. Villous proliferation with extensive lymphocytic and plasma cells.

synoviocytes): type A (macrophage-like cells) and type B (fibroblast-like cells). Type C cells are synovial dendritic cells. In contrast, rheumatoid joint synovium becomes thickened, with more than three layers of synoviocytes. In addition to the synoviocytes, cell infiltrates including neutrophils, lymphocytes, and plasma cells also contribute to the synovial hypertrophy. The synoviocytes, neutrophils, and lymphocytes together constitute synovial cells, which produce numerous pathogenic molecules leading to the disease process in

the rheumatoid synovium. Among the molecules are numerous cytokines that play important pathogenic roles. Proinflammatory cytokines, including tumor necrosis factor-α (TNF-α), interleukin-1β (IL-1β), and interleukin-6 (IL-6), have been extensively studied and confirmed to be pathogenic. On the basis of these proinflammatory cytokines, several biologic agents that target these cytokines have been developed and have been approved to treat rheumatoid arthritis. These agents include TNF-α inhibitors or blockers such as

Plate 5-2   Rheumatic Diseases

EARLY AND MODERATE HAND INVOLVEMENT IN RHEUMATOID ARTHRITIS

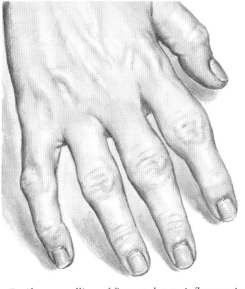

Fusiform swelling of fingers due to inflammation of proximal interphalangeal joints is typical of early involvement.

Moderate involvement of proximal interphalangeal, metacarpophalangeal, and wrist joints

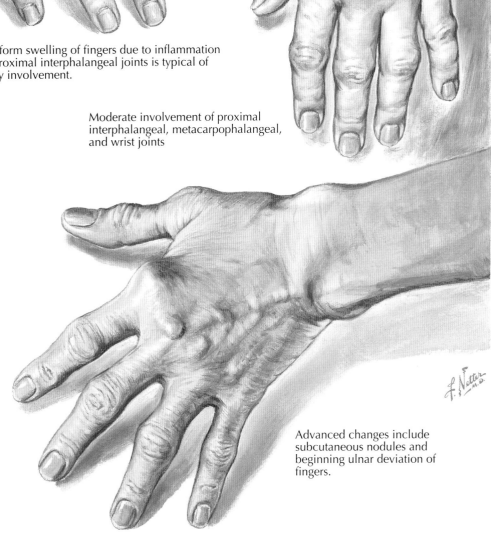

Advanced changes include subcutaneous nodules and beginning ulnar deviation of fingers.

RHEUMATIC DISEASES (Continued)

etanercept (Enbrel), adalimumab (Humira), infliximab (Remicade), and golimumab as well as the IL-1 antagonist anakinra (Kineret) (see later section on therapy for rheumatoid arthritis). In the rheumatoid synovium there are other cytokines, such as IL-17, IL-18, and lymphotoxin-β that could be potential therapeutic targets in the future. In addition, other molecules such as chemokines are found to be involved in the rheumatoid disease process. These chemokines bind to their receptors CXCR3 and CCR5 to recruit inflammatory cells to the sites of the joint inflammation.

The evolution of the pathologic changes in the joint provides the key to understanding the clinical nature of the disease (see Plate 5-1). In the rheumatoid joint, synovitis, the inflammation occurring in the synovium, represents a basic inflammatory disease. The synovial membrane becomes edematous and infiltrated primarily with neutrophils and mononuclear cells. This produces diffuse synovial proliferation, and synovial fluid accumulates. In this early stage, the articular cartilage and subchondral bone are not involved. As the disease progresses, the inflamed synovium continues to proliferate and villous projections grow into the joint cavity (villous synovitis). The villi become infiltrated with lymphoid cells, which may form follicular collections. The proliferations spread along the cartilage surface (pannus formation), eroding and thinning the cartilage. The proliferative inflammation often invades the subchondral bone. Osteoporosis develops in the metaphyseal bone, weakening it, sometimes enough to cause erosion of the supporting cortical bone and thus disrupt the joint.

As the disease becomes more chronic, fibroblasts infiltrate the inflamed joint capsule, which becomes thickened and boggy. The pannus progresses, causing more destruction and joint deformity. The progressive inflammation causes irreversible destructive changes in cartilage and bone. After months or years of periods of active disease and partial remissions, even if the inflammation subsides, fibrous tissue has often increased and further restricts motion, leading to *fibrous ankylosis*. The stiffened, deformed joint may become solidly fused by

bony bridges across the joint space; this final stage is thus called *bony ankylosis*, clinically manifested as advanced secondary osteoarthritic change. Pain lessens as the inflammation subsides, but the joint damage persists, accounting for the stiffened and deformed joints, disability, and incapacitation.

The synovial proliferation along with the microvascular process called angiogenesis may behave like a benign tumor, which is partly caused by defects of some apoptotic genes and their molecules. Based on these

molecules, researchers have studied intra-articular gene delivery of vectors carrying such apoptotic molecules as *P53*, *FasL*, and *TRAIL* to mimic surgical synovial ablation, termed *molecular synovectomy*.

CLINICAL MANIFESTATIONS

Early in the course of the illness, joint involvement is characterized by signs and symptoms of polyarthritis in the limbs, usually in a symmetric distribution. In

Plate 5-3

Musculoskeletal System: PART III

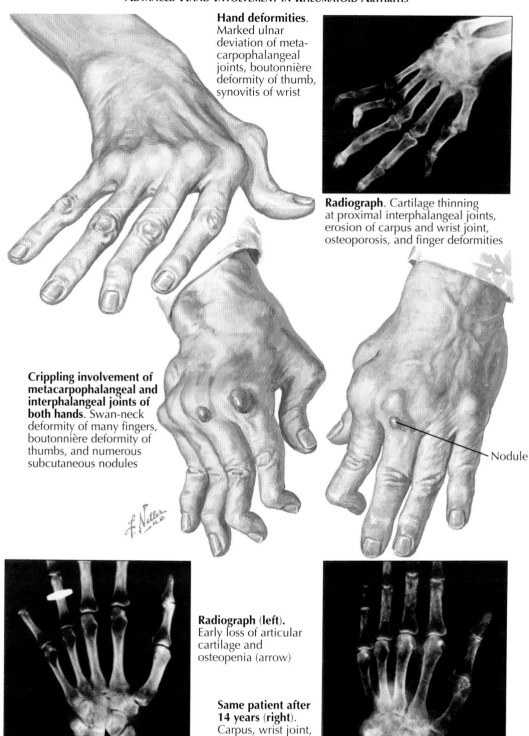

ADVANCED HAND INVOLVEMENT IN RHEUMATOID ARTHRITIS

Hand deformities. Marked ulnar deviation of meta-carpophalangeal joints, boutonnière deformity of thumb, synovitis of wrist

Radiograph. Cartilage thinning at proximal interphalangeal joints, erosion of carpus and wrist joint, osteoporosis, and finger deformities

Crippling involvement of metacarpophalangeal and interphalangeal joints of both hands. Swan-neck deformity of many fingers, boutonnière deformity of thumbs, and numerous subcutaneous nodules

Nodule

Radiograph (left). Early loss of articular cartilage and osteopenia (arrow)

Same patient after 14 years (right). Carpus, wrist joint, and ulnar head completely eroded (arrow)

RHEUMATIC DISEASES (Continued)

pauciarticular (oligoarticular)-onset rheumatoid arthritis, only one or a few joints are involved. The affected joints become diffusely swollen, warm, and tender. Joint movement is painful, and the swelling of the joint capsules creates a feeling of stiffness. Generalized stiffness is also noted after long periods of inactivity, especially on arising in the morning. Depending on the severity of the illness, morning stiffness may last 1 to 2 or even longer hours, making routine daily activities difficult. Even early in the illness, the patient may be partially incapacitated.

Although the progression of joint inflammation follows no fixed pattern, usually several pairs of joints in the limbs are affected first. After months or even years, other joints may become involved, including the acromioclavicular, sternoclavicular, and temporomandibular joints, and even tiny joints such as the cricoarytenoid articulations. It is common, however, for some joints to be spared even if the disease remains active for many years and the joints involved early undergo severe crippling changes. The factors that determine the distribution of the disease and the severity of the inflammatory process in any joint remain unexplained.

EARLY AND MODERATE HAND INVOLVEMENT

The joints of the hands and wrists are among the most frequent sites of involvement (see Plate 5-2). In the fingers, some or all of the proximal interphalangeal joints are often bilaterally affected whereas the distal interphalangeal joints are seldom involved. Because the inflammatory swelling occurs only at the middle joints, the affected fingers become fusiform in the early stages of disease. The metacarpophalangeal and wrist joints may also become inflamed. At first, there is little restriction of motion in the involved joints, but stiffness, swelling, and pain prevent the patient from making a

tight fist, thus weakening grip strength. Except for soft tissue swelling, radiographs reveal no abnormalities.

ADVANCED HAND INVOLVEMENT

As the disease progresses and the inflammation invades the joints, destroying articular cartilage and bone, joint motion becomes severely limited and joint deformities develop (see Plate 5-3). Flexion deformities frequently

occur at the proximal interphalangeal and metacarpophalangeal joints. The patient cannot fully extend or flex the fingers, and the grip becomes progressively weaker. Radiographs reveal cartilage thinning, manifest as joint space narrowing, bone erosions at the joint margins, and metaphyseal (periarticular) osteoporosis. After years of chronic inflammation, joint damage becomes severe; the joint capsule stretches; muscles atrophy and weaken; and tendons stretch, fray, and even

Plate 5-4

Rheumatic Diseases

FOOT INVOLVEMENT IN RHEUMATOID ARTHRITIS

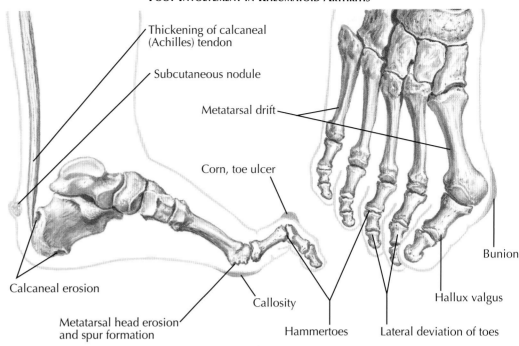

Thickening of calcaneal (Achilles) tendon

Subcutaneous nodule

Metatarsal drift

Corn, toe ulcer

Bunion

Calcaneal erosion

Hallux valgus

Metatarsal head erosion and spur formation

Callosity

Hammertoes

Lateral deviation of toes

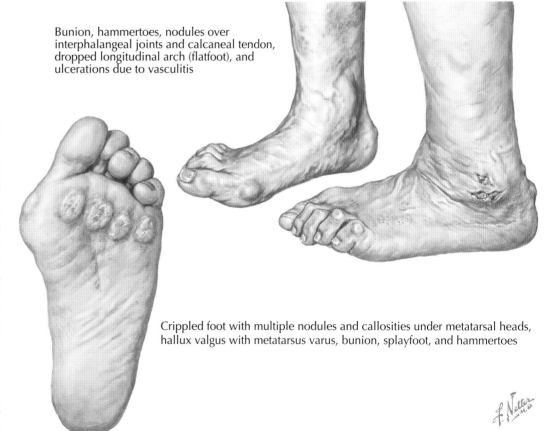

Bunion, hammertoes, nodules over interphalangeal joints and calcaneal tendon, dropped longitudinal arch (flatfoot), and ulcerations due to vasculitis

Crippled foot with multiple nodules and callosities under metatarsal heads, hallux valgus with metatarsus varus, bunion, splayfoot, and hammertoes

RHEUMATIC DISEASES *(Continued)*

rupture. All of these changes result in severe, incapacitating deformities.

A number of hand deformities are seen in the late stages of rheumatoid arthritis. For example, the muscles on the ulnar side of the fingers and wrist may overpower those of the radial group, causing ulnar deviation of the fingers at the metacarpophalangeal joints; the wrists may also be affected. The swan-neck deformity of the finger is common, as is the boutonnière deformity of the thumb, which is caused by hyperextension of the proximal interphalangeal joint and flexion at the metacarpophalangeal joint. The long extensor tendon may rupture near the distal interphalangeal joint, leaving the distal phalanx permanently flexed. Prolonged disease may lead to permanent subluxation or dislocation of the finger joints, and severe cartilage and bone erosion at the wrist may literally destroy the carpus. In this late stage of the disease, radiographs help to define the severity of the structural damage and deformities.

FOOT INVOLVEMENT

Joint involvement in the foot resembles that in the hand, except for deformities that are determined chiefly by the foot's weight-bearing function (see Plate 5-4). The toes usually become hyperextended, or cocked up, at the metatarsophalangeal joints and flexed at the proximal interphalangeal articulations (hammertoes). The joint capsules, fasciae, and tendons become stretched and weakened, and the metatarsal and longitudinal arches flatten. Standing and walking exert great pressure on the osteoporotic metatarsal heads, causing severe erosion of the metatarsals. Frequently, plantar callosities develop under the metatarsal heads. Hallux valgus with bunion formation is also common. Cartilage thinning of the intertarsal joints is usually so severe that the tarsus becomes quite rigid, adding strain to the

inflamed ankle joint. These structural changes make walking both difficult and painful.

KNEE, SHOULDER, AND HIP INVOLVEMENT

Inflammation of the large joints of the limbs causes a boggy and diffuse swelling of the soft tissues of the joints. In the elbows and knees, this swelling is easily observed on physical examination (see Plate 5-5).

Involvement of the hip and shoulder joints, on the other hand, cannot be detected by inspection and palpation because the hips and, to a lesser degree, the shoulders lie deep beneath the skin and are well covered by fleshy muscles. Examination for range of motion elicits pain and restricted movement if the joints are inflamed. In these large, well-covered joints, radiographs are required to evaluate the damage to the articular cartilage.

Plate 5-5

Musculoskeletal System: PART III

RHEUMATIC DISEASES (Continued)

Flexion deformities can develop quickly at the knees and hips, making walking and arising from a sitting position difficult and painful. Extensive damage to the large joints in the limbs may cripple the patient, necessitating use of a cane, crutch, or walker or confinement to a wheelchair or a bed.

EXTRA-ARTICULAR MANIFESTATIONS

Rheumatoid arthritis is a systemic illness, not just a disease of the joints, and thus has a variety of nonarticular, or extra-articular, manifestations (see Plates 5-6 and 5-7). Some of these features are occult, with little clinical importance, but others are clinically significant. In some cases, extra-articular features are the dominant clinical signs.

Rheumatoid inflammation may be nodular or diffuse and may occur in parenchyma and connective tissues throughout the body. It therefore produces a variety of pathologic lesions in many locations. The inflammation of the nonarticular connective tissue has the same characteristics as the synovitis: it is a proliferative inflammatory reaction containing lymphocytes, macrophages, and plasma cells. The lymphocytes often cluster in a follicular pattern.

Rheumatoid Nodules. In about 15% of cases, nodules develop in connective tissue along tendons, at tendon sheaths, in bursa and joint capsules, and in the subcutaneous connective tissue around bony prominences (see Plate 5-6). A common place for nodules to occur is a few centimeters distal to the olecranon process of the ulna. The nodules in subcutaneous tissue are freely movable, whereas those that originate in the periosteum are firmly attached to the underlying bone. Rheumatoid nodules occur singly or in aggregate in clusters, and they vary from 1 mm to more than 2 cm in diameter.

When surrounded by soft tissue, rheumatoid nodules are painless, but nodules located over bony prominences are often painful when pressure is exerted on them. For example, nodules around the ischial tuberosity cause pain when the patient sits on a firm seat and nodules over spinous processes or the occipital protuberance make lying supine on a firm surface painful. Similarly, those occurring on the plantar surface of the foot cause discomfort when standing or walking. Nodules located over the knuckles, toes, or knees may restrict motion in the underlying joint.

The presence of rheumatoid nodules greatly aids in the diagnosis of rheumatoid arthritis because they occur with no other form of chronic arthritis. However, nodular swellings near joints and along the border of the ulna are associated with other illnesses (e.g., urate deposits, or tophi, in gout). If the nature of the nodular swelling and the diagnosis of rheumatoid arthritis is not clear, excision and microscopic study of the tissue is advised. Characteristic histopathologic features of rheumatoid nodules are (1) a central zone of fibrinoid degeneration surrounded by (2) an intermediate zone of palisading epithelioid cells and (3) an outer coat of granulation tissue infiltrated with lymphocytes and plasma cells.

Pulmonary Involvement. Rheumatoid nodules may develop in the parenchyma of the lung (see Plate 5-6). On radiographs, a solitary nodule often cannot be differentiated from a neoplasm, nodules are generally located in subpleural areas or in association with

interlobular septa, but histologic study of the lesion reveals the pathologic features of a rheumatoid nodule. Medications such as methotrexate can cause pulmonary nodules, which are usually located in the middle zones of the lungs. TNF-α inhibitors, used to treat rheumatoid arthritis, can rarely cause lung nodules. Other parenchymal lung diseases (e.g., interstitial fibrosis, pulmonary nodules, and bronchiolitis obliterans/ organizing pneumonia) can occur. Caplan syndrome is

a unique form of pneumoconiosis that may be a granulomatous response to chronic exposure to silica dust. It is especially prevalent in coal miners. Widely distributed and particularly prevalent in the periphery, the nodules usually appear abruptly, with little or no evidence of prior pneumoconiosis. They may occur before, during, or after the onset of arthritis. Patients with Caplan syndrome usually have a high serum titer of rheumatoid factor. Progressive interstitial fibrosis and

KNEE, SHOULDER, AND HIP JOINT INVOLVEMENT IN RHEUMATOID ARTHRITIS

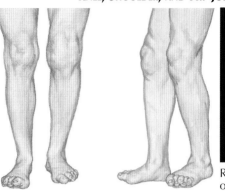
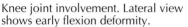

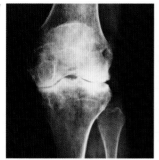

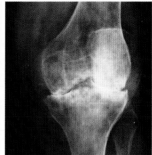

Knee joint involvement. Lateral view shows early flexion deformity.

Radiograph shows thinning of cartilage in both compartments of knee joint.

Same patient 4 years later. Progression of bone erosion and marked osteoporosis.

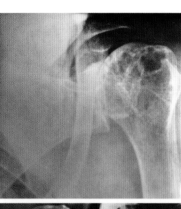

Shoulder joint involvement. Severe osteoporosis cysts in head of humerus and thinning of cartilage at glenohumeral joint.

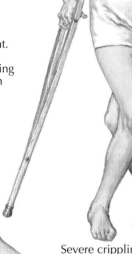

Hip joint involvement. Thinning of articular cartilages and flattening and medial migration of femoral head.

Severe crippling deformities of multiple joints

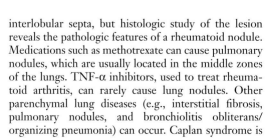

Flexion contracture of hip joint

Plate 5-6

Rheumatic Diseases

RHEUMATIC DISEASES *(Continued)*

pleurisy with or without effusion are other pulmonary manifestations of rheumatic disease.

Cardiac Involvement. In the myocardium, rheumatoid nodules may cause cardiac conduction defects. Pericarditis may occur but is rarely symptomatic; if effusion develops, the fluid, like rheumatoid pleural effusion, has a very low sugar content. This characteristic effusion is a helpful diagnostic finding. Constrictive pericarditis and valvular granulomatous lesions (usually aortic) are rare.

Ocular Changes. About 30% patients with rheumatoid arthritis have features of Sjögren syndrome, called secondary Sjögren syndrome. Keratoconjunctivitis is commonly associated with rheumatoid arthritis. Granulomatous scleritis occurs less often but may lead to scleromalacia perforans (see Plate 5-6).

Nervous System Involvement. The dura mater is another site of rheumatoid nodules. A more frequent clinical manifestation, however, is peripheral neuropathy due to inflammation in the arterioles supplying the nerve. Peripheral nerve compression from localized articular or nonarticular inflammation surrounding the nerve (e.g., compression of the median nerve in carpal tunnel syndrome) is also common. Ulnar neuropathy and radial nerve palsy are seen less often.

Periarticular Fibrous Tissue Manifestations. In many cases, the inflammation affects specialized periarticular fibrous tissue structures, most commonly, tendons, tendon sheaths, and bursae (see Plate 5-7). The periarticular inflammation has the same proliferative and invasive characteristics as synovitis. Tendonitis and tenosynovitis may cause the tendon to rupture; and in some patients, the periarticular inflammation causes as much pain, stiffness, and disability as the arthritis. Muscle weakness and atrophy occur in late stages of rheumatoid arthritis.

Rheumatoid Vasculitis. Now recognized as a major manifestation of rheumatoid arthritis, vasculitis is classified by pathologic changes into three main categories: (1) intimal proliferation of digital arteries causing ischemic areas in the nail fold, nail edge, or digital pulp; (2) subacute lesions in small vessels of muscles, nerves, heart, and other tissues; and (3) widespread fulminant necrotizing arteritis of medium-sized and large vessels. Leukocytosis, scleritis, neuropathy, mesenteric infarction, and ischemic skin ulceration or gangrene are commonly associated with occlusive or necrotizing arteritis.

Rheumatoid arthritis complicated by vasculitis is associated with severe and long-standing joint inflammation, elevated serum titers of rheumatoid factor, diminished serum complement levels, rheumatoid nodules and other extra-articular manifestations, and a poor prognosis. The detection of IgG, IgM, and complement components in the inflamed arterial wall supports the hypothesis that rheumatoid vasculitis is due to the deposition of soluble immune complexes in the vessel wall (see Plate 5-8).

Other Manifestations. Mild-to-moderate anemia is typical of active disease, with the exception of mild cases, and is largely due to a relative failure of bone marrow production because of increased uptake and abnormal storage of iron by the reticuloendothelial system and the phagocytic cells of the inflamed, hyperplastic synovial membrane. Unless an iron deficiency supervenes, the erythrocytes are normocytic and only slightly hypochromic. Impaired absorption of iron from

EXTRA-ARTICULAR MANIFESTATIONS IN RHEUMATOID ARTHRITIS

Crippled hand with subcutaneous nodules over knuckles, swan-neck deformity of middle finger, ulnar deviation of fingers, and muscle atrophy

Nodular episcleritis with scleromalacia

Subcutaneous nodule just distal to olecranon process, and another in olecranon bursa

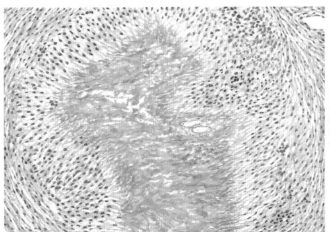

Section of rheumatoid nodule. Central area of fibrinoid necrosis surrounded by zone of palisading mesenchymal cells and peripheral fibrous tissue capsule containing chronic inflammatory cells.

Radiograph shows rheumatoid nodule in right lung. Lesion may be misdiagnosed as carcinoma until identified by biopsy or postsurgical pathologic analysis.

the gastrointestinal tract and, in some cases, bleeding into the gastrointestinal tract caused by nonsteroidal anti-inflammatory agents or other therapeutic drugs also contribute to the development of anemia.

Osteoporosis in the metaphyses of bones adjacent to inflamed joints begins early and is termed *periarticular osteopenia*. This manifestation is caused by inflammatory cells and cytokines in the bone marrow that result in decreased bone formation. In advanced disease,

especially when weight-bearing activity is curtailed, the osteoporosis becomes generalized and often severe.

Although generalized lymphadenopathy is a frequent finding, splenomegaly occurs in only about 5% of patients. When accompanied by leukopenia, the disorder is known as Felty syndrome. Leukopenia, if severe, may lead to serious infection. Other manifestations of Felty syndrome include rheumatoid nodules, chronic leg ulcers, peripheral neuropathy, thrombocytopenia,

Plate 5-7   Musculoskeletal System: PART III

EXTRA-ARTICULAR MANIFESTATIONS IN RHEUMATOID ARTHRITIS (CONTINUED)

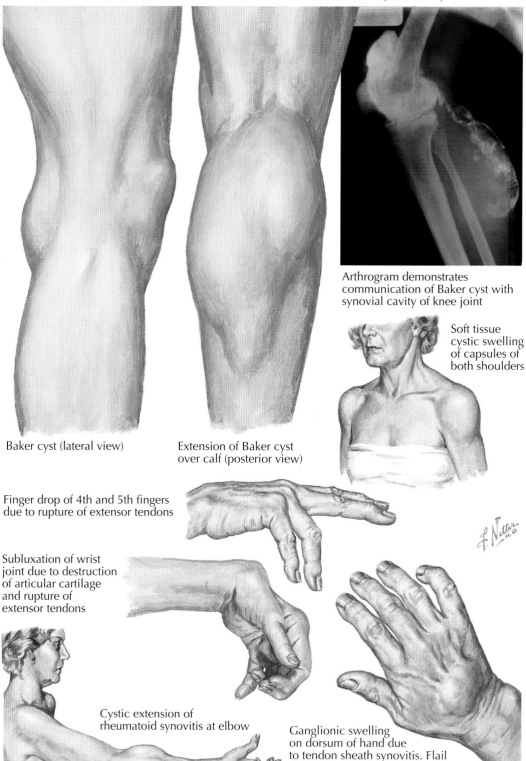

Arthrogram demonstrates communication of Baker cyst with synovial cavity of knee joint

Baker cyst (lateral view)

Extension of Baker cyst over calf (posterior view)

Soft tissue cystic swelling of capsules of both shoulders

Finger drop of 4th and 5th fingers due to rupture of extensor tendons

Subluxation of wrist joint due to destruction of articular cartilage and rupture of extensor tendons

Cystic extension of rheumatoid synovitis at elbow

Ganglionic swelling on dorsum of hand due to tendon sheath synovitis. Flail terminal phalanx of 5th finger caused by rupture of long extensor tendon at insertion.

RHEUMATIC DISEASES (Continued)

anemia (often severe), keratoconjunctivitis sicca, as well as increased myeloid activity and very high titers of rheumatoid factor. Felty syndrome should be differentiated from large granular lymphocyte syndrome. In the latter, peripheral blood analysis and bone marrow biopsy demonstrate typical large granular cells. T-cell receptor recombination studies can provide additional diagnostic evidence.

In the late stage of rheumatoid disease, secondary amyloidosis may occur, but this is relatively uncommon.

IMMUNOLOGIC FEATURES

The serum of most patients with rheumatoid arthritis contains immunoglobulins, or antibodies. The autoantibodies to gamma globulin (IgG) are called *rheumatoid factors*. The latex fixation tests commonly used in the diagnosis of rheumatoid arthritis detect only the IgM class of rheumatoid factor, which is most prevalent; however, IgG and, to a lesser extent, IgA rheumatoid factors are also found. All classes of rheumatoid factor act as antibodies to IgG (which acts as antigen) to form immune complexes. In rheumatoid arthritis, some rheumatoid factor is produced in the synovium. Some of the IgG and IgM shown in plasma cells (see Plate 5-8) consists of rheumatoid factor. Immune complexes containing rheumatoid factor, IgG, and complement are prominent in vacuoles of synovial fluid cells as well as in synovial macrophages and interstitium. The immune complexes also appear to be important in extra-articular disease because they deposit in vessel walls and cause vasculitis. The *latex agglutination test of rheumatoid factor* has been replaced by the enzyme-linked immunosorbent assay (ELISA) in current clinical practice.

Citrullination is the term used for the post-translational modification of the amino acid arginine into the amino acid citrulline. Cyclic citrullinated peptides (CCP) are post-transcriptionally modified peptides, and their antibodies are called anti-CCP antibodies, which were introduced into clinical use in 1997. As with

rheumatoid factors, anti-CCP antibodies aid in the diagnosis of rheumatoid arthritis and may be present before the appearance of symptoms of rheumatoid arthritis. Their presence is an indicator of rheumatoid disease severity. ELISA is widely used to detect the anti-CCP antibodies, and the sensitivity and specificity of the anti-CCP antibodies are 50% to 75% and over 90%, respectively. The newer-generation assays, including the second-generation anti-CCP antibody

assays (anti-CCP2), have improved sensitivity and specificity compared with the original anti-CCP assays.

A genetic predisposition is an important factor in determining the immune response to the still-unknown initiating factors. The major histocompatibility complex class II antigen HLA-DR4 (HLA-DRB1*0401 and HLA-DRB1*0404/0408 by new nomenclature) is associated with an increased incidence of rheumatoid arthritis in many populations, but it is not present in all

Plate 5-8   Rheumatic Diseases

IMMUNOLOGIC FEATURES IN RHEUMATOID ARTHRITIS

Immunofluorescence studies of synovium

Plasma cells containing IgG

Plasma cells containing IgM

Amorphous deposits of IgG in synovium

Amorphous deposits of complement in synovium (immune complex deposits)

Latex agglutination test for rheumatoid factor

Latex particles coated with human IgG (commercially available) are agglutinated by serum or joint fluid containing rheumatoid factor

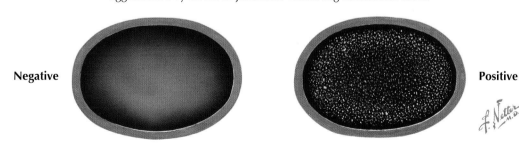

Negative   Positive

RHEUMATIC DISEASES (Continued)

patients with rheumatoid arthritis. PTPN22 (protein tyrosine phosphatase N22) has been associated with rheumatoid arthritis as well, although about 17% of the normal white population also have this missense gene mutation.

Analysis of synovial fluid shows pathologic changes characteristic of rheumatoid arthritis: increased volume and increased leukocyte count (>10,000/mm^3), with a preponderance of mononuclear or polymorphonuclear cells at different stages of disease and in different patients. Activated T lymphocytes are commonly present. There is poor viscosity due to diluted and denatured hyaluronate and low complement levels. Synovial fluid leukocytes often contain inclusion particles that are made up of IgG, rheumatoid factor, and complement. Many of the modulators of inflammation discussed earlier can be identified in joint fluid in rheumatoid arthritis but are not routinely measured.

Thrombocytosis, elevated erythrocyte sedimentation rate (ESR), and C-reactive protein (CRP) usually correlate with the rheumatoid disease activity rather than disease severity. These laboratory tests are thus of some value in monitoring the course of the illness.

ETIOLOGY AND PATHOGENESIS

Although the etiology of rheumatoid arthritis is not yet understood, the following four factors—genetic background, abnormal immunity, environmental, and sex hormones—may play a role in concert with one another. Many causative factors have been proposed, including infectious microorganisms such as bacteria, mycobacteria, *Mycoplasma*, and their components and Epstein-Barr virus, parvovirus, and other viruses. Tobacco smoking has been shown to increase the citrullination of proteins and is associated with an increased risk of developing rheumatoid arthritis.

It is widely believed that rheumatoid arthritis develops in a person with a genetic predisposition following exposure to an unknown infectious agent (possibly viral). It is also possible that the illness results from an inappropriate immune response to a ubiquitous

pathogenic agent. In the absence of an established cause, physicians can only evaluate each clinical and laboratory abnormality in relation to the disease and speculate on its etiologic significance.

Results of numerous studies have clarified the major role of immunologic reactions in the pathogenesis and perpetuation of rheumatoid inflammation.

Synovial T Lymphocytes. In the synovium of chronic rheumatoid arthritis, T lymphocytes constitute about

50% of the synovial cells and are mostly CD4$^+$ T lymphocytes with an activated surface phenotype, and high expression of HLA-DR antigens and CD27. CD4$^+$CD27$^+$ T lymphocytes provide B-lymphocyte help, resulting in antibody production in the synovium.

Synovial B Lymphocytes. Many rheumatoid synovial tissues exhibit a diffuse infiltration with mononuclear cells. There are discrete lymphoid follicles populated by B lymphocytes in the sublining region. B

VARIABLE CLINICAL COURSE OF ADULT RHEUMATOID ARTHRITIS: PROGNOSIS DIFFICULT IN EARLY STAGE

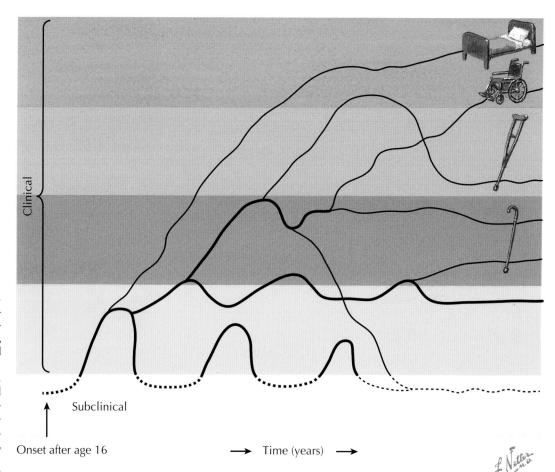

Clinical

Subclinical

Onset after age 16   → Time (years) →

RHEUMATIC DISEASES *(Continued)*

lymphocytes and plasma cells constitute only about 5% of the rheumatoid synovium; however, their hyperactivity is viewed as a key player in the initiation and perpetuation of the early rheumatoid arthritis. As a result, rheumatoid factor and anti-CCP antibodies are detected in the synovial fluid and serum.

Cytokines and Their Network in Rheumatoid Joints. There are numerous cytokines involved in the synovial pathology that form a network to contribute to pathogenesis of rheumatoid arthritis. Type A, B, and C synovial lining cells are major source of various cytokines. The proinflammatory cytokines include TNF-α, IL-1, II-6, IL-17, IL-18, and others.

These studies have proposed a sequence of events in the development of rheumatoid arthritis: (1) An unknown causative factor (antigen), carried to the joint by the circulation, initiates synovitis. (2) The antigen is processed by antigen-presenting cells such as macrophages, dendritic cells, and even B lymphocytes to interact with T and B lymphocytes to stimulate the local production of antibodies. (3) The antigen and antibody interact, forming immune complexes, and the interaction of the resulting immune complex with rheumatoid factor in the synovium and fluid stimulates a sequence of events that generates chemotactic factors. (4) These chemotactic factors attract cellular elements of the blood into the perivascular space. (5) New blood vessels are generated in the rheumatoid synovium. (6) Large amounts of proinflammatory cytokines are produced. All of these events together lead to release of various enzymes such as matrix metalloproteinases (MMPs) to participate in the extracellular matrix degradation of the joint, cartilage damage, and, eventually, whole joint destruction.

CLINICAL COURSE AND PROGNOSIS

The clinical course of rheumatoid arthritis is characterized by remissions and relapses. In the first few months after onset, the course of the disease cannot be predicted because it is so variable (see Plate 5-9). Only repeated observation of the patient with active disease allows the physician to determine the prognosis. Factors associated with a poor prognosis include persistence of active illness for longer than a year, presence of rheumatoid nodules, high serum titers of rheumatoid factor, anti-CCP antibodies, and extra-articular manifestations.

Early and prolonged remission is more likely if the disease is mild at onset. Although partial or even complete remission may occur at any time and continue for a long time, complete remission is seldom seen after 3 or 4 years of continuously active disease.

Appropriate therapy can slow down or arrest the disease process, can relieve joint pain, allows patients to be more active, and helps to avoid disability and incapacitation. Before the early 1990s, it was true that the amount of joint damage and disability was greater after 10 years of continuously active disease than after 5 years and was greater still after 15 years. Thanks to the introduction of newer therapeutic agents, particularly biologic agents since 1998, the frequency of joint damage has been significantly reduced and joint deformities have become less prevalent, as has the need for joint replacement surgery.

DIAGNOSIS

Early in the course of the disease, when synovitis and mild systemic illness are the only clinical manifestations, it is often very difficult to distinguish rheumatoid arthritis from other rheumatic diseases. Because there is no reliable laboratory test for rheumatoid arthritis, diagnosis depends on the judgment of a well-informed physician, usually based on frequent physical examinations and laboratory studies performed over many months. The most significant diagnostic findings are synovitis in many joints (especially paired joints in the limbs); systemic signs and symptoms; elevated ESR;

circulating rheumatoid factor in serum; and rheumatoid nodules. However, circulating rheumatoid factor may not be detected for many months after the onset of illness, and many patients remain seronegative. Likewise, radiographic changes become visible only after months of persistent joint inflammation.

Diagnosis is not difficult after the illness has become chronic or when any of the following manifestations are present: rheumatoid nodules; rheumatoid factor in serum; characteristic joint deformities; and radiographic evidence of articular cartilage thinning, subchondral bone destruction, joint deformity, or ankylosis.

Criteria. The following criteria, formulated by the American Rheumatism Association (ACR) in 1987, are a reliable basis for accurate diagnosis:
- Morning stiffness
- Arthritis of three or more joint areas
- Arthritis of hand joints
- Symmetric arthritis
- Rheumatoid nodules
- Serum rheumatoid factor
- Radiographic changes

A patient could be classified as having rheumatoid arthritis if at least four of these criteria were satisfied; four of the criteria must have been present for at least 6 weeks. In 2010, ACR/EULAR (European League Against Rheumatism) classification criteria were introduced to make a diagnosis of early rheumatoid arthritis among patients newly presenting with undifferentiated inflammatory synovitis. The differential diagnoses includes many other inflammatory conditions.

Plate 5-10

Rheumatic Diseases

TREATMENT OF RHEUMATOID ARTHRITIS

Rheumatoid arthritis is a heterogeneous disease, and there is recognition that treatments will vary among individuals. Early consultation with a rheumatologist is advised to confirm the diagnosis and to outline a treatment plan with the patient. Factors that will influence the therapeutic options include the disease's duration, prognosis, severity, and activity. The simplified goals of therapy, however, remain the same among all patients.

These goals include:

- Education of the patient
- Relief of pain
- Preservation and restoration of function
- Modification of disease progression and damage

With the acquired understanding of the early onset of damage and the ultimate impact on the debility and disability of the rheumatoid arthritis patient, the algorithms of treatment have changed focus to a more aggressive and early approach. The concept of treating to a target of remission or low disease activity state is now widely accepted.

NONPHARMACOLOGIC TREATMENTS

The physician will need to enter into a treatment partnership with the rheumatoid arthritis patient. The education of the patient as to his or her disease features, course, prognoses, and medication adverse effects is the key to a successful treatment program.

Exercise with stretching and strengthening of the involved joints is beneficial in the majority of cases, and patients should be encouraged to stay active (see Plates 5-10 and 5-11). Patients may benefit from a consultation with an occupational and/or physical therapist to help guide and outline an exercise plan. Rest and/or splinting of an acutely inflamed joint may be necessary in some cases. Bed rest and hospitalization is rarely needed in the present era.

Rheumatoid arthritis patients should be encouraged to eat a healthy and balanced diet. Overweight patients should be encouraged to lose weight because excess weight placed on inflamed joints may hasten the damage. There are very little data to support a specific diet in rheumatoid arthritis. An exception may be the increase in dietary or supplemental fish oils, which may provide an anti-inflammatory effect.

Many patients are curious about alternative and complementary pathways of treatments. Unfortunately, there are little data to support the efficacy or ensure the safety of these therapies.

PREVENTATIVE TREATMENTS

The rheumatoid arthritis patient should be encouraged to discontinue tobacco use because there are good data to support the poor prognostic implications of smoking.

Rheumatoid arthritis and other inflammatory and autoimmune diseases appear to be independent risk factors for cardiovascular disease. In addition to cessation of smoking, the individual patient should be assessed for other cardiovascular risk factors, and these should be modified as deemed indicated.

Decreased bone mineral density is common in rheumatoid arthritis patients. Other risk factors including postmenopausal state and corticosteroid use may contribute. Patients should be assessed by bone densitometry testing, and then treatment directed toward bone health should be rendered as indicated.

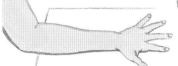

Place hand and forearm flat on table, palm down. Spread fingers apart and bring together.

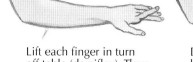

Lift each finger in turn off table (dorsiflex). Then lift all fingers together.

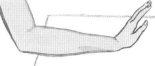

Dorsiflex entire hand at wrist, keeping forearm on table.

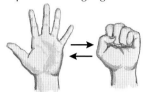

Open and clench hand successively, spreading fingers widely on opening.

Touch each finger in turn to thumb, pinching firmly.

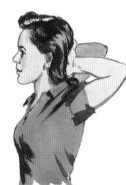

Grasp hammer firmly by handle, holding arm snugly to side. Rotate forearm so that hammerhead swings from side to side. Degree of resistance can be varied by gripping closer to or farther from hammerhead.

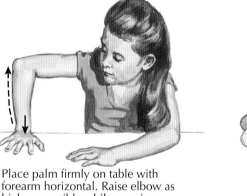

Place palm firmly on table with forearm horizontal. Raise elbow as high as possible while pressing down on table.

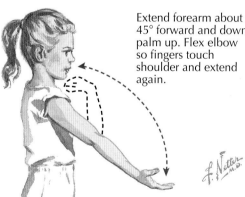

Place hands behind head. Draw elbows back as far as possible, simultaneously pulling chin in and pushing head back.

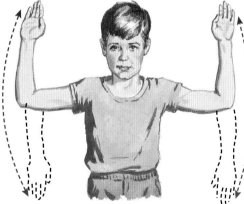

Extend arms sideways with elbows flexed 90°. Swing hands and forearms down and up, thus rotating shoulders.

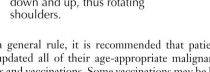

Extend forearm about 45° forward and down, palm up. Flex elbow so fingers touch shoulder and extend again.

As a general rule, it is recommended that patients have updated all of their age-appropriate malignancy screens and vaccinations. Some vaccinations may be less effective or contraindicated while certain immunosuppressive medications are being used.

PHARMACOLOGIC TREATMENTS

Pharmacologic treatment for rheumatoid arthritis is divided into five categories:

- Analgesics
- Nonsteroidal anti-inflammatory drugs (NSAIDs)
- Corticosteroids
- Nonbiologic disease-modifying antirheumatic drugs (DMARDs)
- Biologic DMARDs

As outlined previously, aggressive and early treatment regimens are now the standard of care for rheumatoid arthritis, and most patients will warrant being started on one or more DMARDs at their initial diagnosis. All other medications, including analgesics, NSAIDs, and corticosteroids, are considered adjunctive or bridge therapies. The treatment options will be initiated and further adjusted based on the patient's disease

Plate 5-11

Musculoskeletal System: PART III

TREATMENT OF RHEUMATOID ARTHRITIS (Continued)

duration, prognosis, severity and activity. Both the ACR (in 2008) and EULAR (in 2010) have put forth recommendations for the pharmacologic management of patients with rheumatoid arthritis. The goal of such treatment is to have the patient reach a state of low disease activity or preferably remission.

Analgesics. Pain is the typical chief complaint of the rheumatoid arthritis patient. In spite of aggressive DMARD treatment, many patients will require adjunctive treatment for pain. NSAIDs may fill this role, but for many patients these drugs may be contraindicated or inadequate. Topical agents, such as capsaicin or diclofenac, may be successful. Examples of oral agents include acetaminophen, tramadol, and more potent opioids.

Nonsteroidal Anti-inflammatory Drugs (NSAIDs). NSAIDs interfere with the production of prostaglandins and thus are effective in the reduction of inflammation and, therefore, pain. Many patients will require these agents along with DMARDs for pain management, but NSAIDs should be considered adjunctive and not be used alone for rheumatoid arthritis. There are no data to support NSAIDs as DMARDs. They can also be helpful as a bridge therapy while DMARDs are being initiated. Gastrointestinal adverse effects, including peptic ulcer disease and gastrointestinal bleeding, are the most common reason for discontinuation of these agents. These drugs will be contraindicated or receive limited use in those patients with backgrounds of gastrointestinal bleeding and chronic kidney and liver disease. Cyclooxygenase (COX)-selective NSAIDs (celecoxib) have the advantage of decreased gastrointestinal toxicity, but there remains concern about increased cardiovascular risk in this class compared with the nonselective NSAIDs.

Corticosteroids. As with NSAIDs, systemic corticosteroids can be a beneficial adjunct or bridge therapy (when starting a DMARD) in patients with rheumatoid arthritis. These drugs are very effective in reducing inflammation and, likewise, the signs and symptoms of the disease. Their side effects, including weight gain, cataracts, hypertension, diabetes, infection, and osteoporosis, typically limit their more long-term use; however, some patients may require longer-term use with lower dosages to retain joint function. Intra-articular corticosteroids can be useful when one or two joints remain inflamed in the presence of DMARD therapy or during a flare of the arthritis.

Nonbiologic Disease Modifying Anti-Rheumatic Drugs (DMARDs). DMARD therapy is the cornerstone of the treatment of rheumatoid arthritis. These drugs inhibit inflammatory responses, suppress synovitis, and, in studies, have been shown to improve the signs and symptoms of rheumatoid arthritis and to slow the natural progression of the joint damage. Unless contraindicated or refused, all patients should be started on a DMARD at diagnosis. Patients may not respond to DMARD therapy for up to 3 months after a therapeutic dose is achieved. The evaluation of efficacy requires frequent monitoring of disease activity.

The most common DMARDs are:
- Methotrexate
- Leflunomide
- Sulfasalazine
- Hydroxychloroquine

Methotrexate has become the most commonly used member of this group. It is given either orally or subcutaneously at dosages of 7.5 to 25 mg a week. Common

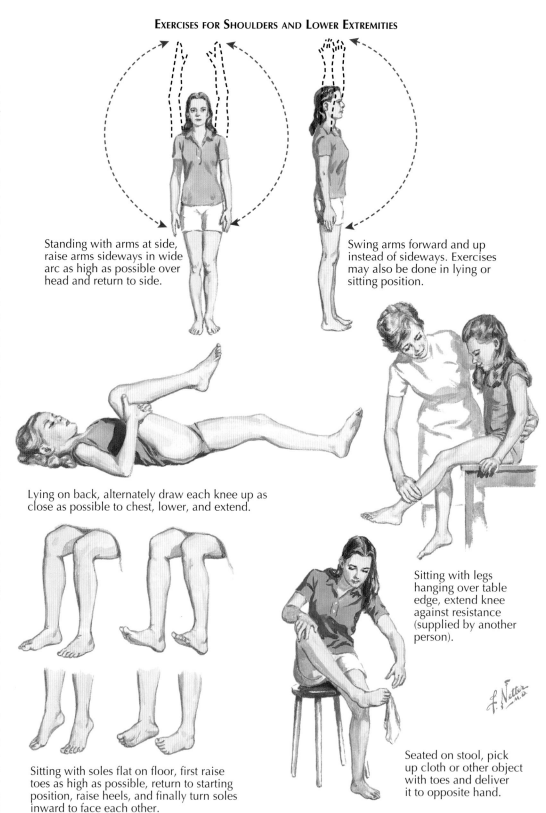

EXERCISES FOR SHOULDERS AND LOWER EXTREMITIES

Standing with arms at side, raise arms sideways in wide arc as high as possible over head and return to side.

Swing arms forward and up instead of sideways. Exercises may also be done in lying or sitting position.

Lying on back, alternately draw each knee up as close as possible to chest, lower, and extend.

Sitting with legs hanging over table edge, extend knee against resistance (supplied by another person).

Sitting with soles flat on floor, first raise toes as high as possible, return to starting position, raise heels, and finally turn soles inward to face each other.

Seated on stool, pick up cloth or other object with toes and deliver it to opposite hand.

side effects include rash, oral ulcers, nausea, and hair loss. More serious side effects including significant cytopenias, cirrhosis, and pulmonary fibrosis are quite rare with these low dosages and close monitoring. Methotrexate is contraindicated in patients with chronic kidney and liver disease, with moderate alcohol use, in pregnancy, and in women and men actively attempting conception.

Leflunomide is given orally at 10 to 20 mg/day. Common side effects include rash, diarrhea, and alopecia. Elevated liver transaminase levels and cytopenias

can be observed. This drug is also contraindicated in pregnancy and in women and men actively attempting conception.

Sulfasalazine is given orally at divided dosages from 1000 to 3000 mg a day, typically starting at lower dosages. This drug is rarely used alone in a patient with a poor prognosis or high disease activity. Adverse effects include abdominal pain, diarrhea, nausea, rash, and, rarely, cytopenias and renal or hepatic dysfunction.

Hydroxychloroquine is likewise recommended for patients with better prognosis and less severe disease.

Plate 5-12

Rheumatic Diseases

TREATMENT OF RHEUMATOID ARTHRITIS *(Continued)*

Typical dosages are in the range of 200 to 400 mg/day. It is the best tolerated of all of the DMARDs and rarely will cause rash or gastrointestinal upset. The well-described retinal toxicity is extremely rare when used at dosages of less than 6 mg/kg/day. Routine eye examinations (tangent screen) are required and can detect early toxicity, which is reversible on discontinuation.

Biologic Disease-Modifying Anti-Rheumatic Drugs. Biologic DMARDs target certain pathways in cell signaling that lead to the inflammatory responses. In the current algorithms, these biologic agents are traditionally reserved for those patients who have not had an adequate response (either remission or low disease activity state) with a nonbiologic DMARD. However, as of this writing, there is a growing movement to consider starting biologic agents at the initial diagnosis, either alone or in combination with nonbiologic DMARDs. In studies, these drugs have been shown to decrease symptoms, improve function, and slow radiographic progression of rheumatoid arthritis.

The first agents in this category were inhibitors of TNF-α (anti–TNF-α agents). Currently, five of these drugs have been approved by the U.S. Food and Drug Administration:

- Adalimumab (fully human monoclonal antibody)
- Certolizumab (pegylated humanized Fab' fragment of TNF monoclonal Ab)
- Etanercept (fusion protein: TNF receptor attached to the Fc region of human IgG)
- Golimumab (fully human monoclonal antibody)
- Infliximab (chimeric monoclonal antibody)

Anti–TNF-α drugs are usually the first biologic agent used in patients with rheumatoid arthritis. These agents are subcutaneous injections, except infliximab, which is an intravenous preparation. The side effects are similar among all and include injection or infusion reactions, infections, and, rarely, demyelinating diseases and malignancies. Patients need to be screened for latent infections, including tuberculosis, before treatment.

Anakinra, an IL-1 inhibitor, is available but has lost favor over time. It is injected subcutaneously daily. It has not shown as robust of a response as other biologic agents in treating rheumatoid arthritis.

Abatacept is a fusion protein of CTLA4-Ig and blocks T-cell co-stimulation. The drug is delivered intravenously once a month. Side effects have included infusion reactions and infections.

Rituximab depletes B lymphocytes as a monoclonal antibody against CD20. It is also given intravenously in two infusions separated by 2 weeks. Treatments may be repeated at 6-month intervals. Infusion reactions and infections remain the most significant risks.

Tocilizumab is an IL-6 receptor antagonist given intravenously every 4 weeks. Risks have included infusion reaction, infections, and elevated liver transaminase levels.

Combinations of DMARDs. Controversy exists on the proper use of combination DMARD therapy. Strategies have included the following:

- Sequential monotherapy
- Initial combination therapy
- Step-up combination therapy
- Step-down combination therapy

Nonbiologic DMARDs can be combined together. The combination of methotrexate and leflunomide carries the increased risks of hepatic and hematologic toxicity. In patients who have had an inadequate response to methotrexate, a biologic agent (most commonly an anti–TNF-α drug) is commonly added. Most agree that biologic DMARD agents should not be combined, owing to the increased infectious risks.

SURGICAL TREATMENT

The benefits of surgical approaches to rheumatoid arthritis are pain relief and restoration of function. Surgical options include synovectomy, arthroplasty, and arthrodesis (see Plate 5-12). Synovectomy of joint and/ or tendons is available for almost all joints. Arthroplasty

is a well-accepted treatment strategy for arthritis of the hands, shoulders, and especially the hips and knees. However, advances in elbow, wrist, and ankle joint arthroplasty are also being made. Arthrodesis, or joint fusion, can be helpful for intractable disease of the fingers, wrists, toes, or ankles. Although surgical options are typically postponed for medical therapies, one should not ignore the pain relief and functional benefits afforded the appropriate patient by these techniques. Technologic advancements in the field of orthopaedics will improve surgical outcomes and replacement longevity.

SURGICAL MANAGEMENT OF RHEUMATOID ARTHRITIS

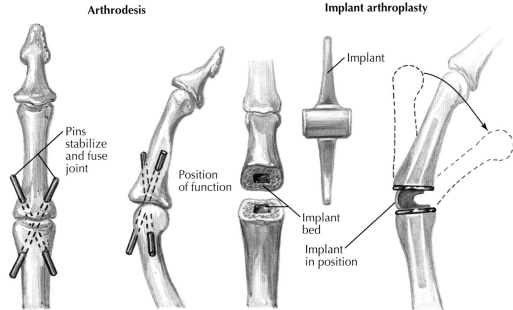

Arthrodesis

Pins stabilize and fuse joint

Position of function

Arthrodesis stabilizes and fuses arthritic joint in position of function.

Implant arthroplasty

Implant

Implant bed

Implant in position

Implant arthroplasty restores functional movement to arthritic joint.

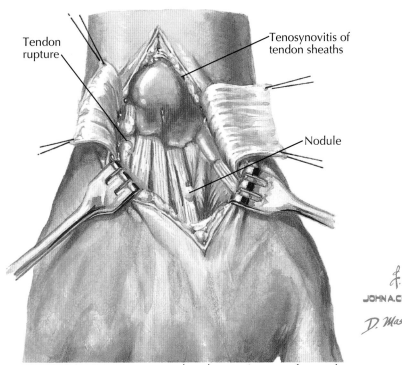

Synovectomy and tendon repair

Tendon rupture

Tenosynovitis of tendon sheaths

Nodule

In some joints, synovectomy and tendon repair or transfer may be required to restore function.

Plate 5-13

Musculoskeletal System: PART III

TECHNIQUES FOR ASPIRATION OF JOINT FLUID

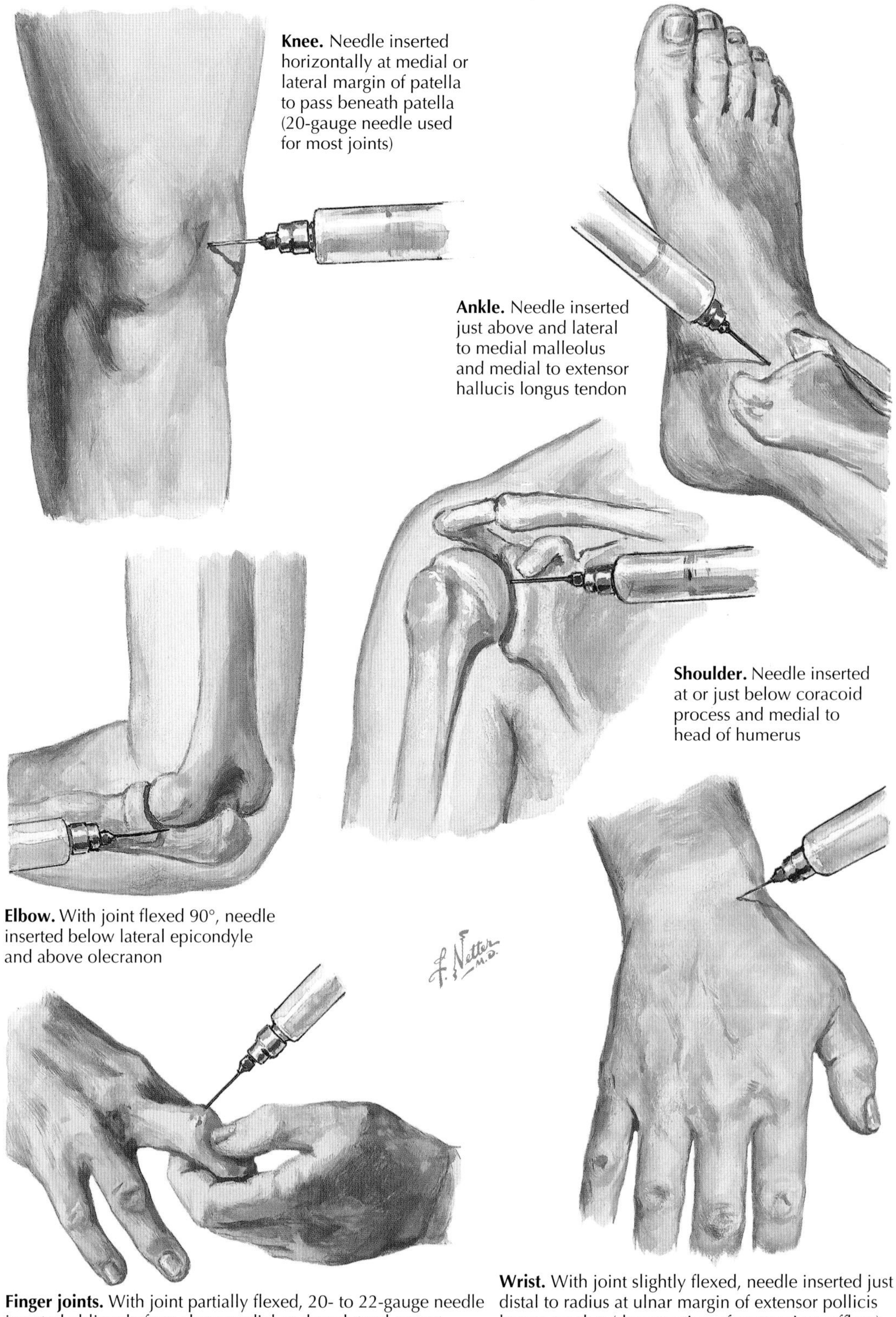

Knee. Needle inserted horizontally at medial or lateral margin of patella to pass beneath patella (20-gauge needle used for most joints)

Ankle. Needle inserted just above and lateral to medial malleolus and medial to extensor hallucis longus tendon

Shoulder. Needle inserted at or just below coracoid process and medial to head of humerus

Elbow. With joint flexed 90°, needle inserted below lateral epicondyle and above olecranon

Finger joints. With joint partially flexed, 20- to 22-gauge needle inserted obliquely from dorsomedial or dorsolateral aspect

Wrist. With joint slightly flexed, needle inserted just distal to radius at ulnar margin of extensor pollicis longus tendon (demarcation of anatomic snuffbox)

SYNOVIAL FLUID EXAMINATION

TECHNIQUES FOR ARTHROCENTESIS

Synovial fluid analysis is necessary for the definitive diagnosis of acute crystal-associated and infectious arthritis. Analysis of joint fluid for culture, cell count and differential, and the presence of crystals is also useful in the evaluation of patients with chronic, unexplained inflammatory arthropathy. In a study of 180 consecutive patients with knee effusions, 20% of the initial diagnoses suggested by clinical signs and history were changed after analysis of joint fluid.

Although arthrocentesis can be performed by experienced clinicians using clinical landmarks, aspiration and injection of deeper joints (hip), complicated joints (wrist), and even large joints such as the knee and shoulder can be performed with far greater accuracy utilizing ultrasound guidance. Some joint aspirations are shown on Plate 5-13. The knee is probably easiest to aspirate because simply positioning the needle beneath the patella suggests that it has penetrated the joint, but this is not ensured without fluid return or visualization of the needle position using ultrasound or alternative imaging.

The joint aspirated should be one that is symptomatic and swollen. The area is cleaned, and the site for needle puncture marked on the skin; this can be done with the wooden tip of a cotton swab. The skin and deeper tissue is infiltrated with a solution of 1% lidocaine for anesthesia. The aspiration needle should be at of least 20 gauge (22-gauge needles may be needed for finger or toe joints) to avoid plugging of the orifice with fat or other soft tissue.

Universal safety precautions should be practiced. One hand is used to identify the anatomic landmarks, with care not to touch the actual site. The initial thrust should be decisive; if fluid is not readily obtained, the position of the needle can be readjusted a little without withdrawing it. A small amount of fluid can be obtained from almost any joint. Only 1 mL of fluid is required for a thorough synovial fluid analysis, but more fluid may be removed, if needed, to relieve symptoms in a distended joint. Even a drop of fluid in the hub of the aspirating needle can allow identification of crystals or infectious agents (if seen on Gram stain), and an estimate of the white blood cell count.

The same procedure is used for intra-articular injections of depot corticosteroids. This treatment may provide temporary relief for some patients with osteoarthritis and more marked relief in patients with crystal-associated and other inflammatory arthritis. Synovial fluid should always be examined as part of the injection procedure and injection avoided if there is any suspicion of joint infection.

Based on the clinical signs and the symptoms reported by the patient, the specific tests and stains needed are determined before aspiration (see Plates 5-14 and 5-15). If infection is suspected, some fluid should be promptly delivered to the laboratory for culture.

Complications from joint aspiration/injection are extremely rare. To help avoid infection, the route of aspiration should not be through areas of cutaneous infection or a rash like psoriasis. Hemarthrosis resulting from a traumatic arthrocentesis ("bloody tap") is a rare complication, and aspiration can be done even in patients being treated with anticoagulants. No

Plate 5-14

Rheumatic Diseases

SYNOVIAL FLUID EXAMINATION

Gross appearance
A. Normal. Clear to pale yellow, transparent
B. Osteoarthritis. Slightly deeper yellow, transparent
C. Inflammatory. Darker yellow, cloudy, translucent (type blurred or obscured)
D. Septic. Purulent, dense, opaque
E. Hemarthrosis. Red, opaque. Must be differentiated from traumatic tap

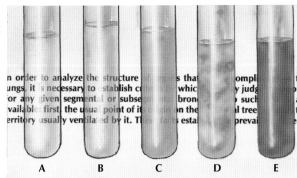

SYNOVIAL FLUID EXAMINATION
(Continued)

special care is needed after the procedure, but rest for 1 to 2 days may increase the efficacy of injected corticosteroids.

GROSS INSPECTION

Analysis of joint fluid begins with gross inspection. The fluid's appearance—clarity and presence of blood—may provide initial clues to the diagnosis and thus influence the physician's selection of laboratory tests.

The clarity of the fluid is assessed by experienced clinicians in the syringe but more reliably can be done by expressing a small amount of fluid out of the plastic syringe into a glass tube. (Plastic tubes have a slight opacity that may confuse the results; see Plate 5-14). Cloudy fluid is not typical of uncomplicated osteoarthritis and suggests an inflammatory process. An opaque, pasty fluid is most often due to pus, thus indicating the presence of infection, but a thick, purulent-appearing fluid occasionally results from massive numbers of crystals, amyloid, or, in rheumatoid arthritis, from degenerated synovial villi (rice bodies). Most infections do not produce pus; cloudy nonopaque fluids can also be due to infection.

Bloody fluid in the joint (hemarthrosis) suggests numerous diagnostic possibilities, including trauma (with or without fracture), pigmented villonodular synovitis, tumors in or near the joint, hemangioma, severe joint destruction (i.e., neuropathic), hemophilia, and, rarely, other bleeding disorders.

MICROBIOLOGIC CULTURES AND LABORATORY STUDIES

If joint infection is suspected, the aspirated fluid should be promptly transported to the microbiology laboratory. Some studies have suggested increased yield with the use of blood culture vials, but different laboratories have different collection guidelines. Unless there is specific clinical concern for mycobacterial, anaerobic, or fungal infection, it is appropriate and cost effective to send the initial fluid only for routine bacterial cultures. There is no purpose in sending the fluid for protein or

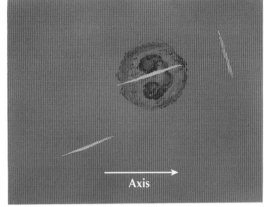
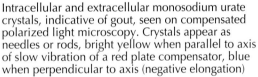

Intracellular and extracellular monosodium urate crystals, indicative of gout, seen on compensated polarized light microscopy. Crystals appear as needles or rods, bright yellow when parallel to axis of slow vibration of a red plate compensator, blue when perpendicular to axis (negative elongation)

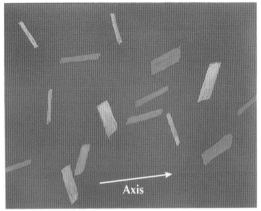

Calcium pyrophosphate dihydrate (CPPD) crystals, indicative of pseudogout, appear as rhomboids or rods, blue when parallel to axis, yellow when perpendicular to it (positive elongation)

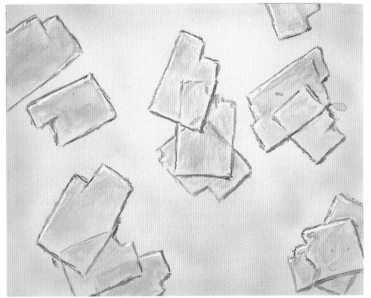

Cholesterol crystals, occasionally found in synovial or bursal fluids of patients with rheumatoid arthritis. Crystals are plate-like, with characteristic notched corners

glucose. Determination of lactate dehydrogenase in the fluid is not usually of value. Polymerase chain reaction may be beneficial when specific infections are suspected.

MICROSCOPIC EXAMINATION

Crystal-induced arthritis is definitively diagnosed only from examination of joint fluid for the presence of intracellular or extracellular crystals (2 to 20 μm).

Occasionally, crystals are also found in tissue or tophi. One or two drops of fluid are expressed onto a clean slide, which is promptly covered with a coverslip. Fluid on a slide can be preserved for a few hours, or a fresh drop preparation can be taken for each examination from fluid kept in a tube. The fluid should ideally be examined promptly because small numbers of calcium pyrophosphate dihydrate (CPPD) crystals may dissolve overnight and, with time, artifactual urate-like structures can form from degenerating cells; but this is not

Plate 5-15

Musculoskeletal System: PART III

SYNOVIAL FLUID EXAMINATION (CONTINUED)

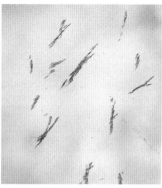

Cartilage fragments, may appear in synovial fluid taken from osteoarthritic joint (unstained, wet preparation)

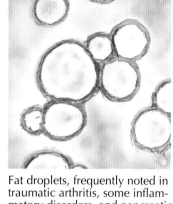

Fat droplets, frequently noted in traumatic arthritis, some inflammatory disorders, and pancreatic disease with synovial fat necrosis (unstained, wet preparation)

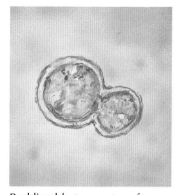

Budding blastomycete, a fungus that rarely appears in synovial fluid of fungal infections and is diagnostic of blastomycosis (unstained, wet preparation)

SYNOVIAL FLUID EXAMINATION
(Continued)

likely a common problem. Anticoagulants in collecting tubes are generally avoided because they may also produce confusing artifacts.

The fluid can be examined with a light microscope, and crystals can be reliably visualized by experienced observers; however, easier and more definitive identification is done utilizing a compensated polarized light microscope (see Plate 5-15). Urate crystals are usually shaped like needles; CPPD crystals are rods or rhomboids. The presence of depot corticosteroid crystals, even from an injection performed many days earlier, may confuse the diagnosis because they can appear similar to CPPD. Cholesterol crystals (i.e., plates with notched corners) are seen most frequently in chronic rheumatoid effusions and have an unclear role in joint inflammation.

The leukocyte count helps determine if the joint effusion reflects an inflammatory or noninflammatory process. Synovial fluid is usually heparinized before the cell count to reduce clumping.

Leukocyte counts greater than 2,000/mm³ usually result in loss of transparency in the fluid, but confirmation that this is due to leukocytosis is important. A classification of joint effusions based on leukocyte counts has been developed. Counts over 75,000/mm³ suggest the presence of infection, but very high counts (including those that are neutrophil predominant) can occur in psoriatic and crystal-induced arthritis and less commonly in rheumatoid arthritis.

Noninflammatory effusions usually contain three or fewer leukocytes per high-power field. Not all noninflammatory effusions are due to osteoarthritis. Some other causes include traumatic arthritis, acromegaly, hemochromatosis, hyperparathyroidism, ochronosis, Paget disease of bone, aseptic necrosis, amyloidosis, hypertrophic pulmonary osteoarthropathy, pancreatitis, and apatite-associated arthritis.

The wet preparations that had been examined for crystals can be used to provide a rough estimate of the leukocyte count. Other findings may also be noted (see Plate 5-15). For example, fat droplets, which usually indicate trauma, a result of marrow fat leaking into the synovial space, can also occur in pancreatic disease with synovial fat necrosis. Crystals of apatite deposition disease, seen in calcific tendonitis or in patients with Milwaukee shoulder/knee syndrome, create irregular, shiny, often nonbirefringent intracellular or extracellular chunks (of 2 to 20 μm) visible on wet preparations; individual crystals can be seen only on electron microscopy.

Single drops of joint fluid can be placed on a glass slide and smeared out into a thin preparation as for a blood smear. Air-drying preserves the cells for staining later in the day. If infection is being considered, smears should be stained with Gram's stain. Identification of pathologic organisms can guide the choice of initial

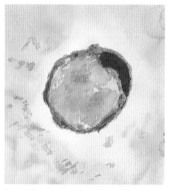

LE cell, seen virtually only in systemic lupus erythematosus (Wright's stain)

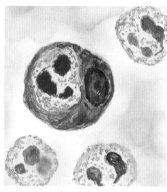

Monocyte that has phagocytized a necrotic neutrophil

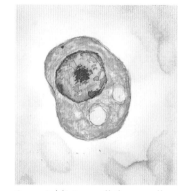

Synovial lining cell (large cell with nucleus usually filling less than 50% of cytoplasm), often seen in noninflammatory aspirates

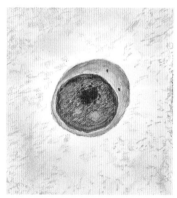

Activated T lymphocyte (large cell with prominent nucleus and nucleolus), most common in rheumatoid arthritis

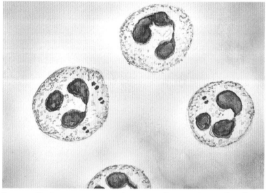

Intracellular gram-negative cocci, seen in only about 25% of cases of gonococcal arthritis (Gram's stain). Gram-positive organisms such as staphylococci seen more often. Diagnosis of tuberculous, gonococcal, or anaerobic infections may require culture on special media.

antibiotic therapy, but failure to find bacteria on a Gram-stained preparation does not exclude infectious arthritis because positive stains for bacteria are uncommon, even with staphylococcal infection.

A differential count with more than 95% polymorphonuclear neutrophils is consistent with infection or crystal-induced disease (see Plates 5-14, 5-38 to 5-40) even if the leukocyte count is not very high. An inflamed joint space produces an ideal medium for the development of LE cells, which are seen almost exclusively in

systemic lupus erythematosus (see Plate 5-51). Mononuclear cells that have phagocytized necrotic neutrophils may occur in reactive arthritis (see Plate 5-33), other seronegative spondyloarthropathies, or (occasionally) gout or pseudogout (see Plates 5-38 and 5-39). Large cells seen in blood smears include synovial lining cells, most common in noninflammatory disorders, and activated lymphocytes, which are common in rheumatoid arthritis and should not be confused with the rare tumor cell found in joints.

Plate 5-16

Rheumatic Diseases

JUVENILE ARTHRITIS

Because the clinical, laboratory, and genetic features of chronic arthritis in children differ significantly from those of classic adult rheumatoid arthritis, the term *juvenile rheumatoid arthritis* has been discarded in favor of *juvenile idiopathic arthritis* (JIA). The disease has a variable onset and course, making it impossible to develop diagnostic criteria that fit every case. The primary diagnostic criterion for JIA is arthritis in one or more joints that persists for at least 6 weeks in a patient younger than age 16 years after other possible causes have been excluded. In its simplest form, arthritis in children is a physical examination finding based on the observation of swelling within a joint, or limitation in the range of joint movement, joint pain with motion, or joint line tenderness. These findings should not be attributable to mechanical disorders or to other identifiable causes. Furthermore, other systemic manifestation in addition to arthritis may occur in children with JIA, including uveitis, psoriasis, inflammatory bowel disease, and serositis.

In 2004, major changes were made to the classification of children with JIA. Based on expert consensus, children with JIA were subclassified into seven subtypes: oligoarticular (either persistent or extended), rheumatoid factor–negative polyarticular, rheumatoid factor–positive polyarticular; systemic arthritis, enthesitis-related arthritis, psoriatic arthritis, and undifferentiated arthritis. Although these subcategories are useful in identifying populations for clinical trials, it is likely that they represent unique conditions that share arthritis as a cardinal feature.

OLIGOARTICULAR ARTHRITIS

Oligoarticular arthritis occurs in 55% to 60% of children with juvenile arthritis. The arthritis is limited to fewer than five joints during the first 6 months after diagnosis. Those patients whose arthritis remains confined to four or fewer joints 6 months after diagnosis are classified as having persistent oligoarticular JIA. Some children may develop involvement of five or more joints after the initial 6-month period and are classified as having extended oligoarticular JIA. In patients whose arthritis extends beyond a few joints, the disease resembles rheumatoid factor–negative polyarthritis and produces more dysfunction than was predicted from the original, limited involvement. Disease activity may be intermittent and even recur in previously uninvolved joints, even after years of remission.

Oligoarticular disease is most likely to be found in toddlers and in females more frequently than males. It is rare for these children to complain about pain; medical care is typically a result of parental observation of joint swelling or the onset of a new functional disability. The knee is most often affected in oligoarticular-onset disease, and monarticular involvement is common. When the knee is involved, parents will often report their child limps in the morning or wishes to be carried. The ankles are the next most common site of involvement, followed by the wrists, elbows, and hips. The small joints of the hands and feet, the cervical spine, and the jaw are affected less often than in polyarticular-onset arthritis.

In some children, the joint contains only a small amount of fluid, particularly in the early stages. The bulge sign is used to confirm the presence of small amounts of fluid in the knee (see Plate 5-19). The bulge is elicited by compressing or stroking proximally the

medial side of the knee, moving fluid into the suprapatellar bursa and the lateral compartment. Rapid compression of the lateral compartment moves fluid back to the medial side, resulting in a bulging of the medial compartment. The effusion may also be demonstrated by compressing the suprapatellar bursa or by distally stroking the lateral compartment. Other important physical examination findings include muscle atrophy or joint contractures.

In monarticular disease, overgrowth of the involved limb may occur as a result of increased blood supply to

the immature growth plate; this is seen most frequently with arthritis of one knee. With remission or treatment, overgrowth ceases, allowing growth in the uninvolved limb to catch up. If left untreated, persistent inflammation results in premature closure of the growth plate and shortening of the affected limb. If the limb-length discrepancy is predicted to be greater than 2.5 cm, early epiphyseal stapling or epiphysiodesis of the affected side may be indicated.

Uveitis in Juvenile Idiopathic Arthritis. A potentially blinding yet clinically silent uveitis is most likely

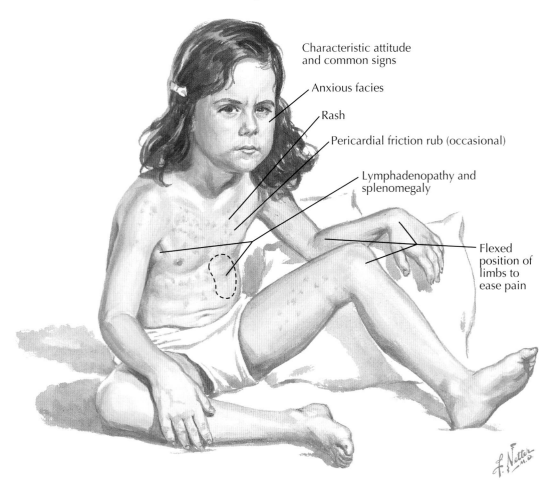

SYSTEMIC JUVENILE ARTHRITIS

Characteristic attitude and common signs

Anxious facies

Rash

Pericardial friction rub (occasional)

Lymphadenopathy and splenomegaly

Flexed position of limbs to ease pain

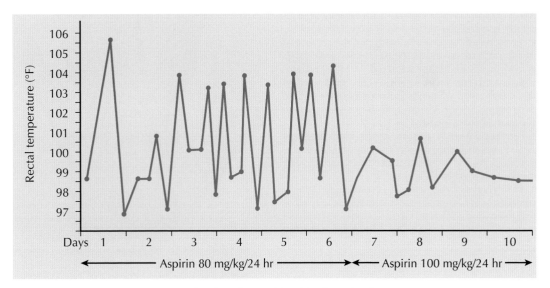

Typical spiking fever with wide diurnal swings

Plate 5-17

Musculoskeletal System: PART III

JUVENILE ARTHRITIS (Continued)

to develop in children with oligoarticular JIA. Only 5% of children with the polyarticular subtype will develop uveitis compared with approximately 20% of children with oligoarticular JIA. This ocular inflammation usually begins within 2 years of the onset of arthritis, and nearly always within the first 4 years. In some children, uveitis becomes evident before the joint manifestations and it is typical for the inflammatory activity in the joints and eyes to occur independent of each other. Patients most at risk for uveitis are girls who are younger than 6 years of age at the onset of arthritis with the oligoarticular subtype, a positive antinuclear antibody (ANA) test, and disease duration of less than 4 years. Periodic slit lamp examination is used to detect ocular inflammation in the early stage and is mandatory in all children with juvenile arthritis. The early changes are not seen readily with the ophthalmoscope.

Uveal inflammation primarily affects the iris and ciliary body, and slit lamp examination reveals white cells and protein in the anterior chamber (see Plate 5-20). Fibrin strands may develop between the iris and the anterior surface of the lens (synechiae), resulting in a fixed or irregular pupil. White blood cells and protein deposited on the surface of the cornea may calcify, resulting in band keratopathy, which can obstruct vision. Cataracts may be caused by a combination of factors, including inflammation, blocked Schlemm's canal, increased pressure, and corticosteroid therapy. Although careful follow-up and aggressive treatment have improved the prognosis for patients with uveitis, uveitis still remains a leading cause of acquired blindness in children.

POLYARTICULAR-ONSET ARTHRITIS

About 20% to 25% of children with juvenile arthritis exhibit polyarticular onset, which is characterized by involvement of five or more joints and the absence of significant systemic manifestations. High serum levels of IgM rheumatoid factor are found in 25% of patients with polyarticular-onset arthritis. This finding led to the classification of polyarticular-onset arthritis into two distinct types: rheumatoid factor–positive and rheumatoid factor–negative.

Polyarticular-onset arthritis affects both large and small joints, including the cervical spine, temporomandibular joints, and growth centers of the mandible. The distribution is generally symmetric.

Radiographs of the involved cervical spine initially reveal a loss of the normal curve; with time, the apophyseal joints (most often at C2 to C3) may narrow and eventually fuse (see Plate 5-21). The fusion may affect the whole cervical spine or only segments. Because limitation of motion is most significant in extension and lateral motion, some children hold the head in a position of fixed flexion (see Plate 5-21). Anterior subluxation of C1 on C2 is a potentially serious complication seen with extensive fusion below C2.

Arthritis of the cervical spine is associated with involvement of the temporomandibular joints, which may result in poor growth of the mandible and crowding of the teeth. Children may refuse to eat breakfast owing to pain and stiffness in this joint, but 80% of children with temporomandibular joint arthritis are asymptomatic. Growth of the maxilla is rarely affected. If temporomandibular joint involvement is unilateral, the lower jaw shifts significantly to the affected side when the mouth is opened. Limitation of intraincisal distance is also a common finding.

SYSTEMIC JUVENILE ARTHRITIS (CONTINUED)

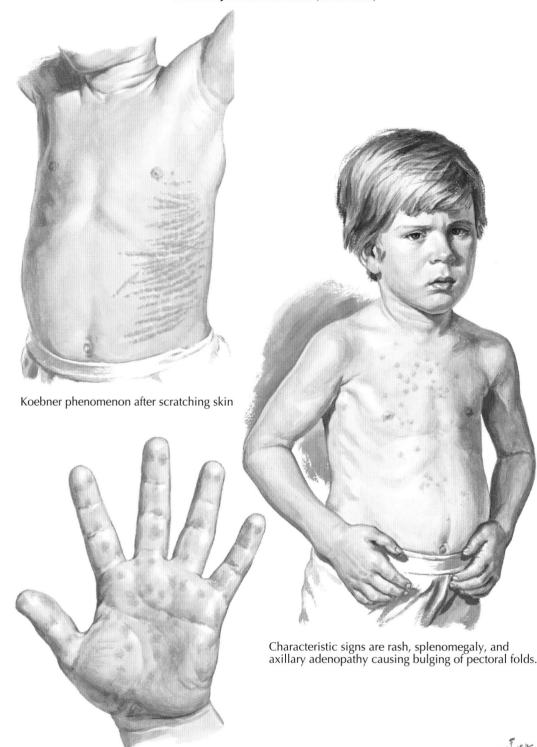

Koebner phenomenon after scratching skin

Palmar rash may be seen. Similar rash occurs in very few other rheumatic conditions.

Characteristic signs are rash, splenomegaly, and axillary adenopathy causing bulging of pectoral folds.

In the hands and feet, the arthritis affects multiple joints in a symmetric pattern. Attenuation of supporting structures and damage to tendons, tendon sheaths, and attachments lead to joint laxity and subluxation. The metacarpophalangeal and proximal interphalangeal joints of the hands are affected first, followed by the distal interphalangeal joints (see Plate 5-18).

Rheumatoid Factor–Positive Polyarthritis. This juvenile version of adult rheumatoid arthritis usually develops in girls older than 10 years of age. The arthritis, which involves multiple large and small joints, is erosive, aggressive, and chronic. Erosions in the small joints may be evident radiographically as early as 6 months after onset of disease, and the destructive synovitis may continue for 10 years or longer.

Subcutaneous rheumatoid nodules may occur, usually developing at or distal to the elbow on the extensor surface. Constitutional manifestations of rheumatoid factor–positive polyarthritis include low-grade fever, easy fatigability, mild-to-moderate anemia, and poor weight gain. Uveitis (iridocyclitis) and episcleritis are rare.

Plate 5-18

Rheumatic Diseases

JUVENILE ARTHRITIS (Continued)

The progressive nature of this disease may lead to significant deformities in the limbs and spine. However, because patients are in late childhood or adolescence at onset, growth of the vertebral bodies is not significantly disturbed even when the spinous processes are fused.

Rheumatoid Factor–Negative Polyarthritis. Approximately 75% of patients with polyarticular-onset arthritis do not have IgM rheumatoid factor in the serum, and the rheumatoid factor test rarely becomes positive 6 months after disease onset. In contrast to rheumatoid factor–positive disease, which primarily affects girls, about 25% of patients in this subgroup are boys.

The arthritis may start at any age, but in about one half of patients onset occurs before age 6. In younger children, parents generally notice only one or two swollen joints, only to have the rheumatologist identify more. The inflammatory process is usually less severe than in rheumatoid factor–positive polyarthritis. Large and small joints are affected, but erosions usually develop later. Early radiographs reveal only osteoporotic changes.

Tenosynovitis on the dorsum of the wrist and tarsus is common, but tenosynovitis in the hand flexors and in tendon structures around the ankle may also be found. Involvement of the finger joints is often symmetric. In young children, swelling of the joints may be partially masked by diffuse swelling of the entire finger (fusiform swelling, see Plate 5-18). Periostitis and widening of the digits are occasionally seen on radiographs. Subcutaneous nodules are uncommon. Chronic, asymptomatic uveitis develops in a small number of patients and is usually associated with a positive ANA test.

The long-term prognosis for patients with rheumatoid factor–negative polyarthritis varies. With treatment, the disease may enter long-term remission, leaving minimal deformities. In others, the course of the disease resembles rheumatoid factor–positive arthritis, only it is less severe. Overall, 70% of children with polyarticular JIA will continue to have some symptoms as adults.

SYSTEMIC-ONSET ARTHRITIS

About 20% of children with juvenile arthritis have the systemic-onset form. The disease may begin at any time during childhood, and both sexes are equally affected. The major signs of systemic-onset juvenile arthritis are a high, spiking fever; characteristic rash; arthritis in one or multiple joints; hepatosplenomegaly; and lymphadenopathy (see Plates 5-16 and 5-17).

The fever in systemic-onset arthritis typically rises above 102°F and falls to normal or below once (quotidian pattern) or twice (double quotidian) during every 24 hours. Although the rise and fall are usually rapid, the pattern of fever may otherwise be quite variable. In some children, the temperature is significantly elevated much of the time, with only short afebrile periods; in others, the duration of the fever spikes is shorter. Single spikes tend to occur in the late afternoon or evening. In patients with a more hectic fever, administration of NSAIDs may change the fever pattern to a once-a-day spike or return the temperature to normal.

The characteristic evanescent rash tends to occur simultaneously with the fever, often disappearing completely during afebrile periods (see Plates 5-16 and 5-17). It may be generalized or develop only in warmer areas such as the axillae and medial thighs or on the palms and soles. The typical rash is macular; individual lesions are pale ("salmon") pink with relatively

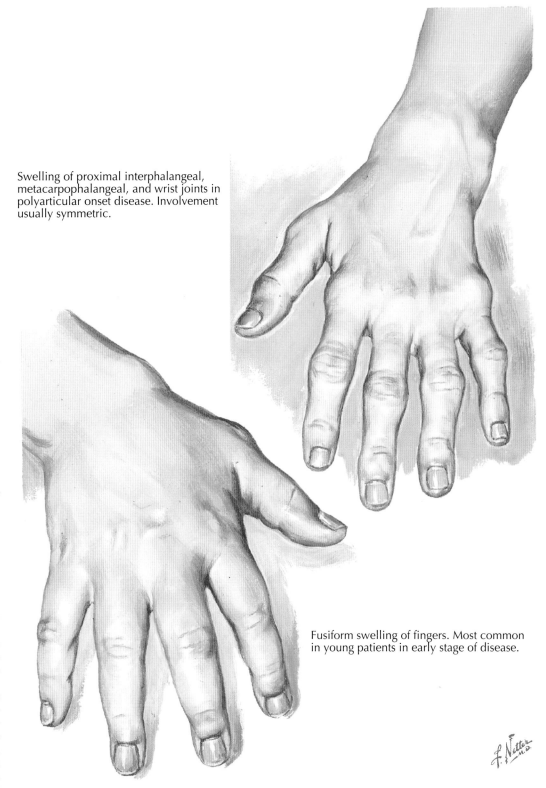

Swelling of proximal interphalangeal, metacarpophalangeal, and wrist joints in polyarticular onset disease. Involvement usually symmetric.

Fusiform swelling of fingers. Most common in young patients in early stage of disease.

indistinct margins and somewhat paler centers. When the rash is extensive, the macules tend to coalesce. About 20% of children with a typical fever pattern have a maculopapular or pruritic rash, and 10% have no rash. In a few children, macules appear along scratch marks made in the skin (Koebner phenomenon). This manifestation, which may not appear immediately, should not be confused with the rapid appearance of the wheal-and-flare response normally seen after scratching.

Severe arthralgia and myalgia are common, particularly during febrile periods. The 30% of children who have no initial evidence of joint involvement may seem to be completely normal during the afebrile periods. During the first 6 months of disease, however, arthritis develops in at least five joints in more than 80% of children with systemic-onset arthritis.

Localized or generalized adenopathy is common; occasionally, the swelling of a single node or groups of

Plate 5-19

Musculoskeletal System: PART III

JUVENILE ARTHRITIS (Continued)

nodes is massive, resembling that of cancer. Biopsy findings usually indicate a reactive hyperplasia. Hepatosplenomegaly is also common.

About 25% of patients with systemic-onset arthritis have symptoms or signs of pericarditis and/or pleuritis. In asymptomatic children, echocardiography may reveal a small amount of pericardial fluid, but this is usually of little clinical significance; rarely, the amount of pericardial fluid is sufficient to cause cardiac tamponade and require aspiration. Pericardial effusions are usually associated with pleural effusions, and myocarditis frequently accompanies pericarditis. A pericardial friction rub may be localized to a small area, usually the lower sternum. Patients with pericardial irritation show a reluctance to lie down because of increased chest pain.

Ocular involvement of any type is uncommon in patients with the systemic-onset form. Central nervous system (CNS) involvement, including seizures, has been reported but is considered rare.

The majority of deaths due to juvenile arthritis have occurred in children with the systemic-onset form. In many countries, the leading cause of death in patients with juvenile arthritis is renal failure secondary to amyloidosis. Amyloidosis appears to be significantly less common in the United States. These regional differences suggest an interplay between genetic and environmental factors in the pathogenesis of secondary amyloidosis.

Laboratory Findings. Laboratory tests may help in the diagnosis of systemic-onset arthritis, but ANA and rheumatoid factor tests are usually negative. Most patients have a modest-to-marked leukocytosis (15,000 to 25,000/mm³); occasionally, the count may be as high as 50,000/mm³. Polymorphonuclear leukocytes predominate, and there is a significant percentage of young cells. In most children, the platelet count is also elevated. Thrombocytopenia is rare. Normochromic, normocytic anemia with a normal mean corpuscular volume develops initially, but with continuing disease activity, the hemoglobin level decreases, followed by a fall in the mean corpuscular volume and development of a microcytic, hypochromic anemia. Serum levels of iron are usually low with a normal-to-high iron-binding capacity. Serum ferritin levels may be normal to significantly elevated and probably reflect the generalized inflammatory disease. Although the anemia is unresponsive to administration of iron, reticulocytosis and a rapid rise in hemoglobin value occur with disease remission. During the febrile phase, urinalysis may reveal intermittent or persistent proteinuria or increased red or white blood cell counts. Liver function may be abnormal, even before treatment with NSAIDs.

Macrophage Activation Syndrome. Macrophage activation syndrome is a potentially lethal complication of systemic-onset JIA. Children with macrophage activation syndrome commonly present with culture-negative septic shock and signs of cardiovascular collapse. Typical laboratory findings include a highly elevated serum ferritin, evidence of disseminated intravascular coagulation with elevated fibrin split products, low ESR due to fibrinogen consumption, elevated serum triglyceride levels, and thrombocytopenia. There is uncontrolled activation and proliferation of macrophages, and T lymphocytes, with a marked increase in circulating cytokines, such as interferon gamma (IFN-γ), and granulocyte-macrophage colony-stimulating factor (GM-CSF). Early recognition and treatment of this condition is necessary to prevent mortality. Macrophage activation syndrome has been described in

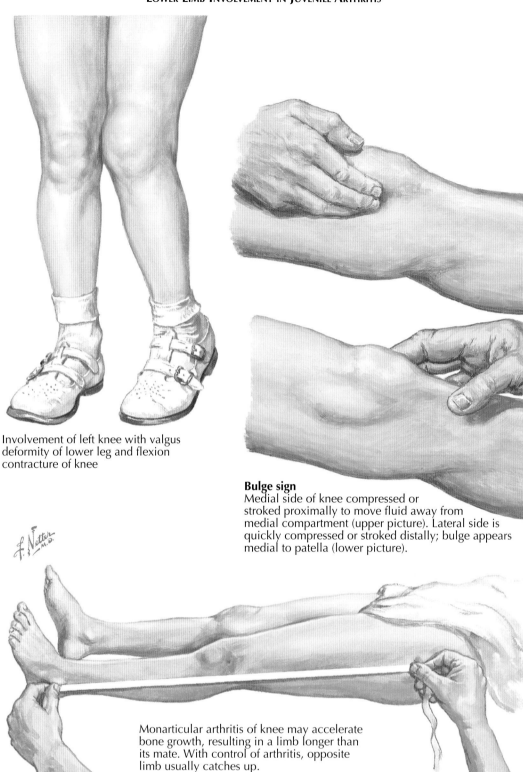

LOWER LIMB INVOLVEMENT IN JUVENILE ARTHRITIS

Involvement of left knee with valgus deformity of lower leg and flexion contracture of knee

Bulge sign
Medial side of knee compressed or stroked proximally to move fluid away from medial compartment (upper picture). Lateral side is quickly compressed or stroked distally; bulge appears medial to patella (lower picture).

Monarticular arthritis of knee may accelerate bone growth, resulting in a limb longer than its mate. With control of arthritis, opposite limb usually catches up.

association with systemic lupus erythematosus, Kawasaki disease, and adult-onset Still disease. It is thought to be closely related and pathophysiologically very similar to reactive (secondary) hemophagocytic lymphohistiocytosis. A bone marrow biopsy or aspirate usually shows hemophagocytosis.

ENTHESITIS-RELATED ARTHRITIS

The subgroup of enthesitis-related arthritis was created to accommodate those children with later-onset asymmetric oligoarticular presentation and a predisposition to develop sacroiliac disease. This subcategory encompasses those patients with the previously categorized seronegative spondyloarthropathies, including those with ankylosing spondylitis. In general, enthesitis-related arthritis tends to strike boys older than age 6 years. Patients may have a family history of ankylosing spondylitis, inflammatory bowel disease, or reactive arthritis. The arthritis has a predilection for the lower extremities, especially the knees, ankles, and hips, and exclusive involvement of the hip is not uncommon.

Plate 5-20

Rheumatic Diseases

JUVENILE ARTHRITIS (Continued)

Enthesitis, inflammation at the insertions of tendons or fascia into bone, commonly effects the insertion of the Achilles, iliotibial, patellar, or triceps tendons. Acute unilateral anterior uveitis with pain and redness, as opposed to the chronic asymptomatic bilateral uveitis seen in oligoarticular patients, affects 20% of patients, but the duration of inflammation is usually short.

In some patients, radiographic changes in the sacroiliac joints, mild back pain, or limitation of motion of the lower spine develops with time. Most children with sacroiliac inflammation will manifest typical inflammatory back pain symptoms, including prolonged morning stiffness, pain reduction with activity, alternating buttock pain, and waking from sleep due to pain in the second half of the night.

The histocompatibility of human leukocyte antigen B27 (HLA-B27) is detected in a large percentage of patients in this subgroup. Children should not be included in this subgroup solely because of the presence of HLA-B27, which is also found in children with other types of juvenile arthritis at the same frequency as in the general population.

DIFFERENTIAL DIAGNOSIS

Systemic-onset arthritis may resemble a number of other diseases. When joint inflammation is absent, it may be confused with infectious, oncologic, or inflammatory diseases. When joint inflammation is present, infectious arthritis, osteomyelitis, and malignancy, especially leukemia, must be ruled out. Other diagnostic possibilities include a variety of systemic autoimmune diseases including lupus, inflammatory bowel disease, various types of systemic vasculitis, and, occasionally, reactions to infections or drugs.

Polyarticular arthritis must be differentiated from other joint diseases such as systemic lupus erythematosus and acute rheumatic fever. Unlike these conditions, however, polyarticular arthritis rarely has significant systemic manifestations.

Oligoarticular-onset arthritis, especially monarticular involvement, can be confused with trauma, joint conditions such as osteochondritis, viral-induced synovitis, Lyme disease, hemarthrosis, vascular malformation, and benign soft tissue tumors such as pigmented villonodular synovitis.

Laboratory studies have no role in the diagnosis of JIA; JIA is a clinical diagnosis, and laboratory studies only aid in the subcategorization of children with arthritis. Up to 30% of the general pediatric population may have a positive ANA, compared with approximately 50% of children with JIA. ANA testing is performed in the diagnostic evaluation of children with JIA only to properly assess their risk for uveitis. Similarly, 3% of healthy children may have serologic evidence of IgM rheumatoid factor whereas up to 10% of patients with JIA manifest similar results. All patients diagnosed with JIA should undergo testing for rheumatoid factor to assist with proper subclassification, but a negative rheumatoid factor test does not rule out JIA. In addition, serologic testing should also include assessment of anti-CCP antibody, an IgG antibody that portends an aggressive and destructive disease course similar to rheumatoid factor–positive disease. Children with JIA may have evidence of systemic inflammation with an elevated ESR, anemia, and thrombocytosis, yet these tests are frequently normal at the time of diagnosis in most patients with JIA.

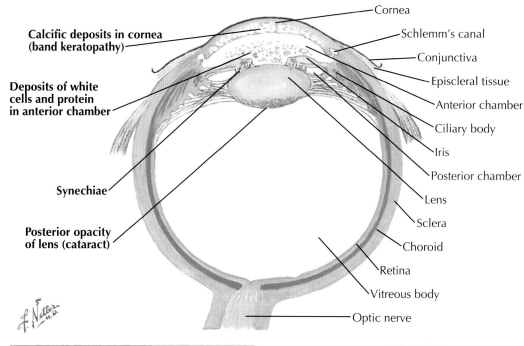

OCULAR MANIFESTATIONS IN JUVENILE ARTHRITIS

Calcific deposits in cornea (band keratopathy)

Deposits of white cells and protein in anterior chamber

Synechiae

Posterior opacity of lens (cataract)

Cornea
Schlemm's canal
Conjunctiva
Episcleral tissue
Anterior chamber
Ciliary body
Iris
Posterior chamber
Lens
Sclera
Choroid
Retina
Vitreous body
Optic nerve

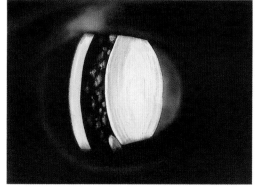

Deposits in anterior chamber viewed with slit lamp

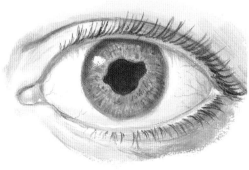

Irregular pupil due to synechiae

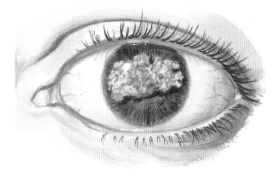

Band keratopathy

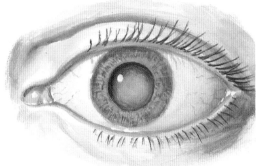

Cataract

Although a promising area of research, genetic sequencing is of little clinical value at present. There is a significantly increased frequency of HLA-B27 in older males with enthesitis-related arthritis and an increased frequency of HLA-DR4 in children with rheumatoid factor–positive polyarthritis, similar to that seen in adult rheumatoid arthritis. Similarly, HLA-DR5 and HLA-DRw8 are often found in patients with oligoarticular-onset arthritis and in those with rheumatoid factor–negative polyarthritis. However, because the same markers are present in many normal people, their demonstration is of value only in population studies, not in individual patients.

TREATMENT

The treatment of juvenile arthritis is multifaceted, requiring a coordinated team approach. Ideally, the primary care physician, rheumatologist, orthopedist, pedodontist, ophthalmologist, and physical therapist should all be involved in the treatment program.

Plate 5-21

Musculoskeletal System: PART III

JUVENILE ARTHRITIS (Continued)

The pharmaceutical options for children with JIA have dramatically increased in the past decade. Although NSAIDs had been a mainstay of treatment in all forms of JIA, they have been relegated to the role of analgesic rather than primary anti-inflammatory agent. For children with persistent oligoarticular disease, intra-articular injections of triamcinolone hexacetonide, a long-acting corticosteroid, are frequently used to control the disease. These injections may be performed blindly utilizing anatomic landmarks to identify the joint space or may be done with radiographic guidance via ultrasound or fluoroscopy. When performed in arthritic knees, these injections will achieve complete remission of the disease for 12 months in 60% of patients. Many joints are amenable to this therapeutic intervention, including the wrist, ankles, hips, elbows, and temporomandibular joints, but with shorter duration of effect.

For children with extended oligoarticular or polyarticular subtypes, weekly administration of methotrexate now stands as the first-line drug of choice. Methotrexate, an antimetabolite, may be administered via the oral or parenteral route with no significant difference in efficacy. Daily leflunomide has been shown to be as effective as methotrexate in controlling JIA symptoms but is associated with increased frequency of gastrointestinal side effects. For patients who fail traditional disease-modifying agents, the development of the biologic response modifiers has represented an important advance in therapy. These agents are a class of medication that selectively inhibits specific proinflammatory cytokines or pathways critical to perpetuating arthritis. Anti–TNF-α agents such as etanercept and adalimumab have been shown to significantly increase the number of children achieving clinical remission with treatment beyond the rates observed with methotrexate. Abatacept, an inhibitor of T-cell co-stimulation, has also been proved to be significantly more effective than methotrexate in controlling JIA symptoms and increasing the likelihood of remission.

Treatment strategies for children with enthesitis-related arthritis are similar to those with polyarticular JIA. However, these children may also respond favorably to sulfasalazine, which is metabolized to the anti-inflammatory 5-aminosalicylic acid. Methotrexate, as well as etanercept, has been successfully used to treat children with juvenile psoriatic arthritis.

The therapeutic approach to children with systemic-onset disease is markedly different than that for other subtypes of JIA. Systemic corticosteroids are used frequently to treat the constitutional symptoms. For those patients who require ongoing systemic corticosteroids to control their disease, the interleukin-1 (IL-1) inhibitors such as anakinra, have been demonstrated to dramatically improve the constitutional symptoms. Methotrexate is often required for patients with polyarticular arthritis. Systemic-onset patients with signs of macrophage activation syndrome respond well to high doses of corticosteroids and anakinra, with the possible addition of cyclosporine.

Children with uveitis related to their JIA also pose unique therapeutic challenges. Frequently, ocular inflammation occurs when joint disease is quiescent. However, given the threat of permanent vision

impairment, these children are aggressively treated with topical prednisolone, methotrexate, and biologic response modifiers such as adalimumab and infliximab.

In addition to pharmacologic treatment, children with JIA will often require care from physical and occupational therapists. These specialists play a critical role in improving the function of those children with functional impairments such as limb-length discrepancy or muscle atrophy. Nutritionists may be required for those

patients on systemic therapy with corticosteroids to design dietary strategies to minimize weight gain. Psychologists may be needed to help patients and families develop strategies to deal with the stress inherent to a chronic illness. JIA patients may require modifications to school activities and schedules requiring a strong advocate, such as a guidance counselor, within their educational system. With the care of a multidisciplinary team and the advances in drug therapy, children with JIA should expect to lead normal and productive lives.

SEQUELAE OF JUVENILE ARTHRITIS

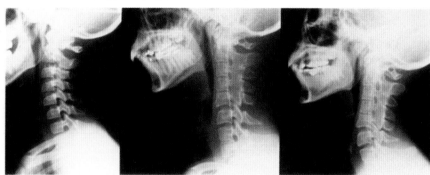

Radiographs show progression of arthritis of cervical apophyseal joints from only upper vertebrae to almost entire cervical spine

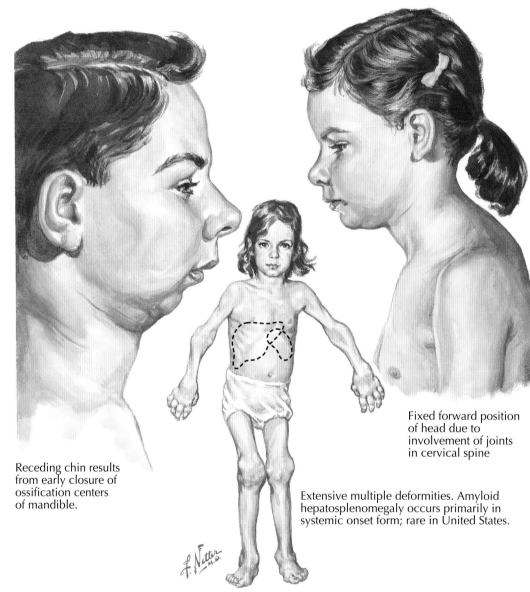

Fixed forward position of head due to involvement of joints in cervical spine

Receding chin results from early closure of ossification centers of mandible.

Extensive multiple deformities. Amyloid hepatosplenomegaly occurs primarily in systemic onset form; rare in United States.

Plate 5-22

Rheumatic Diseases

OSTEOARTHRITIS

The most common joint disease, osteoarthritis, is a progressive disorder characterized by the deterioration of articular cartilage and formation of new bone in the subchondral region and at joint margins. Although commonly termed *degenerative joint disease*, the designation *osteoarthritis* emphasizes the presence of inflammation seen in the synovium in almost all cases as the disease progresses.

Many factors influence its onset and the speed of joint deterioration, including aging, gender, obesity, heredity, trauma (related to sports or occupation), joint overuse, joint instability, and malalignment. Involved basic mechanisms of pathophysiology include "normal" loading on abnormal cartilage versus "abnormal" loading on normal cartilage. *Secondary osteoarthritis*, the term used to designate osteoarthritis appearing as a sequel to other forms of arthritis, injury, internal derangement, or dysplasia of the joint, is not uncommonly seen in younger persons..

Evidence of osteoarthritis has been found in the skeletal remains of prehistoric animals and humans. The true prevalence is difficult to determine because mild or early osteoarthritis may be asymptomatic and is demonstrated primarily radiographically. In asymptomatic persons, osteoarthritis is often discovered accidentally on radiographs performed for other diagnostic purposes.

PATHOLOGY

Unlike rheumatoid arthritis, osteoarthritis is not a *systemic* disease; instead, it is a process that is *localized* in joint structures, with involvement primarily of cartilage, bone, and synovial tissues (see Plate 5-22). Bone marrow lesions and synovitis add significantly to clinical symptoms.

Changes in Articular Cartilage. Pathologic changes in cartilage are characterized by alterations in proteoglycan and collagen. This leads to a softening of the cartilage followed by fraying and fibrillation; cracks develop extending more deeply into the cartilage. Clusters of chondrocytes proliferate in efforts at repair. As degeneration progresses, the entire cartilage becomes thinner and the surface becomes rough from the focal ulcerations. Eventually, the articular surface is denuded of cartilage. Because cartilage has no blood supply, regeneration is limited.

Changes in Bone. New bone forms at two sites: in subchondral bone and at joint margins. In subchondral tissue, the new bone grows chiefly beneath the eroded cartilage surface, thus eventually becoming the articular surface. The new bone becomes smooth, glistening, and sclerotic, or eburnated.

The most characteristic pathologic feature is the growth of osteophytes at the margins of affected joints (spur formation). The osteophyte, which consists of bone growing from the joint margin, usually follows the contour of the articular surface within the capsule and ligamentous attachments.

Changes in Soft Tissue. The synovial and capsular tissues may show mild-to-moderate inflammation and fibrous thickening in joints severely deranged by extensive damage to cartilage and bone. These soft tissue changes are associated with the stress, strain, and mechanical irritation that are secondary to the degenerative changes.

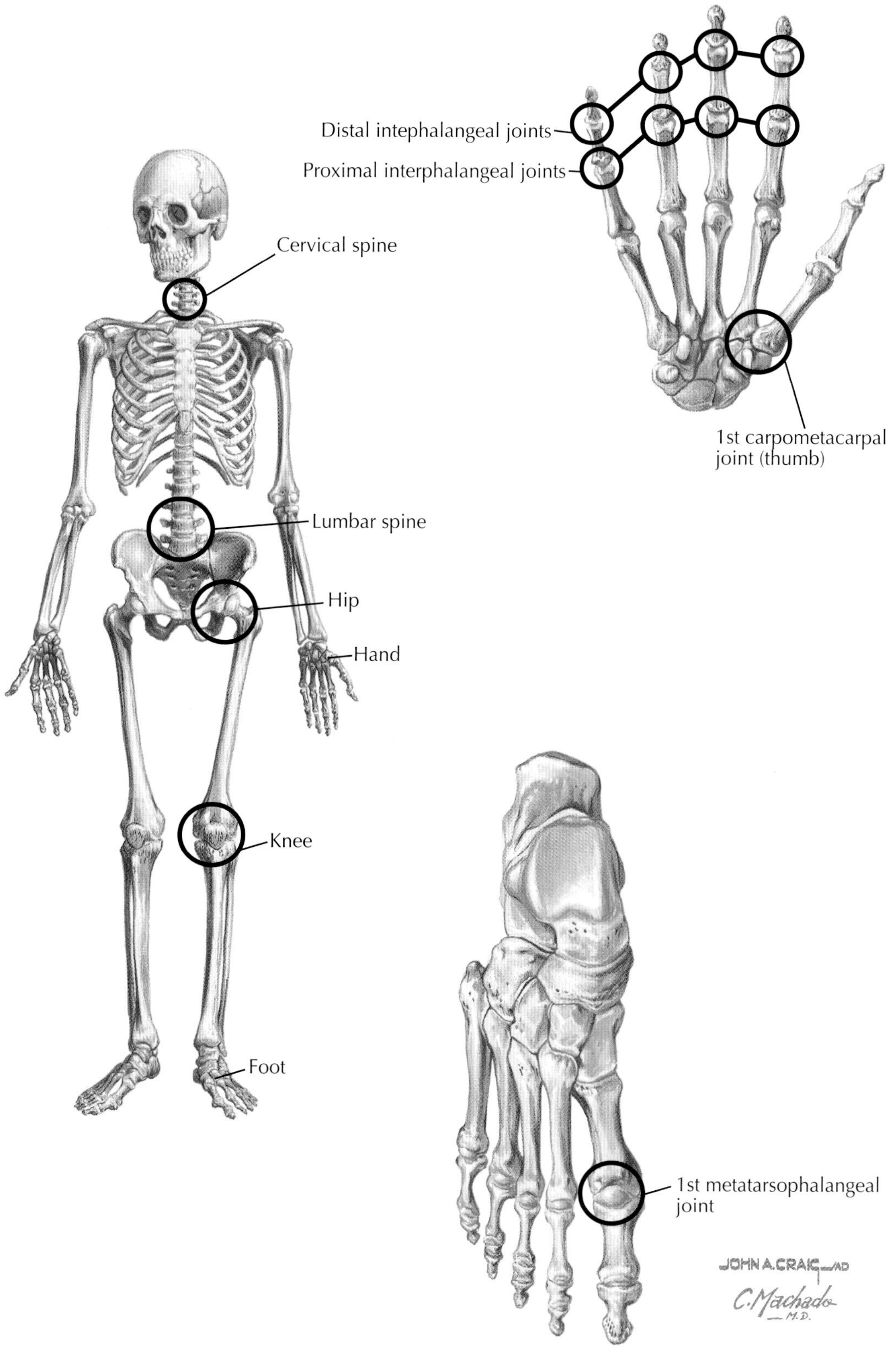

PATHOGENESIS

The pathogenesis of osteoarthritis involves a number of factors, any one or a number of which might be operative in a given patient. As noted, many tissues are involved in the process, including subchondral bone, synovium, cartilage, and bone at the joint periphery, as well as ligaments and muscles. Not well recognized is the presence of synovial inflammation as the disease progresses, related to inflammatory mediators such as IL-1, TNF-α, and prostaglandins. Proteases targeted to proteoglycans and collagen play an important role in joint breakdown. Obesity has a strong relationship to osteoarthritis, especially in the presence of additional factors such as joint instability and malalignment.

DISTRIBUTION OF JOINT INVOLVEMENT IN OSTEOARTHRITIS

Distal intephalangeal joints
Proximal interphalangeal joints
1st carpometacarpal joint (thumb)
Cervical spine
Lumbar spine
Hip
Hand
Knee
Foot
1st metatarsophalangeal joint

JOHN A. CRAIG—MD
C. Machado—M.D.

Plate 5-23

Musculoskeletal System: PART III

CLINICAL FINDINGS IN OSTEOARTHRITIS

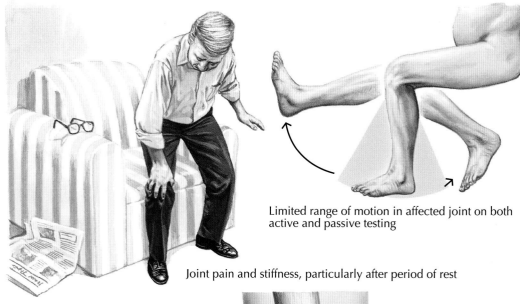

Limited range of motion in affected joint on both active and passive testing

Joint pain and stiffness, particularly after period of rest

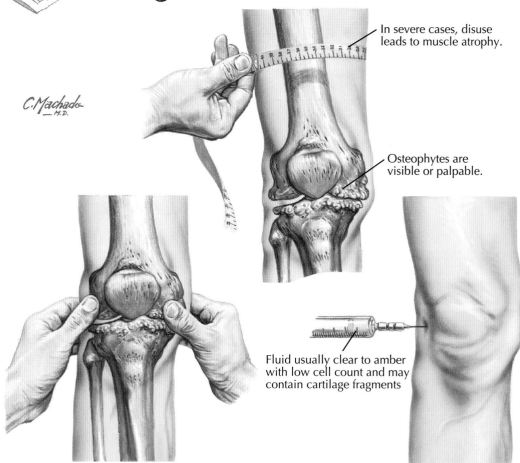

In severe cases, disuse leads to muscle atrophy.

Osteophytes are visible or palpable.

Fluid usually clear to amber with low cell count and may contain cartilage fragments

Joint palpation reveals osteophytes and crepitus (grinding sensation) on joint movement.

Arthrocentesis is most useful for ruling out other joint disorders.

OSTEOARTHRITIS (Continued)

Genetic predisposition to osteoarthritis has been well defined, especially in women with the development of Heberden's nodes, the nodular swellings at the terminal joints (distal interphalangeal joints) of the fingers. There is a suggestion that aging per se may play an etiologic role in the form of advanced glycation end-products that lead to formation of cross-links between sugars and proteins, making the cartilage more susceptible to injury from other risk factors.

Microtrauma caused by daily "wear and tear" on articular cartilage in weight-bearing joints likely contributes significantly to the degenerative process. As noted, mechanical factors that predispose to osteoarthritis are excessive body weight, postural abnormalities, and joint instability. Alterations in joint architecture, such as acetabular dysplasia or pistol-grip deformity of the hip, may play a role in development of osteoarthritis in this joint.

CLINICAL MANIFESTATIONS

The signs and symptoms of osteoarthritis depend on the joint or joints affected (see Plate 5-22). Most commonly involved are the weight-bearing joints (see Plate 5-23) and small joints of the hand.

Pain and restricted movement are the major clinical manifestations. The patient is usually comfortable at rest but finds weight bearing and moving the affected joints painful. Aching during rainy weather, stiffness after inactivity, and crepitation are other frequent complaints.

Physical examination reveals tenderness, pain and crepitation with joint movement, and, usually, a limited range of motion. Although signs of synovitis—warmth and erythema over the joint—are usually limited or absent, swelling exists in association with bony hypertrophy or if there is a joint effusion.

Knee Joint Involvement

Of the large joints, the knee is most often affected. Because the knee is so crucial in the lever action of the leg and in ambulation, osteoarthritis in this joint can be both very painful and disabling, especially when it is bilateral (see Plate 5-24). The medial compartment of the knee is usually more severely damaged than the lateral compartment. The structural damage in the joint causes pain, restriction of motion, and crepitation. Subluxation and angular deformities are late sequelae.

Hand Involvement

Some clinical manifestations are unique to particular joints. Heberden's and Bouchard's nodes, hallmarks of osteoarthritis, develop at the distal and proximal interphalangeal joints of the fingers (see Plate 5-25).

Plate 5-24

Rheumatic Diseases

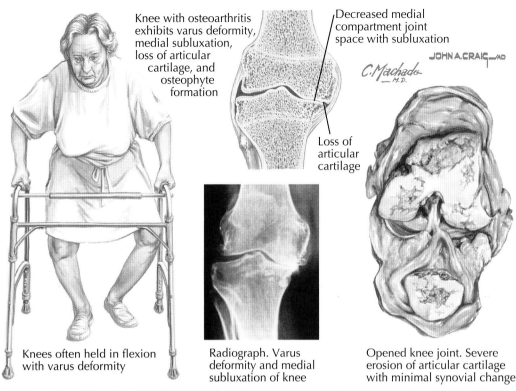

Knee with osteoarthritis exhibits varus deformity, medial subluxation, loss of articular cartilage, and osteophyte formation

Decreased medial compartment joint space with subluxation

JOHN A. CRAIG

Loss of articular cartilage

Knees often held in flexion with varus deformity

Radiograph. Varus deformity and medial subluxation of knee

Opened knee joint. Severe erosion of articular cartilage with minimal synovial change

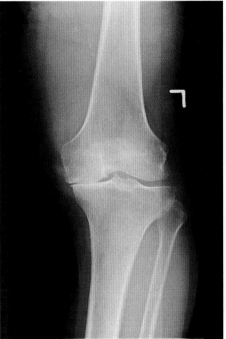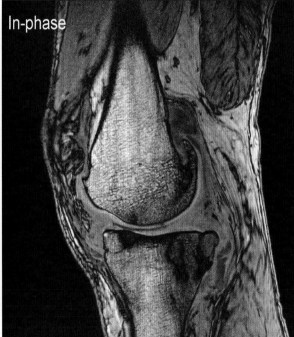

In-phase

Semi-flexed AP view (left) and MRI (right) of left knee. In addition to joint space narrowing (cartilage loss) and osteophyte formation seen on routine X-ray, MRI provides scoring of a number of additional features such as subarticular bone marrow edema, synovitis, and meniscal integrity.
Courtesy of Dr. Steven B Abramson

OSTEOARTHRITIS *(Continued)*

Although the cartilage of the distal and proximal interphalangeal joint is degenerating, osteophytes grow from the dorsomedial and dorsolateral aspects of the base of the distal phalanx to produce these nodular protuberances. Flexion deformity may occur when the pathologic changes are severe. Early in their development, the nodes are tender and painful; when mature, they are often asymptomatic but may have significant cosmetic effects. Heberden's nodes are more common in women and are often familial. Bouchard's nodes, similar to but less common than Heberden's nodes, develop at the proximal interphalangeal finger joints.

At the base of the thumb, the first carpometacarpal joint commonly undergoes the degenerative changes of osteoarthritis. Local tenderness and pain, usually severe, are exacerbated by firm grasping.

Hip Joint Involvement

Osteoarthritis of the hip (malum coxae senilis) is a major crippling and painful form of osteoarthritis. Standing and walking often cause severe localized hip pain that may radiate laterally as well as to the medial aspect of the thigh and knee. The articular cartilage becomes thin, cysts form in the femoral head and acetabulum, the bone softens, and the femoral head flattens. Osteophytes grow from the head of the femur and around the rim of the acetabulum (see Plates 5-26 and 5-27). As a result, joint motion becomes markedly restricted, leading to a fixed deformity of the hip in flexion, adduction, and external rotation. Trochanteric bursitis causing pain at the lateral aspect of the hip is often misdiagnosed as hip osteoarthritis.

Spine Involvement

Degenerative disease of the spine occurs to some degree in almost every person past middle age, but the severity and speed of progression vary greatly. Two types of spinal degeneration are characteristic: one affects the intervertebral discs and their adjacent vertebrae, and the other affects the diarthrodial, or apophyseal, joints. Degeneration of the cartilaginous discs with secondary pathologic changes commonly occur in parallel with facet disease. With aging, the intervertebral discs lose water and the gelatinous central core (nucleus pulposus) becomes hard and brittle. Defects develop in the surrounding fibrous material (anulus fibrosus), which becomes fibrillated. Fissures develop in the anulus fibrosus, through which the nucleus pulposus may herniate. The disc deteriorates and becomes thin, and disc fragments (and sometimes the entire degenerated disc) may become displaced and press on the spinal nerve roots. The vertebrae on either side of the thin disc become closer, putting a strain on the facets (see Plate

Plate 5-25

Musculoskeletal System: PART III

HAND INVOLVEMENT IN OSTEOARTHRITIS

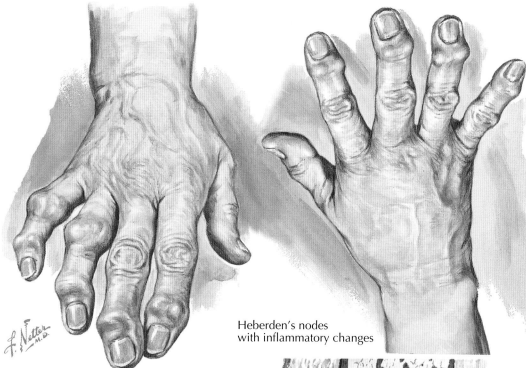

Heberden's nodes
with inflammatory changes

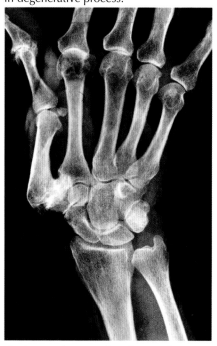

Chronic Heberden's nodes. 4th and 5th
proximal interphalangeal joints also involved
in degenerative process.

OSTEOARTHRITIS *(Continued)*

5-28). Bony spurs grow and protrude from the vertebral margins, sometimes uniting to form a bony bridge between the vertebrae. Intervertebral disc degeneration occurs chiefly where movement is greatest—in the cervical, lower thoracic, and lumbar regions. Movement of the spine causes localized pain, which is intensified by strenuous activity, especially lifting heavy objects.

Degeneration of spinal facets usually occurs in the cervical and lumbar regions in older persons. The degenerating articular cartilage becomes thin, the surface and margins become rough, and spurs grow from the bony edges. Joint motion is restricted and painful, and crepitation is common, especially in the cervical spine.

Neuropathies augment the clinical problems of degenerative disease of the spine. Spurs growing from vertebral margins adjacent to degenerated discs and from facet borders may narrow the foramina through which the spinal nerves exit. Pressure on and irritation of the nerve roots causes neuralgia, paresthesias, or paresis. Neuralgic pain in the occipital region and about the shoulders and arms may result from spurs in the cervical region; sciatic pain is caused by nerve root pressure from a protruding degenerated disc or spurs in the lumbar region. In the cervical spine, compression of the spinal cord from large osteophytes or from displaced degenerated discs may lead to serious neurologic complications manifested by upper motor neuron or long tract signs. The same type of spinal cord compression may result in spinal stenosis in the lumbar spine, leading to claudication and lower limb weakness.

LABORATORY STUDIES

Hematocrits, blood cell counts, ESR, and results of serum protein electrophoresis, blood chemistry studies, urinalysis, and other laboratory tests are usually normal

End-stage degenerative changes in
carpometacarpal articulation of thumb

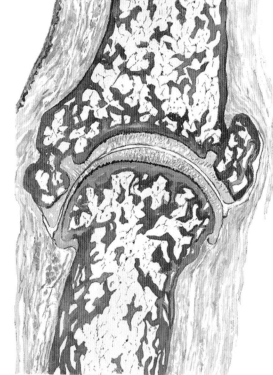

Section through distal interphalangeal joint shows irregular, hyperplastic bony nodules (Heberden's nodes) at articular margins of distal phalanx.

unless other diseases exist. If severe degenerative changes cause a secondary (traumatic) synovitis, the ESR may be slightly elevated. Serum rheumatoid factor may be positive, not as a result of osteoarthritis but due to elevations observed with aging or other disease states that may coexist with osteoarthritis. Synovial fluid analysis of involved peripheral joints reveals limited abnormalities with a slight increase in synovial fluid white blood cell count, usually less than 2000/µL.

Radiographs reveal characteristic diagnostic findings: cartilage thinning, osteophytes (spurs and bony bridging), and bone cysts.

DIAGNOSIS

Diagnosing osteoarthritis and differentiating it from rheumatoid arthritis are usually not difficult. The localization of pathology to one or a few weight-bearing

Plate 5-26

Rheumatic Diseases

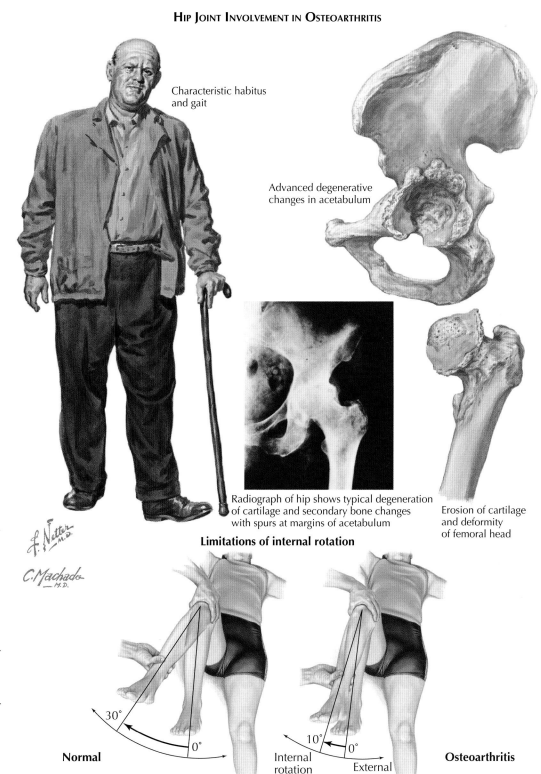

HIP JOINT INVOLVEMENT IN OSTEOARTHRITIS

Characteristic habitus and gait

Advanced degenerative changes in acetabulum

Radiograph of hip shows typical degeneration of cartilage and secondary bone changes with spurs at margins of acetabulum

Erosion of cartilage and deformity of femoral head

Limitations of internal rotation

Normal

30°

0°

Osteoarthritis

10°

0°

Internal rotation

External rotation

Loss of internal rotation with hip flexed is a sensitive and easy test of hip arthritis.

OSTEOARTHRITIS (Continued)

joints of the lower limbs, the spine, the distal and proximal interphalangeal finger joints, and/or first carpometacarpal joints in otherwise healthy older persons, together with normal results of laboratory studies and characteristic radiographs, confirms the diagnosis. However, the abnormalities seen in radiographs of the spine often do not parallel the clinical findings: extensive and severe pathologic changes may be seen in radiographs when the patient has only mild pain and disability. On the other hand, only minor osteophytic or degenerative changes seen in conventional radiographs of the spine may be accompanied by severe arthritic symptoms if the abnormalities are in a critical area. MRI is extremely helpful in delineating details of vertebral and disc alterations occurring in patients with spine involvement and allowing correlations with clinical symptomology. Similarly, MRI is helpful in delineating osteoarthritic changes related to osteoarthritis of the knee or hip joints (see Plates 5-24 and 5-26).

TREATMENT

Treatment is targeted to the following objectives: (1) relief of pain; (2) avoidance of trauma to or excessive use of affected joints; (3) correction of factors that produce strain on involved joints (e.g., overweight, vigorous weight-bearing exercise); (4) prevention or retarding progression of degenerative changes; and (5) maintenance or restoration of joint function. Therapy is benefited by a combination of nonpharmacologic and pharmacologic interventions.

Nonpharmacologic interventions include an umbrella-like group of approaches that should be universally considered in all patients. Advising and educating the patient as to treatment objectives and the importance of exercise, weight reduction, and joint protection is an important baseline initiative.

Joint Rest. Weight-bearing activity should be minimized, without unnecessarily limiting reasonable activities of daily living. Assistive devices such as canes or crutches are helpful in decreasing stresses across weight-bearing joints. Optimally, the cane or crutch should be used in the contralateral hand to the involved joint, although some patients find use of a nondominant hand difficult. Wheeled walkers may be necessary in the presence of bilateral disease. Excess stairs should be avoided if feasible. Knee braces can be helpful in

reducing pain, with simple elastic supports more likely to be used by the patient than metal hinge supports. In patients with spine disc degeneration and facet joint osteoarthritis, a firm mattress or bedboard relieves strain on the back. The use of a high seat is beneficial in protecting the knees from stress in getting in and out of a chair or with toileting.

Physical Therapy. Local heat and appliances to restrict joint motion help to relieve pain and stiffness. Aerobic, muscle-strengthening, and range of motion

Plate 5-27

Musculoskeletal System: PART III

DEGENERATIVE CHANGES

Early degenerative changes

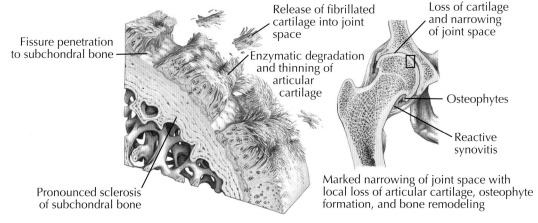

Early disruption of matrix molecular framework (increased water content and decreased proteoglycans)

Surface fibrillation of articular cartilage

Roughened articular surfaces and minimal narrowing of joint space

Superficial fissures

Sclerosis

Sclerosis (thickening) of subchondral bone, an early sign of degeneration

Narrowing of upper portion of joint space with early degeneration of articular cartilage

Advanced degenerative changes

Fissure penetration to subchondral bone

Release of fibrillated cartilage into joint space

Loss of cartilage and narrowing of joint space

Enzymatic degradation and thinning of articular cartilage

Osteophytes

Reactive synovitis

Pronounced sclerosis of subchondral bone

Marked narrowing of joint space with local loss of articular cartilage, osteophyte formation, and bone remodeling

End-stage degenerative changes

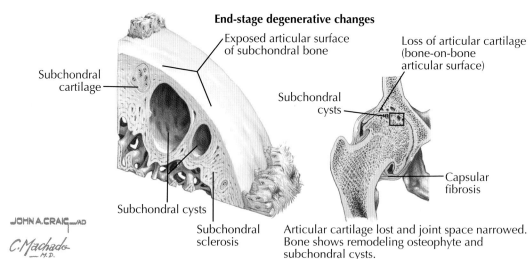

Exposed articular surface of subchondral bone

Loss of articular cartilage (bone-on-bone articular surface)

Subchondral cartilage

Subchondral cysts

Subchondral cysts

Capsular fibrosis

JOHN A.CRAIG—AD
C.Machado
—M.D.

Subchondral sclerosis

Articular cartilage lost and joint space narrowed. Bone shows remodeling osteophyte and subchondral cysts.

OSTEOARTHRITIS (Continued)

exercises are effective in maintaining maximal function. Hip or knee osteoarthritis is benefited by use of appropriate footwear. Lateral wedged insoles can shift weight laterally in patients with medial tibiofemoral compartment knee involvement. Use of traction and a support collar can significantly reduce pain in the cervical region, and a firm corset can be used to support the low back region.

Medications. Although patients will benefit to various degrees from nonpharmacologic approaches, most patients, unfortunately, will require analgesic and anti-inflammatory medicines. Simple analgesics such as acetaminophen can be effective in a number of patients, although not generally as efficacious as NSAIDs. Doses of acetaminophen up to 4 g/day have been recommended in the past, but concern regarding hepatic or renal toxicity with long-term high doses has led to a recommended maximum administration of 3 g/day as the appropriate dose. Alternative analgesics include tramadol and, in selected cases, low-dose opioids.

NSAIDs, either traditional nonselective or COX-2–selective agents, are generally more efficacious than analgesics alone. Although all NSAIDs, selective or nonselective, have the potential for gastrointestinal complications such as peptic ulceration, perforation or obstruction, the COX-2–selective agents appear to be less of a risk in this regard. If nonselective NSAIDS are used, either a proton pump inhibitor or a prostaglandin analog such as misoprostol can be added to protect the gastrointestinal tract.

Of concern was the observation that COX-2–selective NSAIDs were associated with significant cardiovascular side effects, including myocardial infarction. Unfortunately, cardiovascular side effects may be observed with traditional COX-1/COX-2–inhibiting NSAIDs as well. COX-2–selective NSAIDs are specifically contraindicated in the treatment of peripheral pain in the setting of coronary artery bypass surgery. The risk-benefit ratio of any therapeutic agent is key in regard to indications for its use, and a considered balancing of the benefits of diminished pain with improved quality of life versus therapeutic risk is an important consideration in any treatment paradigm.

Weak opioid therapy, carefully considered, is an important therapeutic option in patients with chronic pain related to peripheral joint or spine osteoarthritis not responding to other analgesics. As in all use of such agents, careful assessment for potential abuse is important. Adverse events such as constipation, nausea, and appetite loss, particularly in older individuals in whom osteoarthritis is more likely to be present, may limit their use.

Plate 5-28

Rheumatic Diseases

SPINE INVOLVEMENT IN OSTEOARTHRITIS

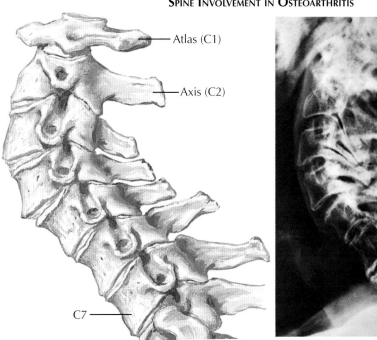

Atlas (C1)

Axis (C2)

C7

Extensive thinning of cervical discs and hyperextension deformity with narrowing of intervertebral foramina. Lateral radiograph reveals similar changes.

OSTEOARTHRITIS *(Continued)*

Topical NSAIDs or chili pepper–derived capsaicin administered locally are helpful in many patients with osteoarthritis and have the advantage of limited potential for toxicity.

Intra-articular corticosteroid administration is extremely helpful for local flares for relief of pain and inflammatory swelling. Too-frequent use should be avoided owing to concerns regarding joint overuse and aggravation of joint breakdown; repeated use more than four times a year is generally to be avoided. Intra-articular hyaluronan injections, approved for injection into the knee, may improve pain and function; these agents are slower than intra-articular corticosteroids with respect to clinical response but may provide a more prolonged duration of effect.

Glucosamine and chondroitin sulfate, available without prescription, have been described as being clinically beneficial, particularly on the basis of studies in osteoarthritis of the knee. Several agents such as diacerein and doxycycline, as well as glucosamine, chondroitin sulfate, avocado-soybean unsaponifiables, and intra-articular hyaluronans, have been described as being disease modifying; additional studies are required before such agents can be definitively identified as having an effect on the disease process. Structure-modifying drugs remain a "holy grail" of osteoarthritis therapy.

Additional Therapeutic Approaches. Acupuncture has been described as being of symptomatic benefit in peripheral joint osteoarthritis, but systematic reviews suggest that although sham-controlled trials show statistically significant benefits, the efficacy is variable.

Surgery. If the patient is otherwise healthy, joint replacement can markedly improve pain and function

Radiograph of thoracic spine shows narrowing of intervertebral spaces and spur formation.

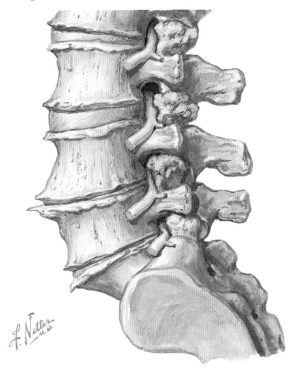

Degeneration of lumbar intervertebral discs and hypertrophic changes at vertebral margins with spur formation. Osteophytic encroachment on intervertebral foramina compresses spinal nerves.

in peripheral joints. Such joint replacement of the hip and knee is now a common procedure with a high success rate, allowing thousands of persons to regain joint movement with limited or no pain. Partial joint replacement (unicompartmental repair) is effective in a number of individuals with knee osteoarthritis, limiting time for rehabilitation with decreased operative risk. Repair of chondral defects using autologous

chondrocyte transplantation or mesenchymal stem cells is undergoing significant evaluation but remains investigational.

Surgery for degenerative spine disease may also be considered to relieve severe pain, eliminate pressure and irritation of spinal nerve roots and the spinal cord, and stabilize the spine, allowing rehabilitation of severely affected patients.

Plate 5-29   Musculoskeletal System: PART III

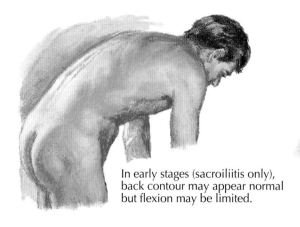

In early stages (sacroiliitis only), back contour may appear normal but flexion may be limited.

In more advanced sacroiliac plus lower spine involvement, back is straightened with "ironed-out" appearance.

ANKYLOSING SPONDYLITIS

Epidemiology. Ankylosing spondylitis is a chronic progressive arthritis that typically affects the joints of the spine and belongs to a group of conditions known as spondyloarthropathies. Spondyloarthritis is a group of several related but phenotypically different disorders that include psoriatic arthritis, reactive arthritis, a subgroup of JIA, arthritis related to inflammatory bowel disease, and ankylosing spondylitis, which is the prototype of the spondyloarthritis group.

The male-to-female ratio is approximately 3 to 1, with prevalence from 0.1% to 6.0% across different populations. The onset of clinical manifestations usually occurs in young adults.

Pathology. The primary pathologic change is an inflammatory process in the apophyseal and costovertebral articulations of the spine and the sacroiliac joints. Initially, the sacroiliac joints become inflamed bilaterally, and the disease can eventually spread up the spine. The speed of progression varies considerably from patient to patient, and the inflammation may stop at any spinal level or encompass the entire spine.

The presence of HLA-B27 in 80% to 90% of patients with ankylosing spondylitis suggests a direct and dominant genetic component. However, only a small group of people who carry the HLA-B27 (5% to 6% in white people) actually develop the disease, which means additional factors may be important. Advances in the genetics of spondyloarthritis have shown that disease association is more complex than with HLA-B27 alone and that there are non–HLA-B27 major histocompatibility complex (MHC) and non-MHC genes important in susceptibility to this disease. Over the past decade, almost 60 subtypes of HLA-B27 have been distinguished, but this has not been accompanied by a great deal of epidemiologic data to evaluate associations with the disease. Understanding of genetics (HLA-B27), the pathophysiology of inflammation (e.g., lesions on magnetic resonance imaging [MRI]), and structural damage is an area of active research and may evolve into new definitions of classification and diagnosis of spondyloarthropathies in the future.

Clinical Manifestations. In the early stage of the disease, patients complain of low back pain, which indicates inflammation of the spine and the sacroiliac joints; this can be accompanied by constitutional symptoms as well. The low back pain is typically worse in the morning and better with activity. Other early signs and symptoms include difficulty in arising from bed because of pain and muscle spasm in the low back, tenderness on pressure and percussion of the sacroiliac joints and lumbar spine, painful restricted motion of the low spine, and flattening of the normal lumbar lordosis (see Plate 5-29). If the cervical spine becomes affected, movement of the head and neck also becomes painful and limited. Chest expansion may be restricted as the costovertebral joints become involved. Some studies

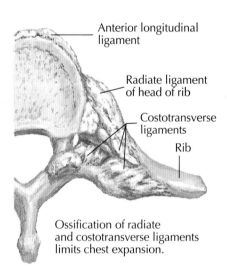

Bilateral sacroiliitis is an early radiographic sign. Thinning of cartilage and bone condensation on both sides of sacroiliac joints.

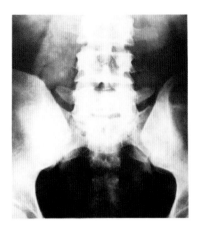

Anterior longitudinal ligament

Radiate ligament of head of rib

Costotransverse ligaments

Rib

Ossification of radiate and costotransverse ligaments limits chest expansion.

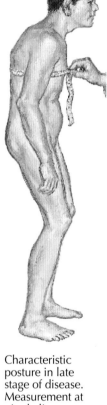

Characteristic posture in late stage of disease. Measurement at nipple line demonstrates diminished chest expansion.

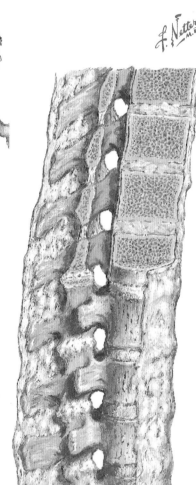

Ossification of anulus fibrosus of intervertebral discs, zygapophyseal joints, and anterior longitudinal and interspinous ligaments

show that half of the patients with ankylosing spondylitis reported temporomandibular joint symptoms when specifically questioned about them. Pain, stiffness, and swelling of peripheral joints may also occur. Enthesitis (inflammation of the enthesis) and dactylitis (diffuse swelling of digit[s] of hands or feet) can also be clinical manifestations of ankylosing spondylitis.

After years of disease activity, the inflammation may subside and pain abate, but because the ankylosis is irreversible, the spine remains rigid with limitation in spine mobility. In advanced disease, the thoracic spine may become kyphotic and the neck and head assume a fixed forward position. Affected hips are also painful, and movement is restricted; a complete, incapacitating ankylosis may result.

The most common extra-articular involvement is acute anterior uveitis. Iridocyclitis in one or both eyes may result in synechiae and impaired vision if it is

Plate 5-30   Rheumatic Diseases

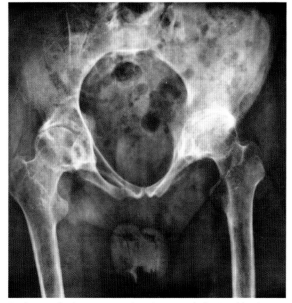

Radiograph shows complete bony ankylosis of both sacroiliac joints in late stage of disease.

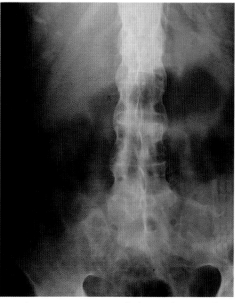

"Bamboo spine." Bony ankylosis of joints of lumbar spine. Ossification exaggerates bulges of intervertebral discs.

ANKYLOSING SPONDYLITIS
(Continued)

severe and untreated (see Plate 5-30). Cardiac involvement in ankylosing spondylitis can also occur in two distinct ways. First, there is an increase in subclinical atherosclerosis in patients with ankylosis spondylitis compared with controls, and early monitoring of possible cardiac involvement along with cardiac risk factor stratification may be helpful. Second, disturbances in cardiac conduction, usually first-degree atrioventricular block, are detected in about 10% of patients and dilatation of the aortic ring and insufficiency of the aortic valve may develop (see Plate 5-30). Less common extraarticular manifestations include pulmonary (apical fibrosis), renal, and bowel mucosal ulcerations.

The diagnosis of ankylosing spondylitis has been based on evidence of structural damage. The modified New York criteria require the presence of radiographic sacroiliitis to give a definite diagnosis. The major disadvantage of this specific criterion is that it can take up to 10 years for these structural changes to become visible on plain radiographs and consequently an early diagnosis cannot be made. Recognition of the drawbacks of these criteria focused on a specific subtype. The Assessment of Spondyloarthritis International Society (ASAS) did a large cross-sectional study to propose new criteria on the basis of the two main clinical features identified in daily practice: axial symptoms and peripheral involvement.

Radiographic Findings. One of the hallmarks of ankylosing spondylitis is involvement of the sacroiliac joints, and this has been the key radiographic finding that is needed to help confirm the diagnosis. In patients in whom ankylosing spondylitis is highly suggested and the plain radiographs do not reveal sacroiliac joint involvement, MRI has become the test of choice because it is more sensitive than plain radiographs to detect early changes of sacroiliac joint involvement. The earliest sign of involvement on MRI is bone marrow edema of the sacroiliac joint.

In the early stage of the disease, the bone on both sides of the sacroiliac joint and the bony borders are indistinct (see Plate 5-31). Later, the cartilage space narrows and erosions appear in the bordering bone. In the late stages, radiographs show complete ankylosis of the sacroiliac joints (see Plate 5-30). After the disease has progressed to involve the lumbar and thoracic spine, the facet borders become indistinct; then the cartilage space appears narrowed, and, later, bony ankylosis is apparent. Ossification of the outer layers of the anulus fibrosus is usually first seen at the L1-2 and T11-12 levels; later, the perispinous calcification spreads upward and downward. In severe, advanced disease, the calcification is continuous throughout the spine, producing a "bamboo spine" radiographic appearance (see Plate 5-30). There are specific

Complications

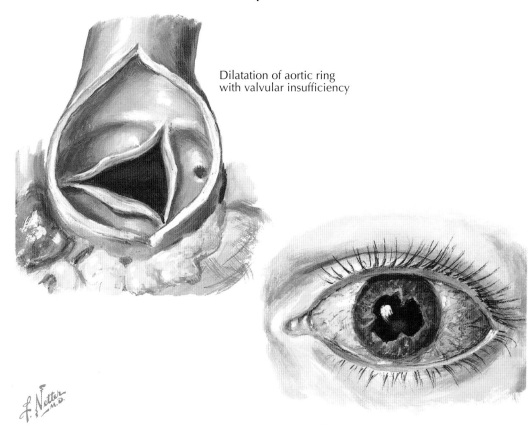

Dilatation of aortic ring with valvular insufficiency

Iridocyclitis with irregular pupil due to synechiae

proliferative changes in the last stages of ankylosing spondylitis, such as syndesmophytes, bridging syndesmophytes, ankylosis of the facet joints, calcification of the anterior longitudinal ligament, and anterior atlantoaxial (C1-2) subluxation, that are characteristic. Fractures can also be seen on radiographs, because minor movements with little trauma in late-stage disease may lead to spinal fractures. In advanced disease, there is radiographic evidence of bony ankylosis in many facets,

together with the perispinous calcification. Axial joints can also be affected in ankylosing spondylitis, which include the hips and shoulders, with radiographic changes that are similar to those seen in rheumatoid arthritis (see Plate 5-30).

Treatment/Prognosis. There has been remarkable advance in the management of ankylosing spondylitis over the past decade. The basis for these updates involves the development and validation of a new

Plate 5-31

Musculoskeletal System: PART III

DEGENERATIVE CHANGES IN THE CERVICAL VERTEBRAE

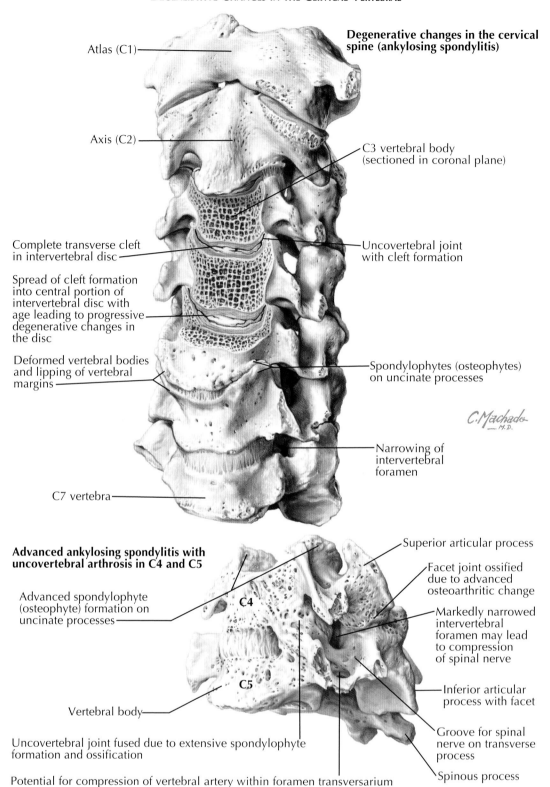

Degenerative changes in the cervical spine (ankylosing spondylitis)

Atlas (C1)

Axis (C2)

C3 vertebral body (sectioned in coronal plane)

Complete transverse cleft in intervertebral disc

Uncovertebral joint with cleft formation

Spread of cleft formation into central portion of intervertebral disc with age leading to progressive degenerative changes in the disc

Deformed vertebral bodies and lipping of vertebral margins

Spondylophytes (osteophytes) on uncinate processes

C7 vertebra

Narrowing of intervertebral foramen

C. Machado
— M.D.

Advanced ankylosing spondylitis with uncovertebral arthrosis in C4 and C5

Superior articular process

Facet joint ossified due to advanced osteoarthritic change

Advanced spondylophyte (osteophyte) formation on uncinate processes

C4

Markedly narrowed intervertebral foramen may lead to compression of spinal nerve

C5

Vertebral body

Inferior articular process with facet

Uncovertebral joint fused due to extensive spondylophyte formation and ossification

Groove for spinal nerve on transverse process

Potential for compression of vertebral artery within foramen transversarium

Spinous process

ANKYLOSING SPONDYLITIS
(Continued)

disease activity score and the new classification criteria for axial spondyloarthritis. New guidelines for the management of ankylosing spondylitis from the 2010 updated consensus of the ASAS/EULAR committee that include evidence-based disease management recommendations have been published. In general, the recommendations include a multidisciplinary approach using both pharmacologic and nonpharmacologic therapies. In addition, tailored approaches to manage ankylosing spondylitis now have included more focused treatment aimed at the predominant symptoms of ankylosing spondylitis, axial involvement, and enthesitis-related or predominantly peripheral arthritis. Extra-articular manifestations should also be treated. Although treatment of ankylosing spondylitis may be similar to that of rheumatoid arthritis in certain aspects, the new recommendations continue to recommend a very restricted role for traditional DMARDs, such as sulfasalazine or methotrexate, and systemic corticosteroids. When peripheral arthritis is predominate, sulfasalazine may be helpful; however, there are few high-quality, controlled trials of methotrexate in the treatment of ankylosing spondylitis. Regarding the recommendation for the use of anti–TNF-α agents, there are two changes. The use of anti–TNF-α agents is recommended for patients fulfilling modified New York criteria for definitive ankylosing spondylitis or the ASAS criteria for axial spondyloarthropathy. The pretreatment period using at least two NSAIDs before biologic therapy is significantly shorter—4 weeks, compared with 3 months. This leads to an earlier initiation of treatment within the ankylosing spondylitis disease spectrum.

- *NSAIDs* are considered the first-line treatment for ankylosing spondylitis using at least two different NSAIDs for 4 weeks. Careful attention should be focused on potential renal and cardiac side effects.
- *DMARDs, preferably sulfasalazine,* may be given along with NSAIDs to slow or stop the progression of the disease in patients with predominant peripheral arthritis.
- *Glucocorticoid* injections can be given in particularly painful and swollen joints that did not respond with other therapies. Systemic corticosteroids should be avoided if possible.
- *TNF inhibitors* are indicated in patients who have active disease in the spine and do not respond to NSAIDs and nonbiologic DMARDs.
- *Exercise and prevention methods* include a program of active, range-of-motion exercises for the spine, hips, and shoulders as well as deep-breathing exercises, abundant rest, especially early in the disease,

use of a firm mattress on a bed board and a firm armchair with a high seat, and application of heat. As the disease activity lessens, medications may be decreased and possibly discontinued, but exercises should be continued to maintain range of motion.
- *Joint replacement surgery* is indicated for pain and functional disability not responsive to medical therapy. Hip replacement is most common and

may cause severe pain and incapacitation, which is relieved by total hip replacement. Hip involvement can occur early in the ankylosing spondylitis disease process.
- *Physical therapy* with supervised exercises that are land or water based should be recommended. Physical therapy is not believed to prevent progression of the disease, but it may minimize the symptoms in some patients.

Plate 5-32

Rheumatic Diseases

PSORIATIC ARTHRITIS

Epidemiology. Psoriatic arthritis is an inflammatory arthritis associated with skin psoriasis. It occurs in approximately 30% of patients with psoriasis, leading to prevalence in the population of 0.3% to 1%. It affects women and men equally.

Clinical Manifestations. Most people who develop psoriatic arthritis have skin symptoms of psoriasis first; however, in 15% of people symptoms of arthritis may appear before the diagnosis of psoriasis. There are various patterns of psoriatic arthritis, and some patients may have overlapping patterns:

- *Distal arthritis*—predominantly affects distal joints of the fingers and toes and can be frequently accompanied by arthritis in a few large joints such as the knee or ankle (5% of the patients)
- *Oligoarthritis*—affecting four or fewer joints, often in an asymmetric distribution (70% of the patients)
- *Symmetric polyarthritis*—affects five or more joints on both sides of the body; may be difficult to distinguish from rheumatoid arthritis (15% of the patients)
- *Spondylitis variant*—affects the joints of the spine as well joints peripherally, which can be similar to ankylosing spondylitis
- *Arthritis mutilans*—destructive and mutilating changes of the phalanges adjacent to the inflamed joints (5% to 25% of the patients)

In addition, there are extra-articular manifestations:

- *Enthesitis*—inflammation at the site of tendon insertion into bone
- *Dactylitis (sausage digit)*—diffuse swelling of the entire finger or toe
- *Tenosynovitis (tendonitis)*—inflammation that may affect the flexor tendons of the fingers, the extensor carpi ulnaris, and other sites
- *Nail lesions* (pitting, onycholysis)

Radiographic Findings/Laboratory Studies. There are no specific laboratory tests for the diagnosis of psoriatic arthritis, but there are some important considerations when a patient with psoriasis presents with inflammatory arthritis:

- Typically the rheumatoid factor and anti-CCP antibody studies are negative, unless there is an overlap with rheumatoid arthritis.
- HLA-B27 is present in some patients.
- The joint pattern often affects distal interphalangeal joints, unlike in rheumatoid arthritis, which usually affects the metacarpophalangeal joints. Osteoarthritis may affect both distal and proximal interphalangeal joints and may be inflammatory.

Typical radiographic features of psoriatic arthritis include a characteristic pattern of bone resorption/erosion, hyperostosis, fusion, enthesopathy, and predilection for the distal phalanx.

Bone resorption/erosion in psoriatic arthritis is not always marginal (as in rheumatoid arthritis) and may involve the entire articular surface, which leads to joint space widening and the late stage of "pencil-in-cup" deformity.

Hyperostosis is a common and distinctive feature of psoriatic arthritis with increased sclerosis of the trabecular bone, fluffy bony productive changes around the erosions or away from the articulation (e.g., radial styloid), and periostitis along the small bones of hands and feet.

Enthesopathy is common at the calcaneal attachments of the plantar aponeurosis and Achilles tendon and is characterized by ill-defined erosion and surrounding hyperostosis.

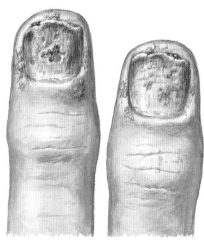

Pitting, discoloration, and erosion of fingernails with fusiform swelling of distal interphalangeal joints

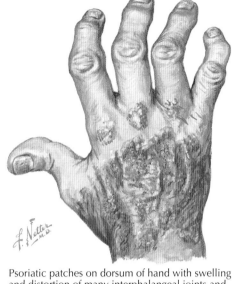

Psoriatic patches on dorsum of hand with swelling and distortion of many interphalangeal joints and shortening of fingers due to loss of bone mass

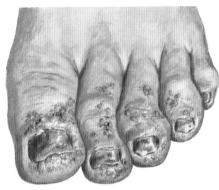

Toes with sausage-like swelling, skin lesions, and nail changes

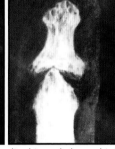

Radiographic changes in distal interphalangeal joint. *Left,* In early stages, bone erosions are seen at joint margins. *Right,* In late stages, further loss of bone mass produces "pencil point in cup" appearance.

Distal phalanx involvement is usually associated with nail disease. Typically seen are osteolysis and hyperostosis. Diffuse hyperostosis of a phalanx is called an ivory phalanx that is virtually pathognomonic of psoriatic arthritis.

Involvement of an entire digit or toe (dactylitis, sausage finger) is due to underlying tenosynovitis and involvement of the periarticular structures.

Involvement of the axial skeleton is common in psoriatic arthritis with radiographic features of spondylitis and sacroiliitis, similar to that in ankylosing spondylitis, but, in general, less diffuse and severe with a propensity for thick, irregular syndesmophytes.

Treatment. There is no cure for psoriatic arthritis, but there have been significant advances in treatment. Treatment can range from physical therapy and NSAIDs to help relieve the joint pain and stiffness symptoms to more aggressive treatment with DMARDs to slow and sometimes halt the progression of the destructive joint disease, especially when treatment is started early in the disease course. Patient screening questionnaires are now available to help diagnose psoriatic arthritis earlier in patients with psoriasis.

- *Physical and occupational therapy* as well as exercise may help to relieve the pain and stiffness and to maintain joint function.
- *NSAIDs* can be used in combination with DMARDs to help to control inflammation and relieve the

pain from psoriatic arthritis. NSAIDs must be taken continuously and at a sufficient dose to have an anti-inflammatory effect. These agents do not slow the progression of the arthritis.

- *DMARDs* should be used early in patients with aggressive and potentially destructive joint disease. DMARDs that should be considered include methotrexate and anti–TNF-α inhibitors (also known as biologic DMARDs).
- *Biologic DMARDs* work primarily by blocking or neutralizing the effects of TNF-α, which is thought to be overexpressed in patients with psoriatic arthritis. These agents usually work rapidly, often within 2 to 4 weeks, and may be used alone or in combination with other DMARDs such as methotrexate.
- *Intra-articular and low-dose glucocorticoids (corticosteroids)* may be used to suppress inflammation and relieve pain until the treatment with DMARDs is established. Oral glucocorticoids should be avoided due to the chance of developing worsening psoriasis.

A family history of psoriasis, extensive skin involvement, disease onset age younger than 20 years, expression of HLA-B27, HLA-B39, or other alleles, and polyarticular and erosive disease may be factors that are predictive of a worse prognosis. It is also important to screen for psoriatic arthritis in patients with psoriasis to help ensure early diagnosis.

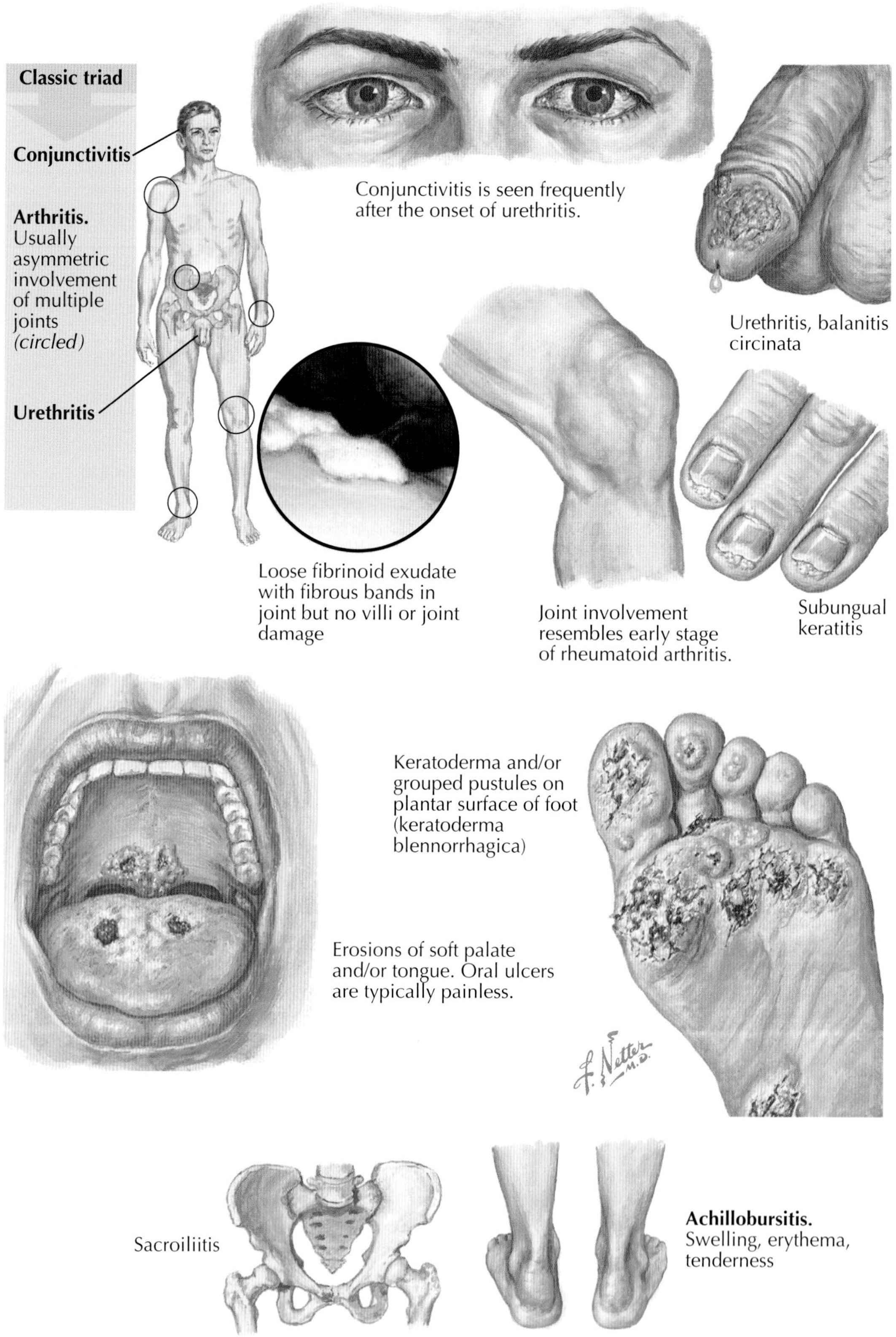

Plate 5-33

Musculoskeletal System: PART III

REACTIVE ARTHRITIS (FORMERLY REITER SYNDROME)

Also classified as a member of the spondyloarthritis group, reactive arthritis is a type of arthritis that manifests as joint pain and swelling after an infection, most commonly in the gastrointestinal tract or genitourinary tract. Traditionally, the presentation includes a triad of postinfectious arthritis, urethritis, and conjunctivitis collectively known as Reiter syndrome. Because diagnostic or classification criteria have not been validated or universally accepted, reactive arthritis is now considered an evolving concept of a spondyloarthritis that develops after an extra-articular infection.

Two types of bacteria cause reactive arthritis in the majority of cases:
- Bacteria that cause bowel infection such as *Salmonella, Shigella, Yersinia, Campylobacter, Clostridium difficile*, and *Chlamydia pneumoniae*
- Bacteria that cause genital infection, such as *Chlamydia*

Reactive arthritis typically occurs in men between 20 and 40 years old. It can appear in women also, usually with milder signs and symptoms. The genetic factor may play a role in the likelihood of developing reactive arthritis; however, HLA-B27 is found in less than 50% of cases. Thus, HLA-B27 testing is reserved for patients with a high to intermediate likelihood of having reactive arthritis and has little diagnostic value in isolation.

Clinical Manifestations. The symptoms of reactive arthritis generally appear 1 to 4 weeks after the triggering infection, with asymmetric oligoarthritis of the extremities as the most common pattern. Other musculoskeletal features include enthesitis, sausage digits (dactylitis), and low back pain.

Genital and urinary symptoms may include genital lesions, pain or burning during urination, rash, redness or inflammation, increased frequency of urination, and urethral discharge. Eye involvement in reactive arthritis can manifest with conjunctivitis and uveitis. Cutaneous signs of the disease include oral and genital ulcers and characteristic keratosis on the palms and soles.

Imaging. The diagnosis of reactive arthritis cannot be established with bone radiographs alone, but they can be used to exclude other types of arthritis with similar presentations. Because enthesitis is common, additional imaging such as ultrasonography, MRI, or bone scanning can be used to document changes suggestive of enthesitis.

Treatment/Prognosis. In general, the prognosis is good. The disease may be self-limiting, lasting only a few weeks or months, although attacks may last as long as a year. A small group of patients may develop

Classic triad

Conjunctivitis

Arthritis. Usually asymmetric involvement of multiple joints *(circled)*

Urethritis

Conjunctivitis is seen frequently after the onset of urethritis.

Urethritis, balanitis circinata

Subungual keratitis

Joint involvement resembles early stage of rheumatoid arthritis.

Loose fibrinoid exudate with fibrous bands in joint but no villi or joint damage

Keratoderma and/or grouped pustules on plantar surface of foot (keratoderma blennorrhagica)

Erosions of soft palate and/or tongue. Oral ulcers are typically painless.

Sacroiliitis

Achillobursitis. Swelling, erythema, tenderness

persistent joint symptoms for years that may be associated with HLA-B27.

Therapy for the arthritic component includes the following:
- NSAIDs to relieve the pain and inflammation are the mainstay of treatment.
- Intra-articular corticosteroid injection may be used if the joint is persistently inflamed.

- DMARDs (sulfasalazine) or anti–TNF-α agents may be used if the symptoms do not improve after therapy with NSAIDs or corticosteroids.
- Physical therapy can help to improve joint function.

Antibiotics to eliminate the documented infection may be prescribed; however, long-term chronic antibiotic therapy is not recommended in reactive arthritis.

Plate 5-34

Rheumatic Diseases

INFECTIOUS ARTHRITIS

Although almost every known bacteria and some viruses, yeasts, and fungi have been implicated, the microorganisms most commonly responsible for acute infectious arthritis in adults are gonococci, staphylococci, and streptococci. The incidence of pyogenic arthritis is higher in children than in adults. Factors that predispose to the development of infectious arthritis are bacteremia, integrity of host immune function, and the tendency of some organisms to attach to the vascular synovial membrane. In addition to being bloodborne, microorganisms may invade the joint tissues from juxta-articular infection or they may be introduced by intra-articular injection, penetrating wound, or surgery.

Pathogenesis. Microorganisms first traverse the highly vascular synovial membrane and subsynovial tissue, where they propagate. This incites an acute inflammatory process characterized histologically by infiltration with polymorphonuclear cells and later with lymphocytes and mononuclear cells, tissue proliferation, and neovascularization. If the inflammatory process spreads into the joint cavity, a purulent exudate develops in the joint space, producing a septic joint. Enzymes released from the bacteria and leukocytes rapidly destroy articular cartilages and bone, causing severe structural damage and joint dysfunction; ankylosis may result.

Clinical Manifestations. Septic arthritis presents as joint pain, with swelling that is evident on examination of peripheral joints. Initially, patients may not have fever, rigors, or even leukocytosis. The presence or absence of these symptoms and laboratory findings thus may not distinguish infection from crystal-induced arthritis. A source for the infection is often not found. Gram-negative infections, other than gonococcal, tend to occur in patients with underlying factors such as malignancy, diabetes, immunosuppression, or gram-negative infection elsewhere.

Diagnosis/Treatment. Prompt identification and treatment of infectious arthritis is essential to prevent irreversible joint damage and mortality. Infectious arthritis should be suspected in all cases of acute articular inflammation in one or two joints, particularly in young adults and children who are far less likely to experience gout or pseudogout. The causative organism should be determined immediately by examination of all mucosal areas, repeated blood cultures, and, especially, analysis of smears and culture of fluid from the inflamed joint. A complete joint examination should be undertaken, including the spine, and alternative disease processes such as psoriasis, reactive arthritis, and inflammatory bowel disease should be sought by history and examination. If a septic joint is suspected, and the causative infectious agent has not yet been identified, initial therapy should be instituted covering staphylococci (including methicillin-resistant staphylococci

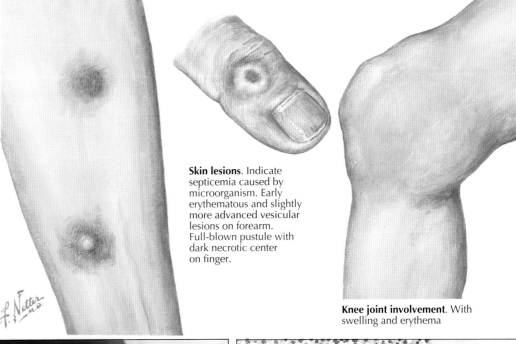

Skin lesions. Indicate septicemia caused by microorganism. Early erythematous and slightly more advanced vesicular lesions on forearm. Full-blown pustule with dark necrotic center on finger.

Knee joint involvement. With swelling and erythema

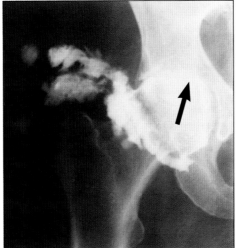

Anthrogram. Shows destruction of cartilage and bone (aspiration yielded purulent fluid)

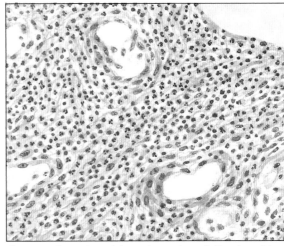

Biopsy specimen. Synovial membrane shows infiltration with polymorphonuclear cells, lymphocytes, and mononuclear cells, and tissue proliferation with neovascularization.

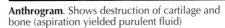
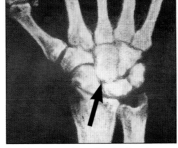
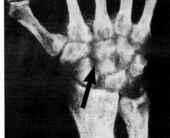
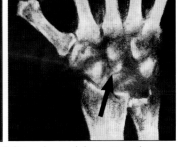

Rapid progression of wrist involvement. Within 4 weeks, from almost normal (left) to advanced destruction of articular cartilages and severe osteoporosis (right)

[MRSA]) and gonococci or gram-negative organism *if* the clinical scenario suggests these are reasonably likely. Infected joint fluid, especially if purulent, should be aspirated daily until the infection is controlled (or infection excluded). As soon as the causative agent is isolated and the antibiotic susceptibilities identified, parenteral antimicrobial therapy should be tailored to culture results and continued until the infection is cured. Septic joints that respond slowly to antibiotic therapy may require arthroscopic or open drainage, and this should be considered early if the joint is not amenable to frequent drainage, the patient is immunosuppressed, there was a delay in diagnosis, or the fluid is extremely thick and adequate drainage is not possible with arthrocentesis. Patients generally require post-treatment rehabilitation.

Plate 5-35

Musculoskeletal System: PART III

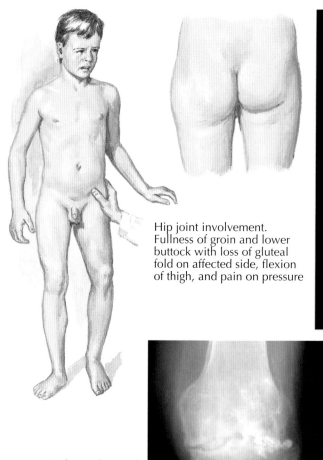

Hip joint involvement. Fullness of groin and lower buttock with loss of gluteal fold on affected side, flexion of thigh, and pain on pressure

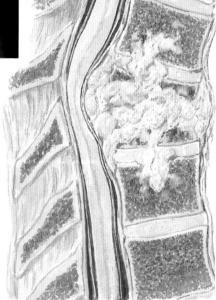

Advanced hip joint involvement shows extensive destruction.

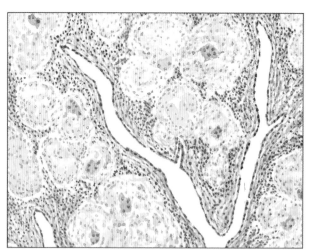

Radiograph reveals degeneration of knee joint and calcified granulomatous material.

TUBERCULOUS ARTHRITIS

The incidence of tuberculous arthritis has declined sharply. However, because of its seriousness, the possibility of tuberculosis should be considered in chronic unexplained proliferative monarticular or oligoarticular arthritis. This is especially true in patients who are immunosuppressed, are on TNF-α inhibitors, or have a history of latent or active tuberculosis.

Clinical Manifestations. Tuberculous arthritis often involves only one joint. In order of frequency, the joints affected are the spine, hip, knee, elbow, ankle, sacroiliac, shoulder, and wrist. The onset of symptoms may be insidious. In children, the first symptom is often a limp or severe muscle spasm that occurs at night. Clinical examination reveals a "doughy" swelling (without erythema) of joints in the limbs, with fluid accumulation and early, severe, localized muscle atrophy. When the spine is involved (Pott disease), walking and negotiating steps are painful. Pott disease often causes anterior wedging of the vertebrae, resulting in an angular kyphosis that is evident on physical examination. Signs of spinal cord compression varying from reflex changes to paraplegia may occur. In late-stage infection, draining sinuses may develop around the affected area.

Radiographic Findings. Radiographs help to establish the diagnosis. The earliest observable change is the decalcification of bone near the diseased joint. Later, marked irregularity and narrowing of the cartilage space indicate subchondral bone invasion. Decreased density of cortical bone is evidence of regional atrophy

Biopsy specimen of synovial membrane shows conglomerate caseating tubercles.

Tuberculous osteomyelitis of spine (Pott disease) with angulation and compression of spinal cord

of bone. In advanced disease, bone necrosis may be extensive, resulting in complete destruction of the joint architecture. Soft tissue shadows of abscesses may be evident.

Laboratory Studies. The tuberculin skin test (or an IFN-γ release assay) is usually strongly positive. In about 50% of patients, chest radiographs show pulmonary tuberculosis. Laboratory tests are usually needed to confirm the diagnosis.

Synovial fluid analysis often reveals a white blood cell count of more than 10,000/mm³ with a high content of mononuclear cells (neutrophils) in early infection. Examination of stained smears of synovial fluid seldom shows acid-fast bacilli, but culture of synovial tissue obtained via biopsy is usually positive.

Treatment. Prolonged chemotherapy is usually curative, even in advanced cases. Surgical drainage, synovectomy, or fusion may be required.

Plate 5-36

Rheumatic Diseases

HEMOPHILIC ARTHRITIS

Hemophilia A is an X-linked recessive disorder that occurs almost exclusively in males (between 1 in 5,000 to 10,000 births). It is caused by factor VIII deficiency. Hemophilia B (Christmas disease) is caused by factor IX deficiency. Morbidity in the hemophilic patient results from hemorrhage and its consequences. The most common site of bleeding in patients is bleeding into the joint (hemarthrosis), which accounts for 80% of bleeding episodes. Hemarthrosis can occur at any stage of life. The age at onset and frequency depend on the degree of factor deficiency. Trauma to the joint is the usual immediate cause of bleeding, although spontaneous hemarthroses may occur in severe hemophiliacs. The injury may be mild and go unnoticed until the hemorrhage is recognized. The most commonly involved joints are those most vulnerable to injury: knees, elbows, and ankles and, less often, shoulders, hips, and small joints of the hands and feet. The arthropathy is believed to be a result of intra-articular bleeding as well as iron deposition in both synovial membrane and articular cartilage. Prothrombin and fibrinogen are absent in synovial joint fluid, which means that the blood does not clot and remains liquid. Synovial lining cells phagocytose red cells, resulting in hemosiderin deposition and creating a proliferative synovitis and pannus, which is destructive (see Plate 5-36).

Hemarthrosis symptoms vary with the severity of the hemorrhage. A larger hemorrhage initiates an acute inflammatory reaction in the joint, which becomes swollen, warm, very tender, and painful to move. Fever and leukocytosis are common associated findings. When joint hemorrhage and synovitis are mild, the arthritis may resolve completely in a few days; if they are severe, the joint inflammation may persist for several months. Excessive iron deposition in synovial lining cells from repeated hemarthroses results in a chronic arthritis that is characterized by villous proliferation of the synovium with few lymphocytes and significant fibrosis. Invasive pannus may develop, leading to cartilage destruction and erosion, creating a secondary osteoarthritis with permanent joint destruction and disability. Extensive bleeding into the muscles around the affected joint may cause hematomas that compress adjacent nerves or blood vessels, or both, further restricting joint motion.

Radiographic Findings. Soft tissue shadows indicate acute hemorrhage into the joint. After repeated hemarthroses, joint radiographs reveal cartilage thinning, narrowing of joint space, rough subchondral bone, marginal spurs, bone cysts, and a thick joint capsule. These same findings are seen in the older patient with osteoarthritis. Radiographic findings unique to hemophilic arthritis are soft tissue densities of hemosiderin deposits, hypertrophy of epiphyses adjacent to the affected joint, enlargement of the radial head, flattening of the articular surface ("squaring") of the patella, slipped capital femoral epiphysis, and, sometimes, deformity or even destruction of the femoral head.

Treatment. Prophylactic clotting factor replacement therapy can decrease the frequency of hemarthroses and help prevent hemophilic arthropathy. Recombinant factor VIII therapy is administered prophylactically to children who have severe hemophilia (factor levels often < 1% of normal). This will reduce the rate of spontaneous bleeding in these patients. Desmopressin, a synthetic analog of vasopressin, can transiently stimulate increase production of factor VIII and can be used in patients with milder forms of the disease. Patients

Swelling of right knee joint and atrophy of thigh muscles in young boy are signs of hemophilic arthritis resulting from repeated hemarthroses. Purpuric patches on left leg and knee are from recent hemorrhages.

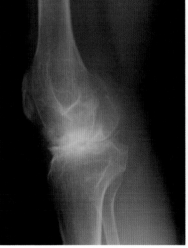

Synovial membrane in chronic disease shows extensive deposits of hemosiderin in lining cells and synovial stroma; reactive fibrosis

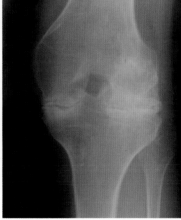

Radiographs of left knee joint show narrowing of joint space (due to loss of articular cartilage), irregular articular surfaces, osteophyte formation, and cyst formation in subchondral bone secondary to multiple hemarthroses.

should make every effort to prevent joint trauma. Children and adults receiving prophylactic therapy may participate in sports with judicious supervision and precautions. High-contact sports should be avoided. Prompt treatment of acute hemarthrosis helps to minimize structural damage that can cause chronic joint disability. On demand factor replacement should be given. The affected joint should be immobilized immediately and ice packs and analgesic drugs used to reduce pain. NSAIDs that inhibit platelets are contraindicated.

After administration of a coagulation factor, blood from the distended joint can be aspirated to relieve pain

and reduce articular damage. After the bleeding and synovitis have subsided, an active physical therapy program is started to restore full joint motion. Intra-articular injections of glucocorticosteroids may reduce joint pain and stiffness. Surgical synovectomy is useful to treat proliferative synovitis and joint damage but has significant morbidity. Arthroscopic synovectomy has fewer complications. Chemical synovectomy (intra-articular injection of osmic acid or other sclerosing agent) and radiation synovectomy (intra-articular injections of yttrium-90 or other agent) demonstrate short-term efficacy. Total joint arthroplasty should be considered for advanced joint disease.

Plate 5-37

Musculoskeletal System: PART III

NEUROPATHIC JOINT DISEASE

Neuropathic joint disease (Charcot joint) is a chronic degenerative disorder caused by a disturbance of the nerve supply to the affected joint. Diagnosis is based on typical clinical and radiographic findings and requires identification of the underlying neurologic disorder.

Many different diseases can cause the arthropathy. The leading cause in Western countries is diabetic neuropathy, and neuropathic arthropathy occurs in approximately 7.5% of diabetic patients but more frequently in those with significant clinical evidence of neuropathy. Charcot joints are also associated with syringomyelia, tabes dorsalis, myelomeningocele, and a group of miscellaneous neurologic disorders, including spina bifida and Charcot-Marie-Tooth disease among others. The loss of proprioception and pain sensation leads to the relaxation of the ligaments and other structures that support the joint. Dysregulation of blood flow to the joint due to abnormalities in the autonomic nervous system contribute to an imbalance between bone formation and resorption. Joint instability results, and, later, injuries related to either daily activities or the neurologic dysfunctions initiate the destruction of bone and cartilage. These changes are similar to those seen in advanced osteoarthritis.

The joints affected depend on the primary neurologic disorder. Diabetic neuropathy most frequently involves the tarsal, metatarsal, and ankle joints. In tabes dorsalis the knee, hip, ankle, and lower thoracic and lumbar vertebrae are most often affected. In syringomyelia, the elbow or shoulder is the site of involvement.

Clinical Manifestations. Patients most often present with a monarthritis. Insidious swelling or instability (or both) of the involved joint is usually the first abnormality noted, followed by effusion and joint destruction. Pain, however, is relatively mild and less than expected based on examination and radiographic findings. Physical examination reveals an enlarged, hypermobile, and slightly tender joint with a large effusion. The effusion and enlargement gradually increase. Late in the disease process, the prominent sign is crepitation, caused by the extensive destruction of cartilage and bone and the accumulation of intra-articular loose bodies. In diabetic neuropathy, the foot widens and the ankle becomes irregularly swollen. Patients may develop spontaneous fractures or dislocations. In the diabetic foot, the toes, midfoot, tarsometatarsal joints, ankle, and calcaneus can be involved. Skin ulcers overlying the areas of joint involvement may occur. Synovial fluid is typically non-inflammatory and may be hemorrhagic.

Radiographic Findings. At first, radiographs may appear basically normal, revealing only joint effusion. Often, soft tissue swelling is massive. Later, loss of cartilage and resorption and fragmentation of bone create a radiographic appearance of numerous loose bodies, bony displacement, and unusually shaped osteophytes at the joint margins. The joint looks like a "bag

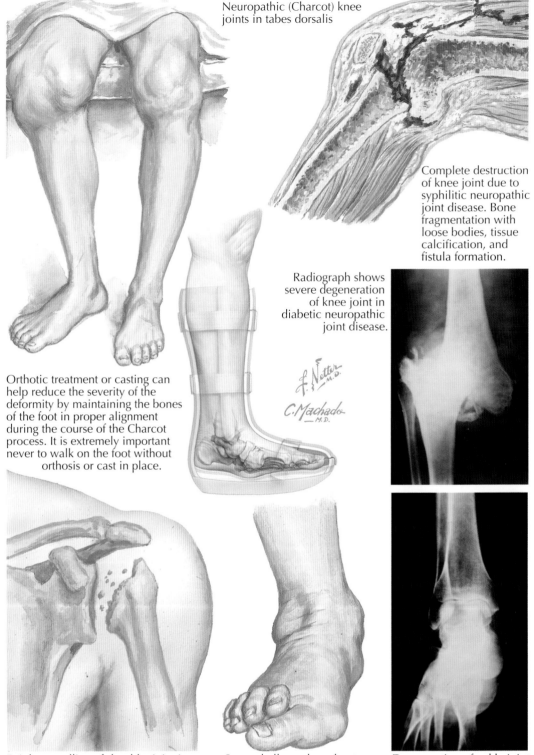

Neuropathic (Charcot) knee joints in tabes dorsalis

Complete destruction of knee joint due to syphilitic neuropathic joint disease. Bone fragmentation with loose bodies, tissue calcification, and fistula formation.

Radiograph shows severe degeneration of knee joint in diabetic neuropathic joint disease.

Orthotic treatment or casting can help reduce the severity of the deformity by maintaining the bones of the foot in proper alignment during the course of the Charcot process. It is extremely important never to walk on the foot without orthosis or cast in place.

Painless swelling of shoulder joint in syringomyelia with extensive loss of bone mass, effusion, and detritus

Severe hallux valgus due to diabetic neuropathic joint disease. Ankle also involved.

Degeneration of ankle joint in diabetic neuropathic joint disease

of bones." MRI may be helpful in diagnosis in the early stages, confirming syringomyelia and differentiating osteomyelitis from neuropathic joint changes.

Treatment. Prompt attention to minor trauma is important to prevent progressive of joint disease. Supportive measures such as the use of braces, splints, orthotics, or casts to stabilize the joint and crutches or a walker may help to decrease the disability. Physical therapy to promote strengthening and occupational therapy to assist in skills of activities of daily living should be considered. Bisphosphonates may be of value in retarding damage in the early phases of Charcot arthropathy. Arthrodesis (joint fusion) may be useful in the foot, ankle, knee, or spine after healing of the active phase. Arthroplasty (total joint replacement) has generally been less effective.

Plate 5-38

Rheumatic Diseases

GOUT AND GOUTY ARTHRITIS

Gout is a disturbance of uric acid metabolism in which the concentration of urate in the blood and body tissues is elevated above its point of solubility (6.7 mg/dL). Acute gouty arthritis is a direct result of the inflammatory response to urate crystals deposited in joint structures. Primary gout, also described as classic or idiopathic gout, is an inherited inborn error of metabolism and is almost always associated with inefficient renal excretion of uric acid. Secondary gout is a consequence of elevated uric acid levels due to systemic illness or drug.

PRIMARY GOUT

Gout is diagnosed mainly in males. Males have higher levels of serum uric acid than women until menopause because estrogen has a uricosuric effect. Although the genetic factors underlying hyperuricemia are presumably present at birth, the disorder produces no clinical signs or symptoms until the hyperuricemia has persisted for years. Clinical manifestations of gout usually appear in middle age in males (age 30 to 50 years) and later in females (see Plate 5-38). Patients with severe hyperuricemia, and some others for unexplained reasons, may develop gout attacks at a younger age.

Pathogenesis. The excessive concentration of uric acid in the blood is responsible for gouty arthritis. Some of the factors contributing to hyperuricemia (in addition to the renal inefficiency in excreting uric acid) include obesity, meat and seafood ingestion, beer and liquor use, and low dairy intake. Factors that can induce an acute attack of gouty arthritis include sudden increase or decrease in the level of (chronically elevated) serum uric acid, surgery, fasting, alcohol ingestion, and joint trauma. The mechanisms of crystal nucleation are not fully understood, but formed urate crystals are phagocytosed by synovial cells and neutrophils, resulting in the release of proinflammatory mediators, including IL-1.

Clinical Manifestations. The first clinical evidence of gout is usually acute arthritis in one or a few peripheral joints. A fulminant synovitis begins abruptly, typically during the night, frequently involving the first metatarsophalangeal joint, midfoot, or other lower extremity joint. The acute involvement of the great toe is known as podagra. The affected joint becomes very swollen, red, hot, tender, and excruciatingly painful (see Plate 5-38). Fever and leukocytosis may accompany the attack, and the ESR may be increased. Hence, acute gout cannot be reliably distinguished from acute septic arthritis. If untreated, acute monarticular gouty arthritis lasts 3 or 4 days; if several joints are severely inflamed, the attack may persist 2 or 3 weeks. The patient may remain asymptomatic until the next attack. After several attacks the gouty episodes tend to be more severe, last longer, and involve several additional joints, tendons, or bursae.

After several years of persistent hyperuricemia, deposits of monosodium urate known as tophi form in joint structures (and other tissues). Tophi are the hallmark of chronic gout, occurring in a significant minority of patients. If tophi are periarticular, the affected joints show irregular knobby swelling and signs of chronic inflammation. Joint motion is limited and painful, deformities develop, and sinuses may form at the swollen joint, from which a chalky exudate drains

Infancy
Inborn metabolic error, but no hyperuricemia or gout

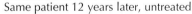

Puberty
In males, hyperuricemia develops, but no clinical signs of gout. In females, hyperuricemia appears later and more rarely.

Adulthood
(30-50 years) Acute gout. Great toe swollen, red, painful

After repeated attacks
Chronic tophaceous arthritis

Early tophaceous gouty arthritis

Same patient 12 years later, untreated

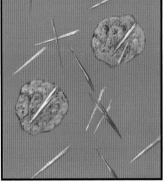

Free and phagocytized monosodium urate crystals in aspirated joint fluid seen on compensated polarized light microscopy

from the underlying urate deposits. Tophi often form in extra-articular structures as well, especially in the extensor tendons of the fingers and toes, the olecranon and infrapatellar bursae, the calcaneal tendon, the cartilage of the external ear, and the parenchyma of the kidney (see Plate 5-39).

Gout in women may initially involve several joints and may include the distal interphalangeal finger joints. This latter pattern of acutely inflamed Heberden's nodes mimics and is often misdiagnosed as

inflammatory osteoarthritis. Thiazide diuretics may predispose to this form of gouty arthritis.

Radiographs show marked destruction of bone and cartilage and "punched-out" areas in the bone with adjacent bone proliferation stimulated by the urate deposits (see Plate 5-38).

Diagnosis. Diagnosis is problematic only in the first or early attacks of acute arthritis. Gout should always be suspected when acute synovitis develops in a few small joints, especially in the great toe of an older

Plate 5-39

Musculoskeletal System: PART III

GOUT AND GOUTY ARTHRITIS
(Continued)

person, particularly a male. A history of gout in close relatives and the finding of hyperuricemia support the diagnosis but are certainly NOT definitive. Additional evidence is a quick and complete resolution of the synovitis after oral colchicine or NSAIDs. The presence of urate crystals in synovial fluid taken from the inflamed joint confirms the diagnosis and is the gold standard for the diagnosis, which should ideally be achieved before initiating lifetime therapy designed to lower serum uric acid levels and reduce attacks.

Late in the disease, the presence of tophi or characteristic radiographic findings makes the diagnosis obvious. A classic radiographic finding is the overhanging ledge, which represents intraosseous tophi that break through cortical bone (see Plate 5-38).

SECONDARY GOUT

Hyperuricemia and gout may be a consequence of the overproduction of uric acid caused by an increased turnover of nucleic acids in myeloproliferative disorders, sickle cell anemia and other hemoglobinopathies, psoriasis, and other chronic diseases characterized by high rates of proliferation. Decreased excretion of uric acid can be a cause of secondary gout with prolonged use of diuretics and in nephritis due to lead poisoning (saturnine gout) or selective tubular dysfunction.

TREATMENT

Acute gouty arthritis can be effectively treated with high-dose NSAIDs, prednisone, intra-articular corticosteroids, an IL-1 antagonist, and, in some patients, with a low dose (1.2 mg followed by 0.6 mg 1 hour later) of colchicine. The choice of agent is usually dictated by comorbidities, patient preference, and cost. In the intercritical period between attacks, if the hyperuricemia is not excessive and the attacks are mild and infrequent, small daily doses of colchicine may suffice as prophylactic treatment. When the serum uric acid concentration is persistently high and attacks are frequent, and in all cases of chronic tophaceous gout, the serum uric acid level should be reduced to a level significantly below the saturation level of 6.7 mg/dL for the rest of the patient's life. In most cases, this can be accomplished with administration of adequate daily dosages of the xanthine oxidase inhibitor allopurinol. Severe gout may require concurrent therapy with allopurinol and a uricosuric drug if the renal function is fairly normal. Frequent determinations of the serum uric acid concentration are required to monitor the effective dosage. This treatment program, which must be continued for the rest of the patient's life, can virtually eliminate acute attacks of gouty arthritis, prevent the deposition of new urate crystals, and reduce existing tophaceous deposits over the course of several months. However, the initiation of hypouricemic therapy quite frequently causes acute attacks of gout. These attacks can be prevented or reduced with the use of low-dose daily colchicine (if renal function is good) for at least several months after initiating uric acid–lowering therapy. With proper treatment and patient compliance, gout can nearly always be controlled.

An uncommon, but severe complication of allopurinol is the risk of systemic hypersensitivity and desquamating skin reactions, which are more common in renally impaired individuals and those with the

TOPHACEOUS GOUT

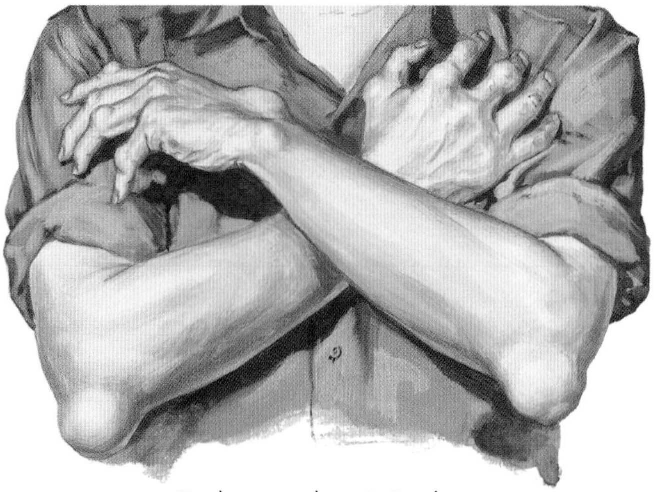

Tophaceous deposits in olecranon bursae, wrists, and hands

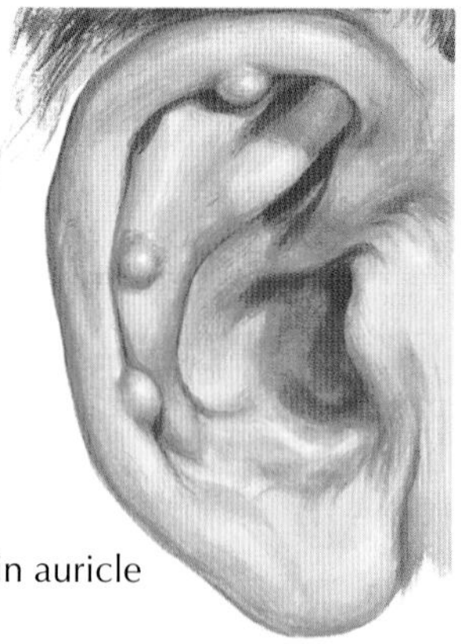

Tophi in auricle

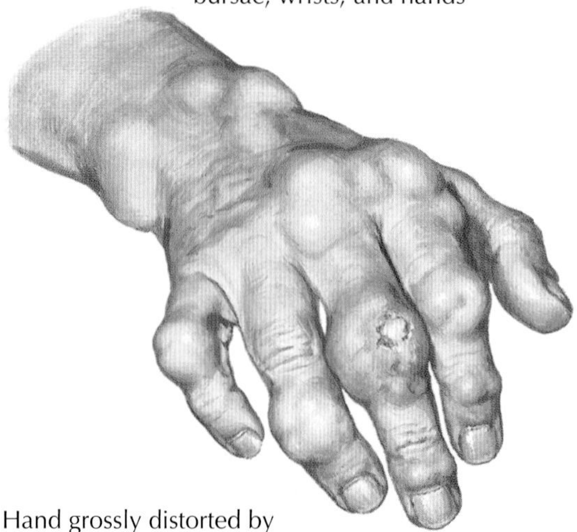

Hand grossly distorted by multiple tophi (some ulcerated)

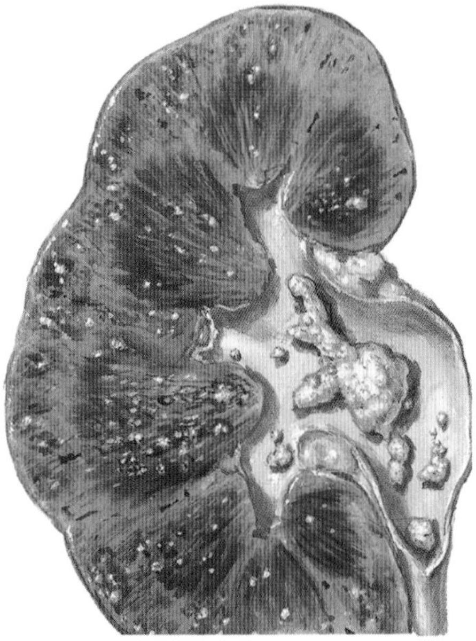

Urate deposits in renal parenchyma, urate stones in renal pelvis

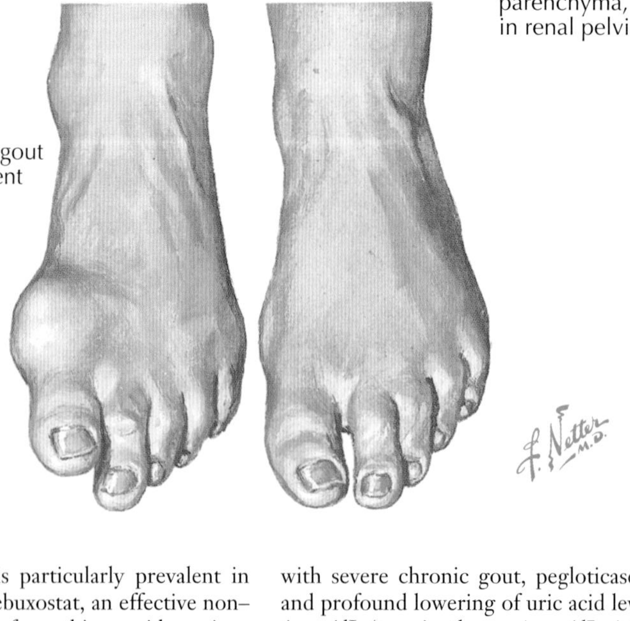

Resolution of tophaceous gout after 27 months of treatment with uricosuric agents

HLA-B5801 gene (which is particularly prevalent in some Asian populations). Febuxostat, an effective non–purine-selective inhibitor of xanthine oxidase, is a potential alternative to allopurinol in these patients, although it is much more expensive in the United States.

Uric acid–lowering therapies may take years to resolve tophi. The speed of resolution is linked to how much the uric acid can be lowered. Pegloticase is a PEGylated mammalian recombinant uricase. In patients with severe chronic gout, pegloticase results in rapid and profound lowering of uric acid levels to well below 4 mg/dL (transiently to ~ 1 mg/dL right after infusion). Pegloticase is a treatment option (biweekly intravenous infusions) that may rapidly resolve tophi, but its use is complicated by anti-drug antibodies that cause significant infusion-related allergic reactions and loss of efficacy. The dramatic uric acid–lowering effect is predictably associated with dramatic and severe flares in gouty arthritis.

Plate 5-40

Rheumatic Diseases

ARTICULAR CHONDROCALCINOSIS (PSEUDOGOUT)

Articular chondrocalcinosis refers to the deposition of calcium-containing salts in the hyaline cartilage and fibrocartilage of joints. The deposition of calcium pyrophosphate dihydrate (CPPD) crystals in the joint causes a symptomatic disorder known as CPPD deposition disease, which is typically manifested as acute arthritis that mimics acute gouty arthritis (pseudogout). Other calcium phosphate salts have been identified in the menisci, but nearly all synovial fluid aspirated from joints affected with pseudogout contains CPPD.

The mechanism of CPPD deposition in articular cartilage is not yet fully understood but may, in part, relate to genetically determined activity of phosphate transporters. Serum calcium, phosphate, and alkaline phosphatase levels are normal, as is urinary calcium excretion. The synovitis of pseudogout is induced by crystals of CPPD in synovial fluid, and trauma to the joint and surgery are two factors that can provoke an attack. Attacks are particularly common after parathyroidectomy as therapy for hyperparathyroidism. Conditions strongly associated with CPPD deposition disease include osteoarthritis, trauma, gout, hyperparathyroidism, hemochromatosis, hypophosphatasia, and hypomagnesemia. Other conditions have weaker associations, including hypothyroidism, Wilson disease, and acromegaly. The crystals may induce inflammation by similar mechanisms to the urate crystal–induced synovitis of gout (see Plates 5-38 and 5-39).

Clinical Manifestations/Radiographic Findings. Pseudogout affects men and women, and patients are generally middle-aged or elderly. One or a few joints of the limbs, most often the knee and wrist, are involved. A self-limiting disorder, an episode of pseudogout lasts from 1 or 2 days to a few weeks. Between attacks, the patient may be asymptomatic.

However, in some patients a subacute or chronic polyarthritis occurs that resembles rheumatoid arthritis. This manifestation occurs either with or without the attacks of acute synovitis typical of pseudogout.

About half of older patients with chondrocalcinosis (mostly women) also exhibit progressive degenerative changes in many joints (osteoarthritis). The knee joint is the most common site of involvement, followed by the wrist, metacarpophalangeal, hip, shoulder, elbow, and ankle joints. Most joints with radiographic signs of chondrocalcinosis are asymptomatic, even in patients with synovitis in other joints. Thus, articular chondrocalcinosis does not necessarily imply the existence of pseudogout. Documentation of synovial fluid crystals remains the gold standard for diagnosis.

On radiographs of the joint, chondrocalcinosis appears as a fine line of CPPD crystals arranged parallel to the cartilage surface. Diagnosis of pseudogout should be suspected in cases of acute synovitis in a large joint of an older person whose serum uric acid level is normal. Diagnosis requires the radiographic demonstration of chondrocalcinosis and the finding of

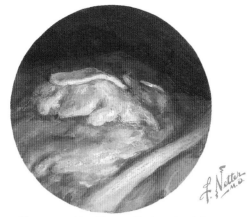

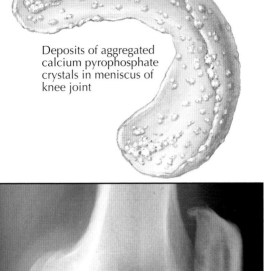

Deposits of aggregated calcium pyrophosphate crystals in meniscus of knee joint

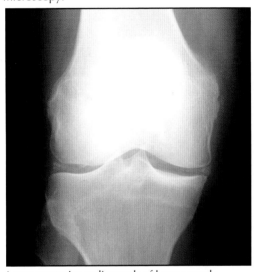

Crystalline synovitis. Biopsy disclosed calcium pyrophosphate crystals seen under polarized light microscopy.

Anteroposterior radiograph of knee reveals densities due to calcific deposits in menisci.

In lateral radiograph, calcific deposits in articular cartilage of femur and patella appear as fluffy white opacities.

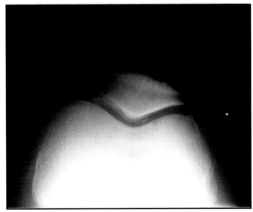

Axial ("skyline") view of knee joint in flexion demonstrates calcinosis of articular cartilages of patella and femur.

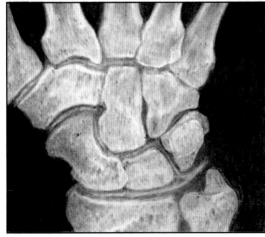

Drawing of radiograph shows calcific deposits in articular cartilages of carpus as fine lines between carpal bones and in radiocarpal joint.

CPPD crystals on microscopic examination of aspirated joint fluid.

Treatment. Aspiration of fluid from the inflamed joint, coupled with intra-articular injection of a corticosteroid, is often sufficient to relieve symptoms of acute pseudogout arthritis. Oral administration of an NSAID is helpful. The response to treatment with colchicine is unpredictable but occasionally dramatic; the efficacy of low-dose colchicine is not as well tested in pseudogout as it is in gout. Some patients may benefit from a short-term course of oral corticosteroid therapy. Treatment of chronic arthritis associated with chondrocalcinosis is the same as that for osteoarthritis. It is not possible to halt the progressive deposition of CPPD crystals in articular cartilage or to remove CPPD crystals that have already been deposited.

Plate 5-41

Musculoskeletal System: PART III

NONARTICULAR RHEUMATISM

Nonarticular rheumatism today can be referred to as a group of nonarticular rheumatic pain syndromes classified into different broad categories, including tendonitis and bursitis, structural disorders, neurovascular entrapment, regional myofascial pain syndromes, and generalized pain syndromes. The incidence of these conditions has been estimated at about 4000 per 100,000 of the U.S. population. Although not life threatening, these disorders can have a significant effect on functional disability. Racial differences have not been documented, and sexual predilection of localized nonarticular rheumatism is fairly evenly distributed.

The nonarticular pain syndromes have been demonstrated to have definite associations with a group of conditions including nonrestorative sleep, irritable bowel syndrome, chronic fatigue, various mood disorders, chronic and migrainous cephalgia, morning stiffness, tender points as well as temporomandibular joint, carpal tunnel syndrome, plantar fasciitis, and cervical neuralgia.

Nonarticular rheumatic disorders can be differentiated from arthritis by accurate localization of tenderness and pain by the absence of clinical and radiographic signs of joint pathology and systemic disease. However, we have learned that, especially in the case of fibromyalgia, the mechanistic characterization of pain including peripheral, neuropathic, and central types can, in combination, be present in a given individual. Thus, our ability to differentiate these different types of pain in a given individual will also aid our diagnosis and treatment.

Tendonitis and bursitis virtually always present as local pain and inflammation, although bursitis affects the synovial fluid–filled saclike structures protecting soft tissues from underlying bone. Both disorders can be associated with overuse, infection, and systemic disease as well calcium apatite and pyrophosphate deposition disorders, but, in addition, gout frequently causes olecranon and prepatellar bursitis.

Structural conditions can be associated with local pain, but disorders such as lateral patellar subluxation, scoliosis, and flatfeet may not necessarily be the primary source of pain or dysfunction.

Neurovascular entrapment can occur centrally or peripherally, and whether this is secondary to carpal or tarsal tunnel syndrome or spinal stenosis, bony enlargement from osteophytes, inflammation, or muscular spasm can add to narrowing of a neurovascular canal and cause discomfort and paresthesias distal to the point of entrapment.

Fibromyalgia is a condition seen most commonly in women in their fifth decade of life with a female-to-male ratio of 8:1. It presents as a form of allodynia, in which painless stimuli are perceived as painful, and hyperalgesia, in which normally painful stimuli are amplified. There appears to be a familial predisposition, suggesting a greater than 8 odds ratio for first-degree relatives and much less familial aggregation with major mood disorders but stronger associations with bipolar and obsessive-compulsive disorders. Levels of substance P, glutamate, excitatory amino acid (EAA), and nerve growth factor can all be elevated, as well as abnormalities of the serotonin system. The cause of fibromyalgia remains unclear, but a recent study links a little known retrovirus to chronic fatigue syndrome. Whether this retrovirus can be associated as well to fibromyalgia remains in question. A host of associated conditions that can occur in association with fibromyalgia but are not necessarily etiologic factors include physical trauma, chronically disturbed sleep, emotional trauma,

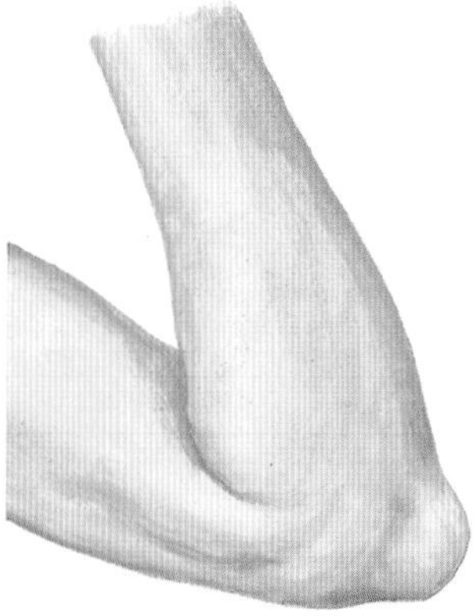

Olecranon bursitis
(student's elbow)

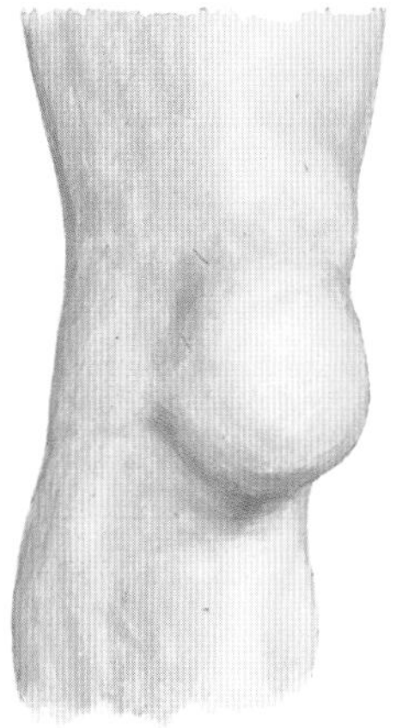

Prepatellar bursitis
(housemaid's knee)

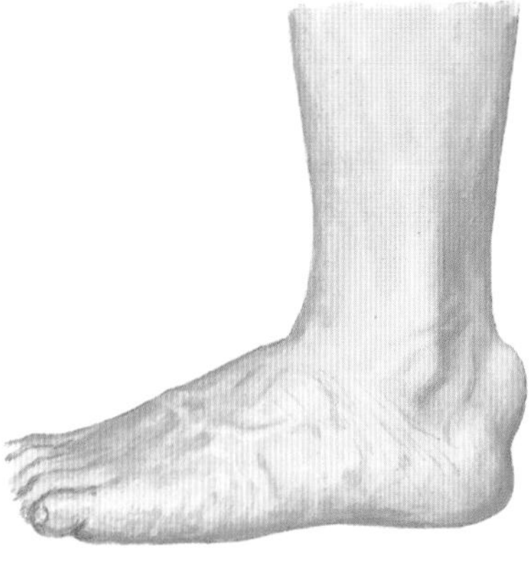

Achillobursitis

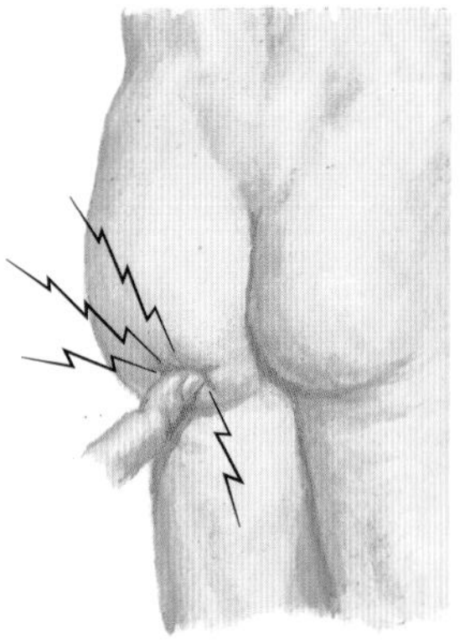

Ischial bursitis
(deep pain and tenderness over ischial tuberosity)

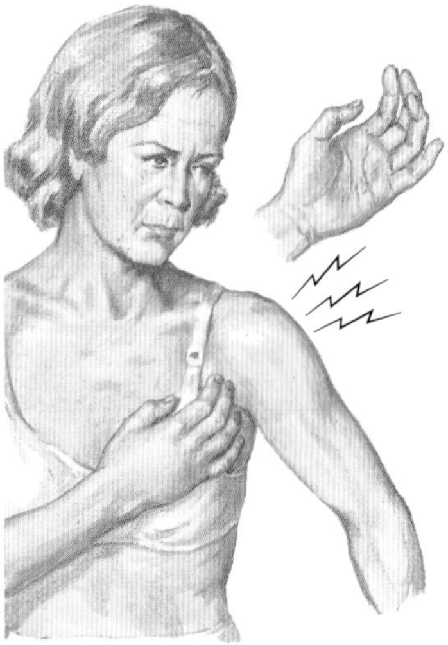

Shoulder-hand syndrome
Pain on shoulder abduction, rotation contracture of fingers due to palmar fasciitis, and swelling of dorsum of hand

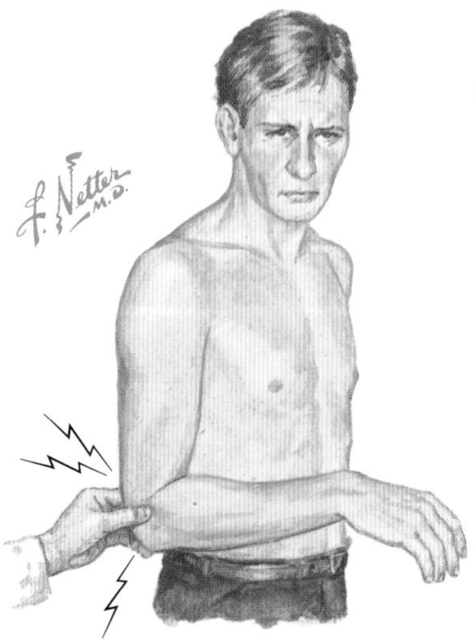

Epicondylitis (tennis elbow)
Exquisite tenderness over lateral or medial epicondyle of humerus

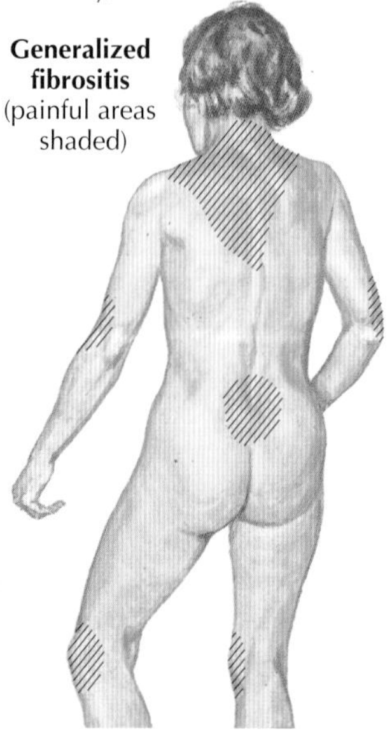

Generalized fibrositis
(painful areas shaded)

autoimmune disease (rheumatoid arthritis and systemic lupus erythematosus), female sex, defined infections such as Lyme disease, hepatitis C or human immunodeficiency virus infection, and a family history of fibromyalgia. Tender point examinations for fibromyalgia are performed using digital thumb pressure at nine bilateral upper and lower extremity sites. Control points including the forehead, midanterior thigh, mid deltoid, thumb, and big toe are useful regarding the patient's sense of general hyperesthesia.

Treatment of nonarticular rheumatism can be very broad and often involves multiple pharmacologic, procedural, and patient-generated approaches guided it is hoped by a single physician source. The pivotal key for appropriate treatment is to understand the various mechanisms that may be contributing to chronic pain and which of the three types, including nociceptive, neuropathic, and nonnociceptive, may be present in combination in a given individual.

Plate 5-42

Rheumatic Diseases

POLYMYALGIA RHEUMATICA AND GIANT CELL ARTERITIS

Polymyalgia rheumatica and giant cell arteritis (GCA) are related conditions that occur in the elderly. Polymyalgia rheumatica coexists with giant cell arteritis in 30% to 55% of patients, and 10% to 20% of patients with polymyalgia rheumatica will develop giant cell arteritis. Both disorders probably represent two extremes of the same disease.

POLYMYALGIA RHEUMATICA

Polymyalgia rheumatica is characterized by *proximal* symmetric limb girdle pain and stiffness that may be accompanied by systemic inflammatory features. The disease responds in dramatic fashion to low-dose corticosteroids. The lack of response to corticosteroids raises the possibility of an alternative diagnosis.

Epidemiology. Polymyalgia rheumatica is extremely uncommon in persons younger than 50 years old. Mean age at onset is 73; women are affected three times more often than men. Whites of northern European or Icelandic descent have a higher incidence of the disease than other ethnic groups.

Pathophysiology. The etiology of polymyalgia rheumatica and giant cell arteritis is unknown. Aging produces dramatic changes in immune, as well as, tissue substrate (e.g., vascular and other tissues). Although such changes are universal in aging, giant cell arteritis and polymyalgia rheumatica remain relatively uncommon, suggesting that additional factors, beyond aging, are at play.

What is the argument for polymyalgia rheumatica being a mild form of giant cell arteritis? The patient demographics for both diseases are identical, and giant cell arteritis is commonly associated with polymyalgia rheumatica. In both diseases, two thirds of patients have the HLA-DRB1*04 allele, and, apart from INF-γ, have similar mRNA for cytokines in temporal artery biopsies. This suggests that in polymyalgia rheumatica there are small but significant numbers of type 1 T-helper (Th1) lymphocytes within the vessel wall but that IFN-γ may be necessary to enhance that response so that it appears as vasculitis.

Clinical Manifestations. Most patients have subacute onset of symptoms. Seventy to 95 percent report neck and symmetric shoulder girdle pain and morning stiffness. Fifty to 70 percent report hip girdle pain and stiffness. Fever, malaise, anorexia, or weight loss may occur in about one third of patients.

Diagnosis. The diagnosis of polymyalgia rheumatica is primarily clinical. The ESR is greater than 40 mm/hr in 90% of cases. Limb girdle pain, morning stiffness, elevated ESR, and a rapid response to low-dose corticosteroids are compatible with this disease. Elevated CRP, normocytic normochromic anemia, thrombocytosis, and elevated alkaline phosphatase may also be present. Muscle enzyme levels are normal.

Conditions that can mimic polymyalgia rheumatica include malignancies, myositis, and proximal-onset rheumatoid arthritis.

Treatment/Prognosis. Corticosteroids are the only consistently effective intervention. Prednisone or prednisolone is usually started in doses of 15 to 20 mg/day. A dramatic response, with near-total relief, should occur within days. After improvement is sustained for 2 weeks to 1 month, a slow taper should begin. The goal is to achieve the lowest effective dose that provides a symptom-free state. Disease flares with corticosteroid

CLINICAL MANIFESTATIONS OF POLYMYALGIA RHEUMATICA AND GIANT CELL ARTERITIS

Pain on chewing

Loss of weight, weakness

Temporal cephalalgia, scalp tenderness

Visual disturbances **Blindness may develop rapidly.**

Low-grade fever, malaise

Symmetric pain and stiffness of shoulder and hip girdle muscles

Anterior ischemic optic neuropathy

Elevated sedimentation rate

Rigid, tender, nonpulsating temporal arteries may be visible or palpable

Hypochromic anemia

tapering are common and often require temporary increase in therapy. Adverse events from corticosteroids occur in almost every patient. The role of immunosuppressive agents other than corticosteroids is of doubtful utility.

Careful follow-up to assess possible drug-related toxicities and expression of the features of giant cell arteritis is essential. New-onset atypical headache, visual changes, murmur of aortic insufficiency, or features of large vessel ischemia should lead to immediate evaluation and institution of higher doses of corticosteroids. Bilateral upper and lower extremity blood pressures should be obtained periodically. Differences between contralateral extremity pressures of more than 10 mm Hg may be an indication of subclavian, iliac, or femoral artery involvement. The finding of bruits over large vessels may be due to atherosclerosis and/or

giant cell arteritis and will require vascular imaging evaluation.

GIANT CELL ARTERITIS

GCA is due to a granulomatous inflammatory injury to medium-sized and large arteries. The most frequently affected vessels are the extracranial branches of carotid arteries and other primary branch vessels of the aortic arch. Less often, internal branches of the carotid are affected, most notably the ophthalmic and posterior ciliary arteries, which when stenotic or occluded may cause visual ischemia or blindness. An exhaustive postmortem study demonstrated that all patients have large vessel inflammation. However, clinically apparent large vessel sequelae occur in only about 25% of cases. This is most often the result of stenoses (especially of the

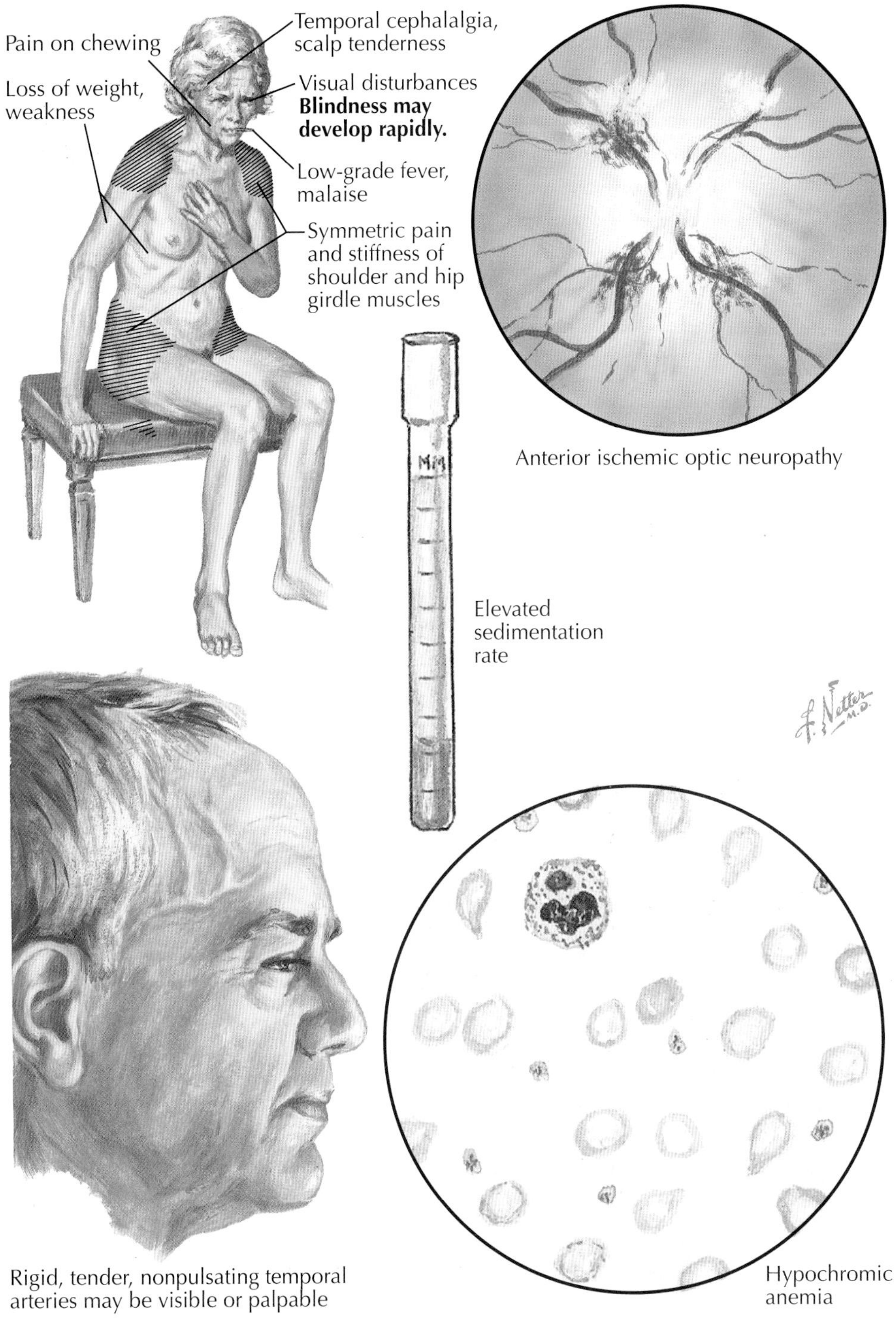

Plate 5-43

Musculoskeletal System: PART III

POLYMYALGIA RHEUMATICA AND GIANT CELL ARTERITIS

(Continued)

subclavian artery) or aneurysms of the aorta (with the thoracic aortic root affected much more often than the abdominal aorta) or its branch vessels.

Giant cell arteritis is the most common vasculitis in whites older than the age of 50 (prevalence = 1 in 500). It has a predilection for people of northern European heritage. Women are affected at least three times more often than men.

Pathophysiology. The cause of giant cell arteritis is unknown. The dominant force in vascular injury is cell-mediated immunity. Resident "sentinel" vascular dendritic cells are thought to present antigen. Migrating dendritic cells, macrophages, and Th1 and Th17 lymphocytes enter the vessel wall via the adventitial vasa vasorum and also play critical roles. Mononuclear cells spread from the vasa vasorum to the media. A small proportion of activated T lymphocytes become clonally expanded. The stimulus for clonal expansion is unknown but may be from an unidentified endogenous or exogenous neoantigen. Weakening of the vessel wall may cause an aneurysm. Luminal narrowing is responsible for ischemic events (e.g., visual loss, stroke, and claudication).

Blood samples before treatment of giant cell arteritis have increased concentrations of IFN-γ and IL-17, as well as IFN-γ– and IL-17–producing T lymphocytes. Corticosteroids suppress Th17 but not Th1 (IFN-γ) components of blood and vascular lesions. Future strategies designed to target corticosteroid-resistant Th1 pathways may allow for more sustained remissions.

Clinical Manifestations. Headache is the most common complaint (75%-95%). Systemic symptoms include fever (<50%), weight loss, malaise, and myalgias and occur in less than 65% of patients. Scalp pain (~25%), jaw pain while chewing (15%-60%), and extremity pain (~20%) may also occur. Visual loss is noted in about 25% of patients. Twenty-five percent of patients develop a *clinically apparent* aortic aneurysm or large artery stenosis at some point during their illness. Up to one half of patients with aortic aneurysms will experience aortic dissection or rupture. The worst prognostic markers for visual loss are already having had amaurosis or established giant cell arteritis–related visual loss in one eye and not being treated for giant cell arteritis.

A thorough physical examination may reveal a prominent, tender temporal artery (20%-70% cases). Asymmetric extremity blood pressures or pulses, bruits, or a murmur of aortic insufficiency suggest aortic or primary aortic branch involvement.

Diagnosis. No serologic test is diagnostic for giant cell arteritis. The diagnosis is based on clinical symptoms, abnormal acute phase reactants, and a positive biopsy. More than 90% of patients will have an elevated ESR. Temporal artery biopsy is the most specific diagnostic test. The sensitivity of biopsy, in series from medical practitioners, in detecting giant cell arteritis is approximately 50%. The yield of biopsy is a function of pretest probability, which may explain why some ophthalmology series, in which visual abnormalities are common, have higher yields (~80%). Biopsy of the contralateral temporal artery adds very little to the sensitivity of the test. Vascular imaging with arteriography or magnetic resonance angiography (MRA) may reveal vascular abnormalities. The subclavian arteries, carotid

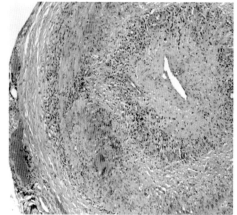

Giant cell arteritis in a temporal artery biopsy stained with H&E. Note the mononuclear cells and giant cells in the infiltrate.

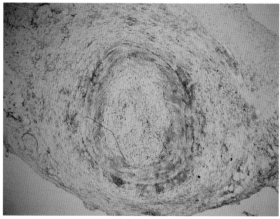

Special stains were used to demonstrate IFN-γ (brown coloring). Other cytokines such as IL17, IL1, IL6, TGF-β, and PDGF are also present but not demonstrated in this example.

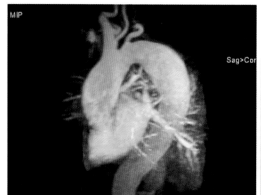

MR angiogram of the aorta and its primary branches in a patient with giant cell arteritis and an aortic root aneurysm

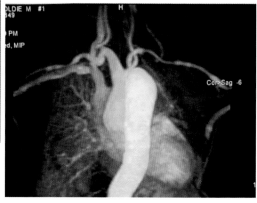

MR image demonstrating bilateral subclavian artery stenosis in a patient with giant cell arteritis

arteries, and ascending aorta are the most commonly affected sites.

Treatment/Prognosis. Corticosteroids are the only drugs of unequivocal value in giant cell arteritis. Therapy should start when the disease is first suspected. Waiting to start corticosteroids after a temporal artery biopsy could result in irreversible visual loss. The optimal, initial dose of prednisone is unclear, but most authorities agree that the initial dose should be between 40 and 60 mg/day. Some advocate the intravenous use of methylprednisolone (1000 mg/day for 3 to 5 days) in patients presenting with amaurosis or blindness. After approximately 1 month, tapering of corticosteroids is begun. The ideal goal is to achieve a corticosteroid-free remission. However, it is not unusual for therapy to extend for many years because of recurrence of symptoms at low doses or after discontinuation is attempted.

Although a variety of adjunctive agents have been evaluated in patients with giant cell arteritis, none has been shown to have clear benefit. Case reports have suggested possible utility of blocking IL-6

(tocilizumab), but before this approach can be endorsed, randomized controlled studies will be required to assess risks and benefits.

Recent data have suggested benefit from the use of low doses of aspirin. Patients so treated appear to have a 3- to 5-fold reduction in visual complications or stroke. Adjunctive low-dose aspirin should be considered in all patients who do not have contraindications for its use.

Although overall mortality in giant cell arteritis is similar to that of matched controls, the subset with aortic aneurysms has increased risk of premature death from aneurysm rupture or dissection. If aortic valve murmurs or bruits are noted, imaging to determine the severity of the aortic lesion should follow. Aneurysm size, rate of change, symptoms suggestive of dissection, and possible congestive heart failure will determine whether surgical intervention is appropriate. Long-term use of corticosteroids is almost always associated with some adverse event, including corticosteroid-induced diabetes, mood changes, infection, avascular necrosis, glaucoma, or osteoporosis/fractures.

Plate 5-44

Rheumatic Diseases

FIBROMYALGIA

Fibromyalgia is best understood as a clinical state of diffuse, chronic pain at rest with fatigue; it is part of a state of generalized perceptual sensory amplification, also *termed central sensitization syndrome*. Interaction of biologic, psychological, and social factors is etiologic and responsible for overall health status and outcome. Therefore, fibromyalgia is best modeled as a biopsychosocial illness in which there is an exaggerated nervous system response.

Pathoetiology. The prevalence and severity of fibromyalgia are determined by impaired slow-wave sleep, the magnitude of mood disturbance, and gene polymorphisms. These factors influence the brain and dorsal horns of the spinal cord, resulting in abnormally low pain thresholds, also known as allodynia. They also activate the stress response, which, in turn, negatively affects the endocrine and autonomic nervous system.

Clinical Manifestations/Diagnosis. Fibromyalgia has a prevalence of about 2%, is more often seen in women, and usually begins as a subacute illness, often with a prior history of related symptoms such as irritable bowel syndrome present before diffuse pain and fatigue become prominent. When it appears after a traumatic event or remembered illness, it is likely that these events marked the onset of the proximate cause of fibromyalgia, which is chronic stress.

The new preliminary diagnostic criteria highlight the core symptoms of fibromyalgia and emphasize the point that fibromyalgia is not just pain. Other symptoms of multisystem amplification responses occur that include increased sensitivity to light, odors, and sound, headache, temporomandibular facial pain, orthostatic hypotension, subjective shortness of breath, intermittent constipation and diarrhea, urinary frequency, subjective weakness, and diffuse paresthesias.

The key finding at physical examination is diffuse articular and nonarticular pain with palpation. Certain tools/questionnaires can be used to better characterize the patient, including the Symptom Intensity Scale and Fibromyalgia Impact Questionnaire, to establish diagnosis and severity. Other tools, including the Brief Patient Health Questionnaire-9, are used to determine the presence and severity of depression; and the Epworth Sleepiness Scale is used to investigate possible sleep apnea.

Serologic testing is unnecessary to confirm diagnosis and is only indicated to test for comorbid disease.

Differential Diagnosis. Some diseases bear superficial resemblance to fibromyalgia but do have their own unique signs and symptoms used to "rule them in" as the correct diagnosis. In real-life situations, many patients carry more than one diagnosis. For instance, a patient is free to have both gout and a fractured tibia. Each separate diagnosis is confirmed using a logical clinical approach, referenced to individual past clinical experience as well as published criteria for each separate disorder. The same is true with fibromyalgia. It is not a "diagnosis of exclusion" but in fact has a distinct phenotype, its own set of highly specific signs and symptoms. These are "unmasked" by using the approach just discussed. When it accompanies other illnesses, fibromyalgia can complicate the diagnosis and determination of disease severity. For instance, comorbid fibromyalgia will falsely elevate the number of tender joints, patient global assessment, and Health Assessment Questionnaire results used in the evaluation of rheumatoid arthritis.

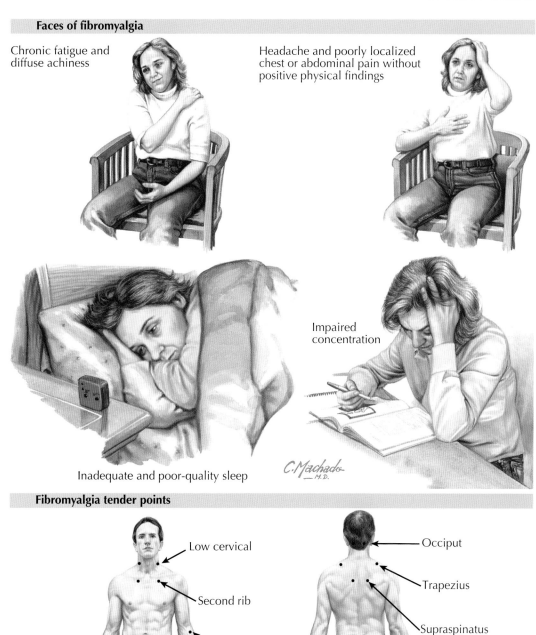

Faces of fibromyalgia

Chronic fatigue and diffuse achiness

Headache and poorly localized chest or abdominal pain without positive physical findings

Impaired concentration

Inadequate and poor-quality sleep

C. Machado — M.D.

Fibromyalgia tender points

Low cervical

Second rib

Lateral epicondyle

Knee

Occiput

Trapezius

Supraspinatus

Gluteal

Greater trochanter

Treatment. Three agents are approved by the U.S. Food and Drug Administration for the treatment of fibromyalgia and include the antidepressants duloxetine and milnacipran as well as the antiepileptic drug pregabalin. Although they have been shown to be more effective than placebo, they are usually not "curative." Other agents that are superior to placebo include fluoxetine, citalopram, and tricyclic antidepressants. Neither corticosteroids nor narcotics are beneficial.

Of at least equal importance are aerobic exercise and education, often combined with some form of cognitive therapy. A discussion of sleep hygiene is often also important.

Fibromyalgia is a syndrome most often associated with distress. Treating underlying depression and anxiety and sleep problems and deconditioning is the basis of therapy. A dismissive attitude on the part of the treating physician can be a major iatrogenic perpetuating factor.

Plate 5-45

Musculoskeletal System: PART III

AUTOINFLAMMATORY SYNDROMES

The autoinflammatory syndromes represent a genetically diverse but phenotypically similar group of conditions characterized by recurrent episodic attacks of fever, rash, serositis, and musculoskeletal pain. Genetically mediated disordered regulation of the innate immune system unifies these syndromes and leads to recurrent and stereotypical attacks of fevers and associated symptoms. Patients typically lack autoantibodies and have no evidence of autoreactive T lymphocytes, thus distinguishing them from the usual rheumatologic conditions.

PRIMER ON THE INNATE IMMUNE SYSTEM

The innate immune system represents the first-line response to immunologic challenges and is composed of cellular defenses (neutrophils, dendritic cells, macrophages, and natural killer cells), proinflammatory signaling proteins known as cytokines, and the complement system. IL-1, IL-6, and TNF-α represent the critical proinflammatory cytokines of the innate immune system. Nearly all mutations found in the autoinflammatory syndromes disrupt normal control of inflammatory signaling and result in generation of a proinflammatory state and inflammatory symptoms.

FAMILIAL MEDITERRANEAN FEVER

Familial Mediterranean fever (FMF) is the most common and best characterized autoinflammatory syndrome. A mutation in the *MEFV* gene disrupts the conformation of pyrin, a protein critical to control of IL-1 production, leading to increased IL-1 levels. Although classically described as autosomal recessive, many patients with FMF have only one abnormal allele. The carrier rate in certain ethnic groups (e.g., Sephardic Jews, Turks, Arabs, Armenians) is very high.

Brief episodes of fever accompanied by intense serositis are the hallmarks of FMF attacks. Approximately 80% of patients will suffer their first attack before age 20 years. Patients have a body temperature that is typically greater than 102°F, with the fever lasting less than 72 hours. Arthritis of predominantly the lower extremities is found in 70% of FMF patients during attacks. Erysipeloid erythema, an intensely erythematous warm, tender, plaquelike lesion on the lower extremities, can be noted in up to 40% of patients. Orchitis also frequently occurs during attacks. Over time, these recurrent episodes of inflammation may result in amyloidosis of the kidneys or liver.

Colchicine is the mainstay of therapy for patients with FMF. Seventy percent of FMF patients treated with colchicine have complete cessation of their symptoms, whereas 25% of patients have a reduction in the severity and frequency of attacks. Only 5% to 10% of FMF patients will not respond to colchicine, usually owing to the gastrointestinal side effects of the drug. In these patients, drugs that inhibit IL-1 activity offer great promise.

The prognosis of FMF is mainly related to genotype and development of amyloidosis. Those patients with genotypes resulting in mild disease have a lower probability of developing amyloidosis, and thus prognosis is favorable. In general, FMF attacks become less frequent and severe over time.

PATHOPHYSIOLOGY OF AUTOINFLAMMATORY SYNDROMES

Innate immune system pathways involved in the autoinflammatory syndromes

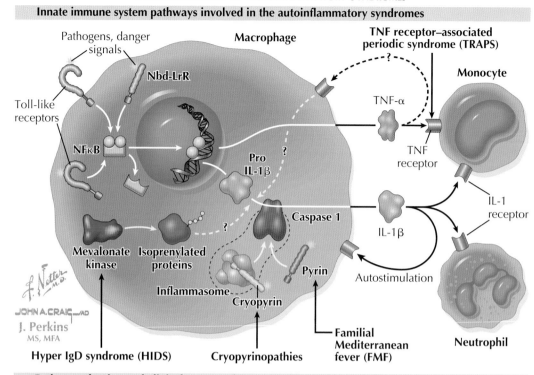

Patient evaluation and clinical presentation

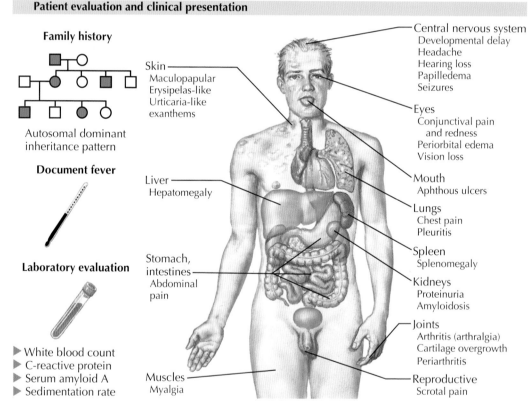

HYPERIMMUNOGLOBULIN D SYNDROME

The underlying genetic abnormality underlying hyperimmunoglobulin D syndrome (HIDS) has been localized to the gene encoding the enzyme mevalonate kinase. Most of these mutations are missense mutations in highly conserved areas of protein resulting in a partial decrease in mevalonate kinase activity. Although classically described as autosomal recessive, many patients with HIDS have only one abnormal allele.

More than 70% of patients will suffer their first HIDS attack before age 2, and the average age at onset is 6 months. Parents may report that routine vaccinations during infancy trigger attacks. Attacks typically last 4 days, and this longer duration can assist in differentiating attacks from FMF. More than 90% of patients will exhibit significant cervical lymphadenopathy, and 80% will develop a nonspecific erythematous rash. Headache, arthritis, and abdominal pain also are found in 70% of patients. As the name implies, serum levels of IgD are elevated in patients with HIDS. However, the specificity of this finding is questionable because elevated IgD levels are found in many children

Plate 5-46

Rheumatic Diseases

AUTOINFLAMMATORY SYNDROMES (Continued)

with chronic inflammatory conditions and levels fluctuate throughout childhood. Assessment of urinary mevalonic acid levels during febrile attacks offers a more reliable method of diagnostic investigation in patients presumed to have HIDS. Genetic sequencing is an alternative method of diagnostic testing in patients with symptoms suggestive of HIDS. However, roughly 30% of patients meeting clinical criteria for HIDS have no definable mutation.

Treatment of HIDS can be quite challenging. Oral corticosteroids are effective, but long-term sequelae from these drugs are undesirable. These patients rarely respond to colchicine, thus differentiating HIDS patients from FMF patients. Etanercept, an inhibitor of TNF-α, has demonstrated success in some patients with HIDS. Inhibitors of IL-1 have been utilized with increasing efficacy in the treatment of HIDS symptoms during attacks.

TUMOR NECROSIS FACTOR RECEPTOR–ASSOCIATED PERIODIC SYNDROME

Tumor necrosis factor receptor–associated periodic syndrome (TRAPS) results from alterations in the gene encoding the TNF cell surface receptor. TRAPS has a widely variable phenotypic presentation. Febrile attacks in TRAPS typically last for 7 or more days, differentiating TRAPS from FMF and HIDS. The median age at onset in TRAPS is 3 years, yet adolescent and adult onset cases have been reported. Intense myalgias are characteristic of TRAPS attacks. TRAPS patients may have an erythematous rash that usually occurs on an extremity and travels in a distal-to-proximal fashion in association with myalgias. Abdominal pain and pleuritic chest pain are common. Painful conjunctivitis and periorbital edema are also frequently observed. Genetic testing can be used to confirm the diagnosis of TRAPS.

Treatment for TRAPS is reliant on use of TNF-α antagonists. Systemic corticosteroids are also effective but require ever-increasing doses and unacceptable systemic adverse effects. Overall, the prognosis of TRAPS is quite good. The risk of amyloidosis is lower than that of FMF.

CRYOPYRIN-ASSOCIATED PERIODIC SYNDROME

The most diverse hereditary autoinflammatory syndrome is the cryopyrin-associated periodic syndrome (CAPS). CAPS encompasses three overlapping phenotypes: familial cold autoinflammatory syndrome (FCAS), Muckle-Wells syndrome (MWS), and neonatal onset multisystemic inflammatory disorder (NOMID). In CAPS, mutations in the *NLRP3* (NOD-like receptor family, pyrin domain containing 3) gene result in increased IL-1β production. Inheritance patterns for CAPS appear to be autosomal dominant, but spontaneous mutations are common.

The physical manifestations of CAPS vary widely. Common findings in CAPS patients include recurrent fevers, urticarial rash, and joint pain. When exposed to sudden drops in ambient temperature, FCAS patients develop symptoms that resolve in less than 24 hours. Patients with MWS have more frequent and prolonged attacks that may or may not be related to changes in ambient temperature. In addition to fever and urticarial

CUTANEOUS FINDINGS IN AUTOINFLAMMATORY SYNDROMES

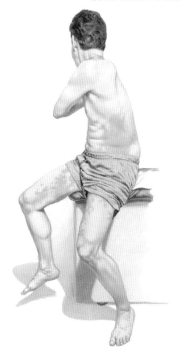

Classic TRAPS rash that migrates in a centrifugal pattern

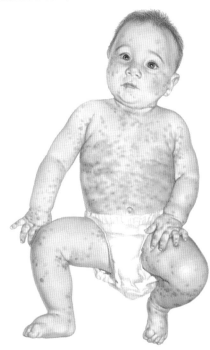

The rash in HIDS can be variable, including maculopapular and urticarial forms.

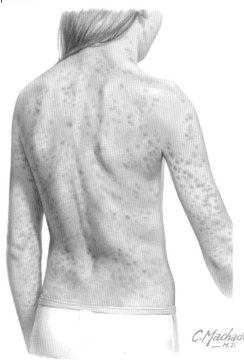

Typical appearance of urticaria-like rash of the cryopyrinopathies

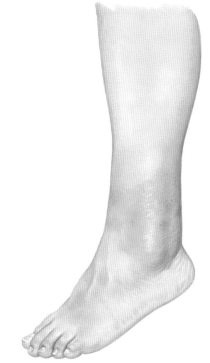

Typical appearance of erysipelas-like FMF rash, often on lower extremities

rash, MWS patients may develop arthritis and headaches due to aseptic meningitis. NOMID is the most severe CAPS phenotype, presenting shortly after birth as fever and persistent urticarial rash. Patients with NOMID suffer from chronic aseptic meningitis, papilledema, and optic nerve atrophy in addition to frontal bossing of the skull. Overgrowth of the epiphyseal regions of long bones and growth delay are characteristic of NOMID (see Plate 5-47).

Control of IL-1β activity is key to successful treatment of CAPS. Many patients with FCAS do not require treatment and may move to warmer climates to avoid the rapid swings in ambient temperature. Patients with MWS and NOMID require therapy with IL-1 antagonists. Overall prognosis for CAPS is largely dependent on phenotype. Patients with FCAS generally have a progressive improvement in attack frequency and severity over time. Patients with symptoms more consistent with MWS also have a relatively good prognosis and low likelihood of amyloidosis and sensorineural hearing loss, especially when treated with IL-1 antagonists. Finally, patients with NOMID carry the greatest risk of sensorineural hearing loss, growth delay, and amyloidosis.

Plate 5-47

Musculoskeletal System: PART III

AUTOINFLAMMATORY SYNDROMES (Continued)

MISCELLANEOUS AUTOINFLAMMATORY SYNDROMES

Patients with deficiency of IL-1 antagonist (DIRA), a naturally occurring antagonist of IL-1β, exhibit a severe pustular rash and osteitis. Patients with pyogenic arthritis, pyoderma gangrenosum, and acne (PAPA) syndrome also have increased IL-1 production owing to a genetic mutation in the *PSTPIP1* gene. Mutations in the *LPIN2* gene result in development of chronic recurrent multifocal osteomyelitis, neutrophilic dermatosis, and dyserythropoietic anemia, termed *Majeed syndrome*. Genetic abnormalities in the *NOD2* gene have been found in patients with Blau syndrome (granulomatosis arthritis and uveitis). Many of these conditions respond favorably to treatment via IL-1 antagonism.

PERIODIC FEVER, APHTHOUS STOMATITIS, PHARYNGITIS, ADENOPATHY SYNDROME

Periodic fever, aphthous stomatitis, pharyngitis, adenopathy (PFAPA) syndrome is a common cause of recurrent fever in children but has also been reported in adults. In this condition, patients develop stereotypical attacks on a predictable schedule. This predictability is unique to PFAPA syndrome and separates it from the hereditary autoinflammatory syndromes, which all occur with irregular and unpredictable frequencies. No single genetic mutation has been associated with PFAPA syndrome.

Age at onset for PFAPA syndrome is typically prior to age 3 years. Febrile attacks on average last 5 days and occur every 4 weeks. During these attacks, PFAPA syndrome patients may experience aphthous stomatitis, nonspecific exudative or nonexudative pharyngitis, and/or enlarged and tender cervical lymph nodes. Between attacks, patients are healthy and exhibit normal growth.

Owing to the self-limited nature of the syndrome, treatment is reserved for those patients with severe disease or those patients whose condition creates difficult socioeconomic circumstances for the family. In patients requiring therapy, one or two doses of systemic prednisone (1 mg/kg) within 6 hours of fever onset is effective in aborting fever in 90% of patients. However, up to 50% of patients may experience an increased frequency of attacks after treatment with systemic corticosteroids. Additional options include daily colchicine or cimetidine, both effective in preventing attacks of PFAPA syndrome in one third of patients. Tonsillectomy represents curative therapy. The prognosis of PFAPA syndrome is favorable. Without intervention, 40% of patients experience a significant reduction in the severity and frequency of fever attacks within 5 years of diagnosis. To date, there have been no reports of amyloidosis or hearing loss in PFAPA syndrome patients.

DIAGNOSTIC EVALUATION OF PATIENTS WITH SUSPECTED AUTOINFLAMMATORY DISEASE

Fundamental historical information and careful physical examination will often lead to the proper diagnosis in patients with autoinflammatory syndromes. Critical historical elements include age at onset of attacks, duration of attacks, presence of serositis, adenopathy, myalgias, arthralgias/arthritis, ocular symptoms, CNS symptoms, orchitis, rash characteristics, family members with similar symptoms, and ethnic background.

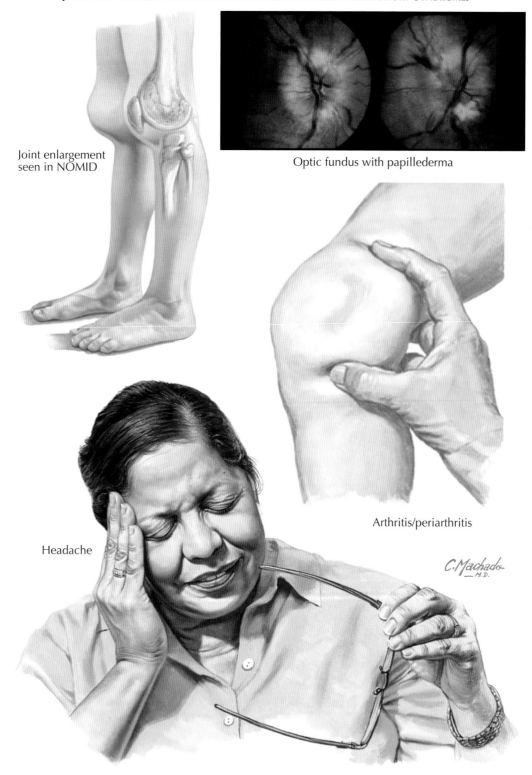

JOINT AND CENTRAL NERVOUS SYSTEM FINDINGS IN AUTOINFLAMMATORY SYNDROMES

Joint enlargement seen in NOMID

Optic fundus with papillederma

Arthritis/periarthritis

Headache

Malignancy and infection should be considered in all patients; however, the repetitive and stereotypical nature of the attacks will differentiate the autoinflammatory conditions. The utility of acute phase reactant assessment in the diagnostic evaluation of patients is limited because all conditions will result in abnormal values. Patients with CNS symptoms should undergo a thorough examination that includes a formal ophthalmologic evaluation, imaging, and possibly lumbar puncture for assessment of intracranial pressure and inflammatory changes in the cerebrospinal fluid (CSF). Dermatologic manifestations should be examined first hand and imaging for fascial inflammation as well as full-thickness biopsy considered at the time of rash occurrence. Gross bony abnormalities should be evaluated with plain radiography, and audiologic testing may also be indicated in the diagnostic evaluation of patients with recurrent fevers. Finally, genetic testing is available commercially for patients with suspected hereditary autoinflammatory syndromes; however, up to 30% of patients with phenotypic manifestations characteristic of a given autoinflammatory syndrome have a normal genetic testing. Genetic testing may ultimately be indicated for proper counseling of reproductive risk.

Plate 5-48

Rheumatic Diseases

VASCULITIS

The vasculitides are a heterogeneous group of diseases that are linked by the presence of blood vessel inflammation. Vasculitis can occur secondary to an underlying disease or trigger or as part of a primary vasculitic disease. Although the etiology and pathogenesis of the primary vasculitides are not known at this time, there is strong evidence to support that these diseases are immunologically mediated. Many forms of vasculitis can be organ and life threatening, which makes early diagnosis with prompt treatment of critical importance. The diagnosis of most forms of vasculitis is typically established by the presence of compatible clinical features combined with histologic and/or arteriographic evidence. These features play a prominent role in differentiating the vasculitides, which can also vary widely with regard to epidemiology, laboratory and imaging features, treatment, and outcome. Each vasculitic disease will tend to predominantly affect a certain vessel size; and although this can be conceptually helpful, most forms of vasculitis can affect a diverse range of vessels. Giant cell arteritis, Behçet disease, and vasculitis of the CNS are discussed elsewhere in this section. The focus here is on polyarteritis nodosa, granulomatosis with polyangiitis (Wegener), microscopic polyangiitis, Churg-Strauss syndrome, and Henoch-Schönlein purpura.

POLYARTERITIS NODOSA

Epidemiology/Clinical Manifestations. Polyarteritis nodosa (PAN) was reported by Kussmaul and Maier in 1866 and was the first vasculitis to be described. The definition of PAN has evolved and, in 1994, PAN was separated from microscopic polyangiitis (MPA). As it is now defined, PAN is an exceedingly rare vasculitis with an annual incidence of 2 to 9 cases per million. PAN occurs equally between men and women with the mean age at onset being 40 to 50 years, although PAN can also develop in children. Hepatitis B or C can be associated with a PAN-like vasculitis and a cutaneous-isolated PAN can also occur, all of which are approached differently.

PAN is predominantly a disease of medium-sized arteries in which the most common clinical manifestations are fever, weight loss, and myalgias (>90%), with vasculitis involving the peripheral nerve (80%), gastrointestinal tract (40%-65%), skin (50%), the nonglomerular renal vessels (40%-50%) that may manifest as hypertension, testis (20%), eye (10%), or heart (5%-10%). CNS involvement is much more common in pediatric PAN, occurring in up to 22% of children.

Diagnosis. There are no laboratory studies that are diagnostic of PAN, and the typical findings are that of a systemic inflammatory process with an elevation in acute phase reactants such as ESR and/or CRP. Dye arteriography is often performed to examine the visceral and renal circulation, in which PAN would be suggested by microaneurysms, stenoses, or a beaded pattern reflecting sequential areas of arterial narrowing and dilation. Computed tomography (CT) and magnetic resonance arteriography do not currently have sufficient resolution to visualize the vessels affected by PAN. Biopsies reveal necrotizing inflammation of the medium-sized or small arteries with neutrophils, fibrinoid changes, and disruption of the internal elastic lamina.

Treatment/Prognosis. Patients with immediately life-threatening PAN involving the gastrointestinal tract, heart, or CNS should be treated with

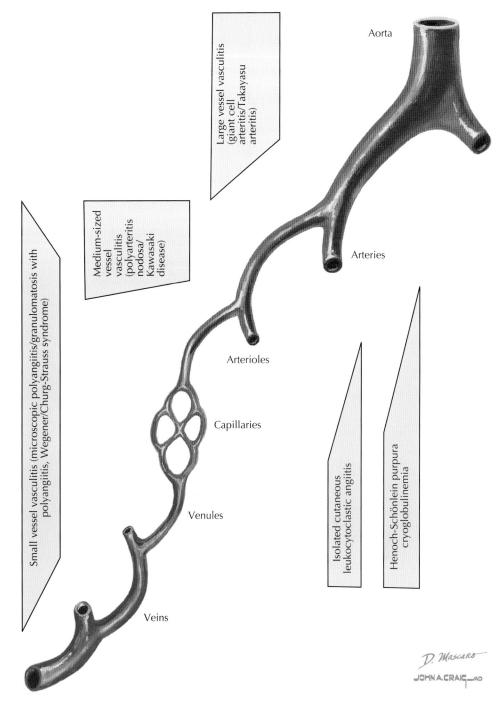

cyclophosphamide and glucocorticoids as outlined later for granulomatosis with polyangiitis (Wegener) (GPA). In patients in whom the disease manifestations do not pose an immediate threat to life or major organ function, glucocorticoids alone can be considered as initial therapy, with cyclophosphamide being added in patients who continue to have evidence of active disease or who are unable to taper prednisone. The estimated 5-year survival rate of treated patients with PAN is 88%, with mortality being influenced by disease severity. Relapses occur in 10% to 20% of patients.

GRANULOMATOSIS WITH POLYANGIITIS (WEGENER)

Epidemiology/Clinical Manifestations. GPA is characterized by clinical involvement of the upper and lower respiratory tracts and kidneys with granulomatous inflammation and vasculitis of the small to medium-sized vessels (see Plate 5-49). GPA is estimated to occur in 3 in 100,000 people and is seen equally between men and women. The average age at onset has ranged from 40 to 65 years.

At initial presentation, more than 90% of patients with GPA seek medical attention for upper and/or lower airway symptoms. Sinonasal disease occurs in more than 95% of patients and may result in nasal septal perforation and/or saddle-nose deformity, with 85% developing pulmonary involvement. Glomerulonephritis, which is present in 20% of patients at the time of diagnosis but manifests in 80% along the disease course, can be rapidly progressive and lead to renal failure. GPA can involve almost any organ site, with other prominent features including arthralgias/arthritis

Plate 5-49

Musculoskeletal System: PART III

VASCULITIS (Continued)

(60%-70%), skin (40%-50%), ocular disease (51%), such as episcleritis/scleritis and orbital involvement, peripheral and CNS disease (40%-50%), and subglottic stenosis (20%).

Diagnosis. The key laboratory studies in GPA include blood cell counts, measurement of renal function and acute phase reactants, and urinalysis. Because renal disease is usually asymptomatic, urine microscopy to look for dysmorphic red blood cells or red blood cell casts is essential in detecting glomerulonephritis. Chest imaging should be performed in all patients because up to one third of patients with pulmonary disease may be asymptomatic. Pulmonary radiographic findings can include single or multiple nodules, infiltrates, or cavities, as well as ground-glass infiltrates that suggest alveolar hemorrhage.

Antineutrophil cytoplasmic antibodies (ANCA) have had important clinical applications in GPA, although their role in pathogenesis remains uncertain. Two types of ANCA have been identified in patients with vasculitis: ANCA directed against proteinase-3 (PR3), which causes a cytoplasmic immunofluorescence pattern (cANCA) on ethanol-fixed neutrophils, and ANCA directed against myeloperoxidase (MPO), which results in a perinuclear immunofluorescence pattern (pANCA). In order to interpret ANCA results, positivity by immunofluorescence should be confirmed with testing for antibodies to PR3 and MPO. In GPA, 75% to 90% of patients have PR3-cANCA, 5% to 20% have MPO-pANCA, and up to 20% may be ANCA negative. Although ANCA has diagnostic utility in settings in which the likelihood of GPA would be high (sinusitis, an active urine sediment, and noninfectious pulmonary disease), for clinical features where GPA would have a lower prevalence, the predictive value of ANCA is insufficient to initiate therapy in the absence of a biopsy-proven diagnosis. ANCA levels do not correlate well with relapse, and a rising ANCA value alone should not be used as the basis to start or increase immunosuppressive therapy.

Biopsies in GPA may demonstrate granulomatous inflammation, necrosis, with necrotizing or granulomatous vasculitis. The highest positive yield of greater than 90% comes from surgical biopsies of affected lung, with biopsies of the upper airways being diagnostic less than 20% of the time. Renal histology is that of a focal, segmental, necrotizing, crescentic glomerulonephritis with few to no immune complexes.

Treatment/Prognosis. Active GPA is potentially life threatening, and initial treatment requires glucocorticoids combined with another immunosuppressive agent. Patients who have active severe GPA should initially be treated with cyclophosphamide in combination with prednisone at 1 mg/kg/day. After 4 weeks of treatment, if there is improvement, the prednisone is tapered with a goal of discontinuation by 6 to 12 months. Cyclophosphamide may either be given orally as 2 mg/kg/day taken all at once in the morning or intravenously as 15 mg/kg every 2 weeks for 3 doses and every 3 weeks thereafter. It has a significant side effect profile that includes infection, cytopenia, bladder toxicity, infertility, and myelodysplasia. To prevent leukopenia, blood cell counts should be measured every 1 to 2 weeks for as long as the patient is taking cyclophosphamide. The drug is given for 3 to 6 months to induce remission, after which time it is stopped and therapy is switched to either methotrexate, 20 to 25 mg/wk, or azathioprine, 2 mg/kg/day, for remission maintenance.

Rituximab (anti-CD20), 375 mg/M²/wk for 4 weeks, combined with glucocorticoids has been found to be as effective as cyclophosphamide to induce remission and represents another treatment option for patients with severe disease. In patients who have active but nonsevere disease, prednisone given together with methotrexate, 20 to 25 mg/wk, can effectively induce and then maintain remission. In the absence of side effects, maintenance therapy is given for at least 2 years, after which time consideration may be made on an individual basis whether to continue the maintenance agent or to taper therapy to discontinuation.

Before the introduction of treatment, patients with GPA had a mean survival time of 5 months. Current regimens induce remission in 75% to 100% of GPA patients and carry the potential for long-term survival.

However, relapse occurs in 50% to 70% of patients and disease-related organ damage is common.

MICROSCOPIC POLYANGIITIS

Epidemiology/Clinical Manifestations. MPA is characterized by necrotizing vasculitis with few or no immune deposits affecting small vessels. It lacks granulomatous inflammation, which differentiates it from GPA. The most common clinical features of MPA include glomerulonephritis (80%-95%), peripheral nerve disease (60%-70%), lung disease, including pulmonary hemorrhage (25%-55%), cutaneous vasculitis (30%-40%), and gastrointestinal disease (30%).

Diagnosis. The essential laboratory studies in MPA, particularly the important role of urinalysis, are similar

CLINICAL AND HISTOLOGIC FEATURES OF GRANULOMATOSIS WITH POLYANGIITIS (WEGENER)

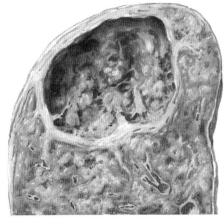

Granulomatosis with polyangiitis (Wegener). Cavity in upper lobe of right lung lined with necrotic material

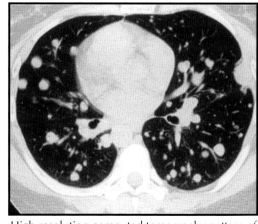

High-resolution computed tomography pattern of multiple, bilateral pulmonary nodules in granulomatosis with polyangiitis (Wegener).

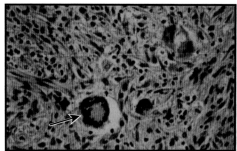

Granulomatosis inflammation. With giant cells (*arrow*)

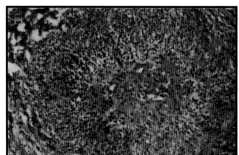

Severe arteritis. With destruction of vessel wall in granulomatosis with polyangiitis (Wegener)

Clinical manifestations of granulomatosis with polyangiitis (Wegener)

Upper respiratory involvement
Ulcerative lesions of nose, sinuses, mouth, pharynx

Lower respiratory involvement
Necrotic areas and cavitation in lungs; cough; dyspnea; hemoptysis; chest pain

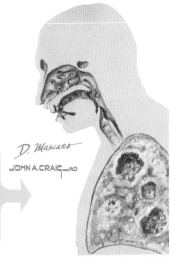

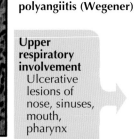

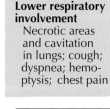

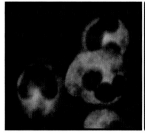

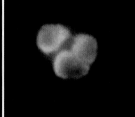

c-ANCA and p-ANCA staining pattern on left and right, respectively

Plate 5-50

Rheumatic Diseases

VASCULITIS (Continued)

to those in GPA. Approximately 75% to 85% of MPA patients have MPO-pANCA, with 5% to 10% being positive for PR3-cANCA and 0 to 20% being ANCA negative. Biopsies in MPA show necrotizing vasculitis of the small vessels or small to medium-sized arteries and the absence of granulomas on immunofluorescence. Like GPA, the renal histology is a focal segmental necrotizing glomerulonephritis with few to no immune complexes.

Treatment/Prognosis. The current treatment of MPA is the same as that outlined for GPA. The estimated 5-year survival rate of MPA is 75% to 80%. MPA is a relapsing disease, with recurrences developing in at least 38% of patients.

CHURG-STRAUSS SYNDROME

Epidemiology/Clinical Manifestations. Churg-Strauss syndrome (CSS) is a rare disease observed in all age groups and occurring equally between sexes with an incidence of about 3 per million people. It is thought of as having three phases: a *prodromal phase*, with allergic rhinitis and asthma, an *eosinophilic phase*, with peripheral and tissue eosinophilia, and *vasculitis* of the peripheral nerve (70%-80%), lung (40%-70%, which includes eosinophilic, granulomatous and vasculitic lung disease), heart (25%-35%), skin (40%-75%), gastrointestinal tract (30%), or kidney (10%-40%). Although these phases are conceptually helpful, they may not be identifiable in all patients and they may not occur in sequence.

Diagnosis. Only about 40% of patients with CSS are ANCA positive, prominently MPO-pANCA. The histologic features of CSS include eosinophilic tissue infiltrates, extravascular granulomas, and small vessel necrotizing vasculitis. Vasculitis can be difficult to definitively establish, making clinical manifestations of greater importance in establishing the diagnosis of CSS.

Treatment/Prognosis. Prednisone, 1 mg/kg/day, is effective for many manifestations of CSS, but asthma often limits the ability for glucocorticoids to be tapered. Patients with life-threatening disease should be treated with glucocorticoids and cyclophosphamide as described for GPA. Prognosis of CSS is influenced by the presence of severe disease involving sites such as the heart, gastrointestinal tract, CNS, and kidney. CSS is characterized by frequent exacerbations of asthma, with relapses of vasculitis occurring in at least 20% to 30% of patients.

HENOCH-SCHÖNLEIN PURPURA

Epidemiology/Clinical Manifestations. Henoch-Schönlein purpura (HSP) is a small-vessel vasculitis in which 75% of cases occur before the age of 8 years, although adults can also be affected. Two thirds of patients report an antecedent upper respiratory tract infection, although no specific inciting organism has been identified.

The four primary features of HSP are cutaneous vasculitis (palpable purpura), arthritis, gastrointestinal involvement, and glomerulonephritis (20%-50%). Gastrointestinal manifestations include colicky abdominal pain, vomiting, and potentially intussusception. Unlike GPA and MPA, glomerulonephritis in HSP is rarely rapidly progressive (and only 2% to 5% progress to end-stage renal failure. HSP in adults may be more

KEY FEATURES OF PRIMARY VASCULITIC DISEASES

Giant cell arteritis	Granulomatous, large vessel vasculitis
	Most commonly affects people > 50 years of age, female > male
	Four phenotypes: Cranial arteritis (headache, jaw claudication, risk of blindness),
	  polymyalgia rheumatica, large vessel vasculitis (aortic aneurysm, subclavian stenosis),
	  systemic inflammation
	Glucocorticoids are proven to reduce risk of blindness

Takayasu arteritis	Granulomatous, large vessel vasculitis, primarily involving the aorta, its major branches, and the pulmonary arteries Characterized by large vessel stenoses and/or aneurysms Most commonly affects women in childbearing years Glucocorticoids are the foundation of treatment Surgical intervention may be required for fixed lesions causing ischemia or for aneurysms
Polyarteritis nodosa	Disease of medium-sized arteries Clinical involvement of nerve, kidney (not glomerulus), GI tract Arteriography (particularly mesenteric-renal) can show microaneurysms and vessel stenoses Severe active disease requires aggressive immunosuppression
Kawasaki disease	Disease of children predominantly < 5 years of age Fever + cervical adenopathy, mucosal disease, rash, conjunctival injection, soft tissue swelling 25% of untreated children develop coronary artery aneurysms Treated with intravenous immunoglobulin
Granulomatosis with polyangiitis (Wegener)	Granulomatous inflammation, vasculitis of small to medium-sized vessels, pauci-immune crescentic glomerulonephritis Frequently affects sinuses, lungs, kidneys Proteinase-3 ANCA seen in 75-90% Severe active disease requires aggressive immmunosuppression
Microscopic polyangiitis	Vasculitis of small to medium-sized vessels, pauci-immune crescentic glomerulonephritis Frequently affects nerve, lungs, kidneys, skin Myeloperoxidase ANCA seen in 75-90% Severe active disease requires aggressive immmunosuppression

Churg-Strauss syndrome	Eosinophilic and granulomatous inflammation, vasculitis of small to medium-sized vessels
	Characterized by asthma, peripheral and tissue eosinophilia, and vasculitis predominantly
	  affecting nerve, skin, heart
	ANCA seen in < 40%, mostly MPO-ANCA
	Many patients can be treated with glucocorticoids alone
	Severe active disease requires aggressive immmunosuppression but many patients can be
	  treated with glucocorticoids alone

Henoch-Schönlein purpura	Immune complex vasculitis associated with IgA-predominant immune deposits Mostly a disease of children < 8 years, but can affect adults Cutaneous small vessel vasculitis, arthritis, GI disease (including intussusception), immune complex glomerulonephritis May not require treatment although glucocorticoids may improve symptoms
Cryoglobulinemic vasculitis	Immune complex vasculitis associated with cryoglobulinemia Mostly secondary to hepatitis C and other causes but can occur as an idiopathic vasculitis Cutaneous small vessel vasculitis, arthritis, neuropathy, immune complex glomerulonephritis Treatment directed at underlying causes when present and also based on severity
Behçet disease	Diverse disease characterized by oral and genital ulcers, inflammatory eye disease, CNS and GI disease, pulmonary artery aneurysms, venous thromboses Vasculitis and venulitis can be seen Treatment based on manifestation and its severity
Primary angiitis of the CNS	Vasculitis exclusively affecting the vessels of the CNS Diverse vessel sizes and histologic patterns can be seen Granulomatous angiitis of the CNS carries the poorest prognosis Almost always associated with an abnormal spinal fluid and brain MRI Treatment based on histology and severity

severe and lead to renal insufficiency in up to 13% of patients.

Diagnosis. The diagnosis of HSP is established by its clinical manifestations. Skin biopsy is not required in most instances but reveals leukocytoclastic vasculitis with a variable degree of IgA deposition in vessel walls. Renal biopsy may have prognostic utility and is an immune complex glomerulonephritis containing IgA.

Treatment/Prognosis. HSP is a self-limited condition that may not require treatment. Glucocorticoids may decrease tissue edema, arthritis, and abdominal discomfort and lower the rate of intussusception. In the hospital setting, a recent study found that early glucocorticoid exposure was associated with benefits for several outcomes in HSP, particularly related to gastrointestinal manifestations of the disease. Glucocorticoids have not been proven to benefit renal disease and do not appear to lessen the likelihood of relapse. Uncontrolled studies suggest that glucocorticoids in combination with a cytotoxic agent may be beneficial in patients with active glomerulonephritis and progressive renal insufficiency.

The outcome in patients with HSP is excellent, with disease-related death occurring in 1% to 3%. Relapse occurs in up to 40% of cases, typically within the first 3 months after the initial episode.

Plate 5-51

Musculoskeletal System: PART III

SYSTEMIC LUPUS ERYTHEMATOSUS

Systemic lupus erythematosus (SLE) is a multiple-organ autoimmune disease with no known cause, extremely variable presentation, and multifactorial pathogenesis. Prevalence rates of SLE in the United States are 51 per 100,000 population.

A positive ANA test alone is not sufficient to establish the diagnosis. Survival rates in SLE are much better today than 50 years ago. Morbidity comes from disease itself, as well as a greater risk of cancer, infections, cardiovascular disease, and osteoporosis.

ETIOLOGY AND PATHOGENESIS

The presence of a large number of autoantibodies against self-constituents indicates a failure of self-tolerance. Several genes have been associated with SLE susceptibility, each of them displaying a small effect, suggesting the need of gene-gene and/or gene-environment interactions. Environmental factors, both external (e.g., infectious agents, exposure to ultraviolet light) and internal (e.g., gender and hormonal profile) may influence disease manifestations. The end result is a defective clearance of chromatin material, which triggers an immune response, facilitated by defective elimination of self-reactive B lymphocytes in the bone marrow.

Family members of patients with SLE have an increased risk of developing SLE. As many as 20% of unaffected first-degree relatives reveal antibodies, and there is a higher rate of concordance (>20%) in monozygotic twins when compared with dizygotic twins (1%-3%).

Almost 80% of SLE patients are women. High estrogen levels have been associated with increased number of autoreactive B lymphocytes, a predominantly Th2 response, and increased antibody production.

CLINICAL PRESENTATION

Manifestations of SLE are protean and can affect any organ system. Typically, the patient is a young woman with some, or more, of the following features: a butterfly rash over the face, fever, joint pain and swelling, pleuritic chest pain, and photosensitivity. It is important to note that many patients, especially women between 20 and 40 years of age, present to their internist or rheumatologist with fatigue, arthralgias, myalgias, slight erythema after sun exposure, light-headedness, and fatigue along with a positive ANA test. These patients feel disturbed by bright lights, which irritate them and make them feel light-headed and cause a brief transient rash. A careful history in these patients will elicit a number of other stress-related symptoms, along with depression, anxiety, and poor sleep. These patients suffer from fibromyalgia and are often misdiagnosed as having SLE. It is important therefore to stress that the diagnosis of SLE relies, besides the findings of a positive ANA test, on objective findings of SLE-related organ involvement, such as (but not limited to): a persistent rash triggered by sun exposure that shows features of interface dermatitis on biopsy, objective swollen joints, objective evidence of pleuritis and pericarditis, and abnormal urine sediment suggestive of glomerular damage.

Mucocutaneous Manifestations. Mucocutaneous involvement is almost universal in SLE. Cutaneous

RENAL LESIONS IN SYSTEMIC LUPUS ERYTHEMATOSUS (SLE)

A. Mesangial type

Glomerulus showing increased mesangial material (PAS stain)

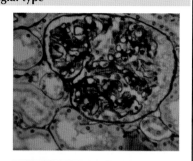

Fluorescence slide*: mesangial deposits of immune complexes

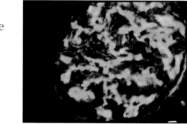

B. Focal proliferative type

Glomerulus showing focal proliferative change and adhesions of glomerular tufts (H & E)

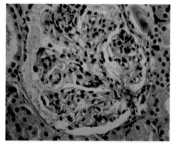

Fluorescence slide: granular deposits of immune complexes in capillary walls

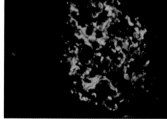

C. Diffuse proliferative type

Glomerulus showing proliferative change, fibrinoid necrosis and hematoxylin body (arrow) (H & E)

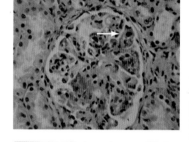

Fluorescence slide: massive deposits of immune complexes

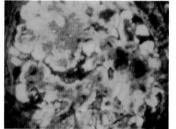

Electron microscopic diagram: massive subendothelial deposits of immune complexes

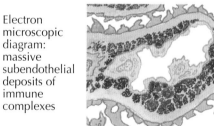

D. Membranous type

Diffuse thickening of basement membrane (PAS stain)

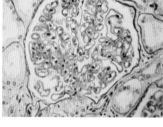

Fluorescence slide: diffuse homogeneous granular deposits along capillary walls

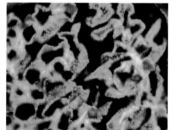

Electron microscopic diagram: diffuse subepithelial deposits

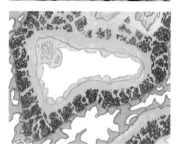

* All fluorescence slides stained with fluorescein-labeled rabbit antihuman gamma globulin

lesions can be further classified as acute, subacute, and chronic lesions. One of the most widely recognized features of lupus is the malar or butterfly rash that can last for several weeks after brief sun exposure. Discoid lupus erythematosus (DLE) lesions are chronic and occur in 25% of patients with SLE but may also occur in the absence of other clinical features of SLE. Patients with isolated DLE have a 10% risk of developing SLE. DLE lesions expand slowly and leave depressed central scars. Other rashes seen in SLE include lupus profundus, lupus tumidus, and livedo reticularis.

Hair loss occurs in most patients with lupus and may involve the scalp, eyebrows, eyelashes, beard, and body hair. Scarring alopecia is a complication of DLE.

Musculoskeletal Manifestations. Diffuse arthralgias and myalgias are extremely common in SLE patients. Some develop Jaccoud arthropathy, a reducible arthropathy due to capsular laxity, involving the same joints as rheumatoid arthritis.

Isolated monarthritis should prompt consideration of other causes such as osteoarthritis, septic arthritis, or avascular necrosis.

Plate 5-52

Rheumatic Diseases

SYSTEMIC LUPUS ERYTHEMATOSUS (Continued)

Corticosteroid myopathy should be considered in the differential diagnosis of muscle weakness. Corticosteroids also contribute to the increased risk of osteoporosis and fractures in lupus patients.

Renal Manifestations. Renal involvement eventually will affect up to 70% to 80% of all patients, but the clinical presentation varies and includes an abnormal urine sediment; nephritis, nephrotic syndrome; or acute or chronic renal insufficiency. Screening the urine for blood and protein is an essential part of each SLE patient's rheumatology visit. Hematuria is usually microscopic. Granular and fatty casts reflect proteinuric states, whereas red blood cells casts or mixed (red and white) cell casts are seen in patients with glomerulonephritis. Renal damage varies as follows: class I—minimal lesions with deposition of immune complexes in the mesangium and seen by immunofluorescence, class II—mesangial hypercellularity, class III—focal lupus nephritis involving less than 50% of all glomeruli with focal subendothelial immune deposits, class IV—diffuse lupus nephritis characterized by diffuse segmental or global endocapillary or extracapillary glomerulonephritis involving more than 50% of the glomeruli, class V—membranous lupus nephritis with global or segmental subepithelial immune deposits. The end result of sustained, untreated renal inflammation is progression to class VI—advanced sclerotic lupus nephritis when 90% or more of the glomeruli are globally scarred.

For an accurate diagnosis, a renal biopsy specimen with 10 or more glomeruli is optimal.

Nervous System Manifestations. Both the central and peripheral nervous system can be affected in SLE. Neuropsychiatric syndromes in patients with SLE include aseptic meningitis, cerebrovascular disease, demyelinating syndromes, headaches, movement disorders, seizures, acute confusional states, cognitive dysfunction, mood disorders, and psychosis. Mononeuropathy, Guillain-Barré syndrome, autonomic disorders, myasthenia gravis, polyneuropathy, and plexopathy have also been reported. These conditions are seen also in patients without SLE; therefore, assigning them to lupus can be a major challenge for the clinician. Non–lupus-related causes such as infections, drugs, electrolyte abnormalities, primary psychiatric disorders, fibromyalgia, and atherosclerosis must be excluded. Vasculitis is rare, whereas a bland vasculopathy involving small vessels is the predominant finding in neuropathologic autopsy studies.

Cardiopulmonary Manifestations. Serositis (pleuritis, pericarditis) is the most common cardiopulmonary complication of lupus. Cardiac tamponade is rare. Myocardial involvement is rare and typically occurs in the setting of generalized SLE activity. SLE patients have an increased risk of death as a result of coronary heart disease and stroke. Diffuse thickening of the mitral and aortic valves, Libman-Sacks endocarditis, valvular insufficiency, and stenosis occur with decreasing frequency. Acute pneumonitis, pulmonary embolism, and alveolar hemorrhage present as acute respiratory symptoms, cough, and dyspnea. Alveolar hemorrhage is an emergency, and these patients should be immediately admitted to a hospital and undergo bronchoscopy while high-dose corticosteroid therapy is initiated. Hemoptysis may be absent; the sole clues to the diagnosis may be a drop in hemoglobin, shortness of breath, and bilateral infiltrates on a chest radiograph.

A. Erythematous malar rash

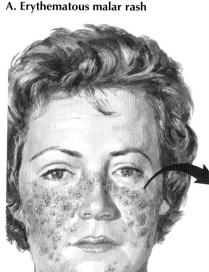
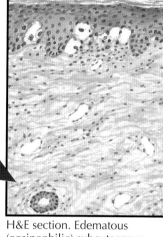
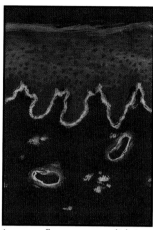

H&E section. Edematous (eosinophilic) subcutaneous tissue with vacuolization of basilar epithelium at the dermal-epidermal junction

Immunofluorescence slide*: bandlike granular deposit of gamma globulin and complement at the dermal-epidermal junction and in the walls of small dermal vessels

B. Normal-appearing (nonlesional and non–sun-exposed) skin of lupus patient

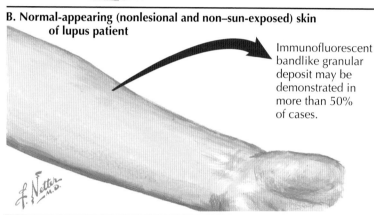
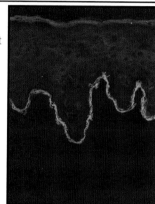

Immunofluorescent bandlike granular deposit may be demonstrated in more than 50% of cases.

C. Discoid lupus

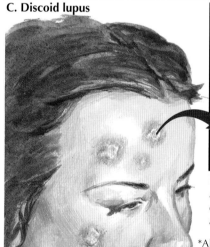
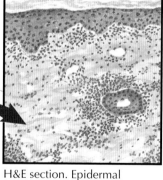
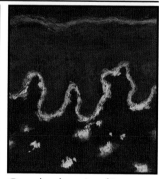

H&E section. Epidermal atrophy, hyalinization of dermis, chronic inflammation around hair follicles

Granular deposits of immune complexes at the dermal-epidermal junction and within dermis

*All fluorescence slides were stained with fluorescein-labeled rabbit antihuman gamma globulin.

Patients with chronic shortness of breath and dry cough should be evaluated for interstitial lung disease and isolated pulmonary hypertension.

Pregnancy in Lupus. Although fertility is not affected by SLE, there is an increased frequency of midtrimester spontaneous abortions, prematurity, and stillbirth. Lupus activity at the time of conception is a predictor of pregnancy outcome.

The use of estrogens in women with active SLE is contraindicated, while their ability to increase flares in stable SLE patients is debated.

Neonatal lupus syndrome may present as rash, transient thrombocytopenia, and complete heart block, which is often irreversible. Screening for complete heart block should be performed in all fetuses whose mothers are positive for IgG anti-Ro/SSA antibodies. These antibodies are able to cross the placenta and injure an otherwise normally developing heart.

LABORATORY TESTING

Antinuclear antibodies are the most sensitive screening test for SLE, but the specificity of this test is very

Plate 5-53

Musculoskeletal System: PART III

SYSTEMIC LUPUS ERYTHEMATOSUS (Continued)

low for SLE. A negative ANA test argues strongly against SLE.

Antibodies to Sm (Smith) antigen are very specific for SLE but found in only 30% of cases. Anti-Ro/SSA and Anti-La/SSB are also found in SLE but are not disease specific. Antibodies to dsDNA are specific and are found in 70% of SLE patients at some point during the course of their disease. Other antibodies seen in patients with SLE are anti-RNP, anti-ribosomal P, and anti-histone antibodies.

Causes of anemia in SLE patients include chronic inflammation, hemolysis, blood loss, renal insufficiency, myelodysplasia, hypersplenism, or marrow aplasia.

A white blood cell count lower than 4500/μL has been reported in 50% of patients. This could be due to lymphopenia, neutropenia, or both and may indicate active SLE but can also be caused by infections, medications, or hypersplenism.

Up to 50% of SLE patients present with mild thrombocytopenia associated with immune platelet destruction or antiphospholipid antibody syndrome. Severe thrombocytopenia should raise the suspicion of thrombotic thrombocytopenic purpura. Other common causes of low platelet count are hypersplenism, drugs, infections, and bone marrow aplasia.

MANAGEMENT AND TREATMENT

The treatment of SLE is tailored to the severity of individual organ involvement and to the degree of disease activity. All patients should be instructed to avoid exposure to ultraviolet light and wear sunscreen at all times. Regular visits to a rheumatologist, even during periods of inactivity, are indicated. Traditional cardiovascular risks should be identified in every patient and measures to correct them should be implemented.

Antimalarial agents are indicated in all SLE patients, not just for the treatment of cutaneous SLE, serositis, and arthritis but also for their immunomodulating and antithrombotic effects. Low-dose aspirin should also be part of the "baseline" treatment of every patient with SLE.

Corticosteroids are the mainstay of treatment for most of the lupus flares. Dosing and route of administration depends on the type and severity of organ involvement.

Corticosteroid toxicity is a major problem in SLE, and the clinician should try to taper the dose as soon as clinically possible. The doses of corticosteroids vary widely from a few milligrams per day to 1 g of Solu-Medrol for 3 to 5 days intravenously in cases of life-threatening or organ-threatening lupus. Protection from osteoporosis is very important, and so is protection against *Pneumocystis jiroveci* pneumonia in patients prescribed moderate and high doses of corticosteroids for prolonged periods of time.

Additional immunosuppressants are frequently used for their corticosteroid-sparing effects and for more severe disease. Drugs in this group include azathioprine, methotrexate, cyclophosphamide, mycophenolate mofetil, and cyclosporine. Potential toxicities make close monitoring mandatory. Contraception is mandatory owing to the teratogenic risk of these medications. Pregnant women with severe active lupus can be treated with high doses of glucocorticoids and azathioprine, and the fetus should be delivered at the earliest time that is deemed safe. Mycophenolate mofetil has emerged

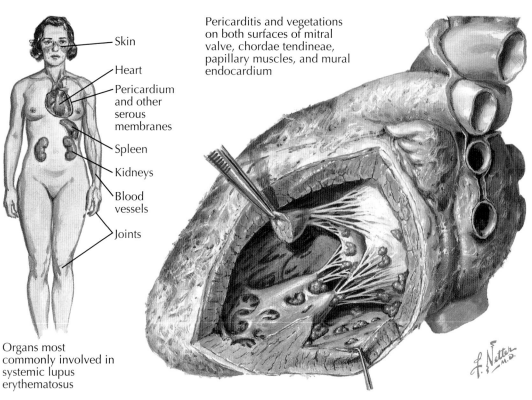

Skin
Heart
Pericardium and other serous membranes
Spleen
Kidneys
Blood vessels
Joints

Organs most commonly involved in systemic lupus erythematosus

LUPUS ERYTHEMATOSUS OF THE HEART

Pericarditis and vegetations on both surfaces of mitral valve, chordae tendineae, papillary muscles, and mural endocardium

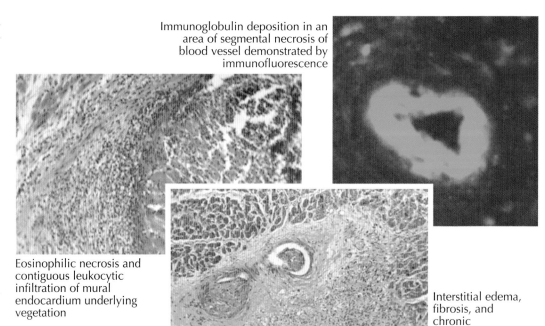

Immunoglobulin deposition in an area of segmental necrosis of blood vessel demonstrated by immunofluorescence

Eosinophilic necrosis and contiguous leukocytic infiltration of mural endocardium underlying vegetation

Interstitial edema, fibrosis, and chronic inflammation in systemic lupus erythematosus myocarditis

as an alternative to cyclophosphamide in some patients with lupus nephritis because studies have shown comparable efficacy and fewer side effects.

Belimumab is a fully human monoclonal antibody that specifically recognizes and inhibits the biologic activity of B-lymphocyte stimulator (BLyS), a factor important for the survival of B lymphocytes. Two studies (BLISS-76 and BLISS-52) have evaluated the efficacy and safety of belimumab plus standard of care in patients with active SLE. Belimumab resulted in a significant improvement in disease activity measures by

week 52 and helped reduce the prednisone dose while increasing the time to the first disease flare and the risk of severe disease flare compared with placebo.

Several new agents are under investigation. Some of these drugs target T lymphocyte co-stimulatory activation (cytotoxic T-lymphocyte–associated protein-4 [CTLA-4]), production of reactive oxygen species (*N*-acetylcysteine), aberrant activation of mTOR (rapamycin), spleen tyrosine kinase (Syk inhibitor), type 1 interferons (anti–IFN-α monoclonal antibody), and IL-6 (tocilizumab).

Plate 5-54

Rheumatic Diseases

ANTIPHOSPHOLIPID SYNDROME

Antiphospholipid syndrome (APS) results from autoantibodies specifically directed against anionic membrane phospholipid-associated proteins and clinically manifests as thrombocytopenia, livedo reticularis, valvular heart disease (Libman-Sacks endocarditis), vascular thromboses (arterial and venous), and pregnancy losses. Antiphospholipid antibodies (aPL) and APS may be idiopathic or secondary. APS is a relatively common form of acquired primary thrombophilia in the general population. Prompt recognition and treatment is imperative to limit associated morbidity and mortality.

CLASSIFICATION CRITERIA

The initial classification criteria for APS (Sapporo, 1998) were revised in 2006. These include clinical (vascular thrombosis and pregnancy-related morbidity) and laboratory (presence and measurement of antibody titers of lupus anticoagulant [LAC], aPL, and β_2-glycoprotein I [β2GPI]) factors.

ETIOLOGY AND PATHOGENESIS

The etiology of primary APS is unknown. The pathogenesis likely involves a primary immunologic defect leading to autoantibody production and the occurrence of clinical manifestations triggered by secondary causes such as infection, malignancy, systemic inflammation, and medications. APS is mediated by multiple components such as endothelial cells, monocytes, platelets, and complement. Organ-specific aPL may not only effect thrombosis but interact directly with the tissue itself. The major targets of these autoantibodies are now believed to be phospholipid-binding plasma proteins such as β2GPI and prothrombin. The exact physiologic function of β2GPI is unknown, but its three-dimensional structure suggests that it is perfectly adapted to interact with negatively charged phospholipids. β2GPI can also bind to other proteins related to coagulation and endothelial cells. Thrombosis results from a complex interaction between aPL, β2GPI, activated endothelium, and activated platelets. APS is also an inflammatory procoagulant process, which includes abnormalities of proteins such as protein C and annexin V. The antibodies are constantly present in circulation, but thromboses are rare and occur only in specific vascular beds.

CLINICAL PRESENTATION

Clinical presentation ranges from asymptomatic with positive aPL serology to severe multiple-organ dysfunction and failure, with resultant mortality.

Thrombotic Events. Thrombosis (arterial and venous) can occur in any vascular location. The most common site of venous thrombosis is the lower extremities and that of arterial thrombosis is the CNS, manifesting as stroke or transient ischemic attacks. Thrombosis probably contributes to manifestations such as nephropathy and obstetric complications.

Pregnancy-Related Morbidity. The most common obstetric manifestation is recurrent miscarriage, defined as three or more consecutive miscarriages before the mid-second trimester (most losses occurring before 10th week of gestation) or one or more unexplained deaths of morphologically normal fetuses of 10 or more weeks' gestation. Other pregnancy morbidity includes fetal growth impairment, oligohydramnios,

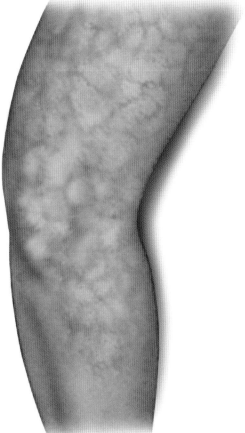

Livedo reticularis

Livedo racemosa

preeclampsia and eclampsia, fetal distress, premature delivery, and postpartum maternal thrombotic events.

Cutaneous Manifestations. Livedo reticularis occurs in 16% to 25% of cases and appears as a lattice ("reticulate") pattern of blue to red subcutaneous mottling. Livedo racemosa is a more open streaklike pattern. Histopathology of livedo reticularis does not show thrombosis. The strongest association of livedo reticularis in patients with SLE is with cerebrovascular ischemia (Sneddon syndrome), but it may be associated with ocular ischemia and seizures. Other cutaneous manifestations include ulcers, skin necrosis, superficial phlebitis, splinter hemorrhages, purpura, digital gangrene, anetoderma, and pseudovasculitis.

Thrombocytopenia. Thrombocytopenia (platelet count < 100,000/mm³) occurs in 16% to 44% of primary APS. aPL are also present in about one third of patients with chronic autoimmune thrombocytopenia. Thrombocytopenia in APS is usually moderate and not associated with hemorrhage.

Cardiac Manifestations. The cardiac valves may be thickened or show noninfective, verrucous vegetations, which may embolize, causing ischemic events. Arterial thrombotic events seem to have the highest prevalence in patients with APS and valvular heart disease. The Task Force on Catastrophic Antiphospholipid Syndrome (CAPS) and Non-criteria APS Manifestations (APS Task Force) recommends a transthoracic echocardiogram in patients with APS and previous arterial thrombosis.

APS Nephropathy. This manifests as new-onset hypertension, proteinuria, hematuria, and decreased renal function. The diagnosis can be made in the right clinical setting without a renal biopsy, but this may be

necessary in other situations. The histopathology shows thrombotic microangiopathy (fibrin thrombi in glomeruli and/or arterioles), intimal hyperplasia, organizing thrombi, and fibrous arterial or arteriolar occlusion. The APS Task Force recommends that "in patients with APS nephropathy lesions and persistently positive aPL, the diagnosis of APS should be considered, provided other conditions resulting in similar renal biopsy lesions are excluded."

Neurologic Manifestations. Stroke is the major neurologic manifestation of APS. Other manifestations include multiple-infarct dementia, TIAs, myelopathy, seizures, chorea, neuro-ophthalmologic syndromes, peripheral neuropathy (including Guillain-Barré–like syndrome), migraine-like headaches, and cognitive dysfunction. The neurologic manifestations are hypothesized to result from thromboses as well as direct interaction between aPL and neurons and glial cells.

Catastrophic Antiphospholipid Syndrome (CAPS). CAPS (Asherson syndrome), a life-threatening syndrome that occurs in 1% patients with APS and associated with high mortality (44%), is characterized by multiple thromboses occurring over a short period of time (days to weeks) involving small vessels in several major organs leading to severe organ dysfunction/failure. SLE is the most common systemic autoimmune condition reported in this complication. The CAPS registry reported this complication as the presenting manifestation in young individuals in 46% of cases and that it was precipitated by infection, surgery, neoplasia, obstetric complications, medications, trauma, SLE flare, and withdrawal of anticoagulant medication. The most common initial organ involvement during CAPS was pulmonary, neurologic, and renal. Large vessel

Plate 5-54

Musculoskeletal System: PART III

ANTIPHOSPHOLIPID SYNDROME
(Continued)

arterial or venous thromboses are less common. Mortality results from thrombotic complications such as myocardial infarction, stroke, and pulmonary embolism.

DIFFERENTIAL DIAGNOSIS

The differential diagnosis involves other causes of thrombophilia and other diagnoses depending on clinical presentation. Recurrent pregnancy loss should be evaluated by a high-risk obstetrician and fertility expert. Inherited thrombophilic disorders may also be associated with recurrent pregnancy loss. CAPS can be mimicked by several conditions, including infective endocarditis, thrombotic thrombocytopenic purpura, and primary medium-sized or small vessel systemic vasculitides.

DIAGNOSTIC APPROACH

APS is diagnosed by clinical and laboratory criteria. The criteria require persistently (12 weeks apart) positive tests for one or more aPL in a patient with a history of arterial or venous thrombosis or recurrent pregnancy loss. International consensus criteria (2006) for classification of definite APS are used for clinical trials but may have limitations regarding diagnosis of individual patients. Identifying the triggering event and a thorough workup for underlying associated systemic disease as well as possible mimics of APS cannot be overemphasized.

Anticardiolipin Antibodies (aCL). Standard solid phase aCL antibody testing by enzyme-linked immunosorbent assay (ELISA) remains the first-line test for APS. Persistently positive medium- or high-titer (>40 U phospholipid antibody titer) tests for IgG or IgM aCL are most likely to be associated with clinical manifestations. Transiently positive and low-titer antibodies have unclear significance. Although IgA aCL have been associated with thrombocytopenia and leg ulcers, and although they may have a role in IgG and IgM aCL-negative APS, testing for IgA aCL and threshold for interpretation are not defined.

Lupus Anticoagulant (LAC). LAC antibodies are detected based on their ability to delay clotting in phospholipid-dependent coagulation reactions. They are strongly associated with thrombotic events and fetal losses. LAC testing is prone to false-positive and false-negative results from variability in laboratory techniques. The key steps in LAC testing involve prolongation of clotting in a phospholipid-dependent assay, evidence of inhibition on mixing studies, demonstration of phospholipid dependence, and, finally, exclusion of coagulation factor–specific inhibitors. It is recommended that LAC should be screened for using at least two tests; the most commonly used are activated partial thromboplastin time (aPTT) optimized for the detection of LAC (lupus aPTT) and dilute Russell viper

venom (dRVVT). The mixing study helps to exclude coagulation factor deficiency. Mixing patient plasma with normal plasma will correct factor deficiency but not inhibitors such as LAC. Correction with cardiolipin suggests the presence of a β2GPI-dependent LAC. Coagulation-based assays for LAC are influenced by anticoagulant therapy, and performing thrombin time or anti–factor Xa assays may be needed.

Protein-Based Immunoassays. Most aPL are directed against β2GPI and prothrombin and not against negatively charged phospholipids. In patients with APS, most aCL antibodies detected are specific for β2GPI. An IgG and/or IgM titer greater than the 99th percentile on two or more occasions at least 12 weeks apart is part of the APS classification criteria. The current consensus statement for diagnosis of APS does not recommend testing for other aPL. Further studies are warranted to establish the significance and test characteristics of anti-prothrombin and anti-annexin A5 antibodies.

High-Risk aPL Profile. The APS Clinical Research Task Force report (2011) concluded that (1) a positive LAC test is a better predictor of clinical events compared with other aPL tests, (2) higher titers of IgG aCL and anti-β2GPI have higher specificity for clinical events, (3) triple aPL positivity (LAC, aCL, anti-β2GPI) is more commonly associated with clinical events compared with double or single aPL positivity, (4) documentation of persistent (≥12 weeks apart) aPL is crucial for diagnostic purposes and to exclude other causes of transient aPL, and (5) thrombotic risk in aPL-positive patients rises with increasing risk factors.

MANAGEMENT AND THERAPY

The management of patients with APS can be thought of as primary prevention (before the clinical event) and secondary prevention (prevention of recurrent clinical events).

Primary Prevention—Asymptomatic aPL. This remains controversial, but risk stratification of patients based on their other risk factors and aPL profile may be useful. Unless contraindicated, low-dose aspirin is commonly recommended for asymptomatic individuals with aPL, including women with a history of obstetric APS who are not pregnant. Low-dose aspirin may lower the thrombotic risk, has a low incidence of adverse side effects, and is inexpensive. Hydroxychloroquine in patients with SLE has been associated with decreased thrombotic events but has not yet become the standard of care for primary prevention of thrombosis in SLE.

Secondary Prevention (for Recurrent Thrombosis). The risk of recurrence for patients with a thrombotic event ranges from 3% to 24%. Long-term anticoagulation is the mainstay of therapy. Warfarin is recommended (after bridging with heparin) and is effective in prevention of arterial and venous thromboses. High-intensity anticoagulation (goal INR 3.0 to 4.0) has not been found to be more effective than moderate intensity (goal INR 2.0 to 3.0) in the prevention of thrombosis. Unfractionated heparin (UFH) or low-molecular-weight heparin (LMWH) may also be used.

In general, anticoagulation is indefinite. Because this is associated with significant bleeding risk, the decision to institute such therapy must be individualized based on the patient's age, compliance, current medications, and comorbidities. The decision to discontinue anticoagulation, and if so, the timing for this, in patients with APS and previous clinical thrombotic events is controversial.

Prevention of Thromboses During Pregnancy. The American College of Chest Physicians (ACCP) guidelines for management of APS in pregnancy recommend antepartum prophylactic UFH or intermediate-dose UFH or prophylactic LMWH combined with aspirin for women with previous pregnancy-related complications, a positive aPL, and no history of venous or arterial thrombosis. Two other indications for aspirin throughout pregnancy are women considered at high risk for preeclampsia and women with prosthetic valves at high risk of thromboembolism. The safety of aspirin during the first trimester remains uncertain, and use should be individualized. The ACCP recommends that, during pregnancy, UFH or LMWH should replace vitamin K antagonists (grade 1A). LMWH is also recommended for prevention and treatment of venous thromboembolism (VTE) (grade 2C). For acute VTE during pregnancy, after using LMWH or UFH (grade 1B), the ACCP guidelines recommend anticoagulation for at least 6 weeks post partum (total minimum duration of therapy = 6 months). For pregnant women with prior VTE on long-term anticoagulation, the ACCP guidelines recommend LMWH or UFH throughout pregnancy followed by resumption of long-term anticoagulation post partum (grade 1C).

Other Therapeutic Approaches. In patients with SLE and aPL, hydroxychloroquine has been reported to lower thrombosis risk. The role of agents such as clopidogrel in APS is unknown. Rituximab may be effective in APS, especially in patients with refractory CAPS. Intravenous immunoglobulin has been used in CAPS in addition to anticoagulation and high-dose glucocorticoids. Statins may have a role, but this has not been formally tested in clinical trials. Cyclophosphamide and plasma exchange have also been used in patients with severe refractory CAPS in addition to anticoagulation and high-dose glucocorticoids, with limited success.

Avoiding Errors. Given the risks of long-term anticoagulation, it is important to determine which patients clearly have APS and require treatment. Ideally, the presence of aPL (LAC, medium- to high-titer aCL or anti-β2GPI antibodies) should be confirmed on two or more occasions at 12 or more weeks apart. A prolonged routine aPTT alone is not sufficient to establish the presence of LAC. Once treatment is initiated, close monitoring is warranted to mitigate toxicity.

In the future, standardized tests for antibodies to other phospholipid proteins may become available, facilitating early recognition and likely timely intervention. A better understanding of APS pathogenesis could grow our therapeutic armamentarium to include therapies targeted against the offending antibodies or downstream pathways such as intracellular protein kinases and complement.

Plate 5-55

Rheumatic Diseases

SCLEROMA

Scleroderma or systemic sclerosis (SSc) is a chronic multisystem, autoimmune disease characterized by a vasculopathy, diffuse fibrosis of skin and various internal organs, and immune abnormalities. The clinical manifestations of this disease are extremely heterogeneous and depend on the presence and degree of involvement of various internal organs.

Scleroderma is categorized into localized and systemic varieties. Localized scleroderma consists of morphea and linear scleroderma, which is manifest as sclerotic lesions of the skin without visceral involvement. Systemic sclerosis, characterized by inflammation and fibrosis in the skin (see Plate 5-55), is also associated with internal organ involvement. It is classified into four major clinical subtypes: limited cutaneous scleroderma (lcSSc) (also called CREST syndrome [Calcinosis cutis, Raynaud phenomenon, Esophageal dysmotility, Sclerodactyly, and Telangiectasia]), diffuse cutaneous scleroderma (dcSSc), systemic sclerosis sine scleroderma, and scleroderma overlap. Limited disease is more common than diffuse disease in a ratio of 2:1.

In addition to the skin, systemic sclerosis involves the blood vessels, joints, skeletal muscle, and, frequently, internal organs such as the gastrointestinal tract, heart, kidney, and lungs. In the United States, the incidence of scleroderma is about 20 new cases per million adults annually, with a prevalence of 240 per million. The female-to-male incidence ratio is 4:1, and the peak age at onset is between 30 and 50 years. White persons develop scleroderma more commonly than black persons (4:1) and more often tend to have limited disease. Afflicted black individuals are more likely to have severe disease (dcSSc) and overall have a worse outcome.

ETIOLOGY AND PATHOGENESIS

The etiology of scleroderma remains unknown. An individual with a susceptible genetic background may encounter an inciting factor such as infection, organic solvents, drugs, or environmental agents.

Clinical expression of scleroderma includes vascular, fibrotic, and immunologic features. Endothelial injury is followed by inflammatory cell extravasation and fibroblast activation. The autonomous activated fibroblasts continue to produce excessive extracellular matrix, which is a self-perpetuating fibrotic process.

CLINICAL PRESENTATION

The clinical subtypes of scleroderma are distinguished from each other primarily on the basis of the extent and degree of skin involvement.

Limited Cutaneous Scleroderma (lcSSc). Skin tightening is restricted, affecting the distal extremities (beyond the elbows and knees) and face. Pulmonary arterial hypertension can be a late manifestation, whereas pulmonary fibrosis develops in about a third of such patients. Symptomatic intestinal pseudo-obstruction can lead to malabsorption. The 10-year survival is more than 70%.

Diffuse Cutaneous Scleroderma (dcSSc). Here widespread skin tightening also involves the upper arms and thighs, trunk, and face. There is rapid progression of skin thickening and early occurrence of visceral disease affecting the gastrointestinal tract, lungs, heart, and kidneys. Palpable tendon friction rubs and flexion contractors develop frequently. The 10-year survival rate is between 40% and 60%.

CLINICAL MANIFESTATIONS OF SCLERODERMA

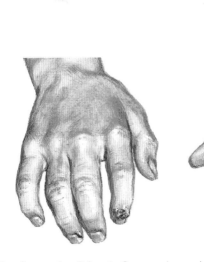

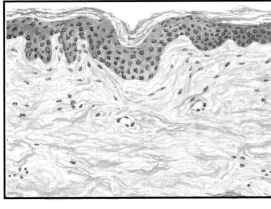

Characteristics. Thickening, tightening, and rigidity of facial skin, with small, constricted mouth and narrow lips, in atrophic phase of scleroderma

Typical skin changes in scleroderma: extensive collagen deposition and some epidermal atrophy

Sclerodactyly. Fingers partially fixed in semiflexed position; terminal phalanges atrophied; fingertips pointed and ulcerated

Scleroderma sine Sclerosis. Some patients with systemic sclerosis may have no detectable skin thickening but present with other features seen in limited scleroderma, such as Raynaud phenomenon, telangiectases, and pulmonary and gastrointestinal disease.

Overlap. Scleroderma-overlap patients concomitantly develop features of one or more of the other autoimmune rheumatic diseases, such as rheumatoid arthritis, SLE, polymyositis, or Sjögren syndrome.

Raynaud Phenomenon. Raynaud phenomenon, an episodic and reversible vasospasm affecting fingers and toes, is precipitated by cold exposure or emotional stress. It occurs in 90% to 95% of patients and is manifested by triphasic color changes: pallor (white), acrocyanosis (blue), and reperfusion hyperemia (red). Ischemic necrosis may occur, leading to ulceration or gangrene of the fingertips.

Cutaneous Manifestations. In lcSSc, skin thickening is confined to distal extremities. Calcinosis from intracutaneous or subcutaneous calcific deposition of hydroxyapatite can develop on the distal digital pads and extensor surface of the forearms, elbows, and knees. Telangiectases can appear on the fingers, face, legs, and

anterior chest. On nail-fold capillaroscopy, dilated nail-fold vessels or capillary "drop outs" can be seen (see Plate 5-56).

In the early phase, patients develop puffy, edematous hands. This is followed by progressive skin thickening and tightening over subsequent weeks to months. Cutaneous hypopigmentation and hyperpigmentation may occur. Often, after 3 to 5 years, the skin starts to soften, and eventually it may revert to normal thickness or even become thin. Perioral involvement leads to thinning of the lips, puckering, and reduced oral aperture.

Musculoskeletal Manifestations. Arthralgias and joint stiffness may affect the small and large joints. Tendon friction rubs commonly palpated over the flexor or extensor tendons due to fibrinous tenosynovitis and tendinitis are specific for dcSSc. Erosive joint disease can develop in some patients. Myopathy can be a result of microvasculopathy and muscle fibrosis, but sometimes there is pathologic evidence of myositis.

Gastrointestinal Tract Manifestations. Esophageal dysmotility eventually develops in about 80% of patients. The most frequent symptoms are heartburn (from gastroesophageal reflux disease) and dysphagia

Plate 5-56

Musculoskeletal System: PART III

SCLERODERMA (Continued)

Gastric antral vascular ectasias (also known as watermelon stomach) is a result of submucosal ectatic vessels in the gastric antrum. These vessels can erode through the gastric mucosa, leading to chronic loss of blood and severe iron-deficiency anemia. Small bowel dysfunction, seen in 20% to 60% of patients, comprises reduced peristalsis, stasis, and bacterial overgrowth. This leads to malabsorption and severe malnutrition. Pneumatosis cystoides intestinales, a condition that results from submucosal or subserosal gas cysts that develop in the wall of the small intestine, can manifest as an acute abdomen, leading to unnecessary laparotomy. Fecal incontinence may develop in some patients due to fibrosis of the anal sphincter. Primary biliary cirrhosis, the liver disorder seen most frequently with lcSSc, is associated with the presence of the anti-mitochondrial antibody.

Pulmonary Manifestations. Pulmonary involvement (interstitial lung disease and/or pulmonary hypertension) occurs in more than 70% of patients with systemic sclerosis and is the most common cause of mortality. The most common symptoms of interstitial lung disease are dyspnea on exertion and a dry cough. Dry, bibasilar end-inspiratory rales are sometimes present. On spirometry, a restrictive ventilatory defect is commonly noted. High-resolution CT of the lungs identifies a ground-glass appearance representing active alveolitis. Alveolitis may progress to fibrosis with irreversible scarring, secondary pulmonary hypertension, and hypoxia. The factors associated with the highest risk for severe interstitial lung disease are black race, male gender, and younger age in patients with dcSSc and the presence of anti-topoisomerase I (Scl-70) antibody.

Pulmonary hypertension, characterized by rapidly progressive dyspnea, occurs in 7% to 12% of patients typically 10 to 15 years after onset of Raynaud phenomenon. The diffusing capacity is disproportionally reduced relative to vital capacity, and the electrocardiogram shows evidence of right-sided heart dysfunction. The prognosis is poor, and the mortality is significantly higher than in patients with idiopathic pulmonary arterial hypertension. The newer classes of novel vasoactive agents may have improved the prognosis of these patients. These agents include parenteral prostacyclin or its analogs, phosphodiesterase-5 inhibitors (sildenafil or tadalafil), or the endothelin receptor antagonists (bosentan or ambrisentan). Many patients require a combination of these therapies.

Cardiac Manifestations. Clinically symptomatic pericardial disease is infrequent (5% to 16%). A large pericardial effusion (>200 mL) can lead to cardiac tamponade and is a marker for poor outcome with an increased risk for impending renal crisis. Symptomatic scleroderma cardiomyopathy, resulting from myocardial microvasculopathy and fibrosis, is rare. Systolic or diastolic dysfunction may develop in this setting. Supraventricular and ventricular arrhythmias are found more frequently in patients with diffuse disease and are strongly associated with mortality.

Renal Manifestations. Twenty-five percent of patients with dcSSc may develop scleroderma renal crisis, which is defined as new onset of accelerated hypertension and rapidly progressive oliguric renal failure. Plasma renin activity is elevated, and mild proteinuria and microscopic hematuria can develop. Microangiopathic hemolytic anemia and thrombocytopenia are prominent hematologic features. Some patients present with congestive heart failure, ventricular arrhythmias, or large pericardial effusions.

CLINICAL FINDINGS OF SCLERODERMA

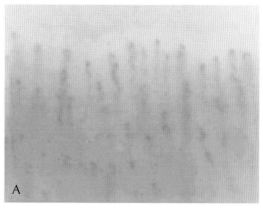

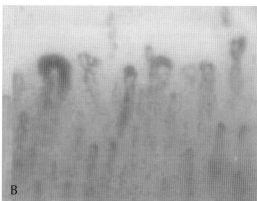

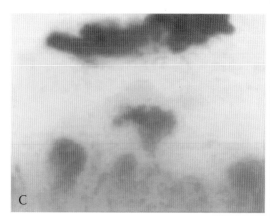

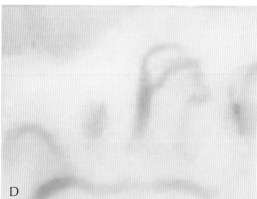

Nail-fold capillaroscopy (×200). **A,** Normal nail-fold capillaroscopy pattern. **B,** Early scleroderma pattern shows well-preserved capillary architecture and density and presence of dilated and giant capillaries. **C,** Active scleroderma pattern shows frequent giant capillaries and hemorrhages, moderate loss of capillaries, and disorganization of capillary architecture. **D,** Late scleroderma pattern shows severe capillary architecture disorganization with dropouts, presence of arborized capillaries, and absence of giant capillaries.

Specific factors associated with a higher risk of developing scleroderma renal crisis include early diffuse disease (<4 years), rapid progression of skin thickening, new cardiac events (e.g., pericardial effusion and/or congestive heart failure), presence of anti-RNA polymerase III antibody, and antecedent high-dose glucocorticoid use (e.g., >20 mg prednisone daily).

DIFFERENTIAL DIAGNOSES

The differential diagnosis of systemic sclerosis requires consideration of several scleroderma-like disorders. Diffuse fasciitis with eosinophilia is associated with swelling, stiffness, and restricted range of motion but usually spares the hands and face. There is sometimes an association with preceding trauma. Sclerodactyly and fibrosis of the palmar fascia occurs in insulin-dependent diabetes mellitus, particularly juvenile-onset type—a condition called *diabetic cheiroarthropathy*. Nephrogenic systemic fibrosis may develop in patients with renal insufficiency after exposure to gadolinium-containing contrast agents administered for MRI procedures. Chronic graft-versus-host disease, particularly after allogeneic bone marrow or stem cell

transplantation, may produce many common clinical and histologic features that mimic scleroderma. Environmental exposures (e.g., inhalation of epoxy resins, vinyl chloride, silica dust, organic solvents, and pesticides; ingestion of toxic rapeseed oil; or injection of paraffin or bleomycin) may produce features of scleroderma.

DIAGNOSTIC APPROACH

The diagnosis of systemic sclerosis is based on a thorough clinical evaluation and supported by the detection of specific autoantibodies and by the detection of major target organ involvement.

Autoantibodies associated with dcSSc are anti-topoisomerase I (Scl 70) or anti-RNA polymerase III antibodies. Anti-centromere antibody is found in 70% to 80% of patients with lcSSc and 5% of those with dcSSc. Additional helpful evaluation includes radiographs of the hands, showing acro-osteolysis and calcinosis cutis (see Plate 5-57). Pulmonary function testing demonstrating a restrictive pattern with decreased forced vital capacity and reduced diffusion capacity (DLco) and high-resolution chest CT showing

Plate 5-57

Rheumatic Diseases

SCLERODERMA (Continued)

ground-glass opacification are sensitive indicators of interstitial lung disease. A skin biopsy from an affected area that demonstrates the typical changes (progressive increase in dermal collagen with loss of appendages) can sometimes establish the diagnosis when the diagnosis is otherwise uncertain.

MANAGEMENT AND THERAPY

There is no proven disease-modifying therapy for scleroderma. The primary focus is preservation of end-organ function to prolong survival and to enhance quality of life. Skin changes in diffuse scleroderma commonly peak in 3 to 5 years and then stabilize. After many years, the skin often softens up and returns to normal tightness, or even thins and atrophies.

Raynaud Phenomenon. The most effective method of preventing Raynaud phenomenon is avoidance of cold exposure. Patients should wear warm protective clothing and avoid tobacco use. Conventional vasodilators, such as long-acting dihydropyridine calcium channel blockers (nifedipine, amlodipine, felodipine), are effective in some patients and are relatively safe. Other vasodilators such as nitrates and prazosin are used alone or in combination with calcium channel blockers in patients who fail to respond adequately to calcium channel blockers alone. One baby aspirin (81 mg) is recommended to inhibit platelet activation and microvascular occlusion. More expensive second-line agents, such as phosphodiesterase-5 inhibitors (sildenafil or tadalafil), endothelin receptor antagonists (bosentan), and intravenous prostanoids (epoprostenol or alprostadil), are reserved for refractory cases with critical digital ischemia leading to ulceration or gangrene. Selective digital sympathectomy has been successful in cases that are not responsive to medical management. Oral antibiotics with good staphylococcal coverage are indicated if lesions become infected. Deeper soft tissue infections or osteomyelitis require treatment with intravenous antibiotics, debridement of devitalized tissue, and, if necessary, amputation.

Gastrointestinal Disease. Esophageal symptoms can be minimized with small, frequent meals, elevation of the head end of the bed, and use of proton pump inhibitors. Patients with persistent symptoms require upper gastrointestinal endoscopy to exclude esophageal stricture and Barrett metaplasia. Small bowel dysmotility symptoms can be managed by increasing dietary fiber, avoiding drugs that affect motility (narcotics), and administering empirical antibiotic therapy cyclically for small intestinal bacterial overgrowth. Octreotide has been used as a small bowel prokinetic agent with variable results. In refractory disease with severe malnutrition and weight loss, parenteral hyperalimentation may be necessary.

Pulmonary Hypertension. Endothelin-1 receptor antagonists (bosentan and ambrisentan) and phosphodiesterase-5 inhibitors (sildenafil and tadalafil) have been approved for treatment of pulmonary hypertension in scleroderma. Inhaled, intravenous or subcutaneous administration of prostanoids is indicated in more advanced cases. Combination therapy is sometimes necessary.

Interstitial Lung Disease. There have been few randomized controlled trials in pulmonary fibrosis in SSc. In double-blind placebo-controlled studies, patients with active alveolitis had stabilization of lung function when treated with oral or monthly intravenous cyclophosphamide for 6 to 12 months. However, the clinical

RADIOGRAPHIC FINDINGS OF ACRO-OSTEOLYSIS AND CALCINOSIS CUTIS

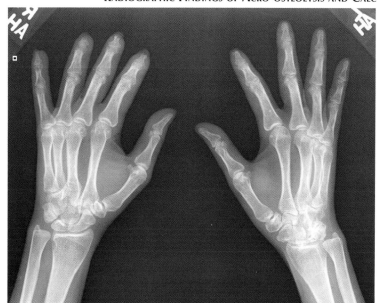

Radiograph from a patient with long-standing systemic sclerosis demonstrating resorption of the tufts of the distal phalanges of left index finger and right index, middle, and ring fingers (acro-osteolysis). In scleroderma, severe and chronic digital ischemia resulting from an occlusive microvasculopathy leads to acro-osteolysis.

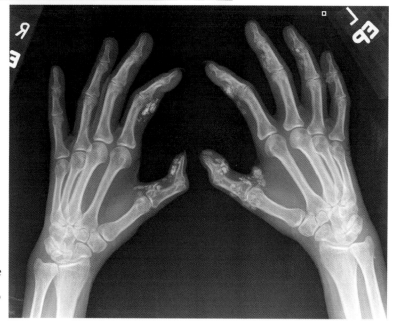

Extensive soft tissue calcification (calcinosis cutis) can be seen in all the fingers of the left hand and the index finger and thumb of the right hand.

relevance of the rather small changes in the forced vital capacity is still in question, and it is debatable whether such a small measurable benefit after 1 year of oral cyclophosphamide is worth the long-term cumulative risk of exposure to this alkylating agent. Mycophenolate mofetil may be effective for interstitial lung disease in scleroderma, and federally funded studies are currently ongoing.

Resting or exertional hypoxia is an indication for supplemental oxygen. Lung transplantation may represent a viable therapeutic option for selected patients.

Renal Disease. Scleroderma renal crisis is a medical emergency. Aggressive antihypertensive therapy with angiotensin-converting enzyme (ACE) inhibitors has considerably improved survival. A rapid-acting ACE inhibitor, such as captopril, should be titrated to normalize blood pressure promptly. Some patients may not respond and progress to renal failure requiring dialysis. However, a subset of patients requiring dialysis may eventually recover renal function after 12 to 18 months if ACE inhibitors are continued.

Cardiac Disease. At present, treatment of symptomatic scleroderma cardiomyopathy is essentially empirical and is similar to the medical treatment of idiopathic dilated cardiomyopathy. Diuretics, ACE inhibitors, β-adrenergic blockers, and vasodilators are routinely used as indicated for cardiac failure. For symptomatic cardiac conduction defects or ventricular arrhythmias, cardiac pacemakers or implantable defibrillators may be required. Cardiac transplant may be a viable option in suitable candidates.

Musculoskeletal Disease. NSAIDs may be used for arthralgias. A regular exercise program can improve joint range of motion and prevent muscle wasting and contractures. Active myositis is treated with methotrexate, azathioprine, or other immunosuppressive agents. Corticosteroid therapy should be avoided or used in precipitating low doses if required, because of the increased risk for scleroderma renal crisis.

Although no cure has been found for scleroderma, the disease is often slowly progressive and manageable, and people who have it can sometimes lead healthy and productive lives. Like many other conditions, education about scleroderma and local support groups can be the greatest tools for managing the disease and reducing the risk of further complications.

Plate 5-58

Musculoskeletal System: PART III

POLYMYOSITIS AND DERMATOMYOSITIS

Polymyositis (PM) and dermatomyositis (DM) are idiopathic inflammatory myopathies (IIM) characterized by inflammation of striated muscle (myositis) and characteristic cutaneous features in DM. These diseases typically present as insidious painless proximal weakness. Extramuscular disease may occur involving the lungs, heart, and musculoskeletal or gastrointestinal systems. PM and DM may present as isolated idiopathic syndromes or may overlap with other autoimmune diseases such as systemic sclerosis.

These diseases are rare, with prevalence rates of approximately 1 per 100,000 in the general population. The annual incidence ranges from 2 to 10 cases per million. Although the disease peak incidence is seen in childhood and adults between ages of 40 and 50, it can occur at any age.

The female-to-male ratio is 2:1. Disease incidence is greater in blacks than whites (3:1).

ETIOLOGY AND PATHOGENESIS

Although the etiology of the idiopathic inflammatory myopathies remains unknown, the pathogenesis is better understood. The major pathologic feature is focal inflammation (myositis), injury, and death of myocytes. Regeneration and hypertrophy, atrophy of myocytes, and replacement of muscle by fibrosis and fat are observed. The inflammatory infiltrate comprises lymphocytes and macrophages and is typically localized and focal.

Both cellular and humoral immune systems are involved in the pathogenesis. In the perivascular regions there is a predominance of B lymphocytes, whereas T lymphocytes are most frequent in the endomysial areas. In DM, perivascular B lymphocytes are numerous with C5b-9 membrane attack complex preceding the inflammatory infiltrate. $CD8^+$ T lymphocytes and macrophages invade the individual muscle fibers, within the fascicle in PM. Expression of MHC Class I is increased in myocytes in both PM and DM. Levels of IL-1 and TNF-α are also elevated in patients with active PM and DM.

Although autoantibodies may be seen in idiopathic inflammatory myopathies, these are more common in patients with an associated connective tissue disease. A group of autoantibodies against cytoplasmic RNA synthetases, other proteins, ribonucleoproteins, and certain nuclear antigens, called myositis-specific autoantibodies, occur in approximately 30% of patients with idiopathic inflammatory myopathies. The pathogenic role of these antibodies is not known, but myositis-specific autoantibodies are associated with specific clinical features and prognosis. The three main autoantibodies include anti-Mi-2, anti–signal recognition particle (anti-SRP), and Jo-1 (anti-synthetase), which is typically associated with interstitial lung disease, fevers, arthritis, Raynaud phenomenon, and mechanic's hands. Anti-SRP is associated with severe PM, and anti-Mi-2 is seen in classic DM.

CLINICAL PRESENTATION

Patients with idiopathic inflammatory myopathies usually present with an insidious progressive painless muscle weakness over a course of several weeks to several months. Acute onset is less common. Patients infrequently report myalgias, and these tend to be mild.

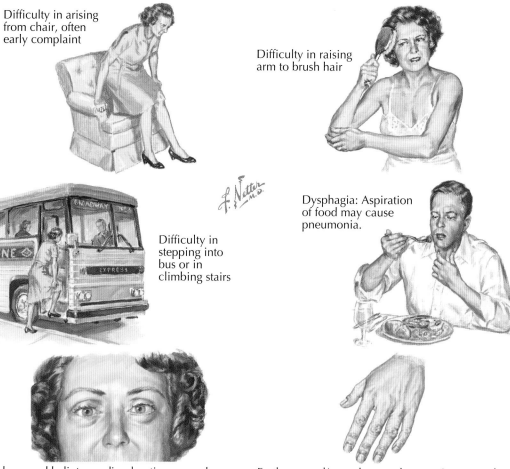

Difficulty in arising from chair, often early complaint

Difficulty in stepping into bus or in climbing stairs

Difficulty in raising arm to brush hair

Dysphagia: Aspiration of food may cause pneumonia.

Edema and heliotrope discoloration around eyes a classic sign. More widespread erythematous rash may also be present.

Erythema and/or scaly, papular eruption around fingernails and on dorsum of interphalangeal joints

Weakness is usually proximal and symmetric, less frequently involving the distal muscles. Rising from a chair, climbing stairs, and combing hair may be difficult. Gait may become unsteady and waddling. Pharyngeal weakness may lead to hoarseness and difficulty swallowing, causing lung aspiration. Fatigue occurs in most patients.

Skin lesions differentiate DM from PM. Cutaneous manifestations typically occur in the upper eyelids, malar areas involving the nasolabial folds, anterior chest, neck, upper back, extensor surfaces of elbows, hands, knees, and periungual areas. Gottron papules are raised plaques over the finger joints, and Gottron's sign is a macular rash over these areas, elbows, and knees. The rash is often photosensitive and may precede, develop simultaneously, or occur after muscle disease. Patients may have DM without muscle involvement, which is referred to as amyopathic dermatomyositis or dermatomyositis sine myositis. In DM, skin lesions may ulcerate and be difficult to heal.

Extramuscular disease may occur, with polyarthralgias or polyarthritis most frequently affecting the hands, wrists, and knees in a rheumatoid-like distribution. The arthritis is usually mild and nondeforming, but in PM associated with anti–Jo-1 antibodies the arthritis may lead to joint damage.

Calcinosis is more common in late stages of chronic DM and can be disabling. Sites of trauma are usually affected, and periarticular calcification can result in joint contractures. Overlying skin may ulcerate and may be complicated by infections and draining sinuses.

Alveolitis or interstitial fibrosis causes dyspnea and cough. Severe alveolitis may be rapidly progressive in patients with anti-tRNA synthetase autoantibodies. Patients with idiopathic inflammatory myopathies usually present with slow progression of lung disease. Dyspnea and cough may also be a result of respiratory muscle weakness or aspiration pneumonia due to pharyngeal weakness.

Dysphagia occurs in up to a third of patients and is due to weakness of the oropharyngeal muscles or striated muscles of the upper third of the esophagus. Patients may have difficulty swallowing, nasal regurgitation, dysphonia, and lung aspiration. In juvenile DM, gastrointestinal bleeding from vasculitic lesions may occur.

Cardiac involvement is frequently asymptomatic with electrocardiographic abnormalities. It rarely causes congestive heart failure, myocarditis, or symptomatic pericarditis.

Raynaud phenomenon may be seen and is often associated with the anti-synthetase syndrome.

An association between idiopathic inflammatory myopathies and malignancy exists, with the risk of cancer appearing to be higher in DM, often occurring within 1 year of diagnosis. Genitourinary sites are more commonly affected, but any neoplasm is possible.

DIFFERENTIAL DIAGNOSIS

The idiopathic inflammatory myopathies are rare diseases that must be distinguished from other conditions

Plate 5-59

Rheumatic Diseases

POLYMYOSITIS AND DERMATOMYOSITIS *(Continued)*

affecting skeletal muscle. Other conditions that cause proximal weakness include the muscular dystrophies, metabolic myopathies, myasthenia gravis, myopathies of endocrine causes, and toxic myopathies. Inclusion-body myositis typically causes distal weakness but may be clinically difficulty to distinguish from PM. Muscle weakness in inclusion-body myositis is asymmetric, is greater in distal than proximal muscles, and occurs at an older age (>50 years).

DIAGNOSTIC APPROACH

A detailed history and a thorough physical examination are essential. Patients may not complain of weakness and frequently describe their symptoms as fatigue. True muscle weakness is evident on physical examination. Patients may have difficulty rising from a seated position without the use of the arms. Strength should be carefully tested and documented. When present, typical cutaneous lesions are helpful in the diagnosis of DM.

Laboratory tests may show anemia, and the ESR sometimes may be elevated. ANA are present in up to 80% of patients. Creatine kinase is the most sensitive and reliable enzyme tested and may be elevated before muscle weakness. Levels increase in periods of disease activity and decrease with response to therapy.

Electromyography is a sensitive, yet nonspecific test for DM/PM. Findings include spontaneous fibrillations, complex repetitive discharges, and early recruitment. The electromyogram is abnormal at presentation in 90% of patients. A normal test makes the diagnosis unlikely. Electromyography may be helpful in the selection of a site for muscle biopsy.

Muscle biopsy is usually performed in all patients with suspected idiopathic inflammatory myopathies. Although percutaneous needle biopsy is less invasive, open surgical biopsy is usually recommended because a larger specimen can be obtained. Histologic features typically reveal chronic inflammatory cells in the perivascular and interstitial areas surrounding myofibrils. Degeneration and necrosis of myofibrils, phagocytosis of necrotic cells, and myofibril regeneration are common features. In DM, perifascicular myofibril atrophy, endothelial hyperplasia of vessels, deposition of immune complexes in intramuscular arteries, and vasculitis can be seen.

The clinical utility of MRI of the muscle has not been well established, but it may be helpful in the selection of muscle biopsy site and in the distinction between active muscle inflammation and fatty infiltration.

Extramuscular involvement should be evaluated by chest radiography, spirometry with diffusion capacity, and electrocardiography. Other tests are obtained if symptoms suggest specific abnormalities such as barium swallow in patients with dysphagia and high-resolution chest CT in patients with dyspnea. Age-appropriate screening for cancer is recommended.

TREATMENT

The severity and prognosis of PM and DM vary, ranging from mild disease to severe disease that may be resistant to multiple therapies. Features that may be associated with a worse prognosis include delay in onset of treatment, severe weakness at presentation, dysphagia, respiratory muscle weakness, and interstitial lung disease. The presence of anti–Jo-1 antibodies may be

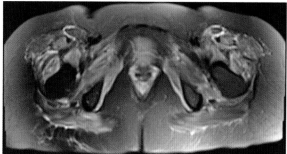
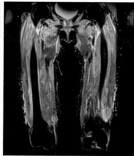

Axial (left) and coronal (right) MR images of femur. Diffuse muscle edema in both anterior and posterior compartments of the thigh, representing inflammation consistent with myositis.

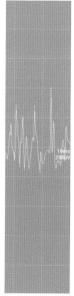
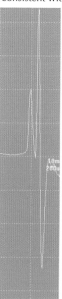
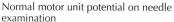

Normal motor unit potential on needle examination

Myopathic motor unit potential changes characterized by polyphasia and reduced amplitude and duration

associated with a poorer response to treatment and prognosis.

Corticosteroids are first-line therapy and should be used in high doses for the first several months, with a very slow taper over a period of 9 to 12 months. Treatment with lower doses and shorter courses may result in incomplete response or disease recurrences. Initial dose is usually 1 mg/kg/day, and pulse intravenous corticosteroids can be given at 1 g/day for 3 days for severe disease.

Immunosuppressive agents such as methotrexate and azathioprine are used for patients who fail treatment with corticosteroids alone or are given at diagnosis in more severe cases. Earlier treatment may limit exposure to corticosteroids. Other medications include mycophenolate mofetil, tacrolimus, and cyclosporine. Cyclophosphamide is used in severe lung disease. Methotrexate is usually avoided in patients with interstitial lung disease because it may be difficult to recognize methotrexate-induced lung toxicity. Studies showed azathioprine use resulted in a lower requirement of prednisone, but response to therapy may take as long as 4 to 6 months. Methotrexate has been studied in retrospective trials, with response rates up to 80%, including patients who had failed corticosteroid therapy.

Most patients require a long course of therapy. An attempt to discontinue the prednisone before stopping other immunosuppressive therapies is preferred. A slow taper of methotrexate or azathioprine after a long period of disease remission can also be attempted. Most patients achieve sustained disease remission on therapy;

however, disease recurrence after discontinuation of treatment is common.

Recurrent and resistant disease pose a major challenge to treatment. Patients who do not completely respond to initial therapy with prednisone, methotrexate, or azathioprine may respond to intravenous immunoglobulin or rituximab. Studies with rituximab are limited by its testing in a small number of patients. Controlled trials with larger number of patients are needed. Intravenous immunoglobulin is an effective short-term therapy for resistant myositis. Cost is an important limitation to this treatment. Cyclosporine, tacrolimus, and mycophenolate mofetil have been evaluated in retrospective studies of patients with resistant disease with positive results, including a reduction in chronic corticosteroid doses.

Response to treatment should be carefully monitored with clinical evaluation and creatine kinase levels. During later stages of disease, with severe muscle atrophy, levels of creatine kinase may not increase significantly and disease flares may be difficult to distinguish from corticosteroid myopathy.

Potential complications from immunosuppressive therapy must be monitored and avoided if possible. Long exposure to corticosteroids has well-known toxicities. Most patients with idiopathic inflammatory myopathies require prolonged exposure to prednisone and therefore should be on prophylactic treatment with bisphosphonates. Patients with new onset of dyspnea and/or cough during therapy should be evaluated for possible lung infection.

Plate 5-60

Musculoskeletal System: PART III

PRIMARY ANGIITIS OF THE CENTRAL NERVOUS SYSTEM

CNS vasculitis is a rare form of vasculitis that causes inflammation of CNS vessels. CNS vasculitis is classified into primary or secondary forms; primary angiitis of the central nervous system (PACNS) is an inflammatory process confined to the CNS, meninges, and spinal cord without any associated systemic disorder. Secondary CNS vasculitis is associated with an underlying systemic disorder. We have witnessed more awareness of PACNS owing to a better understanding of its pathophysiology, advances in neuroradiologic imaging, laboratory findings, and recognition of conditions that mimic PACNS. The diagnostic criteria proposed by Calabrese and Mallek in 1988 remain valuable for evaluation and diagnosis. The incidence rate of PACNS is 2.4 cases per 1 million population. Reversible cerebral vasoconstriction syndrome (RCVS) is the primary mimic of PACNS.

ETIOLOGY AND PATHOGENESIS

Multiple factors such as infection (e.g., herpes simplex virus, varicella zoster virus, and human immunodeficiency virus), immune system dysregulation, and genetics have been implicated in its pathogenesis. Other associated conditions include lymphoma and β-amyloid deposition.

CLINICAL PRESENTATION

PACNS can affect patients at any age but is predominant between the fourth and sixth decades of life. Males are affected twice as often as females. The neurologic signs and symptoms are nonspecific and reflect the diffuse and often patchy nature of the cortical dysfunction. The course of the illness progresses over weeks or months, with insidious course between symptom onset and diagnosis of up to 6 months. However, a remitting-relapsing course has been reported with no new or worsening symptoms of disease at intervals of several months to years. The most common findings include chronic headaches (50%-69%), which are indolently progressive; thunderclap headaches should raise suspicion for RCVS. Cognitive impairment (30%-71%) is subtle, and acute change in mental status and consciousness are very uncommon. Persistent focal neurologic deficits or stroke can occur any time (13%-50%) but rarely at the onset of headache. Stroke secondary to PACNS usually involves multiple vessel territories. Transient ischemic attacks (16%-33%), paraparesis (3%-13%), seizures (7%-11%), myelopathy, or cranial nerve involvement can also occur. Constitutional signs and symptoms such as high-grade fever, weight loss, anorexia, weakness, or visceral target organ disease are atypical. PACNS should be highly considered in patients with the following features: (1) cerebral ischemia involving different vascular territories, distributed over time, accompanied by inflammatory changes in CSF analysis; (2) subacute or chronic headache with cognitive impairment or chronic aseptic meningitis; and (3) chronic meningitis after infectious and neoplastic disorders have been ruled out.

CLINICAL SUBTYPES

Granulomatous Angiitis of the CNS (GACNS). This subgroup predominantly affects males with an insidious headache accompanied by diffuse or focal neurologic

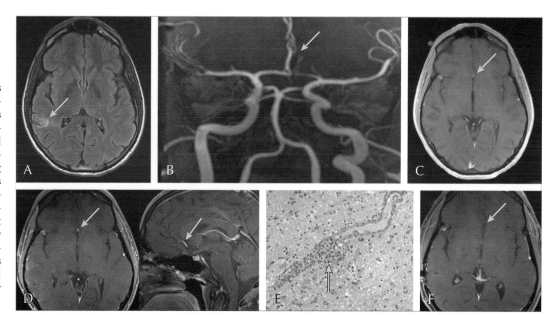

A 23-year-old man was assessed for repeated episodes of left-sided weakness, difficulty speaking, and hearing disturbance along with chronic headaches for 2 months. His medical history was not clinically significant. Blood tests showed a normal erythrocyte sedimentation rate and negative toxicologic screen. His rheumatologic workup did not suggest any systemic vasculitis or autoimmune disease. His stroke assessment included a negative workup for atherothrombotic diseases including a negative transesophageal echocardiogram and hypercoagulable profile. His CSF was notable for raised concentrations of white cells. Brain MRI showed subacute to remote cortical infarcts in the right temporal lobe (**A**). High-resolution magnetic resonance angiography showed a decrease in the size of the left anterior cerebral artery (ACA) compared with the right, with segmental tight stenoses in the A2 segment of the ACA (**B**). Conventional MRI did not show any difference between the right and left ACA (**C**). Postenhancement studies showed thickening and enhancement of the vessel wall in the left A2 segment of the ACA corresponding to the areas of narrowing (**D**). Diagnostic considerations at this stage included PACNS, in view of the negative assessment for thromboembolic disease and other systemic diseases along with the abnormal CSF findings. Hence, brain biopsy was undertaken and revealed lymphocytic vasculitis affecting small vessels of the brain (**E**). The patient was treated with cyclophosphamide and prednisone. Follow-up high-resolution MRI 3 months into treatment showed resolution of the previously noted wall thickening and enhancement of left A2 segment of the ACA (**F**). *Adapted with permission from Hajj-Ali RA, Singhal AB, Benseler S, Molloy E, Calabrese LH. Primary angiitis of the CNS. Lancet Neurol 2011;10(6):561–72.*

deficits. Patients have strokelike symptoms without any other etiology of strokes. Signs and symptoms of systemic vasculitides are absent. CSF analysis reveals an aseptic meningitis. MRI typically shows multiple bilateral ischemic foci. The diagnosis is confirmed by finding small to medium-size vessel granulomatous angiitis with Langhans or foreign body giant cells on the brain biopsy. Treatment with a combination of cyclophosphamide and glucocorticoid is usually required.

PACNS with Lymphocytic Infiltrate by Brain Biopsy. This subclass of PACNS presents as clinical, radiologic, and CSF findings that are similar to those of GACNS. However, brain biopsy reveals the presence of lymphocytic angiitis versus the granulomatous lesions seen in GACNS.

Angiographically Defined PACNS. Medium-sized vessels are affected in this subclass of PACNS, which accounts for a higher frequency of abnormal findings of cerebral angiography. Abnormal CSF analysis is usually present. This is a poorly defined entity; thus, other cerebral arteriopathies such as RCVS, infections, and atherosclerosis should be investigated prior to diagnosis and treatment.

Mass-Lesion (ML-PACNS) Presentation. A rare subset of PACNS with a mass-like lesion has been described. The most common features of patients with ML-PACNS are headache (74%), focal neurologic

deficit (64%), diffuse neurologic deficit (50%), seizures (47%), nausea and vomiting (21%), and constitutional symptoms (12%). MRI findings reveal a mass lesion. CSF analysis shows a distinctive aseptic meningitis picture in approximately two thirds of cases. Cerebral angiography can be abnormal in more than 50% of these patients with features of a mass effect but without signs of vasculitis. The diagnosis of CNS vasculitis is made by the findings of vasculitic changes on brain pathology after ruling out infections and neoplastic conditions.

Amyloid-β–Related Cerebral Angiitis (ABRA). Development of ABRA is attributed to the presence of amyloid β proteins. A higher percentage of ML-PACNS is seen in the amyloid-related angiitis subset and is associated with a poor outcome.

DIFFERENTIAL DIAGNOSIS

A diverse group of disorders has been described that possess clinical and angiographic features similar to PACNS. Atherosclerosis and thromboembolic disorders are likely if a patient has a history of traditional cardiovascular risk factors such as diabetes, hypertension, and hyperlipidemia. Stroke workup should be obtained. Presence of vessel calcifications in CT scans or carotid ultrasound images are suggestive of atherosclerotic disease. Fibromuscular dysplasia, moyamoya

Plate 5-60

Rheumatic Diseases

PRIMARY ANGIITIS OF THE CENTRAL NERVOUS SYSTEM
(Continued)

disease, and radiation vasculopathy can cause angiographic abnormalities that can be mistaken for PACNS. However, they have distinguishing extracranial angiographic features that differentiate them from PACNS.

It is important to differentiate PACNS from its close mimic RCVS. Differentiating these two conditions can be complex, yet is crucial because of contrasting therapy and prognosis. RCVS tends to occur in patients between the ages of 20 and 50 and females are affected more often than males. Presentation includes acute-onset severe headaches, often described as "thunderclap" headaches. Other common findings include focal neurologic symptoms (43%), generalized tonic-clonic seizures (17%), ischemic strokes (39%), convexity subarachnoid hemorrhage (34%), lobar hemorrhage (20%), and brain edema (38%). The presence of clinical cofactors (e.g., Valsalva maneuver, recent childbirth, intake of sympathomimetic drugs) can be identified and may be causal. Major ischemic or hemorrhagic stroke, progressive brain edema, and stroke-related death from severe, sustained cerebral vasoconstriction have also been described. The ESR is normal, and CSF analysis is benign. Angiographic finding for RVCS are those of "string of beads" in multiple vascular cerebral beds with reversibility of vascular abnormalities within 3 months. Brain imaging features include brain infarcts and hemorrhages that are typically located in hemispheric "watershed" regions. Convexity subarachnoid hemorrhage is usually minor and found to be more frequent in women and in patients with migraines.

Brain neoplasm (e.g., Hodgkin and non-Hodgkin lymphoma, leukemia, and lung cancers) and demyelinating diseases (e.g., multiple sclerosis and progressive leukoencephalopathy) may present as neuroimaging features similar to those of PACNS.

Systemic diseases and infections should be ruled out. If CNS infection is suspected, laboratory evaluation for specific pathogens should be guided by epidemiologic analysis and exposure risk factors. Etiologic possibilities include human immunodeficiency virus, syphilis, cytomegalovirus, varicella zoster, herpes simplex, hepatitis, tuberculosis, aspergillosis, histoplasmosis, and cysticercosis. Serologic and microbiologic studies should be requested.

Secondary and autoimmune-related vasculitides, such as rheumatologic diseases (e.g., SLE, Sjögren syndrome, scleroderma), systemic vasculitides (e.g., granulomatosis with polyangiitis, microscopic polyangiitis, polyarteritis nodosa, Behçet syndrome, Cogan syndrome), and other autoimmune disease (e.g., Crohn disease, sarcoidosis), can cause CNS involvement and should be ruled out.

DIAGNOSTIC APPROACH

There are no laboratory markers or radiologic features specific for PACNS. Establishing the diagnosis includes multiple laboratory tests to exclude other diagnoses, particularly infection and malignancy.

Laboratory studies should include serologic tests for rheumatologic disorders and other autoimmune conditions to rule out common mimics of PACNS. Elevation of acute phase markers likely indicates underlying infections or systemic vasculitides because acute phase reactants should be normal in PACNS. Blood cultures and molecular testing for pathogens should be requested when appropriate.

CSF analysis should be performed in all patients with PACNS. CSF analysis is abnormal in 80% to 90% of histologically proven cases of PACNS. CSF findings reflect aseptic meningitis, with modest lymphocytic pleocytosis (median CSF white blood cell count of 20 cells/mL), normal glucose, elevated protein concentration (median CSF protein concentration of 120 mg/dL), and occasionally the presence of oligoclonal bands and increased IgG synthesis. CSF testing including cultures, cell cytology, serologic analysis, and polymerase chain reaction can provide crucial information for detection for other PACNS mimics.

NEUROIMAGING MODALITIES

The most frequently used imaging techniques in the evaluation of PACNS include CT, MRI, MRA, and conventional angiography. However, it is important to remember that none of these neuroimaging studies is specific for PACNS. MRI is abnormal in 90% to 100% cases of PACNS. Common locations of brain lesions are located in subcortical white matter, deep gray matter, deep white matter, and the cerebral cortex. Abnormalities include infarctions, which are detected in up to 53% of patients and can involve variable-size vascular territories. Nonspecific lesions in white matter identified with high-intensity T2-weighted MRI with a fluid-attenuated inversion-recovery sequence (FLAIR) are common. Other causes of T2-hypertintense foci should be ruled out (e.g., hypoxic-ischemic changes, age-related changes, migraine, multiple sclerosis, central pontine myelinolysis, metastasis, metabolic changes, eclampsia, and chemoirradiation).

Visualization of cerebral vessels can be obtained indirectly by MRA or directly by conventional angiography. The typical angiographic abnormalities of cerebral angiography in PACNS include alternating areas of irregular "beadings" (stenosis and dilatation), circumferential or eccentric luminal narrowing, and occlusions of one or more arteries and/or vascular mass effect that can involve single or multiple vessels (see Plate 5-60). Cerebral angiography is limited by its ability to demonstrate vasculitic changes in the small vessels (<500 μm in diameter), which contributes to the low sensitivity. Both sensitivity and specificity of cerebral angiography

are poor; a negative angiogram does not exclude diagnosis of PACNS, nor is a positive angiogram diagnostic for PACNS. Incorporating the clinical information, CSF findings, and pathologic findings in diagnosing PACNS is important.

BRAIN BIOPSY

Brain biopsy is the gold standard for diagnosis of CNS vasculitis. Although this is an invasive procedure, morbidity has been shown to be relatively low. The classic histologic findings typically involve small to medium-sized arteries with segmental granulomatous lesions composed of multinucleated giant cells, predominantly histiocytic cells with variable number of plasma cells, histiocytes, neutrophils, and eosinophils (see Plate 5-60). False-negative biopsies occur in up to 25% of cases, owing to irregular involvement of brain parenchyma and inaccessibility of the lesion. Open-wedge tissue sampling of a radiologically identified area provides the highest yield. If the lesion is not accessible, it is advisable to sample the tip of the nondominant temporal lobe with overlying leptomeninges and underlying cortex. Brain biopsy is helpful in ruling out PACNS mimics, particularly infections and malignancy.

MANAGEMENT AND TREATMENT

Therapeutic strategies are based on retrospective observations and expert opinions. There are no randomized control studies to support the standard therapies.

Cyclophosphamide, in addition to glucocorticoids, has been the mainstay in the treatment of GACNS. The treatment recommendations for PACNS have been adapted from the treatment algorithm used for systemic small vessel vasculitides. A decision on the use of single or combination therapy is usually based on the acuity and severity of neurologic symptoms. Patients with mild neurologic symptoms can be treated with a single regimen of glucocorticoids. Glucocorticoid treatment is typically initiated to achieve rapid suppression of inflammation. Typical regimens include high oral doses of glucocorticoids (1 mg/kg/day) or intravenous pulse methylprednisolone, 1 g/day for 3 consecutive days followed by prednisone 60 mg/day. High-dose prednisone should be continued for 4 weeks until inflammation is well controlled and then followed by a slow tapering regimen. When combination therapy is required, cyclophosphamide is started at 2 mg/kg/day for 3 to 6 months. Patients should be monitored particularly for leukopenia, infections, and bladder toxicity. After achieving remission, alternative immunosuppressive agents such as azathioprine or mycophenolate mofetil should be used as maintenance therapy to limit the toxicity associated with long-term cyclophosphamide therapy. Patients should also be given appropriate preventive measures, including prophylaxis for osteoporosis and *Pneumocystis jiroveci* pneumonia.

Plate 5-61

Musculoskeletal System: PART III

BEHÇET SYNDROME

Behçet syndrome is a rare, systemic inflammatory disorder with an unknown etiology. It was first formally described by Hulusi Behçet, a Turkish dermatologist, in 1937 as a triad of symptoms including aphthae ulcers, genital ulcers, and hypopyon uveitis that could lead to blindness. However, early descriptions of the disease date back to Hippocrates in the 5th century BC. Manifestations of Behçet syndrome are protean and include variable skin lesions, arthritis, thrombophlebitis, and gastrointestinal and CNS involvement. The major causes of mortality are related to vascular involvement and neurologic complications. Genetic studies have shown a strong association with HLA-B51, although this remains an insensitive test for diagnosis. Historically, Behçet syndrome has followed the Old Silk Road trading routes that connected south, east, and western Asia with the Mediterranean world and northeastern parts of Africa. The prevalence of Behçet syndrome is higher in Turkey (up to 420 per 100,000 people) and less frequent in the rest of the world.

DIAGNOSTIC CRITERIA

Many different criteria are used for diagnosis of Behçet syndrome, but the International Study Group criteria are the most used. Recurrent oral ulcers are required along with two other manifestations, including recurrent genital ulceration, eye lesions, skin lesions, and a positive pathergy test.

Mucocutaneous Manifestations. Mucocutaneous manifestations among Behçet syndrome are common. Almost all patients will have oral ulcers frequently as the first symptom of disease. These ulcers are painful and may come in crops. Genital ulcers are less common and may occur only once during the disease course. In males, ulcers tend to occur on the scrotum and less frequently on the glans or shaft. In females, lesions involve both the major and minor labia, usually healing in a period of 2 to 4 weeks. Infectious causes of genital ulcers, such as herpes simplex infections, chancroid, syphilis, granuloma inguinale, and lymphogranuloma venereum, should be ruled out. Other mucocutaneous manifestations of Behçet syndrome include acne-like lesions, papulopustular lesions, and nodular lesions occurring in 80% of patients. Pathergy is an inflammatory reaction manifested by a papule or pustule that forms within 48 hours after intradermal injection of the skin with a 20-gauge needle. A positive pathergy test can be used to aid diagnosis; however, it is less frequently seen in the United States compared with the Mediterranean and Middle East area (see Plate 5-62). Medications effective in the treatment of oral and genital ulcers include azathioprine, etanercept, INF-α_{2a}, dapsone, thalidomide, and colchicine.

Ocular Manifestations. Eye manifestations are estimated to occur in 35% to 70% of patients as anterior or posterior uveitis. Males and young patients tend to have more severe disease. Delays in treatment can result in worse outcomes, including vision loss. Anterior uveitis with intense inflammation can cause hypopyon formation (see Plate 5-61) and be associated with retinal vasculitis. Isolated anterior uveitis is rare. Retinal involvement can be severe, leading to retinal exudate, hemorrhages, venous thrombosis, papilledema, and macular disease. Glucocorticoids should be used initially to quickly decrease inflammation. Both azathioprine and infliximab have been shown to be effective at preventing relapses and maintaining visual acuity. Cyclosporine in combination with colchicine and

INF-α alone have also been used with success. Because of increased awareness and more aggressive treatment, visual loss has decreased from 75% to 20% in this population.

Musculoskeletal Manifestations. Musculoskeletal manifestations include arthritis in 30% to 80% of patients. Arthritis is generally monarticular or oligoarticular and most commonly affects the knees, ankles, and wrists. The arthritis is nondeforming and nonerosive. Synovial fluid analysis during an attack is usually inflammatory. Most patients will respond to colchicine.

Vascular Manifestations. Vascular manifestations carry a poor prognosis. Vascular involvement is less common in the United States than in other parts of the world. It is estimated that 5% to 30% of patients have vascular involvement. What is peculiar about Behçet syndrome is that it is a vasculitis that can affect either veins or arteries of any size. Most common vascular involvement includes thrombophlebitis of either deep

TRIAD OF BEHÇET SYNDROME

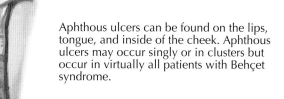

Aphthous ulcers can be found on the lips, tongue, and inside of the cheek. Aphthous ulcers may occur singly or in clusters but occur in virtually all patients with Behçet syndrome.

Behçet syndrome may cause anterior uveitis (inflammation in the front of the eye). Anterior uveitis results in pain, blurry vision, light sensitivity, tearing, or redness of the eye.

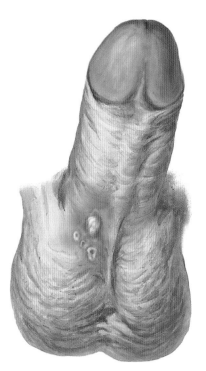

Painful genital lesions may form on the scrotum, similar to oral lesions, but deeper. Lesions appear as red, ulcerated sores. The genital sores are usually painful and may leave scars.

Plate 5-62

Rheumatic Diseases

BEHÇET SYNDROME (Continued)

or superficial veins. Other manifestations include vena cava thrombosis and occlusion of the suprahepatic veins, leading to Budd-Chiari syndrome. It is generally accepted that acute deep vein thrombosis should be treated with immunosuppressive agents such as azathioprine, cyclophosphamide, or glucocorticoids. Thromboembolisms are rare, likely secondary to tight adherence of the thrombosis to the vessel wall; therefore, treatment with anticoagulation is controversial, with most centers advocating for the addition of anticoagulation on top of immunosuppression. Arterial involvement is less frequent (<5%). Any part of the arterial tree can be affected, but most common involvement includes peripheral artery aneurysms. Caution should be used when performing invasive vascular procedures because they place patients at higher risk for pseudoaneurysm development at the puncture site. Insertion of venous catheters may also initiate or aggravate an already developed thrombosis in the peripheral veins.

Pulmonary artery aneurysms, estimated to occur in 1.1% of patients, are associated with a high mortality when present. Nonetheless, mortality rates have improved markedly because of improved recognition and early aggressive treatment, most commonly with cyclophosphamide and glucocorticoids. Pulmonary artery aneurysms typically presents in male patients, with a mean age at onset in the early 30s, commonly with hemoptysis. It is highly associated with other vascular involvement such as thrombophlebitis, with thrombosis of the lower extremities or venae cava. Patients may be mistakenly diagnosed with pulmonary embolism, given the association with peripheral venous thrombosis and the presentation of hemoptysis. Exclusion of pulmonary aneurysms in such a scenario is imperative before starting anticoagulation, which could be detrimental if the diagnosis is erroneous.

Central Nervous System Manifestations. CNS involvement is thought to affect 10% to 50% of patients, with a mortality rate of up to 20%. In general, CNS involvement is one of two presentations: parenchymal or nonparenchymal disease. Parenchymal involvement is a much more common manifestation (81% of CNS involvement). Parenchymal lesions present as recurrent meningoencephalitis involving the brainstem and less commonly the spinal cord and hemispheric regions of the brain. Common symptoms include pyramidal signs, hemiparesis, behavior change, sphincter dysfunction, impotence, and headaches. Nonparenchymal involvement is less common. In this group, intracranial hypertension is the most common manifestation and is frequently caused by a dural sinus thrombosis. Papilledema and arterial involvement are other manifestations. Poor prognostic signs include an abnormal CSF (elevated protein or cell count), parenchymal involvement, recurrent attacks, or a progressive course. There are no controlled trials regarding treatment of neurologic manifestations, but reports support the use of azathioprine, methotrexate, or cyclophosphamide in combination with glucocorticoids. Cyclosporine should generally be avoided in this setting because of the association with a higher rate of neurologic events.

Gastrointestinal Manifestations. Gastrointestinal involvement is present in 5% to 60% of patients. A high prevalence of gastrointestinal involvement exists in Japan, where up to one third of Behçet syndrome patients have gastrointestinal symptoms, but this is rare in Turkey. Symptoms may include anorexia, vomiting,

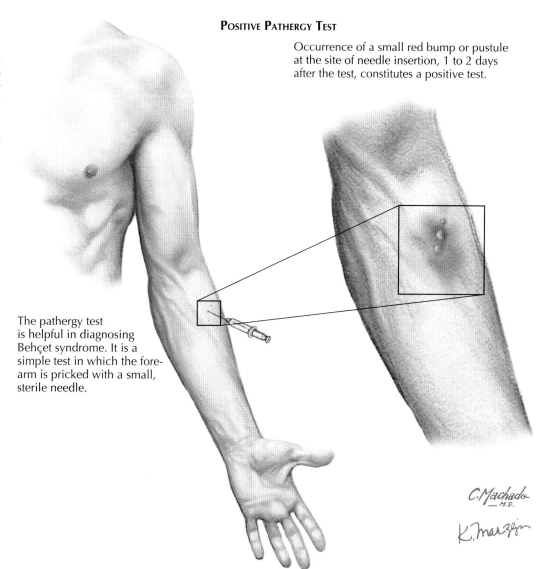

POSITIVE PATHERGY TEST

Occurrence of a small red bump or pustule at the site of needle insertion, 1 to 2 days after the test, constitutes a positive test.

The pathergy test is helpful in diagnosing Behçet syndrome. It is a simple test in which the forearm is pricked with a small, sterile needle.

C. Machado —M.D.

K. Marzęjn

The International Study Group Criteria for Behçet Syndrome

Recurrent oral ulcers (Minor aphthous, major aphthous, or herpetiform ulceration)

Recurrent at least three times in one 12-month period. ***Plus two of following:***

- **Recurrent genital ulceration**
- **Eye lesions**
  - Anterior uveitis
  - Posterior uveitis
  - Cells in vitreous on slit-lamp examination
  - Retinal vasculitis observed by qualified physician

- **Skin lesions**
  - Erythema nodosum-like
  - Pseudofolliculitis
  - Papulopustular lesions
  - Acneiform nodules
- **Positive pathergy test**
  - To be read by a physician at 48 hr, performed with oblique insertion of a 20-22–gauge or smaller needle under sterile conditions

27 countries participated in this effort (2556 BS patients and 1163 controls). Sensitivity is 82.4%. Specificity is 96%. Accuracy of the ISG is 86.7%. *From Lancet 1990;335(8697):1078-1080.*

---

dyspepsia, diarrhea, and abdominal pain. Mucosal ulcerations are most common in the ileum, followed by the cecum and other parts of the colon. In many instances, it is challenging to differentiate it from inflammatory bowel disease. The location, number, and patterns of ulcers as well as a pathergy test may give clues to help differentiate the two disorders because patients with Behçet syndrome tend to have fewer, more focal and rounded ulcers than patients with inflammatory bowel disease. Hepatic involvement is uncommon and should raise suspicion for Budd-Chiari

syndrome. There are no controlled studies regarding treatment of gastrointestinal manifestations, but sulfasalazine, glucocorticoids, azathioprine, tumor necrosis factor antagonists, or thalidomide should be used before considering surgery in most cases. However, situations requiring emergent surgery can arise, such as bowel perforation.

Other Manifestations. Sporadic cases of systemic amyloidosis type AA can occur. Direct bladder involvement can lead to voiding dysfunction. Epididymitis occurs in around 5% of patients.

TUMORS OF MUSCULOSKELETAL SYSTEM

Plate 6-1   Musculoskeletal System: PART III

STAGING OF MUSCULOSKELETAL TUMORS

Stages 1–3. Histologically benign (G₀); variable clinical course and biologic behavior

Benign

Stage 1. Remains static or heals spontaneously with indolent clinical course. Well encapsulated.

Bone tumor   Soft tissue tumor

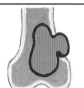
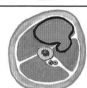

Stage 2. Active; progressive, symptomatic growth. Remains intracapsular. Limited by natural boundaries but may often deform them.

Stage 3. Aggressive; locally aggressive but not limited by capsule or natural boundaries. May penetrate cortex or compartment boundaries. Higher rate of recurrence.

Stage I. Histologically low grade (G₁); well differentiated; few mitoses; moderate nuclear atypia. Tends to recur locally. Radioisotope uptake moderate.

Malignant

IA — Intraosseous or intracompartmental

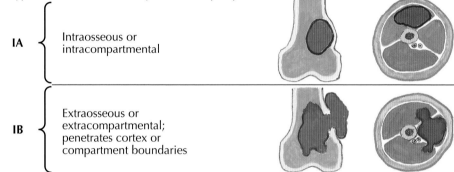

IB — Extraosseous or extracompartmental; penetrates cortex or compartment boundaries

Stage II. Histologically high grade (G₂); poorly differentiated; high cell-to-matrix ratio; many mitoses; much nuclear atypia, necrosis, neovascularity; permeative. Radioisotope uptake intense. Higher incidence of metastases.

IIA — Intraosseous or intracompartmental

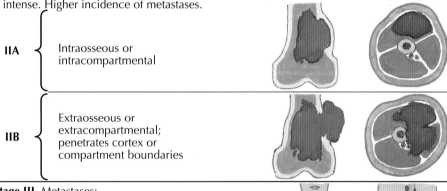

IIB — Extraosseous or extracompartmental; penetrates cortex or compartment boundaries

Stage III. Metastases; regional or remote (visceral, lymphatic, or osseous)

INITIAL EVALUATION AND STAGING OF MUSCULOSKELETAL TUMORS

An understanding of the tumors of the musculoskeletal system requires a thorough knowledge of clinical presentation, natural history, staging characteristics, histopathology, and response to treatment of these tumors. Common bone tumors include myeloma, lymphoma, and metastases from primary breast, lung, kidney, thyroid, and prostate cancers; and these are, in fact, the most common malignant bone lesions in patients older than 40 years of age. Much less common are primary lesions of bone. Osteosarcoma is the most common primary bone tumor, followed by Ewing sarcoma and chondrosarcoma. A classification of primary (musculoskeletal origin) benign and malignant tumors of bone and soft tissue is presented in the table.

Staging studies may be needed to determine the local extent of lesions or distant metastases and histologic diagnosis of the disease.

Radionuclide bone scans are performed to assess multiple sites of involvement, the extent of local intraosseous involvement not apparent on radiographs, and tumor activity.

Computed tomography (CT) of the lesion is employed for determining bone destruction, intrinsic density of the lesion, and cortical extension. Metastases of primary musculoskeletal sarcomas are most commonly found in the lungs. Chest radiographs and chest CT are used for chest surveillance to provide information about metastatic disease. The role of combined positron emission tomography and computed tomography (PET/CT) is unclear, but it has been most useful in delineation of neurofibromas from sarcomas in patients with neurofibromatosis.

Magnetic resonance imaging (MRI) delineates the precise location and extent of tumor involvement. Specifically, MRI is the primary study used to delineate compartmental involvement, intra-articular involvement, and proximity of neurovascular structures; MRI provides superior resolution and sensitivity in depicting abnormalities and is particularly useful in determining the extent of soft tissue lesions and the subtle involvement of the bone marrow in bone lesions.

Staging. The staging system for musculoskeletal tumors shown in Table 6-1 represents an assessment of the surgical grade, local extent of disease, and presence

or absence of metastases. It is based on the stratification and interrelationship of these three factors and is used to predict the prognosis, response to surgical treatment, risk of local recurrence, and metastatic potential.

The *surgical grade (G)* reflects a tumor's aggressiveness based on its histologic pattern: benign (G₀), low-grade malignant (G₁), and high-grade malignant (G₂).

The *local extent of disease (T)* defines the primary lesion as intracapsular (T₀, surrounded by an intact capsule of fibrous tissue or reactive bone); extracapsular

but intracompartmental (T₁, remaining within an intraosseous, intrafascial or intramuscular, periosteal, or paraosseous compartment or potential compartment); and extracapsular and extracompartmental (T₂, extending beyond its compartment of origin or arising within incompletely bounded spaces, such as the popliteal fossa, axilla, or groin).

The designation *M* indicates the presence or absence of *metastases:* no known metastases (M₀) or metastases present (M₁).

Plate 6-1

Tumors of Musculoskeletal System

Surgical Staging System for Musculoskeletal Tumors

		Stage	Grade	Site	Metastasis
Benign	1	Latent	G_0	T_0	M_0
	2	Active	G_0	T_0	M_0
	3	Aggressive	G_0	T_{1-2}	M_{0-1}
Malignant	1A	Low grade, intracompartmental	G_1	T_1	M_0
	1B	Low grade, extracompartmental	G_1	T_1	M_0
	IIA	High grade, intracompartmental	G_2	T_2	M_0
	IIB	High grade, extracompartmental	G_2	T_2	M_0
	IIIA	Low or high grade, intracompartmental, with metastases	G_{1-2}	T_1	M_1
	IIIB	Low or high grade, extracompartmental, with metastases	G_{1-2}	T_2	M_1

Primary Musculoskeletal Tumors and Usual Presenting Stage

Tumors of Bone

Tissue type	Benign	Malignant
Osseous	Osteoid osteoma (2) Osteoblastoma (2–3) Osteoma (1)	Classic osteosarcoma (IIB) Parosteal osteosarcoma (IA) Periosteal osteosarcoma (IIA)
Cartilaginous	Enchondroma (2) Exostosis (2) Periosteal chondroma (2) Chondroblastoma (2–3) Chondromyxoid fibroma (2–3)	Primary chondrosarcoma (IIB) Secondary chondrosarcoma (IA)
Fibrous	Nonossifying fibroma (1–2) Desmoplastic fibroma (2–3) Fibrous dysplasia (NA) Ossifying fibroma (2–3)	Fibrosarcoma of bone (IIB) Malignant fibrous histiocytoma (IIB)
Reticuloendothelial	Eosinophilic granuloma (NA) Hand-Schüller-Christian disease (NA) Letterer-Siwe disease (NA)	Ewing sarcoma (IIB) Reticulum-cell sarcoma (IIB) Myeloma (III)
Vascular	Aneurysmal bone cyst (2) Hemangioma of bone (2)	Angiosarcoma (IIB) Hemangioendothelioma (IA) Hemangiopericytoma (IA)
Unknown origin	Simple bone cyst (NA) Giant-cell tumor in bone (2–3)	Giant-cell sarcoma (IIB) Chordoma (IB) Adamantinoma (IA)

Tumors of Soft Tissue

Tissue type	Benign	Malignant
Osseous	Myositis ossificans (NA)	Extraosseous osteosarcoma (IIB)
Cartilaginous	Chondroma (2) Synovial chondromatosis (2)	Extraosseous chondrosarcoma (IB)
Fibrous	Fibrous (1–2)	Fibrosarcoma (I–IIB)
Fibromatosis (3)	Malignant fibrous histiocytoma (IIB)	
Synovial	Pigmented villonodular synovitis (2) Ganglion cyst (1)	Synovial sarcoma (IIB)
Vascular	Hemangioma (2–3)	Angiosarcoma (IIB) Hemangioendothelioma (IB) Hemangiopericytoma (IB)
Fatty	Lipoma (1) Angiolipoma (3)	Atypical lipoma/low-grade liposarcoma (IA) High-grade liposarcoma (IIB)
Neural	Neurolemmoma (2) Neurofibroma (2–3)	Neurosarcoma (IIB) Neurofibrosarcoma (IIB)
Muscular	Leiomyoma (2) Rhabdomyoma	Leiomyosarcoma (IIB) Rhabdomyosarcoma (IIA)
Unknown origin	Giant-cell tumor of tendon sheath (2)	Epithelioid sarcoma (IB) Clear cell sarcoma (IB) Undifferentiated sarcoma (IIB)

NA = not applicable

Plate 6-2

Musculoskeletal System: PART III

BENIGN TUMORS OF BONE— OSTEOID OSTEOMA

Osteoid osteoma is a benign osseous tumor that occurs primarily in adolescents and less often in children and young adults. The most common site is the proximal femur; and although osteoid osteoma typically involves the diaphysis of long bones, it may also occur in the foot (talus, navicular, or calcaneus) and in the posterior elements of the spine, where it can lead to a secondary scoliosis. The typical presenting symptom is well-localized pain that is most severe at night and is relieved by aspirin and other prostaglandin inhibitors. The lesion typically has a nidus, but this can be difficult to locate on radiograph. CT or MRI can be helpful in locating the nidus and increasing the certainty of diagnosis.

Diagnostic Studies. An intense bony reaction to a small nidus is the radiographic hallmark of osteoid osteoma. Radiographs reveal an oval radiolucent nidus only 3 to 5 mm in diameter and surrounded by a disproportionately large, dense reactive zone. Although usually located in the cortex, a nidus may occur in the subperiosteal and endosteal regions. CT scans at 5-mm intervals are used to confirm a cortical nidus and to help direct the therapeutic approach. The bone scan usually shows increased radioisotope uptake.

The radiographic differential diagnosis includes osteomyelitis (chronic sclerosing osteomyelitis), Brodie's abscess, and stress fracture.

Histologic examination reveals a nidus composed of thick, vascular bars of osteoblastic tissue surrounded by a thin zone of vascular fibrous tissue, in turn surrounded by a dense shell, or margin, of mature reactive cortical bone. The histologic differential diagnosis primarily includes osteoblastoma (see Plate 6-3). Although osteoblastoma is similar to osteoid osteoma in many respects, it is usually larger and has some subtle but distinct histologic differences. Distinguishing osteosarcoma (see Plates 6-15 and 6-16) from the small osteoblastic nidus of osteoid osteoma is rarely problematic.

Treatment/Prognosis. Although osteoid osteoma may eventually resolve spontaneously, with spontaneous ossification and the subsequent relief of pain, most patients prefer not to wait for resolution, owing to severe pain. Percutaneous radiofrequency ablation of the osteoid osteomas can be performed with up to 90% success and can be done under local anesthesia with CT

scan guidance; thus, this is the current initial treatment of choice. When the nidus is located in a low-stress area such as the metaphysis, en bloc excision with a surrounding small block of reactive bone can be performed but has increased morbidity relative to percutaneous ablation. Alternatively, the overlying margin of reactive bone may be shaved until the nidus is visible as a cherry-red spot; this spot then can be removed with curettage. Although intracapsular curettage is

associated with a higher recurrence rate than other types of excision, it minimizes the risk of postoperative fracture in high-stress areas such as the femoral neck. Most recurrences result from fragmentation of the lesion, partial excision, or inaccurate localization of the lesion in an inaccessible place.

After radiofrequency ablation, complete excision, or even spontaneous resolution, prognosis is excellent. No cases of malignant transformation have been reported.

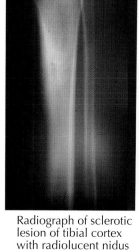

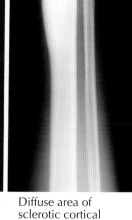

Adolescent indicates site of pain on tibia; bony prominence only slight. Pain often dramatically relieved by aspirin.

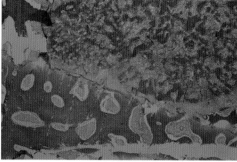

Radiograph of sclerotic lesion of tibial cortex with radiolucent nidus (difficult to see)

Diffuse area of sclerotic cortical thickening apparent during healing phase

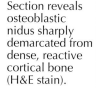

Section reveals osteoblastic nidus sharply demarcated from dense, reactive cortical bone (H&E stain).

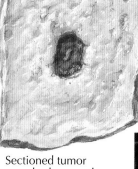

Sectioned tumor reveals cherry-red nidus surrounded by dense, reactive cortical bone.

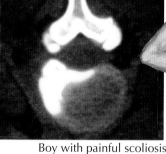

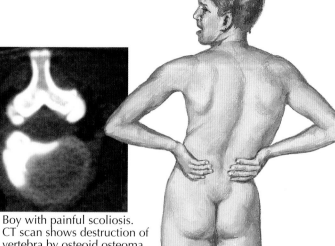

Boy with painful scoliosis. CT scan shows destruction of vertebra by osteoid osteoma.

Plate 6-3   Tumors of Musculoskeletal System

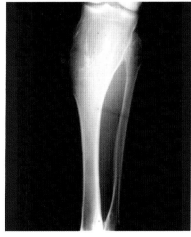

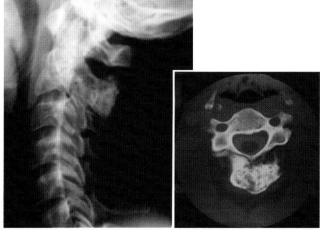

Lateral radiograph of large osteoblastoma of proximal tibia shows
bulging, radiolucent zone with thin
margin of reactive bone.

Radiograph of large osteoblastoma of posterior elements of
upper cervical spine. CT scan (right) reveals involvement of
spinous process of vertebra with encroachment on lamina.

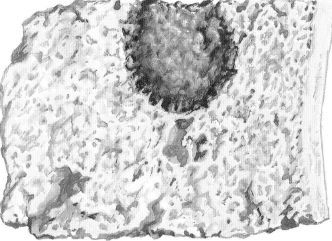

Specimen from neck of scapula,
including glenoid margin, shows
granular appearance of amorphous
ossification in osteoblastoma plus
loose, reactive trabecular bone.

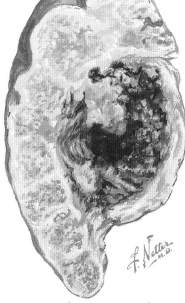

BENIGN TUMORS OF BONE—OSTEOBLASTOMA

Osteoblastoma is a rare benign osseous tumor. Because of its many similarities to osteoid osteoma but larger size (generally > 2 cm), it was at one time called giant osteoid osteoma. Osteoblastoma can be seen in slightly older people than osteoid osteoma. Osteoid osteoma is most common in older adolescents, and osteoblastoma is most common in older adolescents and young adults. There are also important clinical, radiographic, and histologic differences between osteoid osteoma and osteoblastoma. For example, osteoblastoma does not cause well-localized night pain that is relieved by aspirin and it occurs more often in the posterior elements of the vertebrae (transverse and spinous processes and pedicles) and jaw.

Diagnostic Studies. Plain radiographs show a relatively radiolucent, bone-forming (osteoblastic) lesion that is osteolytic and often has an aneurysmal, or blown-out, appearance. It is surrounded by a thin margin of reactive bone that frequently extends into adjacent soft tissue. The intense bony reaction around osteoid osteoma does not occur with osteoblastoma.

The radiographic differential diagnosis includes osteoid osteoma (see Plate 6-2), aneurysmal bone cyst (see Plate 6-11), eosinophilic granuloma (see Plate 6-10), giant cell tumor of bone (see Plate 6-13), and osteosarcoma (see Plates 6-15 and 6-16).

Bone scans demonstrate an intense radioisotope uptake, but MRI helps to determine the surgical approach.

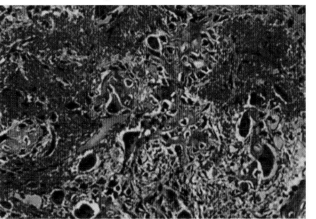

Section shows many plump, hyperchromatic osteoblasts
(chiefly lining spicules of bone and osteoid), numerous
giant cells, and vascular background (H & E stain).

Specimen of recurrent pseudo-
malignant osteoblastoma that
filled hollow of sacrum 14 months
after intracapsular curettage

The histologic appearance of osteoblastoma is quite similar to that of osteoid osteoma but the former has a more prominent vascular component. In addition, osteoblastoma has more stromal tissue and giant cells and broader osteoid seams than osteoid osteoma. These characteristics also distinguish osteoblastoma from osteosarcoma. However, the distinction of osteoblastoma from osteosarcoma is not always clear. For example, osteoblastomas often contain scattered mitotic figures and a proliferation of immature osteoblasts.

Treatment/Prognosis. Osteoblastomas can recur after intracapsular procedures, which are usually done to preserve joint function particularly in the spine.

Some cases of malignant transformation of osteoblastoma into osteosarcoma have been reported, and it is not clear whether this is due to the difficulty in initial diagnosis or genuine transformation. Regardless, patients with osteoblastoma must be observed not only for recurrence but also for malignant transformation.

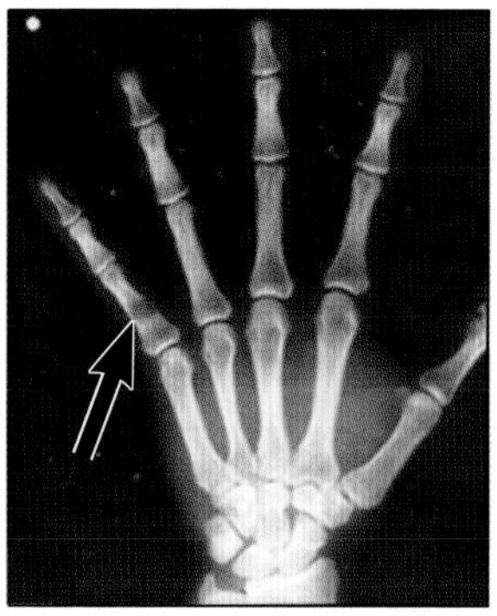

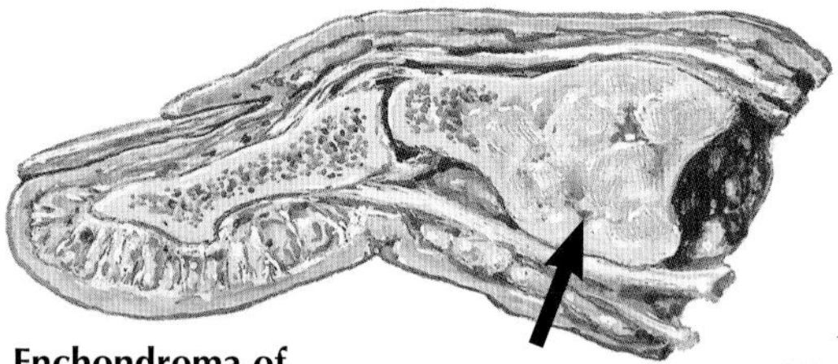

Plate 6-4

Musculoskeletal System: PART III

Sagittal section of middle phalanx. Digit disarticulation at proximal interphalangeal joint (arrow)

Enchondroma of 5th proximal phalanx. Seen as radiolucent lesion with margin of reactive bone (arrow)

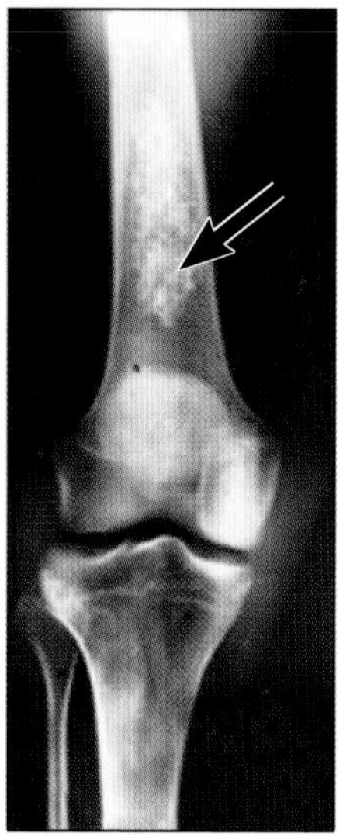

Involvement of distal femur with calcification. Benign enchondromas usually asymptomatic (arrow).

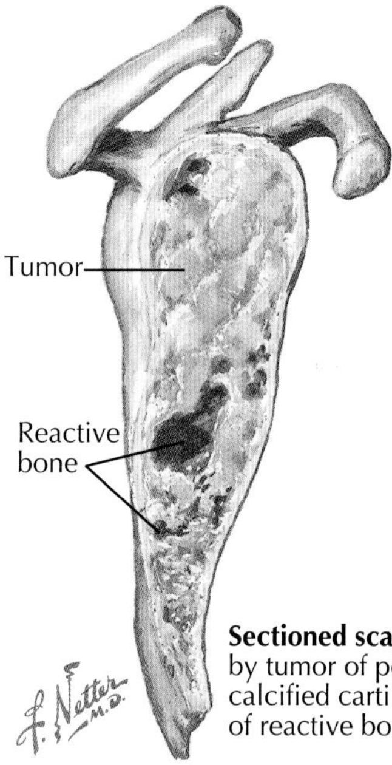

Enchondroma

Tumor

Reactive bone

Sectioned scapula. Blade thickened by tumor of pearly gray, calcified cartilage with margin of reactive bone.

BENIGN TUMORS OF BONE—ENCHONDROMA

Enchondroma is a benign primarily asymptomatic cartilaginous tumor of the intramedullary aspect of bone usually in the metaphysis (see Plate 6-4).

Enchondromas can occur anywhere in the skeleton. In very rare cases, a benign enchondroma undergoes malignant transformation into secondary chondrosarcoma (see Plate 6-17). However, aggressive appearing lesions in the hands are still nearly always benign. The uncommon occurrence of multiple lesions is known as enchondromatosis, or Ollier disease, and these patients more commonly have malignant degeneration of their enchondromas so they require surveillance of their lesions (see Plate 6-17).

Diagnostic Studies. Radiographs show a central radiolucent lesion with a well-defined but minimally thickened bony margin. During the active phase in adolescence, the lesion may slowly enlarge. In the inactive, or latent, phase in adulthood, the cartilaginous tissue may calcify in a diffuse punctate or stippled configuration. These calcifications sometimes appear on the radiograph as subtle "smoke ring" or "ring and arc" images. As the lesion matures, it develops a more reactive margin.

Bone scans can demonstrate radioisotope uptake. CT or MRI may be used to assess cortical erosion, intralesional calcification, and exact location. CT is also useful to rule out a soft tissue mass, which is indicative of chondrosarcoma. There are parathyroid hormone receptor-1 *(PTHR1)* mutations in about 10% of patients with enchondromatosis.

Biopsy is usually not needed to confirm the diagnosis of enchondroma, because its cartilaginous nature is evident radiographically and it is not destructive of the cortex, although these benign lesions can scallop the inside of the cortex. It can be difficult to distinguish

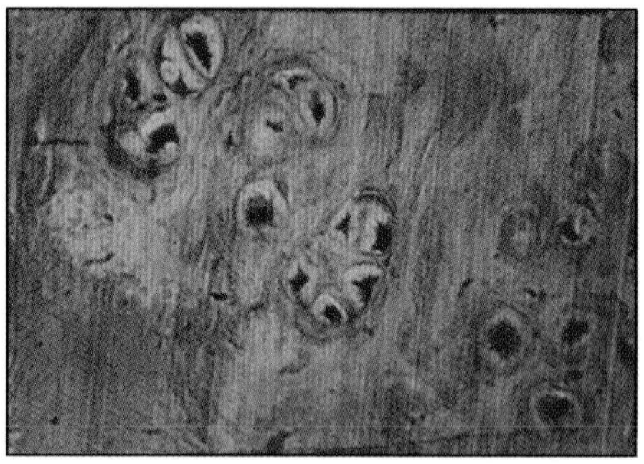

Microscopic section of malignant cartilage. Disorganized cartilaginous tissue with excessive matrix. Nuclear atypia, mitoses, and multiple nuclei not significant in children but suggest malignancy in adults (H & E stain).

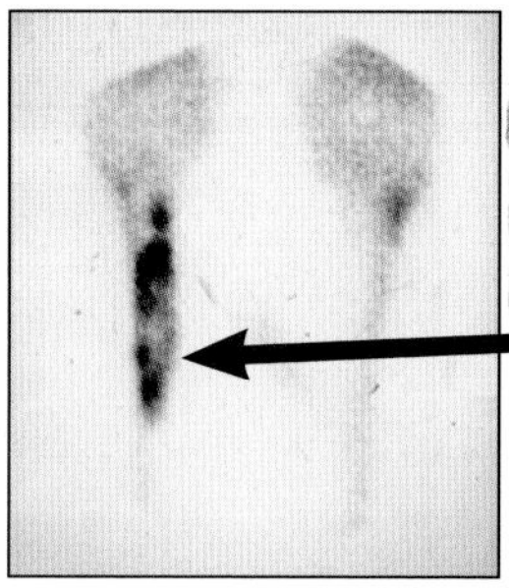

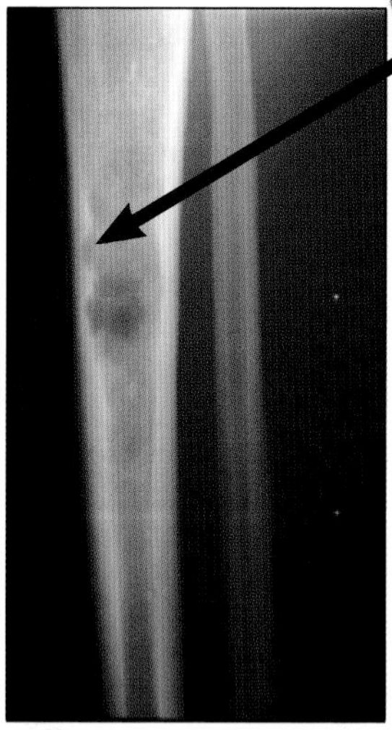

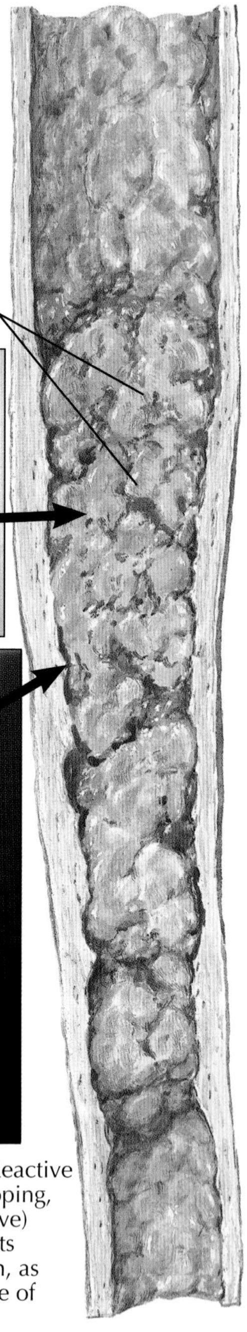

Enchondroma of tibia. Reactive cortical bone with scalloping, seen on radiograph (above) and in specimen, suggests malignant transformation, as does progressive increase of radioisotope uptake on bone scan (top).

between an active benign enchondroma and a low-grade malignant chondrosarcoma on the basis of histologic examination alone. Therefore, if there is radiographic evidence of full-thickness cortical destruction (not just endosteal scalloping from within) or MRI appearance of a soft tissue mass, this may provide evidence that the lesion is a chondrosarcoma.

Treatment/Prognosis. Asymptomatic solitary enchondromas are presumed benign and require only follow-up if pain develops or there is an increase in size.

If solitary or multiple enchondromas become symptomatic and begin to enlarge, staging studies with radiographs (and if still indeterminate then MRI) are indicated to rule out malignancy.

The prognosis for benign enchondroma is excellent. The lesion usually becomes latent in adulthood, and less than 1% of asymptomatic solitary enchondromas become malignant. In enchondromatosis, however, the risk of malignant transformation is much greater (approximately 10% of cases).

Plate 6-5

Tumors of Musculoskeletal System

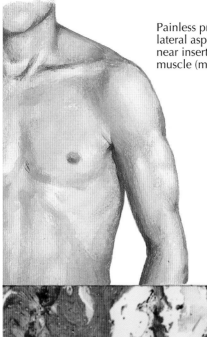

Painless prominence over
lateral aspect of humerus
near insertion of deltoid
muscle (most common site)

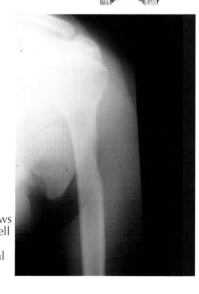

Sectioned humerus shows
pearly, translucent subperiosteal
deposits of cartilage over
eroded and reactive cortical
bone. (Resection of complete
bone segment shown here
only to depict tumor. En bloc
marginal excision usually
suffices.)

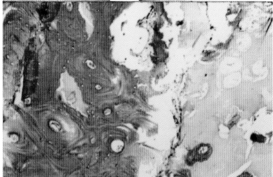

Section reveals cartilaginous component at right
overlying reactive bone at left, with partially
intervening thin zone of calcified cartilage
(H & E stain).

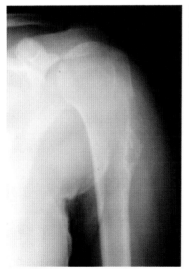

Radiograph
demonstrates
bulging radiolucent
lesion of shaft of
humerus.

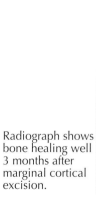

Radiograph shows
bone healing well
3 months after
marginal cortical
excision.

BENIGN TUMORS OF BONE— PERIOSTEAL CHONDROMA

Periosteal chondroma is a cartilaginous dysplasia that arises beneath the perichondrium and produces a broad-based, hemispheric cartilaginous mass that bulges from the cortex into the soft tissues. Typically seen in adolescents and young adults, the tumor manifests as a painless mass on the surface of a major long bone, most commonly the lateral cortex of the proximal humerus just proximal to the insertion of the deltoid muscle (see Plate 6-5).

Diagnostic Studies. Periosteal chondromas appear on radiographs as a radiolucent oval or oblong defect visualized as a crater-like deformity of the periphery of the cortex. The lesion is underlined by a thin, distinct cortical reaction. The tumor has little or no calcification. MRI can identify the density of the cartilage as high on T2-weighted sequences.

The radiographic differential diagnosis includes osteocartilaginous exostosis in younger patients (see Plate 6-6), juxtacortical chondrosarcoma (see Plate 6-17), as well as juxtacortical (parosteal and periosteal) osteosarcomas (see Plate 6-16).

On gross examination, the lesion has the consistency of mature cartilage without evidence of ossification or calcification. Histologic examination reveals hypercellular cartilage, and nuclear atypia may be present.

Treatment/Prognosis. Periosteal chondromas are active benign stage 2 tumors that require marginal excision to prevent recurrence. Because of their peripheral location and their cortical rim, this can usually be achieved without bone grafting or extensive reconstruction. There is a risk of recurrence after excision. Sarcomatous transformation has not been documented, and rare reports of such transformation probably reflect the resemblance of periosteal chondroma to juxtacortical chondrosarcoma.

Plate 6-6

Musculoskeletal System: PART III

BENIGN TUMORS OF BONE— OSTEOCARTILAGINOUS EXOSTOSIS (OSTEOCHONDROMA)

Osteocartilaginous exostosis (osteochondroma) is a common developmental dysplasia of the peripheral growth plate that results in a lobulated outgrowth of cartilage and bone from the metaphysis. The classic presentation is a hard excrescence of bone capped by a thin zone of proliferating cartilage. An exostosis may develop in any bone but is usually seen in the long bones. The most common locations are the proximal or distal femur, proximal humerus, proximal tibia, pelvis, and scapula. The tumor develops in adolescence and continues to enlarge during skeletal growth.

The initial clinical sign is a hard, painless mass fixed on the bone. Symptoms, when present, are usually due to irritation of the overlying soft tissues that may or may not be associated with a fluid-filled bursa. Variations in the fluid content in the bursa create a fluctuating, palpable mass.

In most patients, the lesion is solitary; however, polyostotic tumors occur in a small subset of patients. These multiple hereditary exostoses produce significant deformities, such as short stature and angular deformities. In multiple hereditary exostoses as with enchondromatosis there is an increased incidence of malignant degeneration.

Diagnostic Studies. The radiographic appearance of an exostosis is either a flat, sessile lesion or a pedunculated (stalklike) cortical-sharing process. The lesions are called cortical sharing because they share the same cortex as the adjacent normal cortical bone. It is usually a well-defined metaphyseal projection of bone with mottled density; the cartilaginous cap displays irregular areas of calcification. The radiographic hallmark is the blending of the tumor into the underlying metaphysis. Although a diagnosis is seldom problematic, the presence of a painful and enlarging lesion in an adult may necessitate staging studies to assess the risk of secondary malignant transformation to chondrosarcoma (see Plate 6-17).

Evidence of malignant transformation includes confirmation by CT or MRI of a soft tissue mass with cortical destruction and a sudden increase in size of the mass and pain. The radiographic differential diagnosis is periosteal chondroma (see Plate 6-5) and parosteal osteosarcoma (see Plate 6-16). In an adult, a symptomatic "exostosis" that increases in size could be a malignancy, although benign osteochondromas may develop a reactive bursa that increases in size, simulating tumor growth. About 70% of patients with multiple exostoses have germline *EXT1* or *EXT2* mutations.

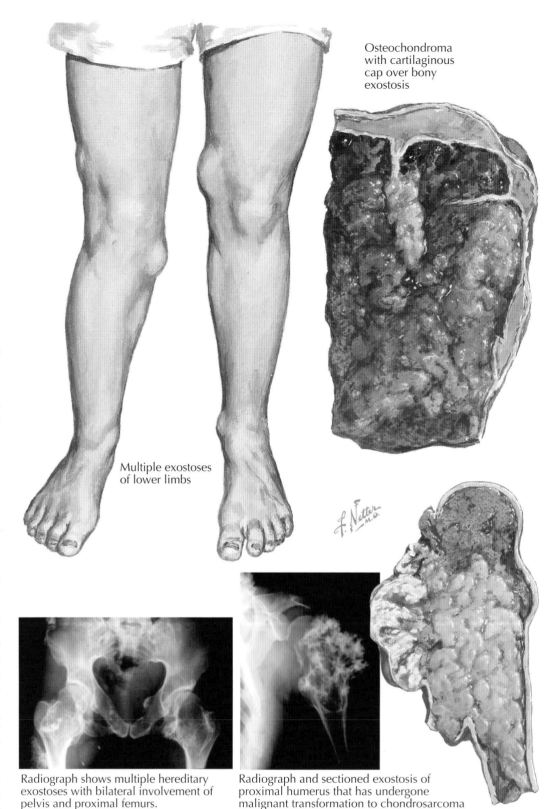

Osteochondroma with cartilaginous cap over bony exostosis

Multiple exostoses of lower limbs

Radiograph shows multiple hereditary exostoses with bilateral involvement of pelvis and proximal femurs.

Radiograph and sectioned exostosis of proximal humerus that has undergone malignant transformation to chondrosarcoma

Exostoses on gross examination reveal an overlying cartilaginous cap with no growth plate but separated from the underlying bone by an irregular, chalky white line (zone of calcification). The mass of trabecular bone that makes up the main portion of the exostosis merges into the underlying normal trabecular bone of the metaphysis.

On microscopic examination, the cartilaginous cap does not have the tidemark characteristic of articular cartilage.

Treatment/Prognosis. Marginal excision of an active exostosis, including the cartilaginous cap and the overlying perichondrium, minimizes the risk of recurrence. The deep bony base has minimal activity and may be removed piecemeal (in more than one piece). The prognosis for a solitary exostosis is excellent (<5% recurrence after marginal excision). The risk of sarcomatous transformation in solitary exostosis is about 1%, but in multiple hereditary exostoses, this risk approaches 10%.

Plate 6-7

Tumors of Musculoskeletal System

Chondroblastoma

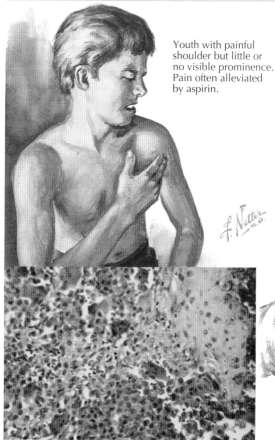

Youth with painful shoulder but little or no visible prominence. Pain often alleviated by aspirin.

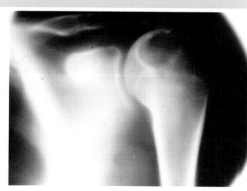

Radiograph reveals ovoid defect in humeral epiphysis extending into metaphysis with fine calcifications.

BENIGN TUMORS OF BONE— CHONDROBLASTOMA AND CHONDROMYXOID FIBROMA

CHONDROBLASTOMA

Chondroblastoma is a painful, benign cartilaginous tumor that arises during adolescence in the epiphysis close to the joint surface and most commonly in the proximal humerus, proximal tibia, or distal femur.

Diagnostic Studies. The radiographic hallmark is an epiphyseal radiolucent lesion with fine punctate calcifications suggestive of a cartilaginous lesion. The tumor is usually bordered by a well-defined margin of reactive bone. Chondroblastomas are more epiphyseally based than the more common epimetaphyseal giant cell tumor. The radiographic differential diagnosis includes aneurysmal bone cyst (see Plate 6-11) and giant cell tumor of bone (see Plate 6-13). Inflammatory lesions such as osteoarthritic cysts also are epiphyseal but are nearly always in older patients, and chondroblastomas are generally in young patients frequently with open growth plates. Giant cell tumors are more common in young adults with closed growth plates.

Histologic examination reveals the characteristic "cobblestone" or "chicken-wire" pattern: areas of round, plump chondroblasts (the stones) are enmeshed in a sparse chondroid matrix (the mortar between the stones). Clumps of giant cells are seen in areas that contain primarily a spindle cell stroma. Unique to chondroblastoma is the fine microscopic pattern of calcifications, usually in a "chicken-wire" arrangement, in and around the islands of cartilage.

Treatment/Prognosis. Curettage is the treatment of choice of chondroblastomas. Curettage near the growth plate must be undertaken with great care in the younger patient to prevent late angular deformities, and curettage near the articular cartilage must be undertaken with great care in all patients.

The prognosis for chondroblastoma is good; most are active stage 2 tumors; however, there is a significant risk of recurrence after curettage similar to that of giant cell tumor.

CHONDROMYXOID FIBROMA

Chondromyxoid fibroma is a rare painless, benign cartilaginous lesion of bone. It occurs in adolescents, most often in the metaphyses of major long bones.

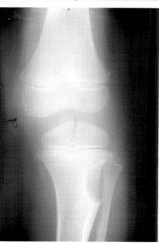

Section shows mixture of chondroblasts and fibrovascular stroma with occasional giant cells (H&E stain)

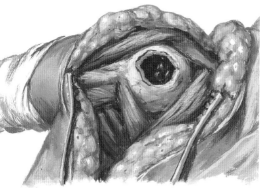

Curettage of cavity before reconstruction with trabecular bone graft

Chondromyxoid fibroma

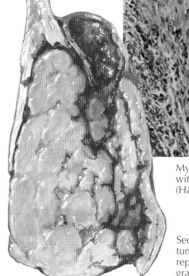

Anteroposterior radiograph shows eccentric radiolucent lesion in proximal tibia with thin margin of reactive bone.

Myxomatous cartilage combined with benign fibrous stroma (H&E stain)

Sectioned cartilaginous tumor. Surgical defect repaired with cortical bone graft from iliac crest.

This lesion most often presents as an active stage 2 lesion and is not known to undergo malignant transformation.

Diagnostic Studies. Radiographs reveal an eccentric metaphyseal radiolucent defect with no evidence of the usual calcification of a cartilaginous tumor. The radiographic differential diagnosis includes nonossifying fibroma (see Plate 6-9) and aneurysmal bone cyst (see Plate 6-11).

Histologic examination shows immature myxoid cartilage with stellate chondrocytes enmeshed in lightly staining myxomatous chondroid matrix. Intertwined throughout the lesion are strands of benign fibrous tissue and small multinucleated giant cells.

Treatment. Curettage carries a low risk of recurrence in well-encapsulated stage 2 lesions, but the size of the defect often necessitates bone grafting (see Plate 6-30).

Plate 6-8

Musculoskeletal System: PART III

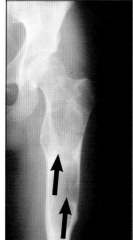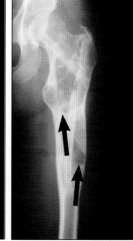

Radiographs of severe monostotic fibrous dysplasia of femur. Treated for fracture prophylaxis with cortical autograft from fibula. Preoperative (left) and postoperative (right) views.

BENIGN TUMORS OF BONE— FIBROUS DYSPLASIA

Fibrous dysplasia is a developmental abnormality of bone that results in a haphazard mixture of immature fibrous tissue and small fragments of immature trabecular bone. The lesions may occur in one bone (monostotic) or in many (polyostotic), and they are sometimes accompanied by precocious puberty and café-au-lait pigmentation in females, making up the triad known as McCune-Albright syndrome.

Monostotic lesions generally occur in the proximal femur, proximal tibia, mandible, and ribs. Polyostotic disease, which usually presents earlier, may be unilateral or widespread, affecting long bones, hands, feet, facial bones, and pelvis. Extensive involvement of the proximal femur results in the distinctive "shepherd's crook" deformity that is characteristic of fibrous dysplasia.

The result of this dysplastic process is a weakened bone that becomes deformed by normal stress or sustains frequent pathologic fractures. Painful stress fractures are especially common in the proximal femur. Although dysplastic bone heals at a normal rate after fracture, the resulting callus is also dysplastic, and the disease persists.

Diagnostic Studies. The classic radiographic feature of fibrous dysplasia is a hazy, radiolucent, or "ground-glass" pattern resulting from the defective mineralization of immature dysplastic bone; it is usually strikingly different from the radiographic appearance of normal bone, calcified cartilage, or soft tissue. A small monostotic lesion may be difficult to distinguish from other benign lesions, but extensive polyostotic involvement is likely to produce the characteristic ground-glass density and significant deformity. The lesion is primarily diaphyseal or metaphyseal and has been described as a "long lesion in a long bone."

Bone scans demonstrate intense radioisotope uptake, and CT scans help visualize the ground-glass density of the lesion. MRI can delineate the extent of involvement and show the characteristic fat or cystic nature of some of the lesions. Fat in the fibrous dysplasia lesions may be present on MRI and is reassuring that the lesion is benign.

The typical histologic pattern is an irregular collection of small pieces of immature bone within a matrix of fibrous tissue. The overall histologic appearance has been likened to that of alphabet soup. The immature trabeculae are not lined with osteoblasts (as in ossifying fibroma), do not contain cement lines, and are obviously not aligned according to stress. The fibrous

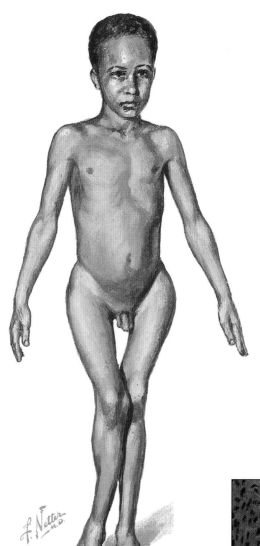

"Shepard's crook" deformity of both femoral necks. Note also deformity of right tibia.

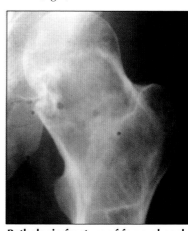

Pathologic fracture of femoral neck. Typical ground-glass appearance of bone

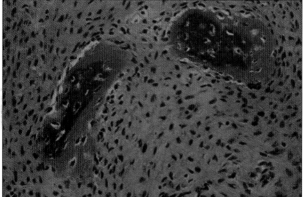

Bone section. Dense fibrous tissue with islands of trabecular bone without osteoblastic rim (H & E stain).

stroma is loosely arranged and immature, replacing the normal marrow. A variable degree of capillary vasculature is seen within the stroma.

The histologic differential diagnosis includes osteoblastoma (see Plate 6-3), osteosarcoma (see Plate 6-15), ossifying fibroma, hyperparathyroidism, and Paget disease of bone. Specific *GNAS* activating (gain-of-function) mutations have been described in fibrous dysplasia and McCune-Albright syndrome.

Treatment. Because more dysplastic bone usually forms and pain does not predictably resolve after curettage, the goal of management should be conservative and prevention of deformity and fracture. This is best accomplished using cortical bone allografts (taken from the fibula), which minimally remodel after incorporation. Treatment methods for severe bony involvement are reconstruction with joint replacements or internal metallic fixation.

Plate 6-9

Tumors of Musculoskeletal System

BENIGN TUMORS OF BONE—NONOSSIFYING FIBROMA AND DESMOPLASTIC FIBROMA

NONOSSIFYING FIBROMA

Nonossifying fibroma (fibrous cortical defect, metaphyseal fibrous defect) is the most common bone lesion. It results from a developmental defect of periosteal cortical bone that leads to a failure of ossification during the normal growth period. This lesion, of fibrous origin, typically develops in childhood with a slightly higher incidence in males. Although usually asymptomatic, nonossifying fibroma can be an active lesion that persists or enlarges throughout childhood. When the tumor occupies a large portion of the bone, fracture can occur. Fractures through nonossifying fibromas will usually heal, but open reduction may be necessary depending on the location. With skeletal maturation, a nonossifying fibroma becomes latent and ossifies.

Diagnostic Studies. The lesion commonly develops in the metaphysis of the distal femur or distal tibia and is eccentrically located, usually within or adjacent to the cortex. Radiographs reveal a well-marginated radiolucent zone, with distinct trabeculation producing a multilocular appearance. In addition, nonossifying fibromas usually cause benign cortical thinning, or erosion. The radiographic pattern is usually diagnostic, and further staging studies are seldom indicated.

Histologic features include a combination of dense collagen arranged in a storiform pattern, a scattering of small, multinucleated giant cells, hemosiderin, and lipid-filled histiocytes. The tissue does not contain the degree of hemorrhage and necrosis or the number of giant cells seen in the giant cell tumor of bone. Although the tissue may resemble the lining tissue of an aneurysmal bone cyst, the lesion does not have a large, central, blood-filled cavity.

Treatment. Reassurance and watchful waiting is usually sufficient except with fracture when closed or open reduction and immobilization with bone grafting is necessary.

DESMOPLASTIC FIBROMA

Desmoplastic fibroma (desmoid tumor) is a rare intraosseous fibroma that typically develops as an aggressive stage 3 tumor. It occurs primarily in young adults but may occur at any age. The long bones—particularly the tibia and the fibula—are the most common sites, although it may occur throughout the skeleton. Its behavior corresponds to that of its soft tissue counterpart, aggressive fibromatosis (see Plate 6-23).

Diagnostic Studies. Radiographs show a centrally located metaphyseal or diaphyseal lesion, poorly or incompletely contained by a thin margin of reactive bone, which frequently has a trabeculated appearance. It may remain within the bone for some time, surrounded by a thin cortical shell, but eventually it extends through the cortex into the soft tissues. The radiographic hallmark is a loculated intraosseous lesion

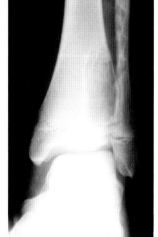

Nonossifying fibroma

Eccentric radiolucent lesion with margin of reactive bone in metaphysis of distal femur

Both distal tibia and fibula involved; fibula fractured.

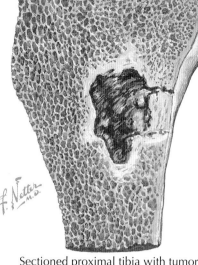

Sectioned proximal tibia with tumor. Reddish tan fibrous core and margin of reactive bone. En bloc excision not usually required as lesions heal eventually, either spontaneously or after curettage.

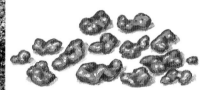

Whorls of fibrous tissue with occasional giant cells seen on histopathologic examination (H&E stain)

Scrapings from curettage

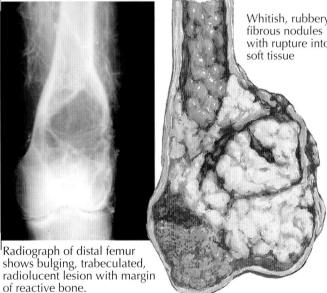

Desmoplastic fibroma

Radiograph of distal femur shows bulging, trabeculated, radiolucent lesion with margin of reactive bone.

Whitish, rubbery fibrous nodules with rupture into soft tissue

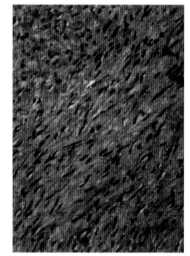

Section shows dense bands of irregularly arranged collagen and mature fibrocytes (H & E stain).

that stimulates very little bony reaction. The radiographic differential diagnosis includes giant cell tumor of bone (see Plate 6-13) and fibrosarcoma of bone (see Plate 6-18). The most characteristic feature is the contrast between the relatively benign findings of the radiographic studies and the tumor's fairly aggressive clinical behavior.

The lesion is composed of dense, white, fibrous tissue with a rubbery consistency and is easily removed with

curettage. The histologic features of dense, irregularly arranged bundles of collagen with an occasional spindle cell closely resemble fibromatosis. Mitoses, vascularity, and necrosis are unusual microscopic findings. The histologic differential diagnosis usually involves low-grade fibrosarcoma of bone.

Treatment. Excision with a wide margin results in local control of the lesion. Recurrence after curettage is frequent, with invasion of the soft tissue.

Plate 6-10

Musculoskeletal System: PART III

BENIGN TUMORS OF BONE— EOSINOPHILIC GRANULOMA

Eosinophilic granuloma belongs to a group of disorders characterized by lesions that occur as a result of metabolic defects in the reticuloendothelial system. This group of disorders, called histiocytosis X, also includes Hand-Schüller-Christian disease and Letterer-Siwe disease. The clinical and radiographic manifestations of histiocytosis X may resemble those of a malignancy, and these lesions can be multifocal, but their clinical course differs from that of malignant reticuloendothelial tumors such as lymphoma, Ewing sarcoma (see Plate 6-19), leukemia, Hodgkin disease, and multiple myeloma (see Plate 6-20).

Eosinophilic granuloma usually occurs as a solitary, symptomatic lesion in children younger than 20 years of age but can occur as multiple tumors at any age and at any site. Low-grade fever, elevated erythrocyte sedimentation rate, and mild peripheral eosinophilia are occasional associated findings. The skull, supra-acetabular region of the pelvis, and diaphysis of the femur are the usual sites of involvement, although any bone can be affected.

Diagnostic Studies. On radiographs, a small lesion may resemble the punched-out radiolucent lesion of multiple myeloma. Involvement of a vertebral body produces the pathognomonic radiographic appearance of vertebra plana ("coin-on-edge" flattened vertebra) after vertebral collapse. A lesion that occurs in the diaphysis or metaphysis of a limb appears as an oval radiolucent area. Because of its variable radiographic characteristics, eosinophilic granuloma has been called the great imitator.

Bone scans are used to document the presence of multiple lesions (<10% of cases); an intense radioisotope uptake indicates an active lesion. MRI is helpful in delineating the lesion, especially in the spine and hip.

Gross examination of an active lesion reveals soft, vascular, granulomatous tissue covered with a mature bony capsule that may be runny and liquefied.

Histologic characteristics are a mixture of Langerhans histiocytes, eosinophils, and occasional giant cells with little background stroma. Birbeck granules can also be seen. The same histologic pattern is seen in each of the forms of histiocytosis X, but the multisystem Hand-Schüller-Christian and Letterer-Siwe diseases have significant morbidity and mortality and are sometimes treated with chemotherapy.

Treatment/Prognosis. The curettage performed to obtain tissue for diagnosis is usually adequate treatment. When the defect is large, bone grafts may be needed to prevent fracture (see Plate 6-30). In a small percentage of patients with a solitary lesion, the visceral manifestations of Hand-Schüller-Christian disease can eventually develop and follow-up or a bone scan should be performed to rule out multifocal disease.

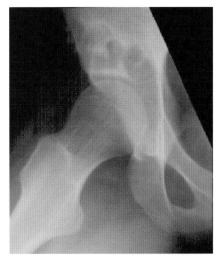

Radiograph shows loculated, bubble-like, radiolucent lesion in supra-acetabular region of right ilium.

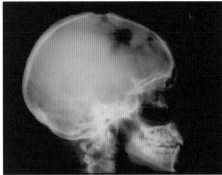

Variegated defects in flat bones of skull

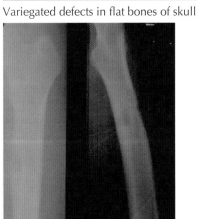

Anteroposterior and lateral views show typical marginated, radiolucent lesions in femoral shaft.

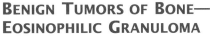

Surgical exploration reveals granuloma eroding through cortex of ilium.

Section reveals pale-staining, foamy histiocytes interspersed with bilobed eosinophilis (H & E stain).

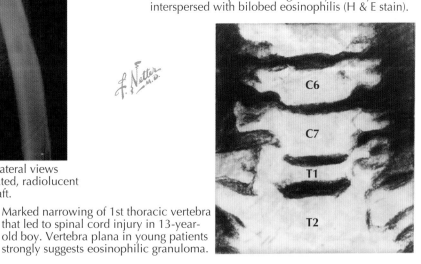

C6

C7

T1

T2

Marked narrowing of 1st thoracic vertebra that led to spinal cord injury in 13-year-old boy. Vertebra plana in young patients strongly suggests eosinophilic granuloma.

Plate 6-11

Tumors of Musculoskeletal System

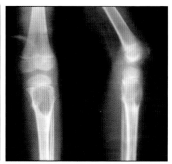

CT scan. Defines margins and density of lesion

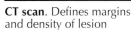

Aneurysmal bone cyst in proximal tibia. Anterior (left) and lateral (right) views

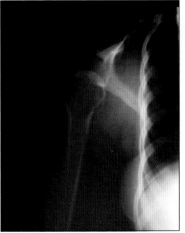

Radiolucent lesion in proximal humerus. Characteristic ballooned, loculated appearance

BENIGN TUMORS OF BONE—ANEURYSMAL BONE CYST

The aneurysmal bone cyst is a tumor-like proliferation of vascular tissue that forms a lining around a blood-filled cystic lesion. Occurring most commonly in adolescents and young adults, it develops in the metaphyseal region of long bones, pelvis, or vertebral body, sometimes secondary to another benign or malignant bone lesion.

Diagnostic Studies. A radiolucent lesion with a ballooned expansion of the bone cortices ("finger in balloon") is the radiographic hallmark of an aneurysmal bone cyst. Although some lesions appear to have an aggressive, expansile quality, they remain contained by a thin rim of reactive periosteal bone. In children, these benign lesions seldom penetrate the articular surface of a joint or the growth plate; therefore, evidence of growth plate penetration by an aneurysmal bone cyst indicates the need for careful staging studies to rule out malignancy. The radiographic differential diagnosis includes simple bone cyst (see Plate 6-12), giant cell tumor of bone (see Plate 6-13), telangiectatic sarcoma, and angiosarcoma (see Plate 6-27).

Bone scans show intense radioisotope uptake in the margin of the lesion. MRI and CT are used to depict the precise anatomic extent and density of the lesion, and especially the thin, limiting margin of reactive bone (which is not well visualized on plain radiographs). A fluid-fluid level seen on the MR image generally confirms the diagnosis and represents the separation between the red cells and serum in the bloody cavity. Other tumors can, however, have fluid-fluid levels and aneurysmal bone cyst–like qualities.

Histologically, the proliferative lining tissue of an aneurysmal bone cyst is often difficult to distinguish from that of a giant cell tumor of bone. It contains a mixture of benign stromal tissue, giant cells, and large amounts of hemosiderin. The tissue usually contains large vascular lacunae lined with giant cells and filled with clotted blood that resembles cranberry sauce. When these histologic features also occur in other lesions (e.g., chondroblastoma, osteoblastoma, osteosarcoma, eosinophilic granuloma, nonossifying fibroma) they are called secondary aneurysmal bone cysts. Because of the preponderance of giant cells, many aneurysmal bone cysts are initially thought to be giant cell tumors of bone, and there is a continuum between giant cell tumors of bone and aneurysmal bone cysts.

Treatment/Prognosis. The majority of active aneurysmal bone cysts are treated with curettage and bone grafting; the recurrence rate, however, is 20% to 30%.

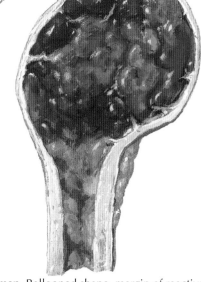

Bone specimen. Ballooned shape, margin of reactive bone, and characteristic multiloculation. Pockets filled with clotted (cranberry sauce–like) blood.

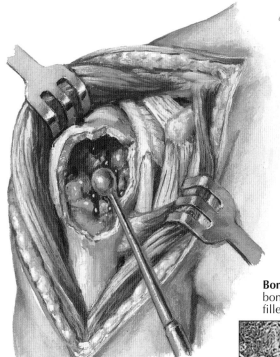

Curettage of cyst. Before reconstruction of cavity with trabecular bone graft

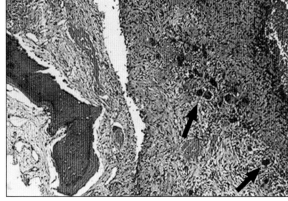

Bone section. Stroma of benign spindle cells, scattered giant cells (arrows), blood, and bone fragments (H & E stain).

After incision of an active cyst, an alarming amount of bleeding may occur until the lining is completely removed. After complete excision of the cyst this bleeding generally decreases. Occasionally, however, there may still be brisk bleeding emanating directly from the bony wall, which can be controlled with coagulation. Curettage may be augmented with cementation with methyl methacrylate, which appears to reduce the risk of recurrence or bone graft, which allows for healing and for a recurrence to be visualized earlier. Lesions in the pelvis and spine have a higher risk of recurrence, where complete surgical exposure and removal are more difficult. Nevertheless, the prognosis for primary aneurysmal bone cyst is excellent and recurrences can usually be managed with more aggressive curettage or excision.

Plate 6-12

Musculoskeletal System: PART III

BENIGN TUMORS OF BONE— SIMPLE BONE CYST

The simple (unicameral) bone cyst is a membrane-lined cavity containing a clear yellow fluid. Occurring most often in children 4 to 10 years of age, the cysts have a predilection for the metaphysis of long bones, particularly the proximal humerus (50% of cases), proximal femur, and proximal tibia. The lesions remain asymptomatic unless complicated by fracture. They enlarge during skeletal growth and become inactive, or latent, after skeletal maturity.

Active cysts usually develop in patients younger than 10 years of age. Typically, the cyst abuts the growth plate and occupies most of the metaphysis; it is expansile with a thin cortical shell, continues to enlarge during observation, and is commonly associated with fracture. The cyst is considered active as it arises and grows adjacent to the growth plate. With growth, it is left behind and becomes increasingly separated from the growth plate and at this point is considered latent.

Latent cysts are usually seen in patients older than 12 years of age. They have a thicker bony wall than active lesions. They remain static or diminish in size, show evidence of healing or ossification, and are less likely to result in fracture.

Diagnostic Studies. Radiographs show a central, well-marginated radiolucent defect in the metaphysis, with a symmetric appearance, usually without bony septations or loculations. The metaphysis is expanded, with marked cortical thinning that predisposes to fracture. After fracture, the eggshell-thin fragments are often displaced into the cystic cavity, thus creating the "falling leaf" sign (Plate 6-12).

The radiographic differential diagnosis is usually limited to fibrous dysplasia (see Plate 6-8) and aneurysmal bone cyst (see Plate 6-11). In some cases, the even radiolucency of the cyst may be difficult to distinguish from the ground-glass density of fibrous dysplasia. However, monostotic fibrous dysplasia is usually eccentric rather than central and diaphyseal rather than metaphyseal; in addition, the periosteal reaction is greater in fibrous dysplasia than in a simple bone cyst. An aneurysmal bone cyst (and even telangiectatic sarcoma) may also appear as a large radiolucent lesion, making it occasionally difficult to distinguish from a simple cyst.

Staging studies are indicated only when radiographs are difficult to interpret. Bone scans show an increased radioisotope uptake around the margin of the cyst, in contrast to the uniform uptake in fibrous dysplasia. The finding of straw-colored fluid on needle aspiration confirms the diagnosis of a simple cyst.

Histologic examination of an active cyst reveals a fibrous membrane lining a thin margin of reactive bone.

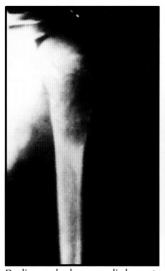
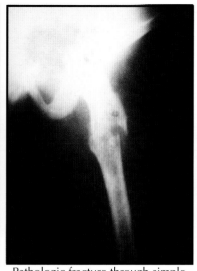
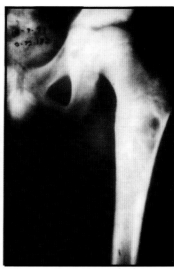

Radiograph shows radiolucent lesion in proximal humerus typical of simple bone cyst abutting growth plate.

Pathologic fracture through simple cyst of femoral neck in 16-year-old boy

Same patient, 7 months later. Fracture healed, cystic cavity becoming obliterated following limb immobilization.

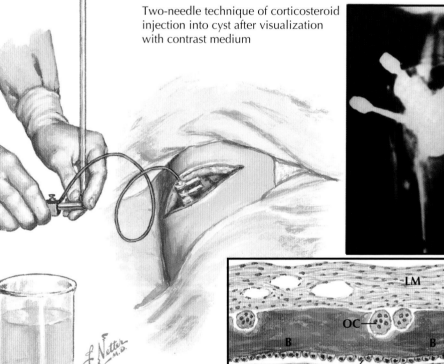

Two-needle technique of corticosteroid injection into cyst after visualization with contrast medium

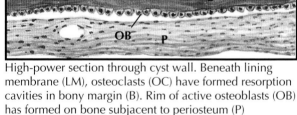

Manometric measurement of intracystic pressure. In active cysts, pressure averages 30 cm H_2O and pulsates with heartbeat. In latent phase, pressure much lower with no pulsation. Note clear, yellowish fluid aspirated from cyst.

High-power section through cyst wall. Beneath lining membrane (LM), osteoclasts (OC) have formed resorption cavities in bony margin (B). Rim of active osteoblasts (OB) has formed on bone subjacent to periosteum (P) (H & E stain).

The inner wall of the margin deep to the membrane is often covered with a network of osteoclasts. Between the membrane and the osteoclastic activity is a layer of areolar tissue containing fibroblastic and multinucleated giant cells. Latent cysts have a thicker membrane with little underlying osteoclastic activity, fewer giant cells, and more reactive bone.

Treatment/Prognosis. Simple cysts are treated with curettage and bone grafting; recurrence is high for active cysts (50%) and low for latent cysts (10%).

Treatment with injection of corticosteroid is based on the theory that corticosteroids stabilize the mesothelial lining and induce healing of the cyst. Cyst fluid is aspirated with sterile percutaneous needle technique; then 80 to 200 mg of methylprednisolone acetate is infused into the cavity. In more than half of patients studied, the cyst healed after this technique, although multiple injections frequently were required. If the lesion fractures, there is a small chance that the fracture can heal and the lesion resolve.

Plate 6-13

Tumors of Musculoskeletal System

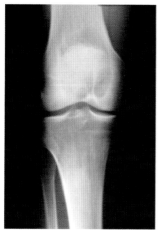

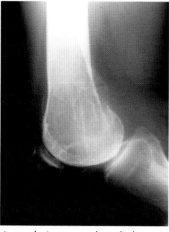

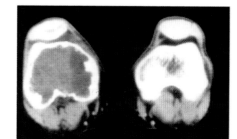

CT scan of right femur reveals marked endosteal erosion by intraosseous lesion.

Pathologic fracture through giant cell tumor of distal femur

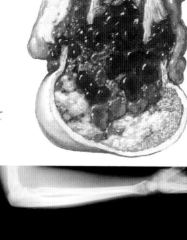

Anteroposterior radiograph shows giant cell tumor of epiphysis and metaphysis of distal femur extending into but not penetrating subchondral plate.

Lateral view reveals radiolucent lesion bulging posteriorly into popliteal fossa.

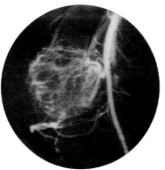

Angiogram demonstrates intense vascularity of tumor area.

Bone scan demonstrates characteristic "doughnut sign" (also typical of aneurysmal bone cyst).

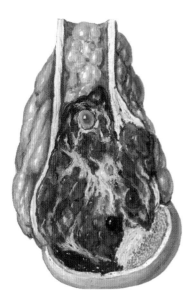

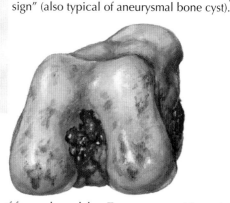

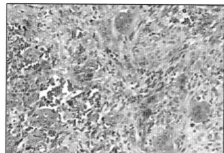

Giant cell tumor of distal radius

Sectioned distal femur shows meaty, hemorrhagic tissue with lighter, dense, fibrous areas, small cysts and blood clots, and thin margin of reactive bone with Codman triangle. Tumor has infiltrated soft tissue.

View of femoral condyles. Tumor apparent in spots through thin subchondral plate and articular cartilage; also in intercondylar notch covered by synovial membrane.

Section shows stroma of spindle-like cells with pale-staining cytoplasm and nuclei, many multi-nucleated giant cells, vascular channels, and free blood (H & E stain).

BENIGN TUMORS OF BONE— GIANT CELL TUMOR OF BONE

Giant cell tumor of bone (osteoclastoma) is a common benign but locally aggressive lesion. It occurs chiefly in persons between 20 and 40 years of age. The lesion is typically located in the epiphysis and metaphysis of the distal femur or proximal tibia. Other common sites are the distal radius, proximal humerus, distal tibia, and sacrum. The tumor usually enlarges to occupy most of the epiphysis and adjacent metaphysis, penetrating and eroding the subchondral bone and even invading the articular cartilage. Patients report a deep, persistent intraosseous pain that mimics an internal derangement of the knee. A pathologic fracture or reactive knee effusion is the initial symptom in about one third of patients; in a small number (<1%), the tumor undergoes pulmonary metastases that are generally but not always benign.

Diagnostic Studies. Radiographs reveal a large radiolucent lesion surrounded by a distinct margin of reactive bone. Cortical thinning, endosteal erosion, and trabecularization, or bony septation, of the cavity are associated findings. CT or MRI discloses the extent of involvement and bony margination. Lesions extend to with 1.5 cm of the adjacent joint space and articular cartilage. A chest radiograph should be performed in all patients with giant cell tumor to rule out metastases.

Gross examination reveals a soft, friable, reddish brown neoplastic tissue with the consistency of a wet sponge. Some areas are gelatinous or fatty, and some are aneurysmal and cavitated. Histologic features include multinucleated giant cells, a proliferative stroma with vesiculated nuclei, areas of aneurysmal tissue, areas of necrosis, reactive peripheral bone, and occasional mitotic figures and intravascular tumor plugs in venous sinuses.

Treatment. The size and stage of the tumor determine the type of treatment. For stage 1 or 2 lesions, curettage is often combined with bone grafting or cementation. Giant cell tumors of bone have a recurrence rate between 5% and 30%; Cementation and adjuvant treatment with phenol or liquid nitrogen may decrease the recurrence rate. For recurrent lesions or articular destruction, extensive joint reconstruction or joint replacement may be required.

Plate 6-14

Musculoskeletal System: PART III

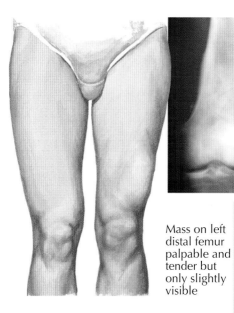

Mass on left distal femur palpable and tender but only slightly visible

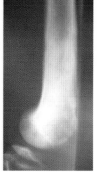

AP and lateral radiograph shows dense lesion and periosteal elevation.

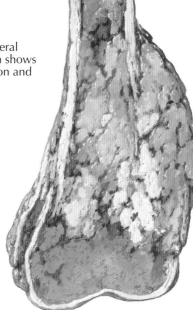

Tumor occupies entire metaphysis of distal femur and has extended into the soft tissues.

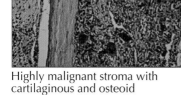

Highly malignant stroma with cartilaginous and osteoid components (H & E stain).

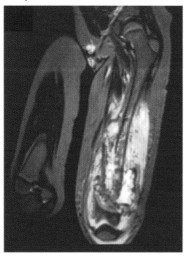

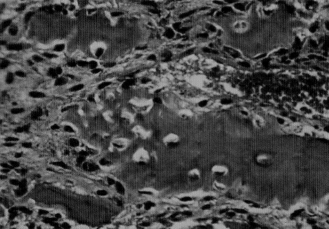

Masses of tumor cells with hyperchromatic nuclei interspersed with foci of malignant osteoid are typical histopathologic findings (H & E stain).

Osteosarcoma
MRI of thigh showing pathologic fracture of distal femur and extensive soft tissue spread of osteogenic sarcoma into both anterior and posterior thigh compartments.

MALIGNANT TUMORS OF BONE—OSTEOSARCOMA

OSTEOSARCOMA

Osteosarcoma (osteogenic sarcoma) is a malignant tumor of bone in which neoplastic osteoid is produced. It is the most common primary malignant bone tumor of mesenchymal derivation (see Plates 6-14 and 6-15). Most osteosarcomas are the classic type; the variant forms, which are distinguished by significant differences in location and/or microscopic appearance and prognosis, include juxtacortical parosteal and periosteal osteosarcomas (see Plate 6-16) and telangiectatic osteosarcoma.

Osteosarcoma usually develops in adolescents and affects males slightly more often than females. Although the lesion may occur throughout the skeleton, in 50% of patients it occurs in the region of the knee. The distal femur is the most common site, and the proximal tibia is the second most common site. Other less common sites are the proximal humerus, proximal femur, and pelvis. Most osteosarcomas originate in long bones in the regions of highest growth, the metaphyses. The initial symptom is pain, and the patients have a tender, bony mass. At the time of diagnosis, most osteosarcomas are stage IIB lesions that have a cortical defect and a soft tissue mass outside the bone. The most common site for metastases is the lungs, and all patients with known osteosarcoma should have chest imaging, preferably with CT.

A small percentage of osteosarcomas in adults occur in association with Paget disease of bone. Severe, unremitting increased pain with or without pathologic fracture is the primary clinical manifestation of sarcomatous transformation in Paget disease. The osteosarcomas may be hard to see within pagetic bone, but on MRI there should be a lack of the normal fatty marrow in Paget disease.

Diagnostic Studies. Radiographs characteristically demonstrate a permeative destructive lesion in which amorphous neoplastic bone can be detected. Typically, the lesion is predominantly dense, or osteoblastic, but may also have a mixed pattern or appear purely osteolytic. Other major characteristics include early cortical destruction, lack of containment by periosteal new bone formation, and a poorly defined margin. On radiographs, the amorphous, neoplastic bone may produce a pathognomonic "sunburst" pattern in which spicules of neoplastic bone arise perpendicular to the long axis of the limb in the periosteum; these spicules have been described as having a "hair on end" appearance. The incompetent periosteal reaction may also take the form of a triangular area of bone at the cortical margins produced by periosteal elevation and reaction

Plate 6-15   Tumors of Musculoskeletal System

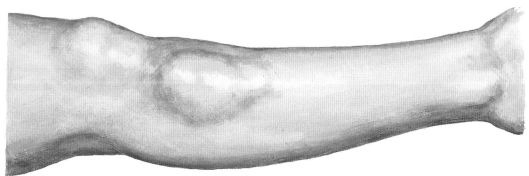

Osteosarcoma of proximal tibia presents as localized, tender prominence.

MALIGNANT TUMORS OF BONE—OSTEOSARCOMA

(Continued)

(Codman's triangle). Any of these periosteal reactions are suggestive of an aggressive bone tumor. Tumors treated with adjuvant chemotherapy can become heavily ossified or necrotic. Satellite nodules of tumor in the bone that may rarely be separate from the main mass can be seen in the peripheral margin.

In most cases, the radiographic differential diagnosis involves Ewing sarcoma (see Plate 6-19) and osteomyelitis; less often, osteosarcoma resembles an aggressive osteoblastoma (see Plate 6-3).

Results of staging studies reflect the tumor's aggressive nature. Bone scans show intense radioisotope uptake and reveal metastatic lesions to other bones. MRI provides more detailed information about intraosseous involvement, skip lesions, and soft tissue extension. Chest CT scans are also needed to detect pulmonary metastases not always seen on chest radiographs. Staging studies are essential to monitor the response to chemotherapy and plan the surgical approach.

Osteosarcomas vary widely in appearance, and it may be difficult to distinguish non-neoplastic, reactive osteoid from trauma or other tumors compared with the immature neoplastic osteoid in osteosarcoma, especially if the tissue sample is small.

Treatment/Prognosis. Forty years ago amputations were routinely performed for patients with osteosarcoma and most patients still eventually died of metastatic disease. However, preoperative (neoadjuvant) chemotherapy has substantially improved the life expectancy from less than 20% to 70% in patients who present without metastases. In addition, most patients now undergo limb salvage procedures compared with the amputations previously performed.

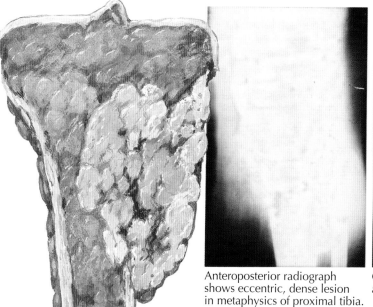

Anteroposterior radiograph shows eccentric, dense lesion in metaphysis of proximal tibia.

Osteosarcoma sometimes appears as radiolucent lesion.

Sectioned proximal tibia. Tumor density fairly uniform with some areas of necrosis and hemorrhage. Neoplasm has penetrated cortex into surrounding soft tissue.

Masses of tumor cells with hyperchromatic nuclei interspersed with foci of malignant osteoid are typical histopathologic findings (H & E stain).

PAROSTEAL OSTEOSARCOMA

Parosteal (juxtacortical) osteosarcoma arises between the cortex and muscle as a low-grade stage IA surface tumor, most commonly in adolescents and young adults (see Plate 6-16). It usually presents as a fixed, painless mass on the posterior aspect of the distal femur (over 50% of cases); other sites include the proximal humerus and proximal tibia. Parosteal osteosarcoma

is distinguished from classic osteosarcoma by its much slower, less aggressive clinical course and broad attachment to the adjacent cortex. Pain is less common with parosteal osteosarcoma than conventional osteosarcoma.

Diagnostic Studies. Radiographs show a dense, heavily ossified, broad-based fusiform mass that appears to encircle the metaphysis. Invasion into the overlying displaced soft tissues is rare. Late in the disease, the

Plate 6-16   Musculoskeletal System: PART III

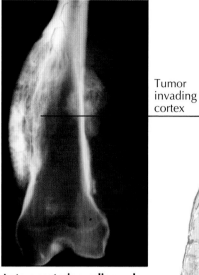

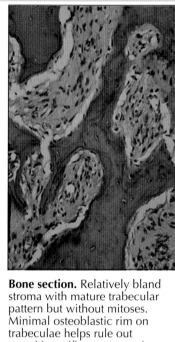

Tumor invading cortex

Anteroposterior radiograph. Densely ossified prominence on anterolateral aspect of distal femur; satellite lesion on opposite side characterizes mass as parosteal osteosarcoma rather than osteoma or osteocartilaginous exostosis.

Sectioned femur. Longitudinal tumor has invaded cortex but not medullary canal. Satellite lesion still separated from cortex by cleft; in early stage, primary tumor is also separated from cortex by uninvolved zone.

Bone section. Relatively bland stroma with mature trabecular pattern but without mitoses. Minimal osteoblastic rim on trabeculae helps rule out myositis ossificans or reactive bone (H & E stain).

MALIGNANT TUMORS OF BONE—OSTEOSARCOMA
(Continued)

tumor extends through the underlying cortex to invade the medullary canal as well, converting to a stage IB tumor; about 10% of these tumors exhibit areas of dedifferentiation into high-grade sarcoma and when dedifferentiated these parosteal osteosarcomas are considered stage IIB lesions.

Differential diagnosis includes osteocartilaginous exostosis (see Plate 6-6), myositis ossificans (see Plate 6-24), and periosteal chondroma (see Plate 6-5), all of which occur in adolescents.

Histologic features consist of mature trabeculae with a peculiar pattern of cement lines similar to that seen in Paget disease of bone. Enmeshed in a low-grade stroma, the trabeculae often contain varying degrees of cartilage that is not obviously malignant. Because of these bland overall features, this tumor is frequently underdiagnosed as benign, leading to inadequate intracapsular or marginal excision and recurrence.

Treatment/Prognosis. Treatment of the parosteal osteosarcoma is wide excision that can usually be accomplished with a limb-salvaging procedure. Unless dedifferentiation (favored by repeated recurrence or prolonged neglect) is present, the prognosis is good and chemotherapy is not indicated because the risks outweigh the benefits in non-dedifferentiated parosteal osteosarcoma.

PERIOSTEAL OSTEOSARCOMA

Periosteal osteosarcoma also is an uncommon variant of osteosarcoma. It primarily affects young adults, usually presenting as an enlarging, often painless mass that grows on the external surface of the bone.

Diagnostic Studies. Radiographs show a largely external, poorly mineralized mass in a crater-like area of cortical erosion with an irregular margin and periosteal reaction. The incidence of pulmonary metastases is higher than in parosteal osteosarcoma, and the prognosis is worse. The radiographic differential diagnosis includes classic osteosarcoma (see Plates 6-14 and

Periosteal osteosarcoma

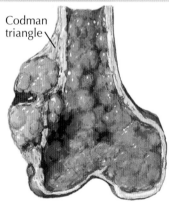

Codman triangle

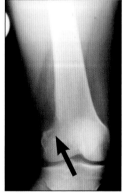

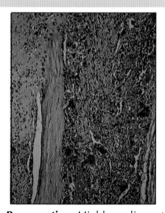

Distal femur. Erosive cartilaginous lesion in periosteum of distal femoral metaphysis. Codman triangles of reactive bone at margins.

Radiograph. Crater-like lesion with margin of reactive bone and faint calcification.

Bone section. Highly malignant stroma with cartilaginous and osteoid components (H&E stain).

6-15), periosteal chondroma (see Plate 6-5), and juxtacortical chondrosarcoma (see Plate 6-17).

Bone scans show a disproportionate increase in radioisotope uptake throughout the tumor, considering its predominantly radiolucent appearance. CT depicts a tumor sitting in a shallow cortical defect with only moderate calcification.

On gross examination, the tumor appears to be composed primarily of cartilage; microscopic examination,

however, reveals areas of malignant mesenchymal stroma containing neoplastic osteoid scattered in and about the lobules of low-grade mature cartilage.

Treatment/Prognosis. Because of its intermediate aggressiveness and accessible location, the lesion is almost always amenable to excision with a wide margin. Adjuvant systemic chemotherapy is indicated only for higher-grade tumors. Prognosis for patients with periosteal osteosarcoma is fair.

Plate 6-17   Tumors of Musculoskeletal System

MALIGNANT TUMORS OF BONE—CHONDROSARCOMA

Chondrosarcoma is a malignant cartilaginous tumor of bone. Primary chondrosarcoma occurs most often in adults and tends to affect the pelvis, proximal femur, and shoulder girdle. A persistent, dull, aching pain, like that of arthritis, is the initial manifestation. Chondrosarcoma can rarely be a secondary malignant transformation of a preexisting enchondroma or osteo-cartilaginous exostoses, although the incidence of degeneration of these benign entities to chondrosarcoma is increased in the multiple lesions seen in enchondromatosis (Ollier disease) or osteochondromatosis. Variants of classic chondrosarcoma are dedifferentiated (high grade), and clear cell (intermediate grade) chondrosarcoma. Dedifferentiated chondrosarcomas have a classic chondrosarcoma component with a higher-grade, more aggressive area superimposed. Clear cell chondrosarcomas are slower growing and primarily occur in the proximal femur.

Diagnostic Studies. Radiographs of chondrosarcomas reveal a lesion nearly always with cortical destruction, and the majority of lesions have calcification or a more discrete "popcorn" pattern. Primary chondrosarcoma may arise centrally in the medullary canal or peripherally on the external surface of the bone, causing the cortical destruction in association with a protruding cartilaginous mass. The pattern of calcification is usually pathognomonic of a cartilaginous process, but the radiographic differential diagnosis includes other cartilaginous lesions. Scalloping of the inner cortex of bone alone without extension into the soft tissues does not generally occur in chondrosarcoma and is more typical of a benign enchondroma.

In the diagnosis of classic chondrosarcoma, radiographs will usually show calcification, and MRI is used to determine if a soft tissue mass is present and to demonstrate the extent of disease. CT can be helpful to prove cortical destruction. This finding is important in the diagnosis of chondrosarcoma because it can be difficult to discern chondrosarcoma from benign cartilage lesions on histologic examination alone. Pain and a soft tissue mass can help to determine the diagnosis when the histology is not clear. High-grade cartilaginous lesions frequently have a soft, viscous, jelly-like consistency, whereas low-grade lesions have a firmer consistency with abundant calcification and distinct cauliflower-like nodules of mature cartilage. In high-grade lesions, including dedifferentiated chondrosarcoma, poorly differentiated areas may be less firm and more gelatinous and can rarely be difficult to identify as cartilaginous.

Treatment/Prognosis. Low-grade tumors rarely metastasize or recur locally after wide limb-salvaging excision, in contrast to high-grade chondrosarcomas, which have a higher rate of recurrence after limb salvage and are prone to pulmonary metastases. Neither chemotherapy or radiation therapy is effective for chondrosarcoma.

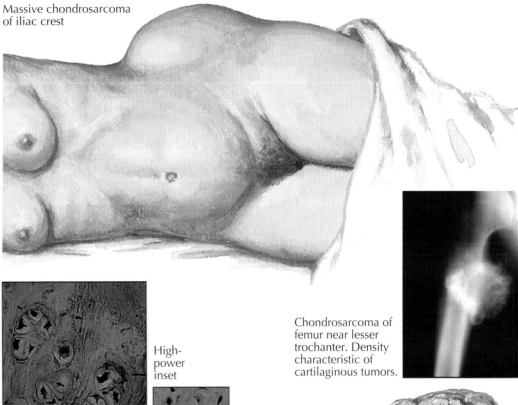

Massive chondrosarcoma of iliac crest

High-power inset

Chondrosarcoma of femur near lesser trochanter. Density characteristic of cartilaginous tumors.

Ratio of cells to cartilaginous matrix, amount of cellular atypia and mitoses, and occurrence of multiple nuclei in lacunae vary with degree of malignancy (H & E stain).

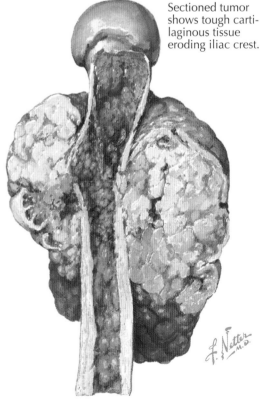

Sectioned tumor shows tough cartilaginous tissue eroding iliac crest.

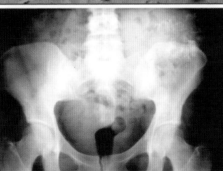

Radiograph of above patient reveals tumor arising in and destroying iliac crest.

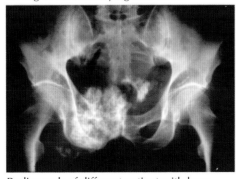

Radiograph of different patient with large chondrosarcoma in region of obturator foramen. Note mottled calcification.

Specimen shows tumor has eroded femoral cortex and invaded surrounding cortex.

Plate 6-18

Musculoskeletal System: PART III

MALIGNANT TUMORS OF BONE—FIBROUS HISTIOCYTOMA AND FIBROSARCOMA OF BONE

These lesions are malignant fibrous tumors of bone and are much less common than their benign fibrous lesion counterparts, nonossifying fibroma, ossifying fibroma, and desmoplastic fibroma in bone.

MALIGNANT FIBROUS HISTIOCYTOMA

Malignant fibrous histiocytoma occurs less often in bone than in soft tissues. It usually presents as an aggressive stage IIB sarcoma; not infrequently, a pathologic fracture is the first clinical manifestation.

Diagnostic Studies. Radiographs show a destructive, radiolucent lesion with cortical erosion and a poorly defined, permeative margin. Extensive bony infiltration by the tumor occurs early in the course of the disease. When associated with a radiodense bone infarct, malignant fibrous histiocytoma may be misinterpreted as a sarcomatous transformation of enchondroma. Staging studies are used to define the extent of extraosseous involvement, and special attention should be directed to ruling out metastases to the regional lymph nodes as well as the chest.

The histologic pattern of malignant fibrous histiocytoma of bone resembles that of a poorly differentiated fibrous tumor. The tumor consists of histiocytic cells that secrete collagen lacking the herringbone pattern of fibrosarcoma. The appearance varies from reddish purple, friable neoplastic tissue to yellowish tan histiocytic tissue. The neoplastic areas are composed of large, bizarre, foamy histiocytes; malignant giant cells; and a loose storiform stroma of spindle cells. In addition, variable areas of necrosis, mitoses, and grossly abnormal histiocytes are present. The fibrous areas may suggest fibrosarcoma.

Treatment/Prognosis. An intraosseous stage IIB malignant fibrous histiocytoma requires resection with a wide margin. Chemotherapy is indicated with these lesions. The overall prognosis is fair.

FIBROSARCOMA OF BONE

Fibrosarcoma is a very rare lesion and usually presents as a painful, tender mass.

Diagnostic Studies. Radiographs reveal a poorly defined, destructive, radiolucent lesion of the metaphyseal region. These tumors are high grade and poorly marginated and produce a permeative, or "motheaten," radiographic pattern of bone destruction.

Treatment/Prognosis. Fibrosarcomas require radical or wide margins with adjuvant chemotherapy. The prognosis for patients with stage II fibrosarcoma is fair.

Malignant fibrous histiocytoma of bone

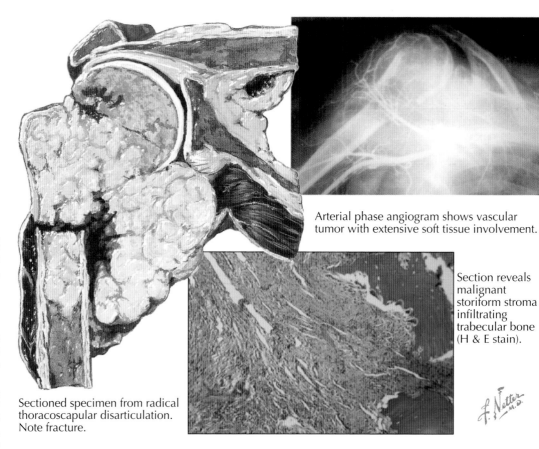

Arterial phase angiogram shows vascular tumor with extensive soft tissue involvement.

Sectioned specimen from radical thoracoscapular disarticulation. Note fracture.

Section reveals malignant storiform stroma infiltrating trabecular bone (H & E stain).

Fibrosarcoma of bone

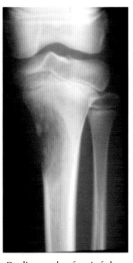

Radiograph of painful, tender mass over proximal tibia shows mottled, radiolucent, poorly defined lesion with penetration of reactive bone, indicative of malignant sarcoma but not specific for type.

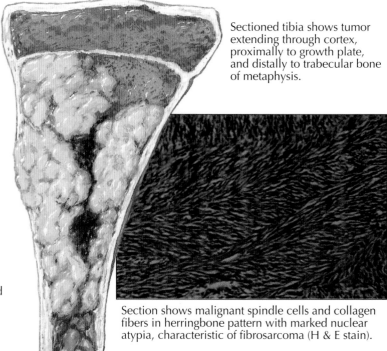

Sectioned tibia shows tumor extending through cortex, proximally to growth plate, and distally to trabecular bone of metaphysis.

Section shows malignant spindle cells and collagen fibers in herringbone pattern with marked nuclear atypia, characteristic of fibrosarcoma (H & E stain).

Plate 6-19

Tumors of Musculoskeletal System

MALIGNANT TUMORS OF BONE—RETICULOENDOTHELIAL TUMORS

EWING SARCOMA

Ewing sarcoma is a highly malignant bone tumor derived from the nonmesenchymal elements of the bone marrow. It represents approximately 7% of all primary bone malignancies and is the fourth most common primary malignancy of bone after myeloma, osteosarcoma, and chondrosarcoma. Onset is primarily between the ages of 5 and 20. Ewing sarcoma almost always presents as a stage IIB lesion. The primary symptom is an enlarging, tender, bony prominence with an associated large, soft tissue mass accompanied by constitutional symptoms (i.e., fever, malaise, weight loss, lethargy). The most common site is the femoral diaphysis, followed by the ilium, and ribs. Tumors in the pelvis are typically detected later and therefore are usually larger at presentation and have a worse prognosis.

Diagnostic Studies. Radiographs show a permeative usually diaphyseal tumor with a mottled, or patchy, density that indicates the tumor's destructive nature. Cortical involvement frequently produces a reactive, "onionskin" appearance of the periosteum, a pattern of layered ossification, or Codman's triangle suggestive of an aggressive lesion. The differential diagnosis includes osteomyelitis, osteolytic osteosarcoma (see Plate 6-14), and eosinophilic granuloma (see Plate 6-10).

Bone scans demonstrate intense radioisotope uptake well beyond the limits seen on radiographs and can reveal multiple skeletal lesions. MRI is used to determine local extent and soft tissue involvement and may reveal extensive areas of bony involvement.

Histologic features are small, round, neoplastic "blue" cells with large, hyperchromatic nuclei that do not make a calcified matrix. These small cells are usually spread out in thick sheets. The diagnosis is supported by the presence of *EWSR1* fusion transcripts from translocation involving chromosome 22.

Treatment/Prognosis. Management of Ewing sarcoma has changed significantly since the effectiveness of various combinations of chemotherapy, radiation therapy, and resection has been demonstrated. Pulmonary metastases have been reduced, and patient survival has improved so that nearly 70% of patients who present without metastatic or multifocal disease survive.

Wide surgical resection is preferred over radiation therapy for local control if (1) the involved bone is reliably reconstructable, (2) the involved bone is expendable (e.g., fibula, rib, clavicle), (3) radiation treatment would cause significant growth deformity (e.g., in young children with growth plate involvement), (4) radiation treatment would cause significant risk of secondary postirradiation sarcoma such as in patients younger than 15 years old, or (5) previous local irradiation was unsuccessful.

EWING SARCOMA

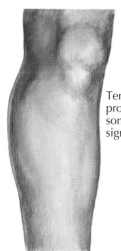

Tender bulge on proximal fibula with some inflammatory signs

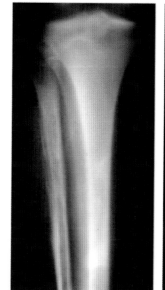

Radiograph reveals mottled, destructive, radiolucent lesion.

Angiogram shows vascular blush extending into soft tissue.

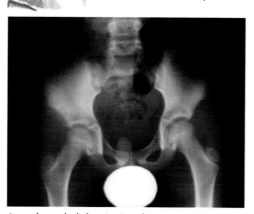

Ewing sarcoma of pelvis. Scarcely visible but palpable mass in right lower quadrant.

Infiltrative, destructive tumor extending into soft tissue seen in sectioned proximal fibula.

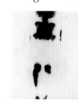

Bone scan shows heavy radioisotope uptake in tumor area. Other hot spots related to normal bone growth.

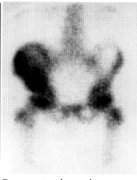

Lesion of mottled density involves anterior superior iliac spine.

Sectioned femur shows highly vascular intraosseous and soft tissue tumor components with much reactive bone.

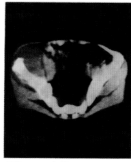

CT scan defines mass filling right iliac fossa.

Bone scan shows heavy radioisotope uptake in right iliac wing.

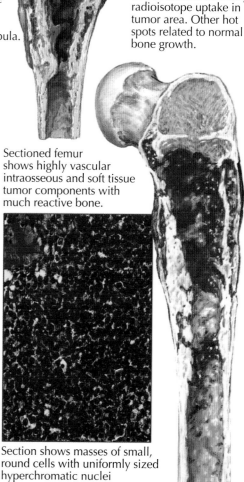

Section shows masses of small, round cells with uniformly sized hyperchromatic nuclei (H & E stain).

Plate 6-20

Musculoskeletal System: PART III

MYELOMA

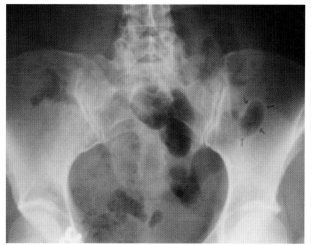

Radiograph of pelvis shows characteristic oval lytic lesion in left ilium.

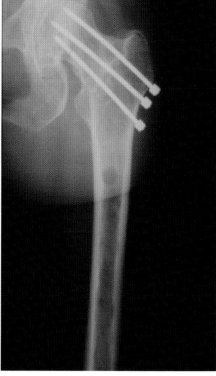

Multiple lesions distal to pathologic fracture of femoral neck (pinned)

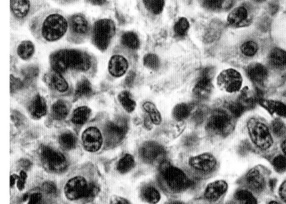

Section shows typical plasma cell composition of myeloma (H & E stain).

MALIGNANT TUMORS OF BONE—RETICULOENDOTHELIAL TUMORS (Continued)

MYELOMA

Myeloma is a malignant tumor of plasma cells. It is the most common malignant primary tumor of bone and usually develops in middle age. Myeloma may arise as a single intraosseous tumor (solitary plasmacytoma), but more often it develops as multiple painful lesions throughout the skeleton (multiple myeloma). Associated findings are constitutional symptoms, anemia, thrombocytopenia, and renal failure.

Diagnostic Studies. The results of most staging studies are the same as for other malignant primary tumors. On bone scans, however, myelomas may not appear as abnormal (cold lesions). Laboratory findings include anemia, hyperuricemia, and hypercalcemia. A serum protein electrophoresis (SPEP) or urine protein electrophoresis (UPEP) usually reveals a monoclonal gammopathy.

Histologic features include aggregates of immature plasma cells with little intervening stroma. The neoplastic plasma cells are hyperchromatic, and the clumps of chromatin give the cell a "clock face" or "spoke wheel" appearance.

Treatment/Prognosis. Myeloma is very sensitive to radiation therapy, and reossification of the tumors often occurs within several months. Large tumors or involvement of high-stress areas necessitate surgical stabilization for fracture prophylaxis; however, myeloma is one of the few malignant bone lesions that can heal, at least in the humerus, even after pathologic fracture (see Plate 6-30). When the disease is disseminated, chemotherapy and even bone marrow transplant may be indicated.

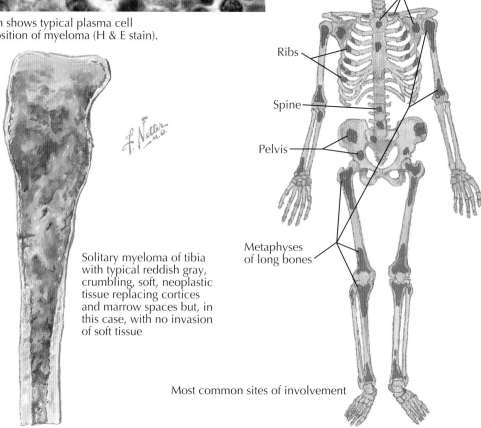

Solitary myeloma of tibia with typical reddish gray, crumbling, soft, neoplastic tissue replacing cortices and marrow spaces but, in this case, with no invasion of soft tissue

Skull

Sternum, clavicle, scapula

Ribs

Spine

Pelvis

Metaphyses of long bones

Most common sites of involvement

Plate 6-21

Tumors of Musculoskeletal System

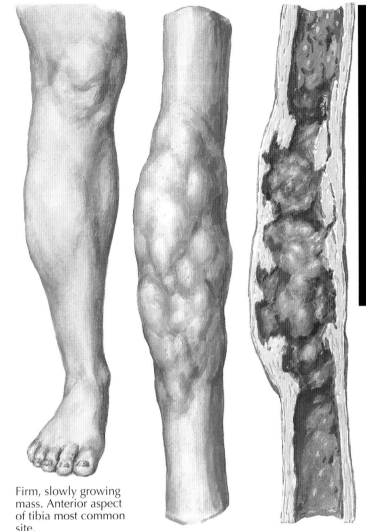

Radiograph shows crater-like radiolucent lesion with "soap bubble" appearance and margins of reactive bone.

Firm, slowly growing mass. Anterior aspect of tibia most common site.

External appearance and section of excised segment of tibia

MALIGNANT TUMORS OF BONE—ADAMANTINOMA

A rare tumor of unknown origin, adamantinoma occurs primarily in young males between 10 and 30 years of age. The tibia is involved in more than 95% of patients.

Diagnostic Studies. The radiographic appearance consists of multiple small, oval, radiolucent cortical defects with a distinct margin of reactive bone and a thickened cortex. Adamantinoma typically has a "soap bubble" appearance with distinct multiloculated lesions that expand the cortex into the soft tissue. The differential diagnosis includes chondromyxoid fibroma (see Plate 6-7), ossifying fibroma, osteofibrous dysplasia (primarily in patients younger than 10 years old), monostotic fibrous dysplasia (see Plate 6-8), and infection.

Definitive information about extension along the medullary canal or into adjacent soft tissue is obtained by MRI.

Histologic examination reveals a classic pseudoglandular appearance with epithelioid cells with nuclear palisading (single file pattern) that may suggest rounded islands of glandular tissue consistent with adenocarcinoma.

Treatment/Prognosis. The treatment of choice is resection where possible, usually with a segmental resection of the tibia that can be reconstructed with autograft bone. More conservative treatment (curettage or marginal excision) is associated with repeated recurrences, which ultimately may require amputation, and occasionally patients develop pulmonary metastases. With adequate local control, the prognosis is good.

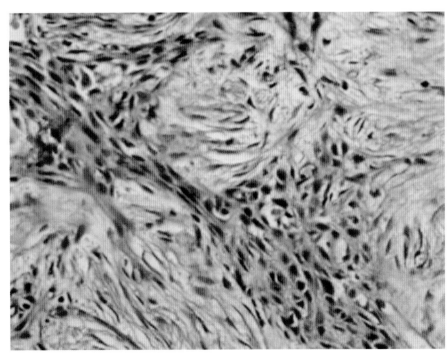

Section shows nests of squamous epithelia-like cells separated by areas of spindle cells (H&E stain).

Plate 6-22

Musculoskeletal System: PART III

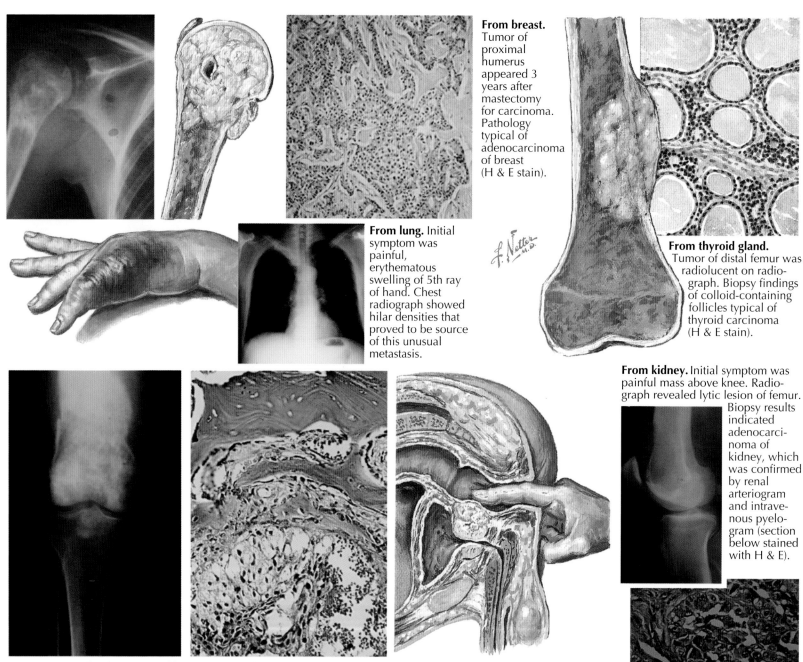

From breast. Tumor of proximal humerus appeared 3 years after mastectomy for carcinoma. Pathology typical of adenocarcinoma of breast (H & E stain).

From lung. Initial symptom was painful, erythematous swelling of 5th ray of hand. Chest radiograph showed hilar densities that proved to be source of this unusual metastasis.

From thyroid gland. Tumor of distal femur was radiolucent on radiograph. Biopsy findings of colloid-containing follicles typical of thyroid carcinoma (H & E stain).

From kidney. Initial symptom was painful mass above knee. Radiograph revealed lytic lesion of femur. Biopsy results indicated adenocarcinoma of kidney, which was confirmed by renal arteriogram and intravenous pyelogram (section below stained with H & E).

From prostate gland. Fracture of femur was initial manifestation. Radiograph revealed destructive lesion suggestive of osteosarcoma, but histologic findings indicated adenocarcinoma. Elevated acid phosphatase level and results of digital rectal examination confirmed origin (H & E stain).

MALIGNANT TUMORS OF BONE— TUMORS METASTATIC TO BONE

Metastatic tumors of the skeleton outnumber primary tumors by 25 to 1. The vast majority occur secondary to carcinoma of the breast, lung, thyroid, kidney, or prostate ("BLT with a Kosher pickle"). Colon cancer is the next most common primary malignancy to metastasize to bone after the aforementioned five. The most common sites of involvement for bone metastases are those containing hematopoietic marrow (e.g., the spine, ribs, skull, pelvis, and metaphyses of the femur and humerus), and metastases are primarily intramedullary. The rare metastasis to cortical bone or to the bones of the hands or feet suggests seeding from a primary lung carcinoma. In children, metastatic skeletal tumors are usually secondary to neuroblastoma in those younger than 2 years old or to lymphoma and Ewing sarcoma in older children. Metastasis after age 40 is usually secondary to the primary carcinomas mentioned earlier.

Purely osteolytic metastases are generally from lung, kidney, thyroid, or colon cancer. Metastatic bone tumors from kidney or thyroid carcinoma are usually hypervascular, and preoperative embolization should be considered. Osteoblastic metastases are most often seen with prostate or breast carcinoma. The primary tumor sometimes may not be known, but it can usually be detected with CT scans of the chest and abdomen. In patients with a history of carcinoma, the presence of a solitary tumor necessitates a search for other sites of skeletal involvement. If there is no history of carcinoma and staging studies do not reveal a primary carcinoma, a needle biopsy is frequently performed to assess the isolated lesion. Even with no known primary tumor, an isolated lesion in someone older than 40 is usually a metastasis and less likely myeloma or lymphoma. Primary sarcomas in patients older than 40 are much less likely than metastatic disease, myeloma, or lymphoma. For multiple metastatic lesions, chemotherapy, hormonal manipulation, and palliative radiation therapy are therapeutic options. Surgery is performed for most pathologic fractures and for some pathologic lesions that are believed to have high likelihood of fracture (impending fractures), such as those with over half of the diameter of the bone destroyed or with bone cortical destruction over 3 cm in length. Prognosis for patients with skeletal metastases is poor, although patients with isolated bone metastases particularly with breast cancer and renal cell cancer can live for a number of years.

Plate 6-23

Tumors of Musculoskeletal System

BENIGN TUMORS OF SOFT TISSUE—DESMOID, FIBROMATOSIS, AND HEMANGIOMA

DESMOID

A desmoid is a solitary, benign fibrous tumor of soft tissue. It may occur at any age, first appearing as an asymptomatic but slowly enlarging soft tissue mass, usually adjacent to fibrous or fascial structures and frequently in extracompartmental soft tissues. The palmar and plantar aspects of the hands and feet are common sites of involvement.

Diagnostic Studies. On MRI, tumor margins are sometimes difficult to distinguish from the normal fascial structures.

Treatment/Prognosis. Treatment of desmoids has historically been by excision or resection, but based on the extremely high recurrence rate other less invasive techniques such as tamoxifen and nonsteroidal anti-inflammatory drugs have met with some early success. Usually nonoperative treatment should at least be attempted with surgery reserved as a last resort.

FIBROMATOSIS

The term *fibromatosis* refers to multiple fibrous tumors that, although benign, are significantly more aggressive than solitary fibroma. These lesions often develop in the proximal limbs or the trunk and are also called abdominal and extra-abdominal desmoid tumors, depending on whether or not they involve the abdominal wall. Although generally superficial, the tumors are locally invasive, frequently involving adjacent neurovascular structures.

Diagnostic Studies. Staging studies are required for fibromatosis because of the lesions' aggressive behavior and the need to exclude low-grade malignancy. Although the lesions usually develop adjacent to or even adherent to bone, bone scans are often cold. On CT and MRI, tumor margins are poorly demonstrated because the lesions infiltrate the surrounding fascial or fibrous structures. Histologic examination reveals scattered spindle cells enmeshed in heavy strands of mature collagen.

Treatment/Prognosis. Because the extent of involvement and the aggressiveness of fibromatosis are often underestimated, the surgical margins achieved may be inadequate as with desmoids tumors. Even if the tumors are excised with a wide margin, recurrence is likely. Recurrences are difficult to distinguish from the scarring of previous excisions, thus making subsequent excision even more difficult. Adjuvant radiation therapy may reduce the recurrence rate after marginal, or even after intracapsular, excision but has its own risk and may even cause malignant degeneration of these benign lesions.

HEMANGIOMA

Hemangioma of soft tissue is a benign, vascular tumor that occurs in children, usually in the limbs or the trunk. Sometimes, hemangioma is congenital, appearing as a solitary tumor that infiltrates local tissue and, like fibromatosis, may involve adjacent neurovascular structures. Capillary hemangiomas are noninvasive and usually smaller and more cellular than cavernous

Fibromatosis

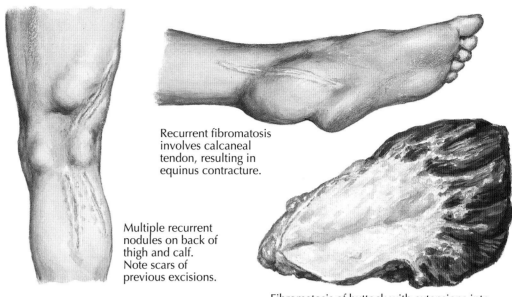

Recurrent fibromatosis involves calcaneal tendon, resulting in equinus contracture.

Multiple recurrent nodules on back of thigh and calf. Note scars of previous excisions.

Fibromatosis of buttock with extensions into gluteus maximus muscle

Hemangioma

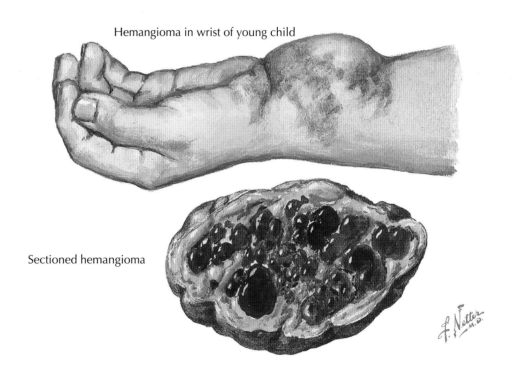

Hemangioma in wrist of young child

Sectioned hemangioma

hemangiomas, which are invasive and frequently contain calcifications or phleboliths that are readily seen on radiographs. The most common form is a tumor with infiltrative margins composed of both large and small vessels.

Diagnostic Studies. On physical examination, elevating the affected body part above the level of the heart may noticeably reduce the size of the mass by emptying venous blood in the lesions. Hemangiomas have a characteristic (bull's-eye) appearance on MRI frequently with feeding vessels, and this appearance along with the findings of the history and physical examination can frequently preclude the need for a biopsy.

Treatment/Prognosis. Despite their vascular origin, hemangiomas do not metastasize or undergo malignant transformation. However, hemangiomas frequently recur after surgical resection; therefore, injection by interventional radiology or vascular surgery has been successful and should generally be attempted, with resection as a last resort.

Plate 6-24

Musculoskeletal System: PART III

BENIGN TUMORS OF SOFT TISSUE—LIPOMA, NEUROFIBROMA, AND MYOSITIS OSSIFICANS

LIPOMA

Lipoma, the most common tumor of soft tissue, is a benign tumor usually composed of lobules of mature fat. It occurs in adults and is usually soft, slowly enlarging, and asymptomatic and usually located superficially in the subcutaneous tissues. However, it can also be deep and in muscle bellies. Lipomas that arise in deep tissues may become remarkably large and have an increased chance of being an atypical lipoma.

Diagnostic Studies. Radiographs may also show calcification in areas of necrosis and metaplastic bone or cartilage inside lipomas. MRI reveals a homogenous fatty tumor that can be quite large.

Treatment/Prognosis. Marginal excision is successful for lipoma, and recurrences are rare. However, recurrences are higher (approximately 25%) in atypical lipomas with MDM2 amplification by fluorescence in-situ hybridization or immunohistochemistry. Lipomas and even atypical lipomas do not metastasize.

NEUROFIBROMA

A neurofibroma is a benign tumor of neural origin. Although it may affect almost any tissue type, it is most commonly found in skin and subcutaneous tissue and is associated with nerve fibers. Whether they are solitary or multiple, neurofibromas can occur in persons of any age. Multiple neurofibromas are a primary manifestation of neurofibromatosis. Neurofibromas also occur in conjunction with scoliosis, congenital pseudarthrosis of the tibia, and gigantism of a limb. (For a discussion of these conditions, see Section 4, Congenital and Developmental Disorders.)

Long-standing neurofibromas, particularly in patients with multiple neurofibromas (neurofibromatosis), may undergo malignant transformation.

Diagnostic Studies. Neurofibroma is frequently seen as a fusiform mass in continuity with a major nerve best demonstrated by MRI. These lesions originate from a nerve, and therefore resection will usually require at least cutting nerve bundles. In contrast, schwannomas are benign tumors of the nerve sheath and can frequently be excised without demonstrable damage to the adjacent nerve. Histologic examination of a neurofibroma reveals a loose, spindle-cell stroma containing wavy eosinophilic fibrillar material and occasional Verocay bodies, which are composed of amorphous eosinophilic material that is surrounded by spindle-shaped or oval cells.

Treatment. Neurofibromas can be excised if painful or they can be followed, since they are benign. If a neurofibroma is excised, the nerve, or at least the nerve fascicle of origin, will need to be excised. If a neurofibroma is rapidly enlarging, a biopsy should be performed to rule out malignant degeneration to a malignant peripheral nerve sheath tumor (MPNST). MPNST occurs primarily in patients with neurofibromatosis.

MYOSITIS OSSIFICANS

Myositis ossificans is a non-neoplastic reparative or reactive ossification of soft tissue that usually occurs after blunt trauma, particularly in conjunction with

Lipoma

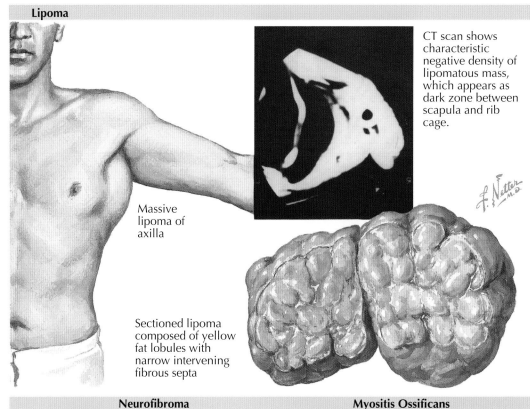

CT scan shows characteristic negative density of lipomatous mass, which appears as dark zone between scapula and rib cage.

Massive lipoma of axilla

Sectioned lipoma composed of yellow fat lobules with narrow intervening fibrous septa

Neurofibroma

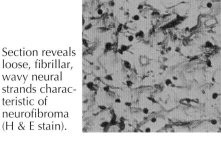

Surgical stripping of large, solitary neurofibroma from sciatic nerve

Section reveals loose, fibrillar, wavy neural strands characteristic of neurofibroma (H & E stain).

Myositis Ossificans

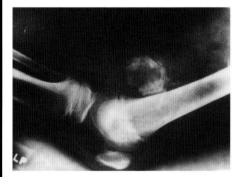

Lateral radiograph shows nodule with peripheral maturation in soft tissue of posterior distal thigh.

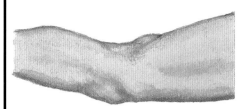

Prominence on posterior distal femur limits flexion.

head trauma. It can occur in adolescents as a painless, enlarging mass in the upper arm, thigh, or buttocks. This clinical presentation may erroneously suggest an extraosseous osteosarcoma or soft tissue sarcoma.

Diagnostic Studies. Radiographs reveal a round mass with a distinct margin of mature ossification and a radiolucent center of immature osteoid and primitive mesenchymal tissue (the reverse of that seen in a malignant tumor). Differential diagnosis includes juxtacortical osteosarcoma; however, the peripheral maturation in myositis ossificans is so characteristic that documentation with CT can resolve fears of malignancy even when suggested by the histologic appearance of the central immature area.

Treatment/Prognosis. Because recurrence is high, early excision of myositis ossificans should not generally be attempted except for diagnostic purposes when diagnostic studies are inconclusive.

Plate 6-25

Tumors of Musculoskeletal System

MALIGNANT TUMORS OF SOFT TISSUE—SARCOMAS OF SOFT TISSUE

The incidence of soft tissue sarcomas is greater than that of bone sarcomas. Most soft tissue sarcomas are palpable or symptomatic, yet they are rarely well visualized on radiographs. As a result, they are frequently managed initially as a benign lesion such as a lipoma, hematoma, thrombophlebitis, cyst, or abscess. Imaging with magnetic resonance is important; and if the lesion is indeterminate with MRI, then a biopsy is indicated. Most of the time with soft tissue sarcomas a needle biopsy is adequate.

Limb-salvage procedures (i.e., local excision) have replaced amputation as the primary treatment of soft tissue sarcomas; however, despite the efficacy of limb-salvage procedures in obtaining local control, pulmonary metastases remain a significant problem and occur in 30% to 50% of patients.

MALIGNANT FIBROUS HISTIOCYTOMA

Malignant fibrous histiocytoma is seen in adults and primarily metastasizes to the lungs.

Diagnostic Studies. Although the extent of soft tissue involvement and the tumor's relationship to the major neurovascular structures can be estimated by CT, MRI is more precise and differentiates normal from neoplastic tissue and shows edema.

Treatment/Prognosis. Treatment with a wide surgical margin of greater than 1 cm is usually adequate. In areas where a 1-cm margin is not possible, irradiation either preoperatively, intraoperatively, or postoperatively should be considered. CT should be obtained to determine if chest metastases are present; if they are, then chemotherapy should be considered, although chemotherapy is not of proven benefit in most soft tissue sarcomas. Amputation is reserved for multiple recurrences in which the tumor bed or previous surgical field cannot be completely resected.

FIBROSARCOMA OF SOFT TISSUE

The diagnosis of fibrosarcoma is rare (see Plate 6-25). Low-grade stage I fibrosarcoma is often difficult to distinguish from its benign but aggressive counterpart of fibromatosis (see Plate 6-23).

Diagnostic Studies. Radiographs show a lesion with a discrete margin. Histologic characteristics are marked cellular atypia and abundant collagen in a herringbone pattern. A low-grade fibrosarcoma can be confused with aggressive juvenile fibromatosis, a diagnostic difficulty that affects treatment choices.

SYNOVIAL SARCOMA

Synovial sarcoma is a tumor of children and young adults and is derived from the synovial tissues found along fascial planes, in periarticular structures, and, rarely, in joints (see Plate 6-26). An enlarging, painful, juxta-articular mass is the primary clinical

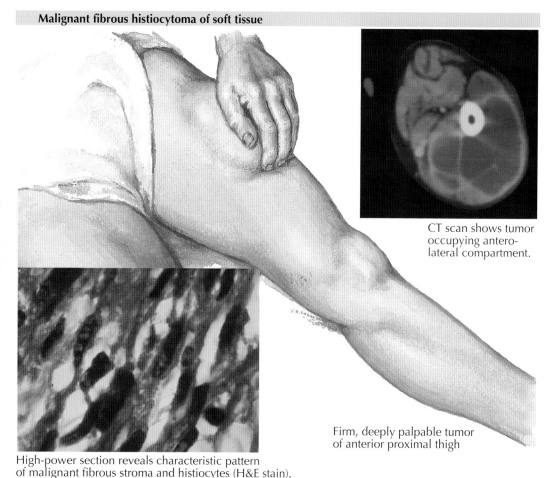

Malignant fibrous histiocytoma of soft tissue

CT scan shows tumor occupying antero-lateral compartment.

High-power section reveals characteristic pattern of malignant fibrous stroma and histiocytes (H&E stain).

Firm, deeply palpable tumor of anterior proximal thigh

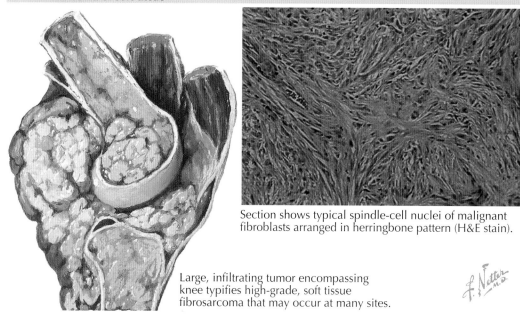

Fibrosarcoma of soft tissue

Section shows typical spindle-cell nuclei of malignant fibroblasts arranged in herringbone pattern (H&E stain).

Large, infiltrating tumor encompassing knee typifies high-grade, soft tissue fibrosarcoma that may occur at many sites.

manifestation. Occurring most frequently as a stage IIB lesion in the lower limbs, it may also appear as a stage I tumor, in which case it may be confused with a ganglion.

Diagnostic Studies. The lesion is often adjacent to major neurovascular structures and adjacent to, but not usually within, joints despite the term *synovial.* Accurate localization is best provided by MRI.

Histologic examination reveals a biphasic pattern, with intermixed areas of epithelial, glandular synovial-like cells and spindle-shaped cells. Depending on the relative prominence of these two components, synovial sarcomas are classified as biphasic, monophasic, and poorly differentiated.

Treatment/Prognosis. Despite adequate local control, the incidence of both regional and pulmonary

Plate 6-26

Musculoskeletal System: PART III

Synovial sarcoma

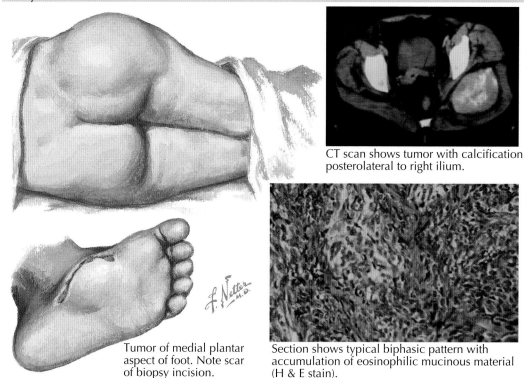

CT scan shows tumor with calcification posterolateral to right ilium.

Tumor of medial plantar aspect of foot. Note scar of biopsy incision.

Section shows typical biphasic pattern with accumulation of eosinophilic mucinous material (H & E stain).

Liposarcoma

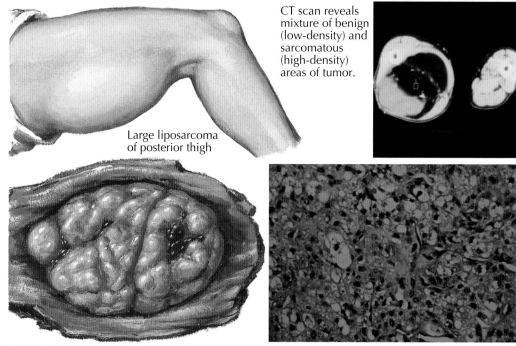

CT scan reveals mixture of benign (low-density) and sarcomatous (high-density) areas of tumor.

Large liposarcoma of posterior thigh

Excised tumor with muscle at margin; tumor darker and firmer than benign lipoma.

Section shows characteristic malignant lipoblasts (H & E stain).

MALIGNANT TUMORS OF SOFT TISSUE—SARCOMAS OF SOFT TISSUE *(Continued)*

metastases is high, and the long-term prognosis for patients with synovial sarcoma is poor. Synovial sarcoma not only metastasizes to the lungs but also has about a 10% incidence of lymph node metastasis, which has led some to recommend sentinel lymph node biopsy as part of the staging. Synovial sarcoma is sensitive to chemotherapy, with a response in 50% of patients.

LIPOSARCOMA

Liposarcoma (see Plate 6-26), a tumor derived from fat tissue, occurs in several forms: myxoid liposarcoma, dedifferentiated liposarcomas, and other liposarcomas. There is another group of borderline malignancies with MDM2 amplification called atypical lipomatous tumors; these lesions have no metastatic potential but a recurrence rate between that of lipomas and liposarcomas.

Diagnostic Studies. Liposarcoma is best imaged by MRI and will have at least some fat with high signal intensity on T1-weighted images. Dedifferentiated liposarcomas will have a large area of fat except in the high-grade areas within the tumor that will be darker on T1-weighted images.

Treatment/Prognosis. Wide resection with a negative margin of greater than 1 cm is the standard of care for liposarcomas. In addition to lung metastases,

liposarcomas have a higher chance of metastasis to the abdomen than other sarcomas.

MALIGNANT PERIPHERAL NERVE SHEATH TUMOR

Malignant peripheral nerve sheath tumor (MPNST) usually arises in a patient with neurofibromatosis. The distinction between the malignant area and the

Plate 6-27

Tumors of Musculoskeletal System

Malignant peripheral nerve sheath tumor (MPNST)

Specimen of sciatic nerve removed after amputation shows large fusiform tumor and smaller, more proximal tumor.

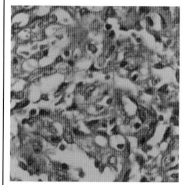

Section reveals round, hyperchromatic nuclei mixed with myxomatous, undulating spindle-cell stroma indicative of neural origin (H&E stain).

Rhabdomyosarcoma and leiomyosarcoma

Angiosarcoma

Leiomyosarcoma. Excised distal femur (F), tibia (T), reflected patella (P), and tumor. Arrow indicates area of cortical penetration. Section (above) shows transversely and longitudinally sectioned malignant smooth muscle cells (H&E stain).

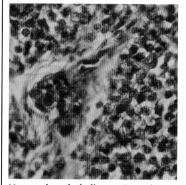

Hemangiopericytoma. Eccentric hyperchromatic nuclei of pericytic cells surrounding vascular spaces (H&E stain).

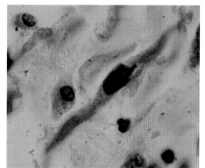

Rhabdomyosarcoma. High-power section demonstrates typical "strap" cells. Cross-striations seen under oil immersion (H&E stain).

Hemangioendothelioma. Central hyperplastic capillary surrounded by malignant endothelial cells (H&E stain).

MALIGNANT TUMORS OF SOFT TISSUE—SARCOMAS OF SOFT TISSUE (Continued)

widespread neurofibromas in the patient with neurofibromatosis is difficult, particularly on imaging. PET/CT may be useful in this differentiation because the neurofibromas are usually of lower intensity on PET/CT than MPNSTs. Other benign tumors such as schwannomas do not have an increased incidence of malignant degeneration into MPNST. Wide resection with a negative margin of greater than 1 cm is the standard of care for MPNST. This will require the sacrifice of the nerve in which the tumor arose.

RHABDOMYOSARCOMA AND LEIOMYOSARCOMA

Rhabdomyosarcomas are sarcomas of skeletal muscle and leiomyosarcomas are sarcomas of smooth muscle (see Plate 6-27).

Diagnostic Studies. MRI is the best imaging modality for both rhabdomyosarcoma and leiomyosarcoma.

Treatment/Prognosis. Rhabdomyosarcomas occur primarily in children, and there has been a significant improvement in survival rates in patients with rhabdomyosarcomas primarily owing to the efficacy of multiple-agent chemotherapy. Leiomyosarcomas occur primarily in adults and are not particularly sensitive to chemotherapy or irradiation. Surgical resection of both of these with a 1-cm margin is the preferred treatment.

ANGIOSARCOMA

Angiosarcomas are high-grade sarcomas of the soft tissue that respond very poorly to surgical resection with a very high rate of recurrence. Many centers do not recommend routine resection of angiosarcomas but rather primarily use chemotherapy. Amputation may be necessary for severe extremity involvement.

Plate 6-28

Musculoskeletal System: PART III

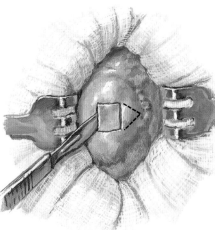

Proposed incision site for tumor removal

Biopsy incision longitudinal (not transverse); placed to permit inclusion of biopsy tract in definitive tumor excision. Neuro-vascular bundle must be avoided and shortest route to tumor used, with least removal of soft tissue.

Wedge-shaped specimen must be of adequate size and include both intraosseous and extraosseous tissue. Contamination of soft tissue with tumor cells must be avoided. Strict hemostasis must be achieved before closure. Bone defect plugged with cement

Multiple cultures

Specimen may be used for frozen section, fixation for histopatho-logic study, electron microscopy and study with special stains.

Wound closed neatly with short sutures

TUMOR BIOPSY

Successful management of a tumor is based on an accurate histologic diagnosis. If a malignant neoplasm is suspected, incisional biopsy is the most reliable technique for obtaining an adequate amount of tissue for histologic study. Needle biopsies are routinely used with or without CT guidance to make the diagnosis of sarcoma. However, open incisional biopsy, which involves cutting into and taking a piece of the lesion, remains the gold standard for diagnosis but does risk contamination of the adjacent tissues. The risk of wound contamination with incisional biopsy can be minimized by a strict adherence to the following surgical principles.

Correct Placement of Incision. In any limb, a straight longitudinal incision is used. The biopsy incision is placed in the line of the planned subsequent resection (if malignant) so that the biopsy tract can be excised en bloc with the lesion at the time of the resection.

Minimal Dissection of Soft Tissue. The surgical approach for biopsy should be direct, with minimal dissection of soft tissue. Muscle, fascia, and capsule or pseudocapsule are preserved for later closure; and an approach through muscle allows for a barrier to avoid contamination of internervous planes.

Avoidance of Neurovascular Structures and Adjacent Joint. The biopsy site should be selected carefully to avoid exposure of major vessels, nerves, and joint capsules, thus preventing their contamination and the necessity of their subsequent sacrifice if surgical resection is required.

Adequate Specimen. During the biopsy procedure, frozen sections should be evaluated to ensure the adequacy of the tissue specimen. Cultures are performed if infection is in the differential diagnosis, and additional tissue may be required for histochemical stains, electron microscopy, flow cytometry, and other special studies.

Strict Hemostasis. If practical, a tourniquet should be used to prevent bleeding and the tumor capsule is closed meticulously. Strict hemostasis should be achieved with electrocautery or even suturing, if necessary, before wound closure. Holes in bone that may leak

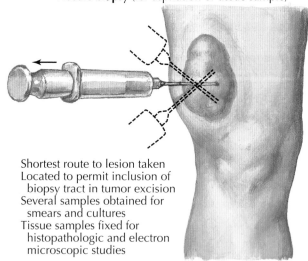

Needle biopsy (for aspiration or tissue sample)

Shortest route to lesion taken
Located to permit inclusion of biopsy tract in tumor excision
Several samples obtained for smears and cultures
Tissue samples fixed for histopathologic and electron microscopic studies

tumor cells can be plugged with methyl methacrylate cement. A drain may be inserted to avoid a hematoma, but it should be inserted in line with and close to the incision.

Tight Wound Closure. The pseudocapsule and fascial layers should be closed meticulously.

Complications. A poorly conceived and executed incisional biopsy may lead to a dissecting hematoma, which may contaminate previously uninvolved tissues with sarcoma cells. Thus, a subsequent excision of the tumor often requires a wider surgical margin. Widespread contamination may preclude a limb-salvage procedure or greatly increase the risk of local recurrence after limb-salvage resection

Alternative Biopsy Procedures. En bloc excisional biopsy is done for accessible clearly benign tumors.

Plate 6-29

Tumors of Musculoskeletal System

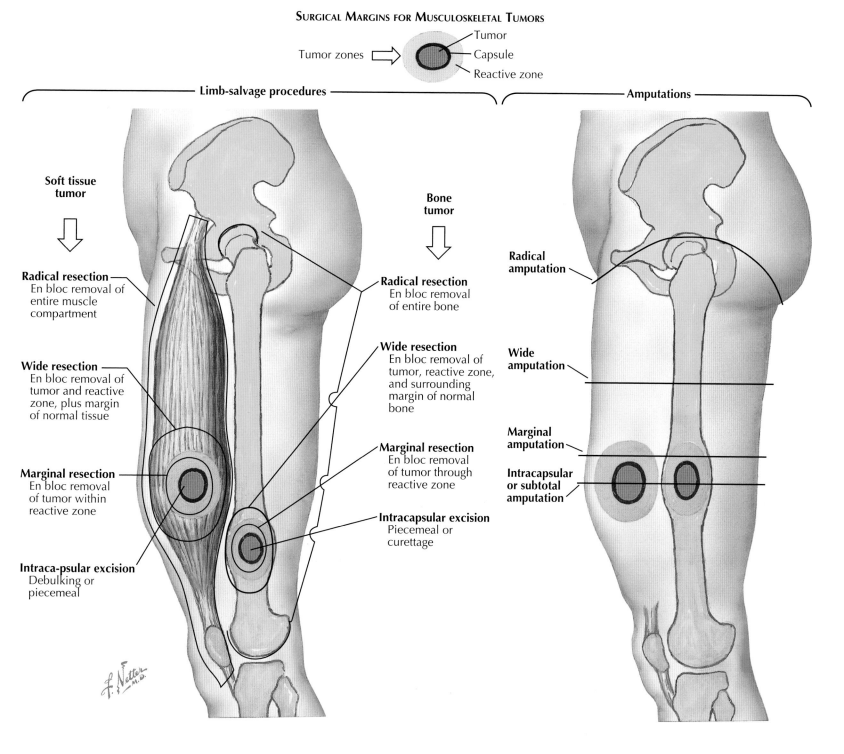

SURGICAL MARGINS FOR MUSCULOSKELETAL TUMORS

Tumor zones — Tumor / Capsule / Reactive zone

Limb-salvage procedures — Amputations

Soft tissue tumor

Bone tumor

Radical resection
En bloc removal of entire muscle compartment

Wide resection
En bloc removal of tumor and reactive zone, plus margin of normal tissue

Marginal resection
En bloc removal of tumor within reactive zone

Intraca-psular excision
Debulking or piecemeal

Radical resection
En bloc removal of entire bone

Wide resection
En bloc removal of tumor, reactive zone, and surrounding margin of normal bone

Marginal resection
En bloc removal of tumor through reactive zone

Intracapsular excision
Piecemeal or curettage

Radical amputation

Wide amputation

Marginal amputation

Intracapsular or subtotal amputation

SURGICAL MARGINS

The surgical removal of a tumor is most accurately described by stating the procedure and the surgical margin achieved—the amount and type of the non-neoplastic surrounding tissue. The four basic surgical margins are intracapsular, marginal, wide, and radical. Each margin may be achieved with limb salvage surgery or amputation.

An *intracapsular margin* is obtained when the surgical dissection extends through the reactive zone and the capsule or pseudocapsule into the tumor itself. A *marginal margin* describes a plane of dissection through the reactive zone just outside the capsule or pseudocapsule.

A *wide margin* is achieved when the dissection plane is through normal tissue outside the reactive zone; thus, the tumor and its pseudocapsule are excised along with an intact "cuff" of normal tissue. A *radical margin* describes removal of the tumor and the entire compartment (the entire bone or muscle compartment) that contains it. Although marginal, wide, or radical margins may all be free of tumor cells, the marginal margin, because of the closer proximity of the surgical margin to the tumor, is more likely to leave behind microscopic fragments of tumor and thus lead to local recurrence. Similarly, a wide margin of less than 1 cm, despite removal of a cuff of normal tissue, usually still has a higher risk for leaving residual tumor cells than does a radical procedure.

The term *contaminated margin* refers to a recognized intraoperative violation of the lesion, followed by closure and subsequent adjustment of the plane of dissection. For example, a contaminated wide excision indicates that the tumor was inadvertently entered during the tumor removal, the exposed tissues were contaminated by leakage from the tumor, the opening was closed, and the contaminated tissues were excised to obtain a wide margin.

The adequacy of the surgical margin is estimated by gross and microscopic examination of the excised specimen. Gross inspection is particularly important in distinguishing whether a wide margin or a radical margin has been obtained, because the microscopic appearance of each is free of tumor cells.

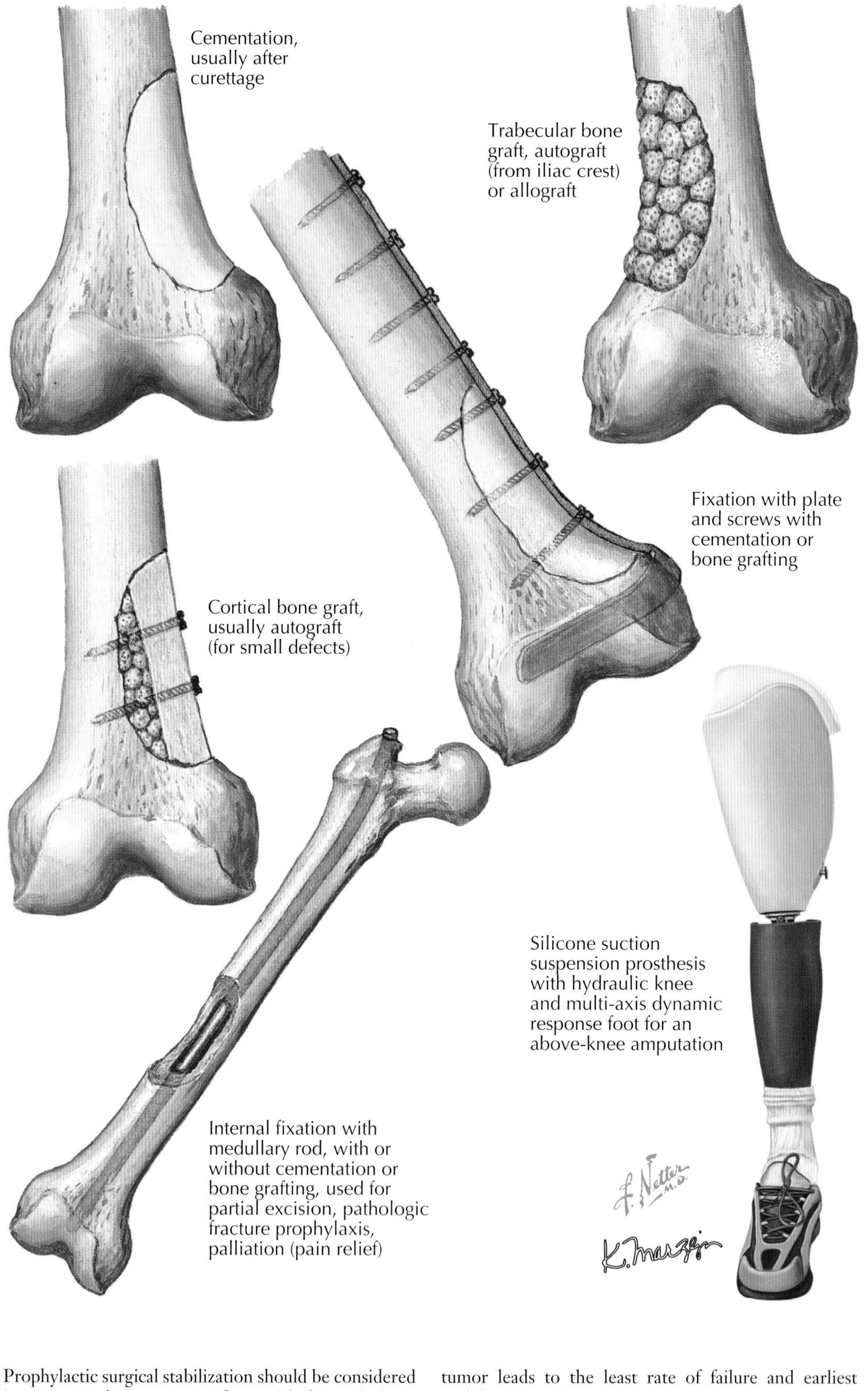

Plate 6-30

Musculoskeletal System: PART III

Cementation, usually after curettage

Trabecular bone graft, autograft (from iliac crest) or allograft

Fixation with plate and screws with cementation or bone grafting

Cortical bone graft, usually autograft (for small defects)

RECONSTRUCTION AFTER PARTIAL EXCISION OR CURETTAGE OF BONE (FRACTURE PROPHYLAXIS)

The excision of a tumor with removal of one cortex (wide fenestration) and curettage of the metaphysis is a common treatment for active or aggressive benign tumors or metastatic bone lesions. Reconstruction of the resulting surgical defect depends on its size and location and the age of the patient. In a child or young adult with a small cortical defect, for example, the weakened bone can be managed with a protective plaster cast while the defect heals. Excision of active or aggressive benign tumors often requires a wide surgical margin, which leaves a large defect that increases the risk of pathologic fracture. In these instances, the defect can be reconstructed with cortical bone autografts or allografts or with methyl methacrylate (cementation). For example, cementation after curettage of an active stage 2 giant cell tumor of bone lowers the risk of tumor recurrence and postoperative fracture. An additional advantage of this technique is the resulting immediate stabilization of the affected joint, which contributes to faster and more effective rehabilitation. However, cementation can make the evaluation of recurrence with follow-up radiographs more difficult and does change the biomechanics of the adjacent articular surface if the cement is applied to the subchondral area. This change in biomechanics may increase the incidence of degenerative joint disease in the adjacent joint. Moreover, cementation blocks healing in the area it is applied to, necessitating healing around the cement. When necessary, curettage plus cementation or bone grafting may be combined with internal fixation to preserve the integrity of a fragile remnant of cortex. Reconstruction of large metaphyseal defects with bone grafting involves the selection of appropriate cortical and trabecular bone autografts or allografts.

The potential for pathologic fracture is a common problem associated with metastatic carcinoma or myeloma. These tumors often present as painful osteolytic lesions in the lower limb, with pain on ambulation reflecting significant intrinsic bone weakness. The risk of pathologic fracture in a tubular bone is significant when the tumor occupies 50% or more of the bone diameter or produces a cortical defect longer than 3 cm.

Silicone suction suspension prosthesis with hydraulic knee and multi-axis dynamic response foot for an above-knee amputation

Internal fixation with medullary rod, with or without cementation or bone grafting, used for partial excision, pathologic fracture prophylaxis, palliation (pain relief)

Prophylactic surgical stabilization should be considered in patients who are at significant risk for pathologic fracture or who have fractures or painful tumors of the diaphysis that prevent ambulation. Stabilization of most diaphyseal bone tumors is best accomplished with intramedullary rod fixation with or without cementation.

When the tumor is located in the proximal femur or distal femur most of the time the use of a tumor prosthesis that takes the place of the bone involved with the tumor leads to the least rate of failure and earliest mobilization. Destructive tumors in the acetabulum may be treated with curettage and cementation in conjunction with a cage prosthesis and total hip replacement, but the remaining proximal, uninvolved ilium requires careful stabilization. Treatment of symptomatic tumors of the humerus also includes surgical stabilization after tumor removal, preferably with an intramedullary rod.

Plate 6-31

Tumors of Musculoskeletal System

LIMB-SALVAGE PROCEDURES FOR RECONSTRUCTION

Limb-salvage procedures for reconstruction of joint after resection for tumor

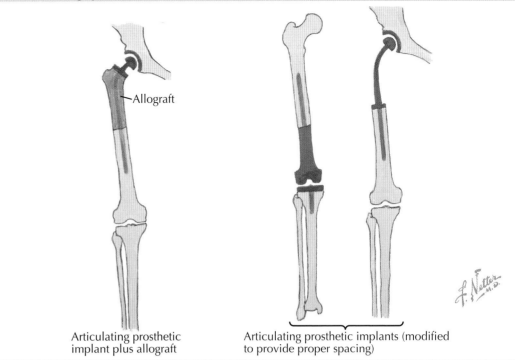

Articulating prosthetic
implant plus allograft

Articulating prosthetic implants (modified
to provide proper spacing)

Limb-salvage procedures for reconstruction of diaphysis after resection for tumor

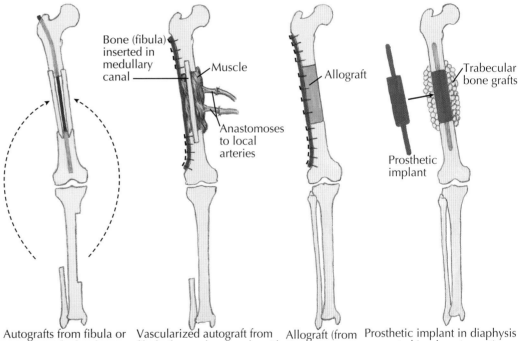

Bone (fibula)
inserted in
medullary
canal

Muscle

Anastomoses
to local
arteries

Allograft

Trabecular
bone grafts

Prosthetic
implant

Autografts from fibula or
segments of other long
bones combined with
internal fixation with
medullary rod

Vascularized autograft from
fibula (bone plus muscle with
vessels anastomosed to local
vessels)

Allograft (from
donor or bone
bank)

Prosthetic implant in diaphysis
cemented in place (sometimes
with trabecular bone autografts
from iliac crest)

LIMB-SALVAGE PROCEDURES

A major development in the management of musculoskeletal tumors in the limbs has been the increasing effectiveness of limb-salvage procedures. In patients with osteosarcoma and Ewing sarcoma, with adjuvant chemotherapy, limb-salvage procedures now do not have a significant increase in local recurrence compared to amputation.

Two principles are recognized in limb-salvage surgery—careful, adequate excision of the tumor followed by optimal functional reconstruction of the limb. Patient lifestyle and expectations should be carefully considered when selecting the reconstructive procedure. Most patients can be successfully treated with limb-salvage procedures, but in some patients with stage IIB tumors, only amputation can minimize the likelihood of recurrence. In addition, amputation may still be needed if the limb-salvage procedure is followed by recurrence, deep infection, or vascular insufficiency.

RECONSTRUCTION AFTER LIMB-SALVAGE RESECTION

After excision of a soft tissue sarcoma, the defect is usually reconstructed with a local tissue transfer to obliterate dead space or a temporary vacuum drain is used to avoid wound complications. Large soft tissue reconstructions after excisions may involve the transfer or rotation of a muscle or skin flap, split-thickness skin grafts, or, in rare situations, a free vascularized muscle or cutaneous muscle flap.

When half of the joint or the whole joint is resected, the reconstructive procedures used are primarily arthroplasties (see Plates 6-31 to 6-33).

Arthroplasty. Successful arthroplasty depends on surrounding musculature that has good power, vasculature, and innervation. The optimal result of arthroplasty is a painless, stable joint with good range of motion.

Arthroplasty may be achieved with (1) implantation of a prosthetic joint or partial joint (in the hip or shoulder) (see Plate 6-31), (2) transplantation of an articulating bone allograft, or (3) a composite technique—a combination of prosthesis plus bone allograft (see Plate 6-31). Use of bone allografts offer the advantage of a biologic implant that has the potential for gradual incorporation and soft tissue attachment. However,

allografts are associated with a high rate of complications such as infection, fracture, and nonunion at the graft-host junction. The risk of a serious complication necessitating removal of the graft or another operative procedure, including amputation, is as high as 30%. In the hip joint the acetabulum can be reconstructed with a cage-type acetabular prosthesis in many cases. Arthroplasty with a combination of prosthesis and

bone allograft (i.e., an allograft prosthetic composite) can be a useful reconstruction particularly in the proximal humerus, allowing for improved elevation and decreased dislocation compared with a prosthetic alone. In the proximal tibia an allograft prosthetic composite can lead to improved patellar tendon insertion and thus improved knee extension and strength (see Plate 6-31).

Plate 6-32   Musculoskeletal System: PART III

RADIOLOGIC FINDINGS IN LIMB-SALVAGE PROCEDURES

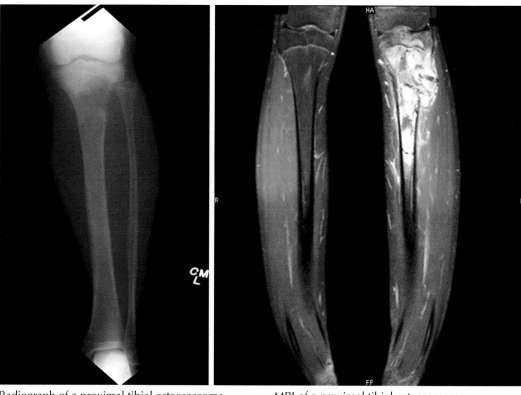

Radiograph of a proximal tibial osteosarcoma   MRI of a proximal tibial osteosarcoma

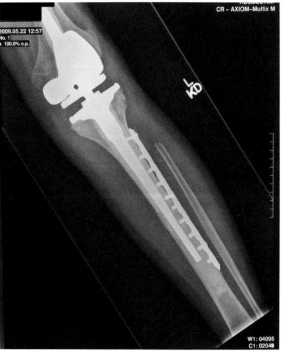

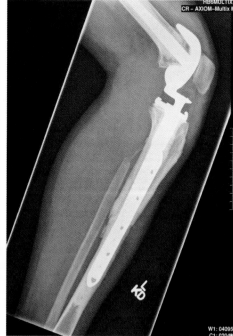

Lateral radiograph after resection and reconstruction with an allograft prosthetic composite reconstruction

Anteroposterior radiograph after resection and reconstruction with an allograft prosthetic composite reconstruction

LIMB-SALVAGE PROCEDURES
(Continued)

Arthrodesis. In this technique, the resected bone is replaced with bone grafts that achieve fusion of the joint. Arthrodesis is most successful in the wrist; and the incidence of delayed union or nonunion is moderate. A successful arthrodesis results in a durable limb that can last a lifetime. Its chief disadvantage is permanent loss of joint motion.

RECONSTRUCTION OF DIAPHYSIS

Reconstruction of the diaphysis (intercalary procedure) after tumor removal is achieved with bone grafts or prosthetic implants, or both (see Plates 6-31 and 6-32). Grafting alternatives include the use of conventional dual fibular autografts, bone allografts, and vascularized fibular autografts.

Fibular Bone Grafts. Fibular autografts, combined with intramedullary rod or plate fixation, offer good stabilization but are weaker than the normal bone. Bone allograft is even more readily available and can also be combined with intramedullary rod or plate fixation. However, the distal osteosynthesis site can be a problem in terms of healing of the allograft to the adjacent host bone.

Transplantation with a vascularized fibular graft with microscopic arterial and venous anastomoses is a complex procedure requiring significantly longer operating time than other bone grafting techniques. It offers the potential of a viable graft that has the ability to heal, remodel, and hypertrophy much more rapidly than a conventional fibular graft. Usually placed within the medullary canal, this type of graft requires rigid fixation.

Prosthetic Implant. A segmental diaphyseal defect may be reconstructed using a porous prosthetic implant inserted into the medullary canal (see Plate 6-31). This reconstructive option is generally used for low-demand and morbid patients who would not tolerate a larger, lengthier allograft procedure or who have decreased life expectancies.

PSEUDARTHROSIS

Reconstruction with a pseudarthrosis (flail joint) can be performed after a radical resection of the acetabulum

Plate 6-33

Tumors of Musculoskeletal System

Tikhoff-Linberg procedure for tumors of scapula and proximal humerus

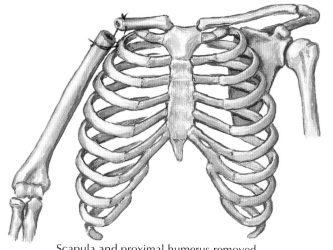

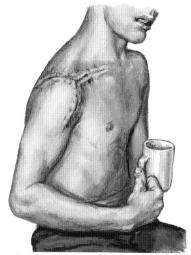

Scapula and proximal humerus removed. Remaining humerus stabilized by suturing to clavicle and 2nd rib.

Patient now has flail shoulder but acceptable elbow flexion and good hand and finger function.

Rotationplasty for sarcoma of distal femur

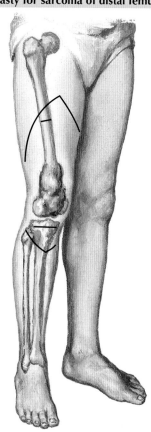

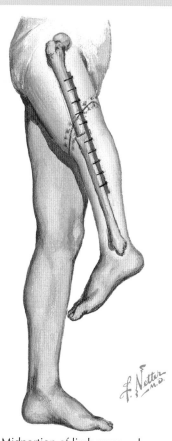

LIMB-SALVAGE PROCEDURES
(Continued)

or scapula. Although functionally inferior to a painless arthroplasty or arthrodesis, it is superior to an arthroplasty or arthrodesis complicated by instability, pain, and infection. A pseudarthrosis requires only soft tissue reconstruction. The resultant joint is excessively mobile and has less stability.

Tikhoff-Linberg Shoulder Girdle Resection. This procedure is a classic example of reconstruction by a pseudarthrosis after en bloc interscapulothoracic resection of the upper humerus and scapula (see Plate 6-33). It has traditionally been used as an alternative to amputation for sarcomas that involve the shoulder girdle but not the brachial plexus and vessels. Although the original procedure involved complete resection of the scapula and the lateral half of the clavicle, later modifications have preserved a greater portion of the clavicle, when appropriate, to support the remaining limb and give it a moderate amount of stability. In the procedure used at present, the proximal humerus is suspended from the remaining clavicle with a heavy suture or the biceps brachii tendon(s). This reconstruction allows normal hand-and-finger function with moderate relief of pain.

ROTATIONPLASTY

This reconstructive procedure is used in a skeletally immature patient after en bloc extra-articular resection

Osteosarcoma of distal femur. Skin incisions and lines of bone resection indicated.

Midportion of limb removed. Distal segment rotated 180°, and tibia united to femur.

of osteosarcoma about the knee (see Plate 6-33). The technique was devised by Van Nes in 1950 for the reconstruction of severe congenital defects of the femur and has been widely used in Europe to treat sarcoma in young children. After resection of the diseased bone, the remaining tibia is rotated 180 degrees to the proximal femur and fixed to it with plates. The redundant vessels are carefully looped in the soft tissues. The length of the newly created limb is adjusted so that the

ankle is positioned at the level that will match the level of the contralateral knee at completion of growth. The rotated ankle functions as a knee joint, and the foot serves as the stump of a below-knee amputation. Rotationplasty provides a better functional result than above-knee amputation, but the patient must be willing to accept the unusual cosmetic appearance. However, this procedure is being used less frequently because there are now prostheses that can be lengthened.

INJURY TO MUSCULOSKELETAL SYSTEM

Plate 7-1

Musculoskeletal System: PART III

INJURY TO SOFT TISSUE

Three basic mechanisms cause soft tissue injuries: blunt trauma, crushing injury, and penetrating trauma. Blunt and crushing injuries are called closed injuries because they do not penetrate the overlying skin. Penetrating (open) injuries violate the protective skin layer, contaminating the wound and thus producing open injuries.

CLOSED SOFT TISSUE INJURIES

Closed injuries are characterized by variable degrees of damage to skin and underlying soft tissue and are an inevitable component of any fracture (see Plate 7-1). Blood vessels are most vulnerable to injury; thus, closed soft tissue injuries usually produce bleeding and swelling beneath the skin. The pathophysiologic process of a soft tissue injury can be broken down into three phases: inflammatory, proliferative, and reparative. The initial trauma injures the blood vessels, causing local bleeding, disruption of the microcirculation, and exposure of subendothelial collagen, which triggers the cellular inflammatory and clotting pathways. Inflammatory mediators increase capillary permeability, leading to edema, further local impairment of perfusion, and local tissue hypoxia and acidosis. Chemotactic factors also attract immune cells; mainly neutrophils and macrophages in the acute stage—neutrophils to defend against bacteria and macrophages for debridement of necrotic tissue. This phase reaches a maximum intensity at 1 to 3 days after the injury. The second, or proliferative, phase involves fibroblast production of extracellular matrix proteins and revascularization via endothelial ingrowth. The third, or reparative, phase involves scarring and fibrosis. Bleeding results from disruption of the blood vessels, and swelling results from damage to the endothelial lining of the blood vessels, which allows plasma to leak into the soft tissue spaces.

The most common soft tissue injury is a contusion (bruise) caused by blunt trauma that damages blood vessels and results in bleeding or swelling into the soft tissues. Usually the blood and the edema fluid dissect between the cells of the soft tissues, causing localized swelling. Bleeding produces the typical black-and-blue discoloration of a contusion. If large vessels are disrupted, the pressure of the escaping blood can induce separation of the tissue planes, leading to the accumulation of a large hematoma beneath the skin or between the deeper layers of soft tissue.

Contusion and hematoma formation may accompany more serious injuries of the limbs, such as fractures, dislocations, and sprains. The clinical examination of a patient with a painful contusion must rule out more serious underlying problems. A simple contusion or hematoma is treated with the immediate application of ice, a gentle compression dressing, and elevation of the injured part. Temporary restriction of activity—voluntary or with the application of a compression dressing or splint—facilitates the body's ability to repair a soft tissue injury. The simple mnemonic *ICES* (Ice, Compression, Elevation, and Splinting) can be used to remember the principles of treatment. Because soft tissue injuries rarely cause significant disruption of important soft tissue structures, the body reabsorbs the extravasated blood and edema fluid within a few days, allowing gradual return of function. A large hematoma may take several weeks to resolve, however.

Soft tissue injuries associated with fractures (closed) can be described according to the classification system of Oestern and Tscherne, which grades soft tissue injuries from 0 to 3:

Contusion

Hematoma

Severe contusions of hand and wrist treated with ice pack, bulky dressing, and elevation.

Note: Both closed and open soft tissue injuries may result in compartment syndrome.

Lying in one position for long time (as in intoxication or coma) exerts persistent pressure on some body parts, such as arm and hand, causing ischemia and tissue necrosis.

Entrapment under heavy load may occlude blood supply, leading to necrosis and even gangrene.

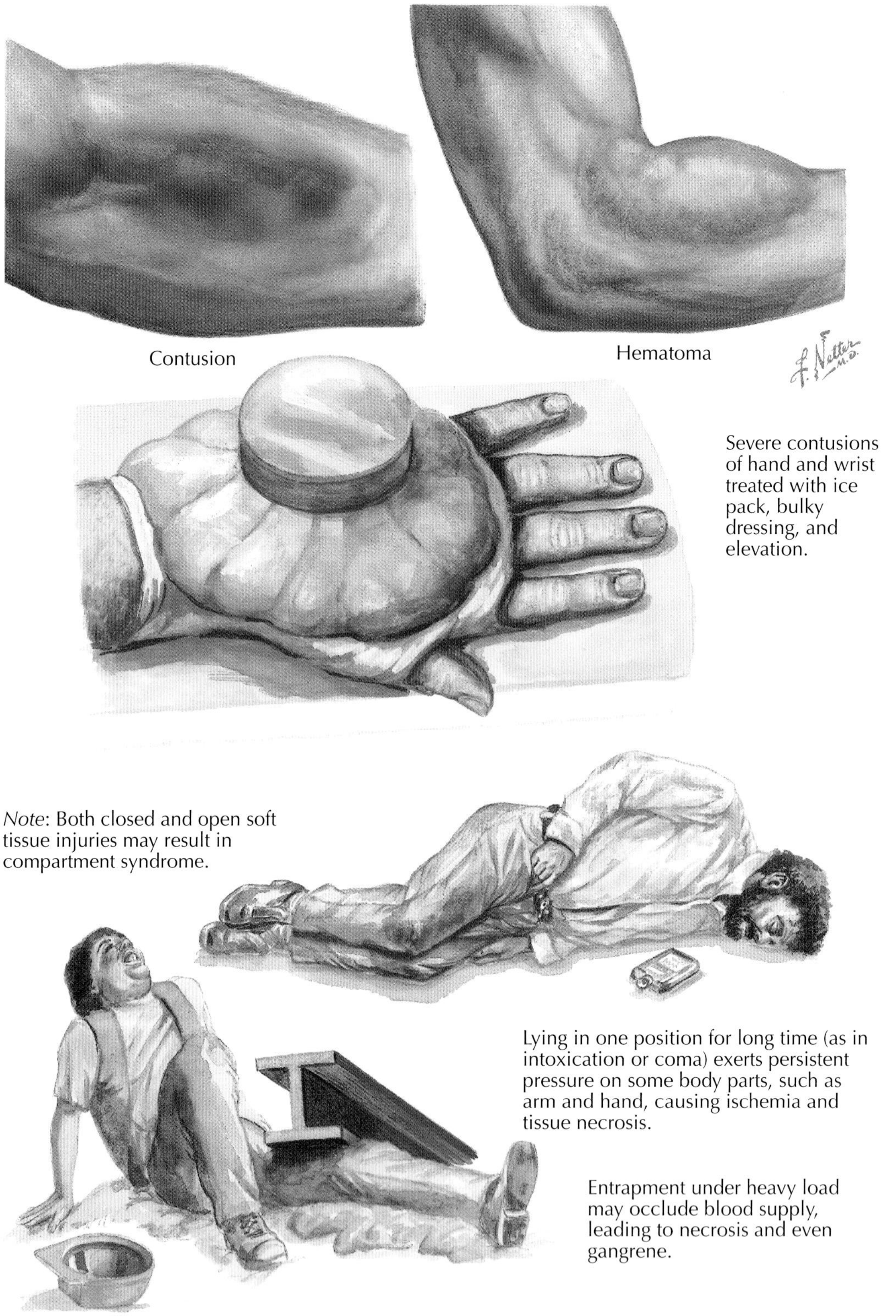

Grade 0: minimal soft tissue damage usually from an indirect injury to the limb and typically associated with a simple underlying fracture pattern

Grade 1: superficial abrasions or contusions typically associated with a mild underlying fracture pattern

Grade 2: deep abrasions with skin or muscle contusion usually from direct trauma to the limb and typically with a severe underlying fracture pattern

Grade 3: extensive skin contusion or crush, severe damage to underlying muscle, subcutaneous avulsion, and compartment syndrome and typically seen with a severe fracture pattern

This grading system is often used to guide timing and surgical planning when operative fixation is needed. It has also been shown to be predictive of the time to return to function.

An internal degloving injury is a unique type of soft tissue injury that may be seen with or without fracture. It results from significant shear forces causing the separation of subcutaneous tissues from underlying fascial or osseous structures with a resultant collection of liquefied fat, blood, and necrotic tissue. It is most commonly seen over the greater trochanter, where it is referred to as a Morel-Lavallée lesion, but can be

Plate 7-2

Injury to Musculoskeletal System

INJURY TO SOFT TISSUE
(Continued)

seen in the flank or lumbodorsal regions as well. These injuries can compromise the overlying skin and soft tissue if not addressed surgically and present a risk for infection and a challenge in planning for operative fixation of underlying fractures.

Soft tissues can also be damaged by the continuous application of force over relatively long periods of time (hours or days). This mechanism of injury, called a crushing injury, causes damage by direct force and also by impairment of circulation to the tissues. Continuous pressure that is in excess of the capillary filling pressure causes the compressed soft tissue to become ischemic and die.

Crushing injury takes many forms. One of the most vulnerable soft tissues is the skin; continuous pressure applied for more than 2 hours can result in ischemia and the development of a pressure ulcer. Pressure ulcers are particularly likely to develop in skin that overlies a bony prominence and is compressed against a firm surface such as a cast, a rigid shoe or brace, or even a firm mattress. Although the initial lesion is closed, when the skin dies, it sloughs and the lesion may become infected.

Another type of crushing injury occurs when a heavy load falls on a limb, rendering it immobile and obstructing the blood flow (venous, arterial, or both) for several hours. The result is a compartment syndrome. If the resulting ischemia lasts for more than 2 hours, it may cause the death of muscle tissue, with associated permanent loss of function. When blood flow is restored to a crushed limb, the necrotic muscle releases myoglobin into the venous circulation. The myoglobin may sludge in the kidneys, producing acute renal failure. The risk of this complication may be minimized by adequate hydration of the patient after a crush injury. Ischemia that persists for a long time leads to gangrene of the entire crushed limb.

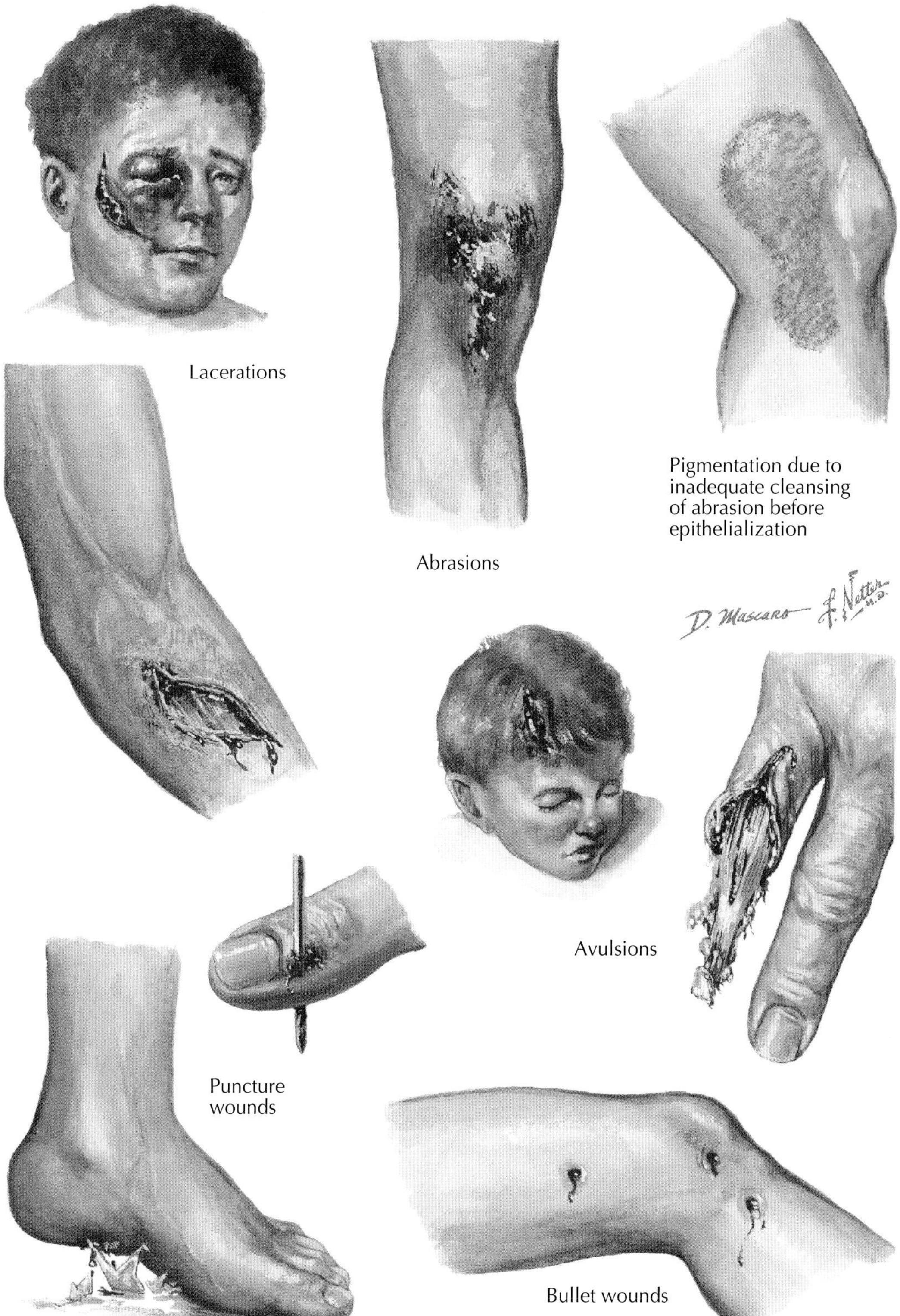

OPEN SOFT TISSUE INJURY

Open soft tissue injuries are, by definition, contaminated (see Plate 7-2). The many different types of open soft tissue injuries—abrasion, laceration, avulsion, puncture, degloving, and amputation—are caused by a variety of mechanisms. Regardless of the particular pattern of injury, the common denominators are penetration of the skin and bacterial contamination of the deeper tissues, which establish the potential for infection. Blood loss in open wounds is usually greater than in closed injuries, because the bleeding is not limited by the tamponade effect created by the encompassing soft tissues.

Treatment of open wounds initially focuses on controlling the bleeding and contamination. Pressure should be applied to the wound at once to stop bleeding, and tetanus prophylaxis must be confirmed or provided and in certain situations (e.g., open fracture) antibiotics should be administered. After the bleeding is controlled, all open wounds must be thoroughly debrided to remove as much contaminating material and nonviable tissue as possible. Whenever the adequacy of the initial debridement is in doubt, wound closure should be delayed until the surgeon is confident that no deep contaminants persist and there is no sign of active wound infection. In patients with severe contamination, or open fractures, antibiotics can be used to help control the onset of infection but should never

OPEN SOFT TISSUE WOUNDS

Lacerations

Abrasions

Pigmentation due to inadequate cleansing of abrasion before epithelialization

Avulsions

Puncture wounds

Bullet wounds

be used as a substitute for surgical debridement. If needed, serial debridements should be performed at 48- to 72-hour intervals until the surgeon is satisfied that all contaminated and necrotic or nonviable tissues have been removed. Often in the case of open fractures or other high-energy injuries it is not possible to determine the full extent of soft tissue injury at the index debridement. Once adequate debridement has taken place, delayed primary closure can be attempted.

Not all wounds are amendable to primary closure, even on a delayed basis. Advancements in wound care

technology have afforded new ways to achieve closure of a wound, decrease the need for flap coverage, and improve survival of split-thickness skin grafts. The most significant advancement is that of "vacuum-assisted wound closure," or the wound VAC. The wound VAC is a closed, negative-pressure system for healing wounds. After a wound has been adequately debrided a reticulated polyurethane sponge is trimmed to fit the wound so that it is in direct contact with all wound surfaces and either packed into or placed on top of the wound. This is then covered with a clear adherent

Plate 7-3   Musculoskeletal System: PART III

INJURY TO SOFT TISSUE
(Continued)

flexible plastic dressing through which passes a plastic tube that attaches to a suction/reservoir device. The VAC is typically changed roughly every 48 hours either at bedside or in the operating room if sedation is required. The pump is typically run at a continuous −125 mm Hg because this has shown to produce the peak improvement in blood flow without the pain from intermittent pressure with wound contraction/expansion.

The negative pressure system removes interstitial edema fluid that grossly decreases swelling. On a micro-circulatory level, it decreases capillary afterload, improving local blood flow and oxygen delivery. The mechanical stress created from the negative pressure and resultant contraction of the "dead space" of the wound may stimulate angiogenesis. Granulation tissue formation and wound contracture are stimulated. Because it is a closed system there is less risk of bacterial contamination, especially for those patients in intensive care unit settings or with wounds in moist or frequently contaminated areas. The wound VAC has shown to be beneficial when applied over the recipient site of a split-thickness skin graft with increased ingrowth rates for which the sponge is applied on top of the graft (sometimes with a petrolatum gauze layer in between to prevent adhesion and liftoff with sponge changes). The VAC has shown promise in helping with persistently draining surgical wounds when applied over the draining incision for a brief period to help decrease local swelling.

With the exception of certain nerve injuries, all soft tissues heal by the formation of collagenous scar tissue. Prompt, careful, and anatomic reapproximation of injured tendon, muscle, and skin provides the best basis for a functional and satisfactory result. Failure to achieve repair of an injured tendon often results in significant functional loss.

Effective repair of a lacerated tendon remains a great surgical challenge because tendons often heal with an excess of scar tissue and loss of their natural gliding function. The principles of tendon repair therefore include thorough debridement of the wound, precise anatomic reapproximation, and protected active range of motion during healing to help maintain the mobility essential for normal function. The range of motion allowed after repair is limited by the particular tendon injured, the location of the laceration along the course of the tendon, and the strength of the surgical repair.

Peripheral nerve injury was described by Seddon as either neurapraxia, axonotmesis, or neurotmesis and later further subdivided by Sunderland. Neurapraxia (Sunderland 1) involves local damage to myelin, often from compression or stretch associated with an injury. There is no disruption in axon continuity, and no distal degeneration takes place so no permanent loss of function is expected; recovery typically takes weeks to months. Axonotmesis involves loss of continuity with varying damage to surrounding connective tissue. Sunderland subdivided this with type 2, retaining intact endoneurium, perineurium, and epineurium, which helps guide healing axons and prevents infrafascicular healing so complete functional recovery may take place, but on the order of months. Sunderland type 3 involves disruption of the endoneurium, and recovery is often incomplete. In Sunderland type 4, the perineurium is disrupted as well, leaving only epineurium, and may require excision and surgical repair of the damaged

segment. Neurotmesis, equivalent to Sunderland type 5 injuries, involves complete disruption of the nerve. Laceration of a peripheral nerve disrupts the axons that normally carry impulses to and from the central nervous system, and restoration of nerve function depends on the effective repair of these axons. The distal segment undergoes wallerian degeneration, leaving the basal lamina of the Schwann cells to serve as guiding structures for the growth cone at the tip of the regenerating axon to it is hoped grow through. Complete nerve lacerations should be referred for surgical evaluation to an

orthopaedic or plastic surgeon trained in microsurgical nerve repair. The principles of peripheral nerve repair include adequate debridement, careful anatomic repair by means of group fascicular repair, and/or simply epineurial repair (controversy still exists between the two). When primary repair cannot be achieved without tension, autografts, allografts, and entubulation chambers are therapeutic options being investigated. Failure to achieve satisfactory repair of a lacerated peripheral nerve results in permanent loss of its function and often produces a painful neuroma at the injury site.

TREATMENT OF OPEN SOFT TISSUE WOUNDS

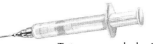

Essentials of treatment for all open wounds

Cleansing
Debridement of nonviable tissue
Antibiotics (local or systemic)

Tetanus prophylaxis

Control of bleeding with local pressure

Methods of wound closure

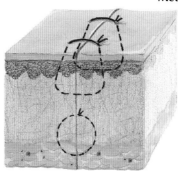

Simple suture. Deep part of suture longer than superficial part to slightly evert wound edges. Deep sutures used to close dead space.

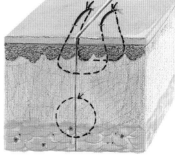

Mattress suture

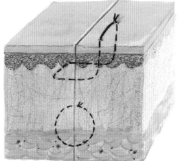

Half-buried mattress suture

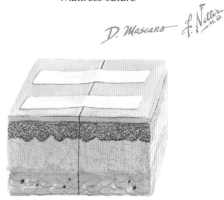

Some superficial wounds may be closed with adhesive strips rather than sutures.

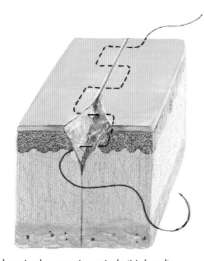

Subcuticular running stitch (Halsted)

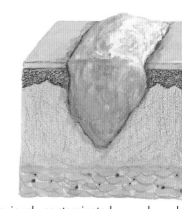

Obviously contaminated wounds are best debrided, packed open for 48–72 hours, debrided again, and delayed primary closure done.

Plate 7-4

Injury to Musculoskeletal System

PRESSURE ULCERS

Pressure ulcers are localized areas of necrosis involving skin and/or deeper tissues usually occurring over a bony prominence (see Plate 7-4). They develop when the soft tissue is compressed between the body and a rigid or firm surface and are common complications of immobilization. Elderly patients are particularly at risk, and in patients older than 70 years of age, pressure ulcers increase the risk of death up to four times. Pressure ulcers, formerly called decubitus ulcers and bedsores, can occur anywhere, but the most common sites are over the sacrum, coccyx, greater trochanter, ischial tuberosity, and heels. Pressure ulcers are caused by a combination of pressure and shear forces. *Pressure* is described as force directed perpendicular to the surface, and *shear* is force directed parallel to the surface. Pressure forces compress the vessels that run parallel to the surface of the skin, and shear forces cause bending and occlusion of those perpendicular to the skin. Studies have shown that pressure in excess of approximately 32 mm Hg will occlude dermal vessels, resulting in local ischemia, interstitial fluid, pain, and necrosis of tissue, and that this may start after as little as 2 hours at such levels. The deeper tissues such as muscle are more sensitive to pressure, and as such the damage may spread over a greater area the deeper it goes. Damage may also be done to soft tissue by friction forces, such as those seen on the skin from sliding or moving patients across bed linens. This causes abrasions and epidermal damage that further decrease the tissue's tolerance to insult from pressure. Necrotic tissue is highly susceptible to bacterial infection, which contributes to further necrosis and destruction of both soft tissue and bone.

In 2007, the National Pressure Ulcer Advisory Panel revised its previous staging scale to include *Suspected Deep Tissue Injury* and *Unstageable Ulcers* in addition to the previously described *Stages I to IV:*

Suspected deep tissue injury: purple or maroon localized area of discolored intact skin or blood-filled blister due to damage of underlying soft tissue from pressure and/or shear. The area may be preceded by tissue that is painful, firm, mushy, boggy, and warmer or cooler as compared with adjacent soft tissue.

Stage I: intact skin with nonblanchable redness of a localized area usually over a bony prominence. Darkly pigmented skin may not have visible blanching; its color may differ from the surrounding area.

Stage II: partial-thickness loss of dermis presenting as a shallow open ulcer with a red pink wound bed, without slough; may also present as an intact or open/ruptured serum-filled blister.

Stage III: full-thickness tissue loss. Subcutaneous fat may be visible, but bone, tendon, or muscle is not exposed. Slough may be present but does not obscure the depth of tissue loss; may include undermining and tunneling.

Stage IV: full-thickness tissue loss with exposed bone, tendon, or muscle. Slough or eschar may be present on some parts of the wound bed; often includes undermining and tunneling.

Unstageable: full-thickness tissue loss in which the base of the ulcer is covered by slough (yellow, tan, gray, green, or brown) and/or eschar (tan, brown, or black) in the wound bed. Unstageable ulcers may be restaged after debridement allows determination of the true extent of the wound.

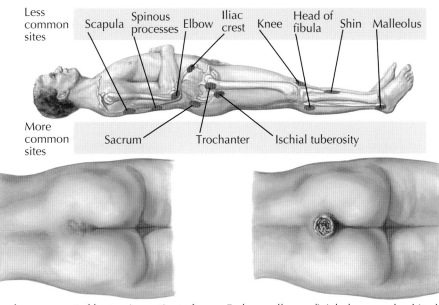

Less common sites: Scapula · Spinous processes · Elbow · Iliac crest · Knee · Head of fibula · Shin · Malleolus

More common sites: Sacrum · Trochanter · Ischial tuberosity

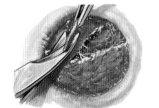

Pressure ulcers prevented by turning patient often, gentle massage with skin lotion, and avoidance of further pressure. Rubor a premonitory sign.

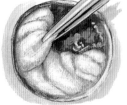

Early, small superficial ulcer may heal itself with relief from pressure and good skin care. More often, specific treatment necessary.

Curled-in edges cleanly debrided, eschar removed, and wound washed

Ulcer packed with moist (not soaked) gauze twice a day

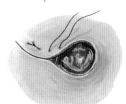

Split-thickness skin grafting or primary closure done if skin condition adequate

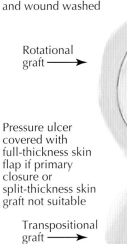

Rotational graft ⟶

Pressure ulcer covered with full-thickness skin flap if primary closure or split-thickness skin graft not suitable

Transpositional graft ⟶

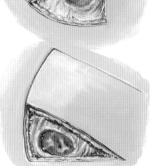

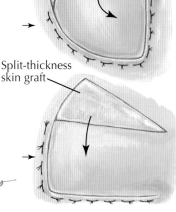

Split-thickness skin graft

Split-thickness skin graft

Risk factors for development of a pressure ulcer include neurologic impairment due to decreased muscle tone, loss of muscle bulk, and diminished or absent sensorimotor abilities. Surgical patients are at risk during surgery from prolonged positioning and hypotensive anesthesia and postoperatively from immobility, sedative medications, and casts/splints. Other factors that contribute to the development of pressure ulcers, particularly in elderly patients, are impaired circulation, poor nutrition, and possibly impaired immune response.

Maceration of the skin, usually due to incontinence, also significantly increases the risk of ulceration. Bedridden and wheelchair-bound patients are particularly vulnerable to the development of pressure ulcers.

A pressure ulcer requires intensive and costly long-term treatment. Therefore, aggressive intervention programs are essential to prevent or abort their formation, particularly in high-risk patients. The most effective means of prevention is the frequent repositioning of patients who are confined in bed, chair, or

Plate 7-5

Musculoskeletal System: PART III

EXCISION OF DEEP PRESSURE ULCER

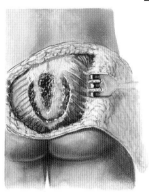

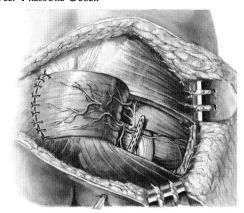

Deep pressure ulcer over sacrum excised, and crests of sacrum removed with wide osteotome. Split-thickness skin graft used to complete coverage of donor site.

Flap of gluteus maximus muscle formed, turned over defect, and sutured in place. Drain passed through puncture wound.

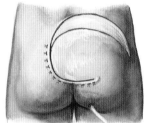

Full-thickness skin flap rotated to cover sacral defect, and split-thickness skin graft applied to cover residual donor site defect.

PRESSURE ULCERS *(Continued)*

wheelchair. Position changes must occur every 2 hours to avoid continues excessive pressure over any single bony prominence. Vulnerable skin areas must be monitored frequently, and pressure on stage 1 lesions must be avoided to prevent further progression. For patients at risk for pressure ulcers, passive (or static) cushioning devices such as supersoft mattresses and wheelchair cushions made of foam, water, gel, or air-filled materials should be used; patients who are severely immobilized require active (or dynamic) pressure-relieving devices such as an alternating pressure, air fluidized, or air suspension mattress. Sedation should be avoided, incontinence controlled, and any nutritional deficiencies corrected in all immobile patients. Several studies have shown aggressive intervention applied by an effective multidisciplinary team can greatly reduce the incidence of pressure ulcers in hospitalized patients.

TREATMENT

Treatment of an established pressure ulcer must be aggressive and persistent. Pressure-relieving strategies are essential during the entire course to facilitate healing. The first step in management is to assess the extent, depth, and stage of the lesion. Local treatment of a specific ulcer begins with removing the source of pressure. Second, any necrotic tissue is removed. Debridement of necrotic and infected tissue is accomplished with frequent changes of wet-to-dry dressings or with surgical excision of the infected necrotic tissue followed by the application of wet-to-dry dressings or negative pressure wound therapy (NPWT). The use of topical disinfectants and antibiotics is controversial. Although such medications effectively decrease the local bacterial count, many also have the disadvantage of causing local tissue necrosis of the ulcer bed. Dilute noncytotoxic solutions of povidone-iodine or sodium hypochlorite may help to decrease the bacterial count without causing tissue necrosis.

Once the ulcer is clean and a granulation tissue bed well established, definitive coverage/closure needs to be addressed. Small superficial ulcers heal by secondary intention as long as pressure is kept off the affected

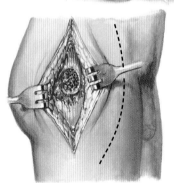

Deep pressure ulcer over trochanter widely excised with sinus tracts and trochanter. Broken line indicates skin-relaxing incision.

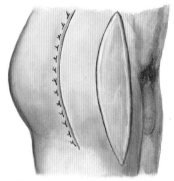

Bipedicle flap of skin and subcutaneous tissue pulled over and sutured to cover defect. Donor site closed with split-thickness skin graft.

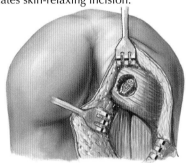

Ischial pressure ulcer removed completely along with ischial prominence.

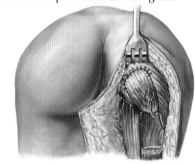

Biceps femoris muscle divided, turned up, and sutured over defect. Skin closed with direct sutures plus skin graft, if needed.

area. Larger lesions can be treated surgically with split-thickness skin grafting; occasionally, primary skin closure is accomplished by mobilization of adjacent skin flaps. Large ulcers occasionally require full-thickness coverage with a local full-thickness rotational skin flap and the assistance of a plastic surgeon. At the time of flap rotation the underlying bony prominences may be removed or remodeled to reduce the potential for recurrent pressure ulcers. Negative pressure wound therapy has been a significant advancement in the

treatment of pressure ulcer wounds. Negative pressure wound therapy can facilitate fibrinous debridement at dressing changes the way wet-to-dry do and also isolates the wound from contamination while removing edema and local moisture. It also encourages contraction of the wound and may limit the extent of coverage needed. In areas that are particularly vulnerable to recurrence, rotation of a myocutaneous flap to provide greater padding over the bony prominence should be considered.

Plate 7-6

Injury to Musculoskeletal System

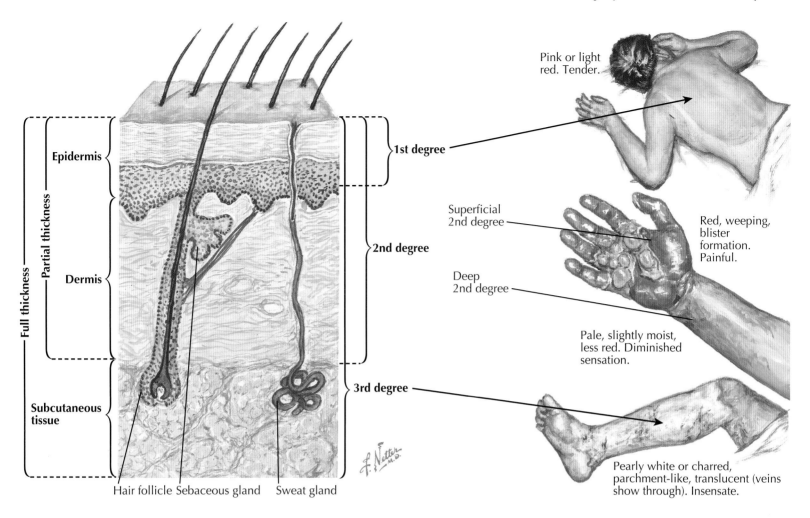

Epidermis

Partial thickness

Dermis

Full thickness

Subcutaneous tissue

Hair follicle Sebaceous gland Sweat gland

1st degree

2nd degree

3rd degree

Pink or light red. Tender.

Superficial 2nd degree

Deep 2nd degree

Red, weeping, blister formation. Painful.

Pale, slightly moist, less red. Diminished sensation.

Pearly white or charred, parchment-like, translucent (veins show through). Insensate.

CLASSIFICATION OF BURNS

More than 2 million people in the United States are burned every year. The severity of tissue damage is related to both the temperature and the duration of exposure. The local effects of a burn, the wound care required, and the ultimate functional and cosmetic results are determined by the depth of cell injury. The outer layer of the skin, the epidermis, is made up of stratified epithelial cells that arise by proliferation of the basal layer and become progressively keratinized as they are slowly elevated to the surface, where they desquamate (see Plate 7-6). The dermis is the inner layer of vascularized and variably dense connective tissue in which arise the skin appendages (hair follicles, sebaceous glands, and sweat glands). Beneath the dermis lies a layer of fatty, loose areolar connective tissue.

Heat of sufficient intensity and duration causes coagulation necrosis and cell death, but the cell damage due to heat of lesser intensity is potentially reversible. The region of immediate cell death caused by a burn is the *zone of coagulation*. Areas of progressively less damaging cell injury are the *zones of stasis*, in which the initially compromised blood flow improves with time, and the *zone of hyperemia*, in which there is marked increase in blood flow as a consequence of burn-induced inflammation. In a full-thickness (third-degree) burn, the zone of coagulation comprises the entire thickness of the dermis. In a partial-thickness (second-degree) burn, a variable portion of the dermis is involved, and in a first-degree burn, only the epidermis is affected.

PARTIAL-THICKNESS BURN

A *first-degree burn* is the most superficial form of a partial-thickness burn, sunburn being the most common. The skin is pink or light red; the surface is usually dry, although small blisters may form. The skin remains soft with minimal edema, with subsequent exfoliation of the superficial epidermis. Such injuries are hypersensitive but heal in 3 to 6 days. They require little treatment other than administration of analgesics and oral anti-inflammatory medications to minimize inflammation. Cool showers help lessen postural hypotension and provide some pain relief. At the time of exfoliation, antipruritic treatment may be necessary.

Second-degree burns, also partial-thickness injuries, can be subdivided into superficial second-degree burns, which heal within 21 days, and deep second-degree burns, which take longer to heal. Second-degree burns are caused by limited exposure to a hot liquid, flash, flame, or chemical agent. Superficial second-degree burns appear pink or bright red with profuse serous exudation from the surface and may form blisters between the epidermis and the dermis. These injuries are hyperesthetic—even a draft of air can cause pain. Deep partial-thickness, or second-degree, burns extend to the lower layers of the dermis. The surface of a deep second-degree burn is moist and mottled in various hues of red. Sensation to pinprick is reduced, but pressure sensation remains intact. If protected from infection, these injuries heal spontaneously in 3 to 9 weeks, although often with scarring. When occurring around joints, they may impair function and require excision and grafting.

FULL-THICKNESS BURN

Third-degree burns result from prolonged exposure to a flame, hot object, or chemical agent or from contact with high-voltage electricity. They involve all layers of the dermis as well as underlying adipose and connective tissue. If deeper structures such as muscle, tendon, ligament, and bone are involved, the injury is considered a *deep full-thickness* or *fourth-degree burn* and may involve more extensive reconstruction or amputation. The surface of the burn appears pearly white, charred, translucent, or parchment-like; thrombosed superficial vessels are often visible. In young children, the initial appearance of third-degree burns can be misleading: they are initially dark red, slightly moist, and pliable; then the wound desiccates and becomes unpliable and dark reddish brown. Chemical burns cause injury by coagulation necrosis, which may take 12 to 24 hours for the full extent to be seen. Strong acid burns produce deep gray to brown coloring of the skin, which may be confused with suntan. Exposure to strong alkali may result in soap tissue necrosis. High-voltage electric injury typically causes loss of tissue and dense charring at contact sites. The majority of the injury occurs to deeper structures so the initial wound/burn on the skin may be deceiving. The wound surface of all full-thickness burns is insensate and always requires skin grafting for closure.

Plate 7-7   Musculoskeletal System: PART III

CAUSES AND CLINICAL TYPES OF BURNS

The incidence and causes of burn injury are related to age, occupation, and economic circumstances, with the economically disadvantaged, the elderly, and the very young at greatest risk of both burn injury and death from that injury.

FLAME BURNS AND SCALDS

Flame burns are the most common burns in adults. They are usually caused by the mishandling of flammable liquids, ignition of clothing, and house fires and result in an injury of variable thickness: charred, leathery full-thickness burns are intermixed with areas of partial-thickness injury. Sometimes focal areas of uninjured skin in the axilla, groin, antecubital space, and palm are found within the burn. In children younger than 5 years of age, spill scalds are the most common form of injury.

ELECTRIC BURNS

The risk of high-voltage electric injury is greatest in electricians, construction workers, farm workers who move irrigation pipes, oil field workers, truck drivers, and antenna installers. The damage to the tissue is due to heat produced by the resistance of tissue to the passage of electric current. The cell damage is greatest at the site of cutaneous contact but also includes the subcutaneous tissues and organs in the path of the electric current flow. Extensive devitalization of muscle may occur beneath deceivingly small cutaneous lesions. Current arcing also causes severe cutaneous injury at the flexor surfaces of joints, such as the wrist, elbow, and axilla. Claw hand deformity with inability to extend the fingers indicates severe and irreversible damage to the tissues of the hand and forearm and commonly predicts the need for amputation.

Formation of edema beneath the investing fascia of injured tissue may result in impaired blood supply to the distal unburned tissue, necessitating a fasciotomy to reduce the fluid pressure in soft tissue and prevent ischemic necrosis of unburned tissue.

CHEMICAL BURNS

Chemical agents cause exothermic reactions, dehydration, liquefaction necrosis (alkalosis), and delipidation in tissue. The severity of a chemical burn is related to the concentration of the chemical and the amount and duration of contact with tissue. In patients with chemical injury, immediate wound care is the priority, unlike treatment of all other burn patients, in whom systemic support takes precedence. All contaminated clothing should be removed immediately and copious water lavage begun to dilute the chemical agent and reduce the heat in the injured tissue. Strong acids may produce profound tanning of the skin, and strong alkalis penetrate tissue rapidly, causing characteristic liquefaction necrosis of soft tissue.

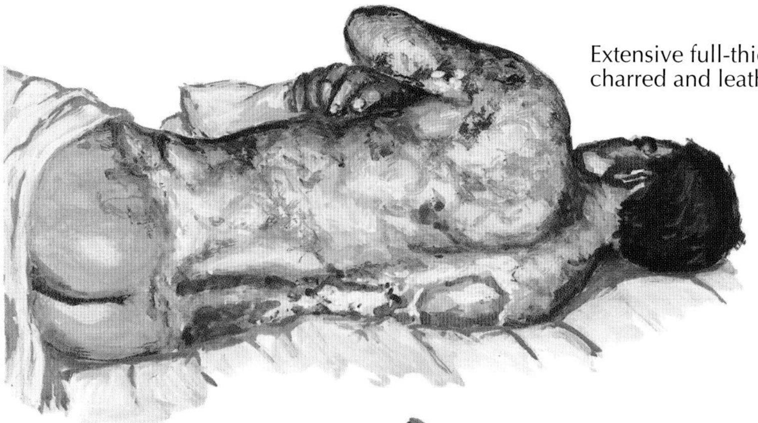

Extensive full-thickness flame burn. Appears charred and leathery. Note sparing of axilla.

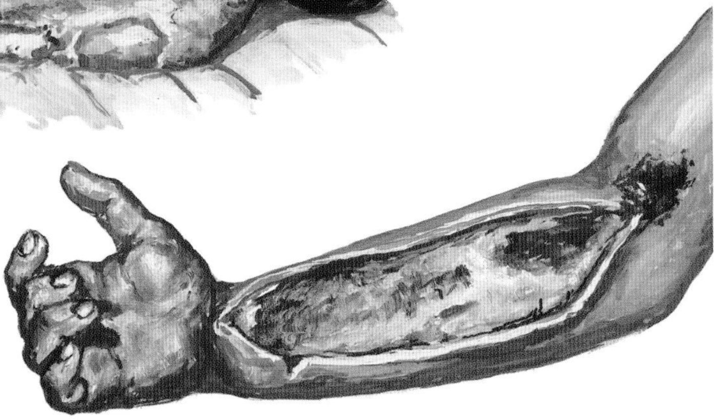

High-voltage electric burn (after fasciotomy). Typical, claw hand deformity and accentuation of burn at wrist and antecubital fossa due to arcing of current.

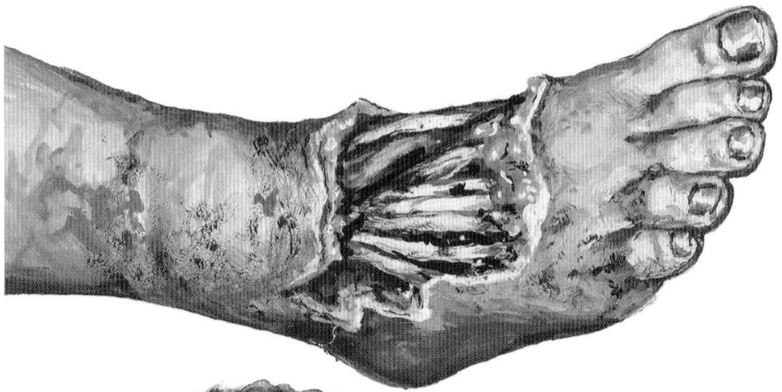

Penetrating chemical burn caused by strong alkali. Characteristic dissolution of soft tissues.

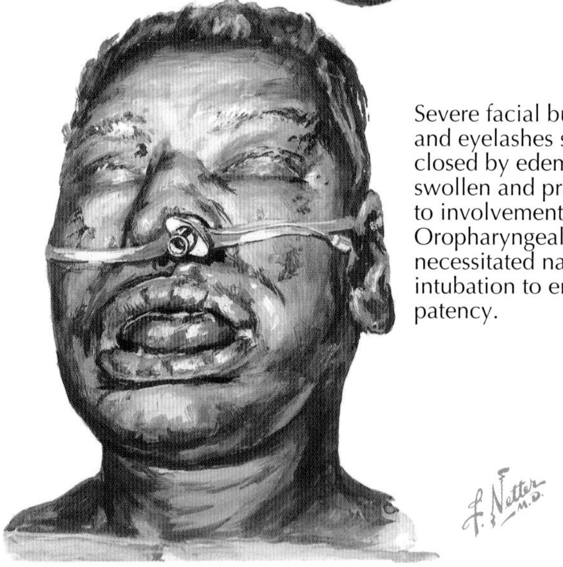

Severe facial burn. Eyebrows and eyelashes singed, lids closed by edema, tongue swollen and protruding owing to involvement of oropharynx. Oropharyngeal edema necessitated nasotracheal intubation to ensure airway patency.

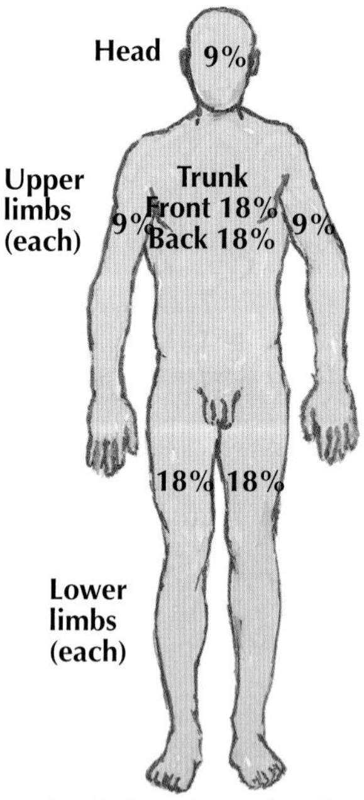

Head 9%

Upper limbs (each) 9%

Trunk Front 18% Back 18% 9%

18% 18%

Lower limbs (each)

Rule of nines for estimating percentage of body surface involved

Formation of edema in the burn area is the result of increased vascular permeability and alterations in the relationships of transvascular pressure. Effects of edema are particularly marked in the loose areolar tissues of the face and oropharynx. The eyelids swell rapidly and may obstruct vision, even though the globe is typically protected by the blink reflex. Swelling of the tongue and other oropharyngeal tissues may compromise the supraglottic airway, necessitating endotracheal intubation to ensure adequate ventilation.

The magnitude and duration of physiologic changes are proportional to the extent of second- and third-degree burns, expressed as a percentage of the body surface. The extent of the burn can be most easily estimated using the rule of nines. In the adult, the surface area of specific anatomic parts represents 9% or a multiple thereof of the total body surface: head and neck, 9%; each upper limb, 9%; each lower limb, 18%; anterior trunk, 18%; posterior trunk, 18%; and genitalia, 1%.

Plate 7-8

Injury to Musculoskeletal System

Escharotomy incision on midlateral aspect of forearm for circumferential 3rd-degree burn

Escharotomy incision on midmedial aspect of upper limb for circumferential 3rd-degree burn

Medial and lateral escharotomy incisions for circumferential 3rd-degree burns of lower limbs

Preferred sites for escharotomy incisions (lines shown thicker over joints to emphasize importance of carrying incisions across involved joints)

Escharotomy incisions for circumferential 3rd-degree burns of lower limbs and trunk in severely burned patient

ESCHAROTOMY FOR BURNS

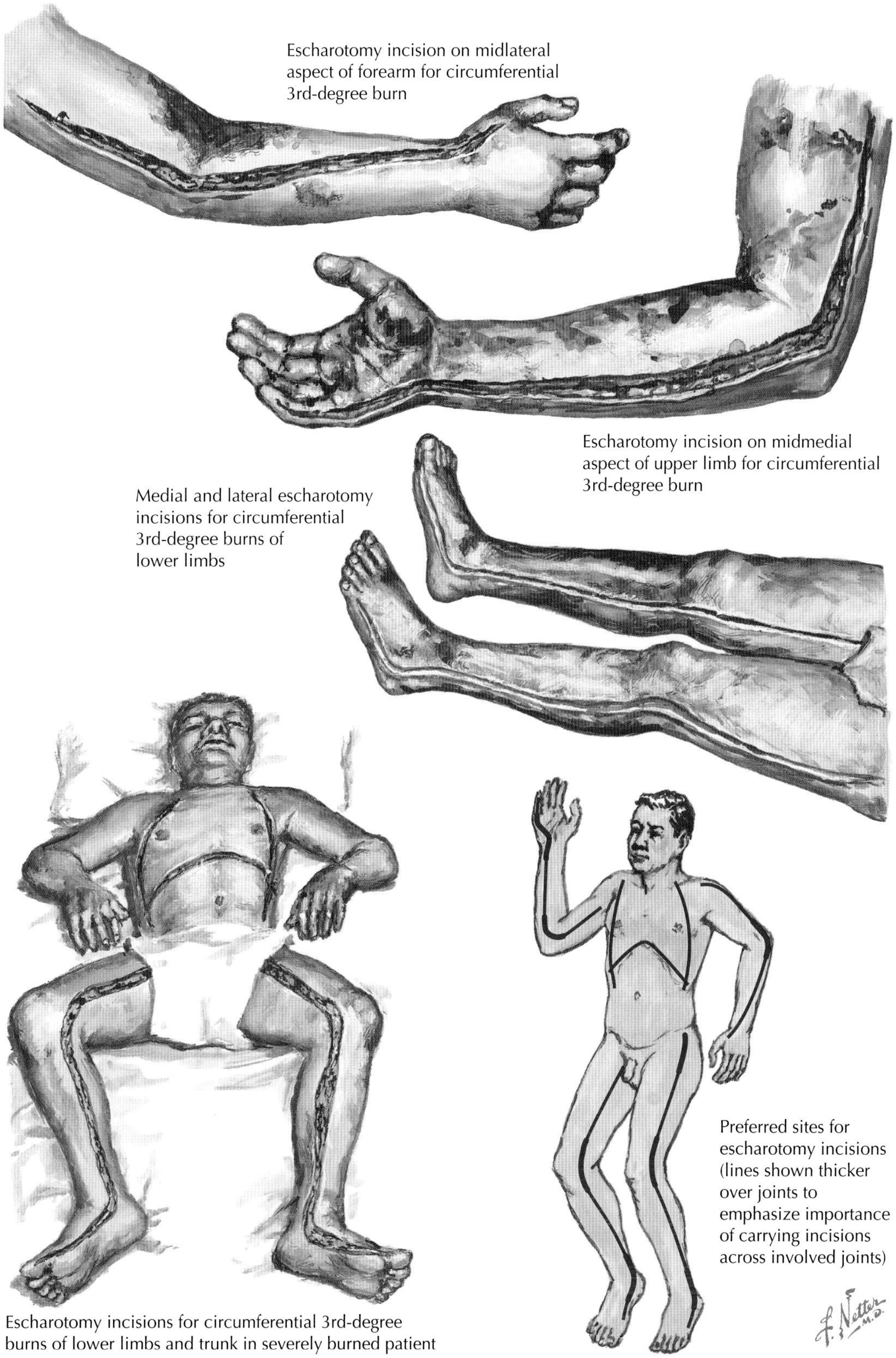

Formation of edema beneath the unyielding leathery eschar of a circumferential third-degree burn on a limb or on the trunk can compromise circulation, ventilation, and nerve/muscle function (see Plate 7-12). As the edema increases, tissue pressure rises to exceed venous pressure and approach arteriolar pressure, impairing blood flow to underlying unburned tissues. In the distal unburned tissue, edema and coolness to touch normally accompany thermal injury. Clinical signs of impaired circulation are cyanosis and delayed capillary refilling of distal unburned skin, as well as neurologic change, particularly progressive paresthesias, and unrelenting deep pain. Neurologic change is the most reliable of the clinical signs that predict the need for escharotomy, but an absence of pulsatile blood flow or progressive diminution of flow detected with serial measurements using an ultrasonic flowmeter is a far more reliable indicator. The palmar arch vessels in the upper limb and the posterior tibial vessels in the lower limb are used for assessment. Because hypovolemia and vasoconstriction can attenuate the flowmeter signal, assessment of blood flow should be made only in patients whose hemodynamic stability has been restored with the administration of resuscitation fluid.

Direct measurement of tissue pressure in muscle compartments using a pressure monitor (e.g., Stryker Pressure Monitor introduced in 1988) may also be useful in determining if escharotomy and fasciotomy are needed (see Plate 7-15). However, use of invasive pressure monitoring increases the risk of infection of the muscle because the needle must traverse the invariably contaminated burn wound.

Evidence of vascular embarrassment mandates immediate escharotomy, which is performed at bedside using either a scalpel or electrocautery device. Anesthesia is not required because the incisions are made in an insensate third-degree burn. The escharotomy incision is placed in the midmedial or midlateral line of the involved limb and must extend from the distal margin to the proximal margin of the encircling eschar. The incision is carried through the eschar and the immediately adjacent superficial fascia only to the depth necessary to permit the cut edges of the eschar to separate. Bleeding, which is minimal in a properly performed escharotomy, is readily controlled with electrocautery or brief application of external pressure. The escharotomy incisions must be carried across involved joints, where there is the least amount of subcutaneous padding and the vessels and nerves are most easily compressed by the edema-generated pressure.

If a midlateral escharotomy does not restore circulation to a circumferentially burned limb, a second incision is placed in the midmedial line. If the circulation remains impaired after the second escharotomy, fasciotomy must be considered. Rarely, encircling burns of the neck require escharotomy in the line of the anterior margin of the sternocleidomastoid muscle and a circumferentially burned penis may require escharotomy in the middorsal line.

If edema formation beneath an encircling third-degree burn on the truck impairs the ventilatory excursion of the chest wall, mild hypoxia may develop and increased pressure may be needed to ventilate the patient. Bilateral escharotomy incisions extending from the clavicle to the costal margin should be made in the anterior axillary line. If the burn involves a significant portion of the anterior abdominal wall, the anterior axillary incisions should be connected by an incision at the costal margin. All escharotomy incisions must be protected by a generous application of a topical chemotherapeutic agent.

Plate 7-9

Musculoskeletal System: PART III

PREVENTION OF INFECTION IN BURN WOUNDS

If a burn wound is not protected by topical agents, initially gram-positive flora proliferate and changes and gram-negative microorganisms predominate (see Plate 7-9). These organisms penetrate the eschar and multiply in the subeschar space (interface between nonviable and viable tissue). If host resistance is inadequate, the microorganisms penetrate viable tissue. Systemic spread to remote tissues and organs may occur when *Pseudomonas* organisms invade the microvasculature.

After resuscitation, management focuses on wound care to limit microbial proliferation, which can convert a partial-thickness into a full-thickness burn, and to prevent invasive infection of underlying tissue. Initial care includes gentle cleansing with a surgical detergent disinfectant, debriding nonviable tissue, and shaving hair from the area. A topical agent such as mafenide acetate cream or solution, silver sulfadiazine cream, 0.5% silver nitrate solution, or newer nanocrystalline silver preparations is applied. Silver nitrate solution is bacteriostatic against gram-negative bacteria including some against *Pseudomonas*, but does not penetrate eschar and has limited antifungal activity. It has the potential to cause electrolyte imbalance because it binds chlorine ions, discolors the wound bed, making visual inspection difficult, and is difficult to apply and maintain, so it is rarely used. Silver sulfadiazine is bactericidal against gram-negative bacilli and sometimes against *Pseudomonas* with minimal toxicity but does not penetrate eschar. Mafenide acetate (Sulfamylon) (10% cream or 5% solution) has broad gram-negative coverage including *Pseudomonas* as well as *Clostridium* species but is ineffective against fungi so concomitant antifungal therapy is needed. The cream is applied to the surface and the wound is left exposed; the solution is applied and soaked in; both formulations penetrate eschar. The solution has been shown to have less pain with application and less inhibition of carbonic anhydrase (leading to metabolic acidosis). Nanocrystalline silver preparations exist in multiple commercial forms; they have broad-spectrum activity, including against *Pseudomonas aeruginosa*, methicillin-resistant *Staphylococcus aureus*, and vancomycin-resistant enterococci. They can be left in place for days at a time if the wound does not have significant exudates and are becoming a popular alternative. Mupirocin is used in centers where methicillin-resistant *S. aureus* is problematic. Nystatin is used as an antifungal agent in conjunction with antibacterial therapy to treat both superficial and deep burn wound infections.

None of the available topical agents sterilizes the burn wound; therefore, protection from invasive infection is not complete. During daily wound care when the topical agent has been removed, the wound must be examined to identify local signs of infection. Common color changes that signal infection are focal, multifocal, or generalized dark brown, black, or violet discoloration. The most reliable sign of invasive infection is the conversion of an area of partial-thickness burn to full-thickness necrosis. Other local signs include hemorrhagic discoloration of subeschar tissue; unexpectedly rapid separation of the eschar (most commonly due to fungal infection); green pigment visible in the subcutaneous fat; edema or violet discoloration, or both, of unburned skin at the margin of the wound; and rapidly expanding ischemic necrosis.

Because noninfectious factors such as minor local trauma can induce similar local changes in the burn

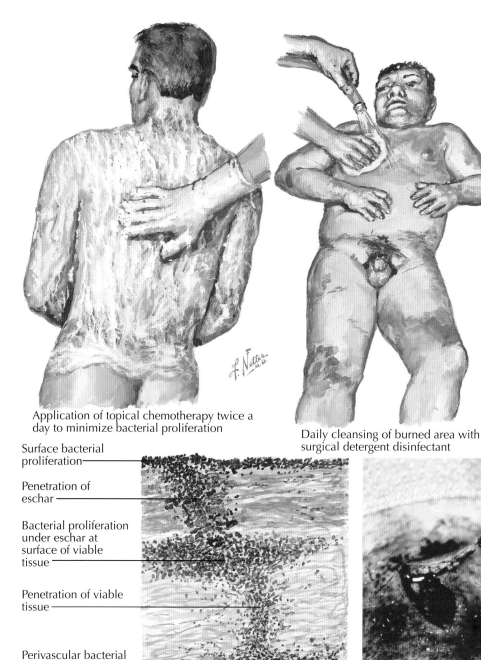

Application of topical chemotherapy twice a day to minimize bacterial proliferation

Daily cleansing of burned area with surgical detergent disinfectant

Surface bacterial proliferation

Penetration of eschar

Bacterial proliferation under eschar at surface of viable tissue

Penetration of viable tissue

Perivascular bacterial pallisading

Systemic dissemination (sepsis)

Schematic section shows bacterial penetration of burn wound.

Lenticular biopsy sample elevated from burn wound, which is insensate. Specimen must include both burned and unburned tissue.

wound, assessment of the microbial status of the wound is needed. A 500-mg lenticular biopsy sample is harvested from the area of most marked changes and must include the eschar and underlying unburned tissue so that the nonviable-viable tissue interface is where invasive infection begins. One half of the specimen is cultured, and the other half is sent for histologic examination.

On detection of microorganisms in unburned tissue, local and systemic therapy is begun. Treatment comprises application of mafenide acetate burn cream if other topical agents have been used; subeschar injection of a broad-spectrum penicillin solution into infected areas, followed by surgical excision of the infected tissue; and systemic antibiotics.

The goal is to promote an environment prone to healing or amenable to definitive coverage. A newer approach called "moist wound healing" has been advantageous in superficial burn wounds, meshed skin grafts, and excised burn wounds. The goal is to maintain a moist environment about the surface that stimulates growth factors, increases proteolytic enzymes to clear devitalized tissue, enhances oxygen delivery and immune response, promotes angiogenesis and fibroblast proliferation, has improved epithelialization, and has less pain associated with moisture retaining dressings. Although topical creams cause desiccation due to their hyperosmolar properties, they are still the standard of care for deep burn wounds.

Plate 7-10

Injury to Musculoskeletal System

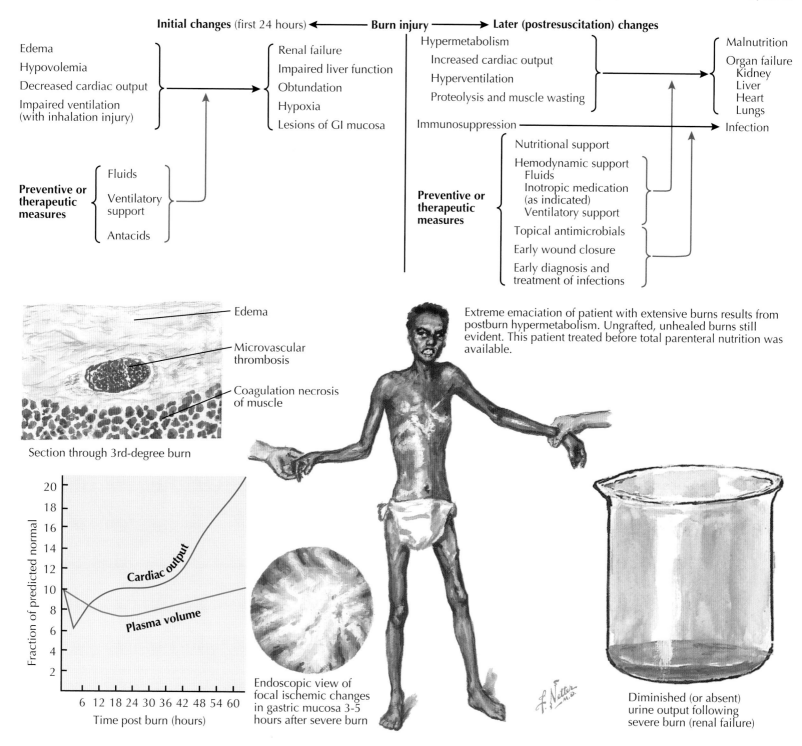

Initial changes (first 24 hours) ◄──── Burn injury ────► Later (postresuscitation) changes

Edema
Hypovolemia
Decreased cardiac output
Impaired ventilation
(with inhalation injury)

Renal failure
Impaired liver function
Obtundation
Hypoxia
Lesions of GI mucosa

Hypermetabolism
Increased cardiac output
Hyperventilation
Proteolysis and muscle wasting

Immunosuppression

Malnutrition
Organ failure
Kidney
Liver
Heart
Lungs

Infection

Preventive or therapeutic measures
Fluids
Ventilatory support
Antacids

Preventive or therapeutic measures
Nutritional support
Hemodynamic support
Fluids
Inotropic medication (as indicated)
Ventilatory support
Topical antimicrobials
Early wound closure
Early diagnosis and treatment of infections

Edema
Microvascular thrombosis
Coagulation necrosis of muscle

Section through 3rd-degree burn

Extreme emaciation of patient with extensive burns results from postburn hypermetabolism. Ungrafted, unhealed burns still evident. This patient treated before total parenteral nutrition was available.

Fraction of predicted normal: 20 18 16 14 12 10 8 6 4 2
Cardiac output
Plasma volume
6 12 18 24 30 36 42 48 54 60
Time post burn (hours)

Endoscopic view of focal ischemic changes in gastric mucosa 3-5 hours after severe burn

Diminished (or absent) urine output following severe burn (renal failure)

METABOLIC AND SYSTEMIC EFFECTS OF BURNS

The deleterious effects of burn injuries on every organ system are proportional to the extent of the thermal injury. The prominence and clinical importance of the various systemic effects are time related. Some systemic effects are evident immediately, whereas others develop only after resuscitation or even far into the convalescent period. The initial and later (postresuscitation) changes and appropriate preventative or therapeutic measures are shown on Plate 7-10. During the first 24 hours, hemodynamic and pulmonary dysfunctions predominate and require therapeutic intervention to minimize complications. During the second 24 hours, functional capillary integrity is restored, plasma volume is reconstituted by continued administration of resuscitation fluid, and cardiac output rises to supranormal levels—the first manifestation of postinjury hypermetabolism. Metabolic and immunologic changes due to the burn injury itself can all be aggravated by superimposed complications, particularly infection and sepsis. Early diagnosis and prompt treatment of infections that do develop minimize the occurrence of sepsis-related kidney, liver, heart, and lung failure. Pulmonary insufficiency due to sepsis predisposes the patient to pneumonia, the most common fatal complication, and may also impair oxygenation of peripheral tissues and increase susceptibility to invasive wound infections. Failure to meet the patient's markedly elevated nutritional needs not only permits erosion of lean body mass but also is associated with delayed healing, impaired take of skin grafts, exaggeration of immunologic deficits, increased risk of infection, and delayed convalescence. Maintaining pulmonary and cardiac functions to provide adequate tissue blood flow and oxygenation ameliorates the incidence and severity of the complications of these late metabolic and immunologic changes, thereby optimizing the resistance of the burn wound and other tissues to infection. Total metabolic support entails maintenance of fluid balance, mechanical ventilatory support, use of topical antimicrobial creams, nutritional support, and early wound closure.

Plate 7-11

Musculoskeletal System: PART III

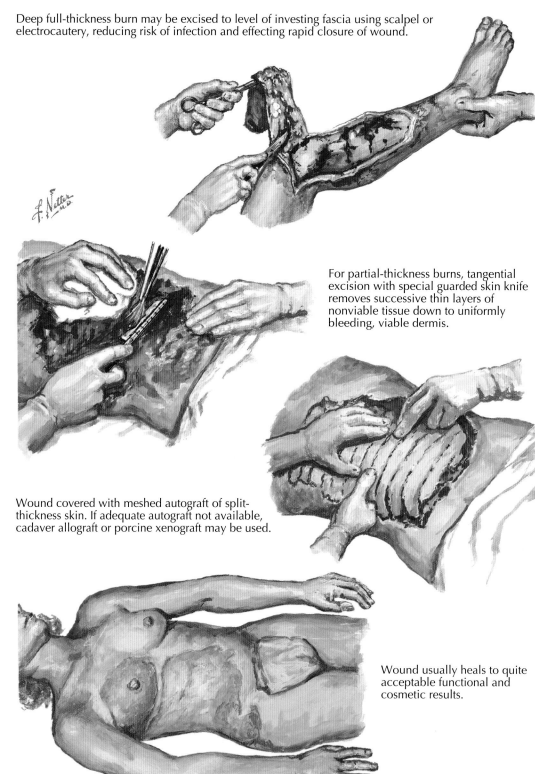

Deep full-thickness burn may be excised to level of investing fascia using scalpel or electrocautery, reducing risk of infection and effecting rapid closure of wound.

For partial-thickness burns, tangential excision with special guarded skin knife removes successive thin layers of nonviable tissue down to uniformly bleeding, viable dermis.

Wound covered with meshed autograft of split-thickness skin. If adequate autograft not available, cadaver allograft or porcine xenograft may be used.

Wound usually heals to quite acceptable functional and cosmetic results.

EXCISION AND GRAFTING FOR BURNS

Surgical excision of burn wounds should be performed as soon after resuscitation as the patient's hemodynamics and pulmonary status permit (see Plate 7-11). Surgical removal of the necrotic tissue contributes to minimizing the risk of infection and the degree and duration of physiologic stress.

Deep, unequivocally full-thickness burns may be excised to the level of the investing fascia using a scalpel, an electrocautery device, or even a laser. The excised wound must be covered with a skin graft to prevent desiccation of the exposed tissue and to effect definitive closure.

Tangential excision is commonly employed in the treatment of partial-thickness burns. Successive thin layers of nonviable tissue are removed until a wound bed of viable tissue, characterized by uniformly dense capillary bleeding, is developed. If the full thickness of the skin is involved, the excision should extend until normal fatty tissue is encountered. The wound is closed with a split-thickness skin graft. Blood loss associated with tangential excision, which can be prodigious, can be minimized by the application of gauzes soaked in a thrombin solution; by subcutaneous injection of ornithine vasopressin; or, if the burn is on a limb, by use of a tourniquet.

In patients with extensive burns but limited donor sites, the use of meshed grafts increases the area of burn wound that can be covered with the skin harvested from a donor site of given size. Although the expansion ratio of meshed grafts can be as great as 9:1, such large grafts are associated with a prolonged time of epithelialization of the interstices and increased scarring. Therefore, expansion should be limited to the commonly used ratios of 2:1 or 3:1. When donor sites are inadequate

because of extensive burns, any of several synthetic or biologic dressings can be used for temporary coverage of the wound. Viable cutaneous allograft is the gold standard of biologic dressings and when obtained through reputable sources such as the American Association of Tissue Banks the risk of disease transmission has been decreased significantly. Cutaneous xenografts (commonly porcine) are alternatives to cadaver allografts, and synthetic products such as Biobrane, a silicone membrane on nylon fabric coated with dermal porcine collagen, and Transcyte, which is Biobrane and

cultured newborn human fibroblasts, may also be used for temporary wound coverage.

The benefits of burn wound excision are realized at specific physiologic costs: blood loss, pulmonary effects of anesthesia and surgery, and sacrifice of any partial-thickness burn within the area of a full-thickness burn. Along with physiologic fluid resuscitation, improved ventilatory support, and effective control of infection, excision has greatly helped survival in burn patients. Improvements in functional and cosmetic therapies further facilitate rehabilitation of patients.

Plate 7-12

Injury to Musculoskeletal System

COMPARTMENT SYNDROME

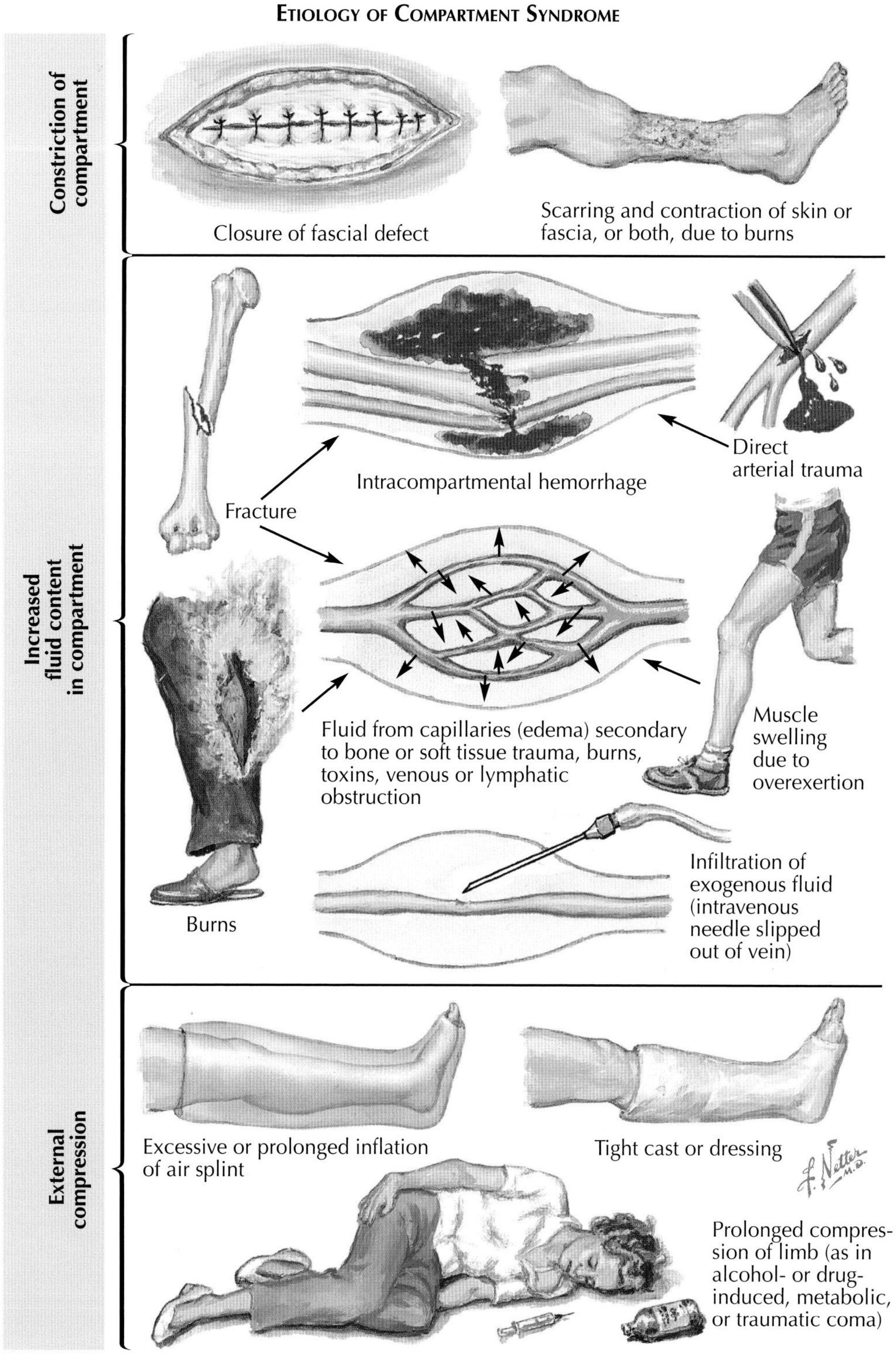

ETIOLOGY/ PATHOPHYSIOLOGY

Compartment syndrome results when fluid accumulates at high pressure within a closed fascial space (muscle compartment), reducing capillary perfusion below the level necessary for tissue viability. It may be initiated by a variety of conditions, such as fracture, vascular injury, burns, exertion, prolonged limb compression, or contusions. These traumatic events cause hemorrhage or edema, or both, in a muscle compartment enclosed in relatively noncompliant osseofascial boundaries (see Plate 7-12). Pressure then builds up within the compartment, producing compartment tamponade. The osseous and fascial structures of the compartments serve as nonyielding boundaries within which the pressure builds around the muscles within them. Studies have shown that in the setting of total ischemia, skeletal muscle retains electrical responsiveness for up to 3 to 4 hours, has variable tolerance of 4 to 8 hours, and after 8 hours suffers complete, irreversible damage. Peripheral nerves have been found to tolerate total ischemia for 1 hour, suffer neurapraxia after 4 hours, and have irreversible damage after 8 hours. Ischemia is seen when the pressure in the compartment exceeds the perfusion pressure of the tissues and is therefore variable based on the patient's blood pressure. The diastolic pressure is an accurate and simple measurement to use for this. Studies have demonstrated that healthy muscle can tolerate pressures up to within 10 mm Hg of the diastolic blood pressure before ischemia is seen, but in damaged tissue this changes to 20 mm Hg below the diastolic pressure. Thus, although prior discussions attempted to establish an absolute critical pressure, the current recommendations are to use a compartmental pressure of anything greater than the diastolic blood pressure minus 20 mm Hg to define a compartment syndrome. Compartment syndrome is seen most commonly in the lower leg after tibia fracture in which the deep posterior and anterior compartments are the most commonly affected but may be seen in any compartment. When a compartment syndrome is missed, the ischemia damage to the muscle and nerves can have devastating effects on the function of the limb; Volkmann contracture is the residual limb deformity that follows untreated acute compartment syndrome or ischemia due to arterial injury. However, prompt diagnosis and early effective treatment can result in a limb with normal function.

If multiple compartments are involved and a significant amount of muscle infarction is present, the patient may develop crush syndrome, which refers to the systemic effects of myonecrosis on the renal and cardiovascular systems. Myonecrosis causes the release of myoglobin, which is deposited in the distal convoluted tubules, ultimately occluding them and causing acute myoglobinuric renal failure. Third-space fluid loss occurs rapidly, leading to further hypotension and shock. The myonecrosis causes acidosis and hyperkalemia. Because the excessive potassium released from the damage muscle is not excreted in the presence of renal failure, cardiac arrhythmias may occur.

The most common cause of crush syndrome is prolonged compression of a limb (>12 hours) after alcohol or drug intoxication and stupor. Occasionally, trauma resulting from entrapment in debris produces the same effects. The presenting signs are hyperkalemia, acidosis, disorientation or coma, possibly cardiac arrhythmias, hypotension, renal failure, and swollen,

tense limbs with pressure sores. Results of laboratory studies are typically very abnormal. Concentration of creatinine phosphokinase is usually greater than 10,000 IU, and serum levels of creatinine, blood urea nitrogen, and potassium are also elevated. The finding of myoglobinuria confirms the diagnosis.

The three main causes of compartment syndrome are increased accumulation of fluid, decreased volume (compartment constriction), and restricted volume expansion secondary to external compression (see Plate 7-12). Although compartment syndrome develops most frequently in the four compartments of the leg, it can also occur in the forearm, hand, arm, shoulder, foot, thigh, buttocks, and back.

ETIOLOGY OF COMPARTMENT SYNDROME

Constriction of compartment

Closure of fascial defect

Scarring and contraction of skin or fascia, or both, due to burns

Increased fluid content in compartment

Fracture

Intracompartmental hemorrhage

Direct arterial trauma

Fluid from capillaries (edema) secondary to bone or soft tissue trauma, burns, toxins, venous or lymphatic obstruction

Muscle swelling due to overexertion

Burns

Infiltration of exogenous fluid (intravenous needle slipped out of vein)

External compression

Excessive or prolonged inflation of air splint

Tight cast or dressing

Prolonged compression of limb (as in alcohol- or drug-induced, metabolic, or traumatic coma)

INCREASED ACCUMULATION OF FLUID

The most common mechanism of compartment syndrome is increased fluid content in the compartment. The most common cause is a fracture, with the tibia the most often fractured bone. It is important to note that compartment syndrome can still occur after open fractures (particularly of the tibia) and that the soft tissue disruption does not offer adequate decompression of the compartment. It can also be seen after severe contusion of the limb with no fracture.

Injury to a major blood vessel may produce compartment syndrome by three mechanisms: (1) bleeding into the compartment, (2) partial occlusion of the artery secondary to spasm or intimal tear with inadequate

Plate 7-13

Musculoskeletal System: PART III

COMPARTMENT SYNDROME

(Continued)

collateral circulation, and (3) postischemia swelling after circulation is restored. Postischemia swelling and compartment syndrome result if repair of the artery and restoration of the circulation are delayed more than 6 hours.

Extreme exertion may initiate acute or chronic compartment syndrome. The more common chronic form is mild, recurrent compartment syndrome associated with exertional pain in the anterior compartment of the leg and frequently a muscle hernia. Symptoms abate when the excessive exercise is discontinued.

Thermal injuries (burns), in addition to decreasing compartment space, are associated with massive edema. Measurement of intramuscular pressure is needed to document the underlying compartment tamponade and the need for treatment with decompressive escharotomy.

Another cause of fluid accumulation is hemorrhage in patients who are receiving anticoagulant therapy after arterial puncture and in patients who have a bleeding diastasis such as hemophilia. Infiltration of exogenous intravenous fluid into the compartment and venomous snakebites may also produce compartment syndrome.

CONSTRICTION OF COMPARTMENT

Compartment syndrome may also result from surgical closure of a fascial defect. For example, a high performance runner may develop a muscle hernia and fascial defect. The hernias are usually bilateral and develop in the lower third of the leg overlying the anterior and lateral compartments, causing pain on exertion and often numbness. Unfortunately, some hernias are treated with surgical closure of the fascial defects, which decreases the volume of the compartment and increases intracompartmental pressure. The treatment of choice for a runner with exertional leg pain and muscle hernia is fascial release, not fascial closure.

Another cause of compartment volume is circumferential full-thickness (third-degree) burns. This injury decreases compartment size and coalesces the skin, subcutaneous tissue, and fascia into one tight, constricting eschar that requires immediate decompression.

EXTERNAL COMPRESSION

Unconsciousness after drug overdose can precipitate not only multiple compartment syndromes but also crush syndrome if the person lies with the limbs trapped beneath the torso or head. Compression of the forearm or leg produces persistent elevation of intracompartmental pressure, which often is greater than 50 mm Hg. Prolonged inflation of air splints and incorrect application of circumferential casts may also produce external compression that limits compartment swelling. Deflating the splint and splitting the cast quickly decrease the compressive pressure. Usually neither device causes compartment syndrome unless there is an underlying injury such as fracture or contusion.

DIAGNOSIS OF ACUTE COMPARTMENT SYNDROME

Clinical Manifestations

The clinical examination findings play an important role in the diagnosis of a compartment syndrome; where invasive pressure measurement formerly played

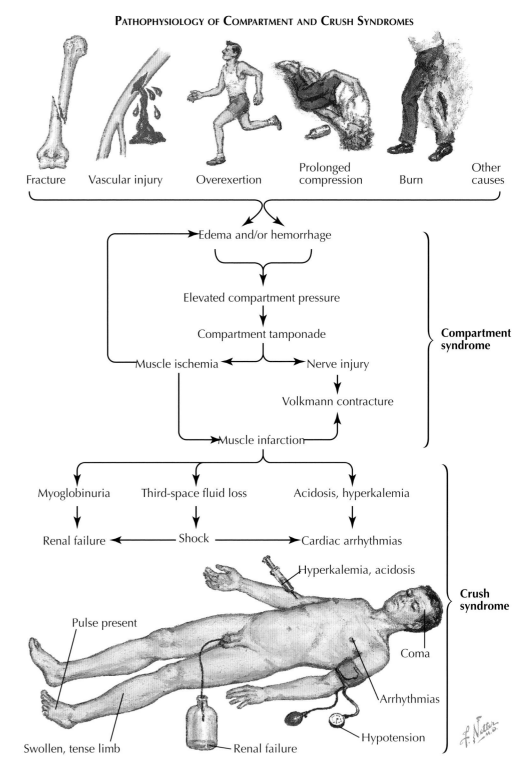

PATHOPHYSIOLOGY OF COMPARTMENT AND CRUSH SYNDROMES

Fracture   Vascular injury   Overexertion   Prolonged compression   Burn   Other causes

Edema and/or hemorrhage

Elevated compartment pressure

Compartment tamponade

Muscle ischemia ← → Nerve injury

Volkmann contracture

Muscle infarction

Myoglobinuria   Third-space fluid loss   Acidosis, hyperkalemia

Renal failure ← Shock → Cardiac arrhythmias

Compartment syndrome

Hyperkalemia, acidosis

Coma

Pulse present

Arrhythmias

Hypotension

Swollen, tense limb   Renal failure

Crush syndrome

a larger role, the diagnosis is now widely considered to be a clinical diagnosis. The most important symptom of an impending compartment syndrome is pain that is out of proportion to the primary problem or injury. However, *pain may be absent* if there is a superimposed deficit of the central or peripheral nervous system or if the process has been present for a sufficient amount of time to cause permanent nerve damage. Other early symptoms are best remembered by the *six P's* of a compartment syndrome (see Plate 7-14).

Pressure. The earliest finding is a swollen, palpably tense compartment. Palpation is difficult to quantify and has poor interobserver reliability. Furthermore, significant subcutaneous edema may mask the underlying pressure.

Pain on Stretch. Passive movement of the digits may produce pain in the involved ischemic muscles, and this is now widely considered the most sensitive clinical finding. Increased tissue pressure (even below the ischemic threshold) causes significant pain with stretching of the involved muscles, and thus this is often the earliest finding. Additionally, the course of pain, that is, pain that is continually worsening, is an important indicator of a potential impending compartment syndrome. Pain will diminish late in the course when nerve conduction is affected by the ischemia.

Paresis. Muscle weakness may be due to primary nerve involvement, muscle ischemia, or guarding secondary to pain.

Plate 7-14

Injury to Musculoskeletal System

COMPARTMENT SYNDROME
(Continued)

Paresthesia or Anesthesia. Sensory and motor changes may be seen after 1 hour of ischemia to the involved nerve. Initially, the sensory deficit may manifest as paresthesia but may progress to hypesthesia and anesthesia if treatment is delayed. Careful sensory examination helps determine the compartments involved.

Pulses Present and Pink Color. Unless there is a major arterial injury or disease, peripheral pulses are palpable and capillary refill is routinely present. Although compartment pressures are occasionally high enough to occlude a major artery, in more than 90% of patients the pulses are intact or can be confirmed with Doppler ultrasonography.

Differential Diagnosis

In patients with limb injuries and neurovascular deficits, the differential diagnosis is limited primarily to compartment syndrome, arterial injury, and nerve injury. Identification of the problem is important because the treatments differ: a compartment syndrome requires immediate decompression; an arterial injury requires immediate restoration of the circulation (either by repair of the artery or by removal of a thrombus); a nerve injury associated with a fracture or contusion (most commonly, neurapraxia) is usually treated with observation.

Compartment syndrome, arterial injury, and nerve injury frequently coexist, and the clinical findings overlap. Each condition may have associated motor and sensory deficit and pain. Arterial injury usually results in absent pulses, poor skin color, and decreased skin temperature, but a pseudoaneurysm and adequate collateral circulation may allow for a distal pulse. In contrast, in compartment syndrome, peripheral pulses are nearly always intact. Nerve injuries usually cause little pain, but the pain caused by antecedent trauma may be difficult to differentiate from ischemia pain. Diagnosis of neurapraxia is by exclusion of the other two entities. Doppler ultrasonography and arteriography are useful in diagnosing an arterial injury, and measurement of intracompartmental pressure may be used to detect or confirm compartment syndrome.

MEASUREMENT OF INTRACOMPARTMENTAL PRESSURE

Several techniques have been used to measure intracompartmental pressure (see Plate 7-15). The needle technique, first described in 1884, was popularized in the United States in the 1970s by Reneman and Whitesides. A variation of the needle technique employs continuous infusion of saline for long-term pressure monitoring.

The wick catheter does not require the injection of saline solution to measure equilibrium pressure. It was designed to prevent the catheter tip from being blocked by soft tissue and to maximize the surface area between the saline in the catheter and the fluids in the soft tissue. The fully automated, fluid-filled wick catheter system is connected to a pressure transducer and to a recording device for constant measurement of tissue pressure.

The slit catheter system is less likely to induce coagulation during long-term measurements, has a faster response time during exercise studies, and is more easily manufactured than the wick catheter.

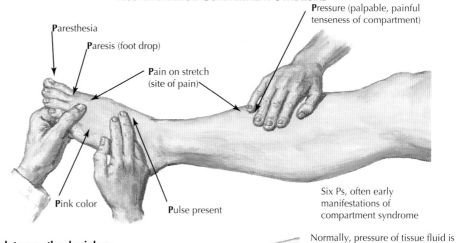

ACUTE ANTERIOR COMPARTMENT SYNDROME

Paresthesia

Paresis (foot drop)

Pressure (palpable, painful tenseness of compartment)

Pain on stretch (site of pain)

Pink color

Pulse present

Six Ps, often early manifestations of compartment syndrome

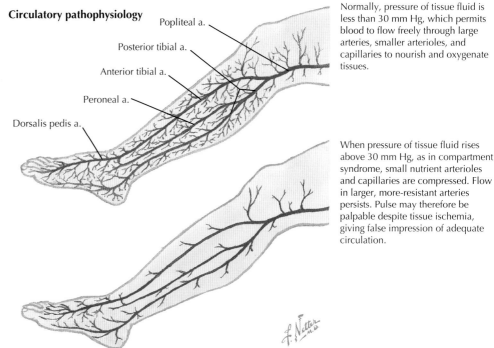

Circulatory pathophysiology

Popliteal a.

Posterior tibial a.

Anterior tibial a.

Peroneal a.

Dorsalis pedis a.

Normally, pressure of tissue fluid is less than 30 mm Hg, which permits blood to flow freely through large arteries, smaller arterioles, and capillaries to nourish and oxygenate tissues.

When pressure of tissue fluid rises above 30 mm Hg, as in compartment syndrome, small nutrient arterioles and capillaries are compressed. Flow in larger, more-resistant arteries persists. Pulse may therefore be palpable despite tissue ischemia, giving false impression of adequate circulation.

Differential diagnosis

	Compartment syndrome	Arterial occlusion	Neurapraxia
Pressure increased in compartment	+	–	–
Pain on stretch	+	+	–
Paresthesia or anesthesia	+	+	+
Paresis or paralysis	+	+	+
Pulses intact	+	–	+

Newer commercial devices have been developed; the most commonly used is the Stryker STIC Device. This device is small, portable, and easy to use and allows for repeat measurements in the same, or multiple, compartments easily.

Regardless of which device is chosen, it is important that it is zeroed and used properly. Studies of tibial fractures have shown a relationship between the distance from the fracture and the recorded pressure, so in the setting of a fracture the pressure measurements should be taken from within 5 cm of the fracture site. With or without an underlying fracture, multiple measurements can be taken and the highest recorded value considered.

INDICATIONS

The diagnosis of a compartment syndrome is now largely based on the clinical signs and symptoms. Invasive pressure measurements are still useful in situations in which the diagnosis cannot be made clinically or if confirmation is desired before surgical intervention:

Uncooperative or unreliable patients: interpretation of clinical findings may be difficult or not possible in adults with alcohol or drug intoxication. Frequently, children with fractures may be so frightened that careful neurologic evaluation is not possible.

Unresponsive patients: clinical evaluation of patients who are unconscious because of head injuries or

Plate 7-15

Musculoskeletal System: PART III

COMPARTMENT SYNDROME
(Continued)

drug overdose is not possible. The only reliable physical finding may be a swollen leg, making confirmation of the intracompartmental pressure mandatory.

Patients with associated neurovascular injury: it is often difficult to differentiate a nerve deficit associated with neurapraxia or with arterial injury from a compartment syndrome without measuring the intracompartmental pressure.

INDICATIONS FOR FASCIOTOMY

Surgical decompression should be performed as early as possible once the diagnosis of a compartment syndrome is made whether clinically or by measurement of compartment pressures. The pressure threshold at which fasciotomy should be performed remains controversial, and currently more authors favor a relative pressure based on the patient's blood pressure versus an absolute pressure. Because a pressure of 20 mm Hg below the diastolic pressure causes ischemia in injured tissue, that number currently serves as a guideline (not an absolute) for intervention. In borderline cases, it is more prudent to decompress the compartment earlier rather than later. Frequently, the duration of the increased pressure is not known and treatment must be based on the patient's systemic blood pressure, overall condition, progression of symptoms and signs, cooperation and reliability, and the type of injury. Late decompression in the setting of necrotic muscle when recovery is not expected should be approached with caution unless it is believed that all of the necrotic tissue can be debrided because otherwise it will result in a wound at high risk for infection. Another situation in which late decompression should be avoided is in the anterior compartment of the lower leg in which the scarring of necrotic muscle helps counteract the foot drop that may result.

DECOMPRESSION OF COMPARTMENT SYNDROME

There are no satisfactory nonsurgical methods for treating compartment syndromes; however, cooling of the tissue may prolong tolerance to ischemia and proper hydration may help avoid the renal damage after decompression. Surgical decompression, which allows the volume of the compartments to increase, is the primary means of relieving pressure. Each of the surrounding envelopes of the compartment may play a role in limiting compartment volume and must be considered, including volume-restricting plaster casts and circular dressings. Splitting and spreading a plaster cast may result in a 65% decrease in intracompartmental pressure. However, if symptoms of neurologic deficit persist more than 1 hour after cast splitting, the top half of the cast and all circular dressings must be removed and the limb examined. The skin may be a limiting envelope if, for example, there is significant subcutaneous edema or thermal injuries that have merged skin and fascia. In these cases, adequate decompression is achieved with a long dermatomy and fasciotomy.

INCISIONS FOR FOREARM AND HAND

The forearm consists of three compartments; volar, dorsal, and the mobile wad with the volar compartment

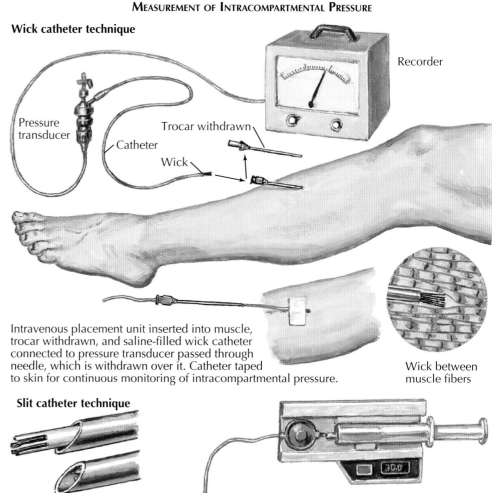

Wick catheter technique

Pressure transducer

Catheter

Trocar withdrawn

Wick

Recorder

Intravenous placement unit inserted into muscle, trocar withdrawn, and saline-filled wick catheter connected to pressure transducer passed through needle, which is withdrawn over it. Catheter taped to skin for continuous monitoring of intracompartmental pressure.

Wick between muscle fibers

Slit catheter technique

Tip of slit catheter protrudes from needle during filling with saline. All air bubbles expressed, and catheter tip withdrawn into needle before insertion into muscle.

Compact device with combined pressure transducer, digital recorder, and saline syringe may be used with slit catheter or wick catheter. Device and catheter may be taped to limb for continuous monitoring.

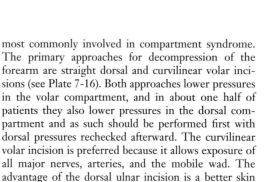

most commonly involved in compartment syndrome. The primary approaches for decompression of the forearm are straight dorsal and curvilinear volar incisions (see Plate 7-16). Both approaches lower pressures in the volar compartment, and in about one half of patients they also lower pressures in the dorsal compartment and as such should be performed first with dorsal pressures rechecked afterward. The curvilinear volar incision is preferred because it allows exposure of all major nerves, arteries, and the mobile wad. The advantage of the dorsal ulnar incision is a better skin coverage over the neurovascular bundles and tendons after decompression. The curvilinear volar incision

begins proximal to the antecubital fossa and extends to the middle of the palm. It is gently curved medially until it reaches the midline at the junction of the middle and distal thirds of the forearm and is continued straight distally to the proximal wrist crease, just ulnar to the palmaris longus tendon. The forearm incision is extended across the volar wrist crease to aid release of the carpal tunnel. It is carried no farther radially than the midaxis of the ring finger to avoid injury to the superficial palmar branch of the median nerve.

Median nerve neuropathy, in addition to carpal tunnel release, requires exploration of the nerves in the proximal forearm. The three main areas of potential

Plate 7-16

Injury to Musculoskeletal System

COMPARTMENT SYNDROME
(Continued)

nerve compression are the bicipital aponeurosis (lacertus fibrosis), the proximal edge of the pronator teres muscle, and the proximal edge of the flexor digitorum superficialis muscle.

After the volar fasciotomy, which is made in the same line as the skin incision from proximal to distal, compartment pressure is checked to ascertain that all the deep flexor muscles have been decompressed. After volar decompression, pressure measurements of the volar compartment, mobile wad, and dorsal compartments are repeated. If the pressures in the mobile wad and dorsal compartments remain elevated, these compartments should also be decompressed. The mobile wad can be approached through the volar curvilinear incision by lifting up the volar flap over that area. The dorsal compartment is approached through a longitudinal incision that is approximately one-third the length of the forearm in line with the lateral epicondyle of the humerus and the distal radioulnar joint. Through this incision, the fasciotomy is performed and final pressure measurements made. The skin incisions for all wounds are not closed at the time of fasciotomy but may be loosely approximated with rubber bands or covered with a wound VAC. If the diagnosis was delayed or some muscle appears necrotic, superficial debridement is carried out and more definitive debridement performed 4 to 7 days later, when muscle viability can be determined more accurately.

Postoperative care of the forearm includes a bulky dressing and splinting. The dressing is changed in 3 to 4 days in the operating room. Split-thickness skin grafts are almost always required, but skin grafting and closure are postponed until all necrotic tissue has been debrided, edema has resolved sufficiently, and wounds are appropriate for skin grafting. Active and active-assisted range-of-motion exercises for the hand are started immediately after surgery. The bulky dressing is usually removed at 3 weeks, and volar splints are then used until full motion is restored.

Compartment syndromes of the forearm associated with fracture of the distal humerus, radius, or ulna are usually treated with open reduction and internal fixation. Treatment of an associated arterial injury must be individualized.

Decompression of the hand may be required after crushing injuries. Diagnosis is made on the increased pressure in the interosseous compartments. There are 10 compartments of the hand. Incisions are made on the radial side of the thumb metacarpal, dorsally over the index and ring metacarpals, and one over the ulnar aspect of the little finger to release the thenar muscles, four dorsal interossei, three volar interossei, hypothenar muscles, and adductor pollicis muscle. Decompression of the arm and shoulder uses longitudinal incisions over the involved muscles. With involvement of the deltoid muscle, where fascia and epimysium form one layer, multiple incisions in the fascia are necessary.

INCISIONS FOR LEG

Current treatment of compartment syndromes of the leg is decompression that avoids fibulectomy while providing adequate decompression to the four compartments of the lower leg (anterior, lateral, superficial posterior, and deep posterior). This can be accomplished through either a single-incision or two-incision technique. The single-incision technique is technically

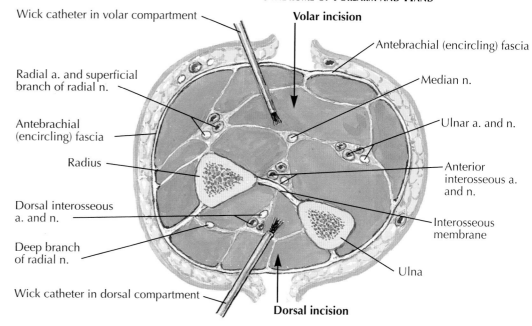

INCISIONS FOR COMPARTMENT SYNDROME OF FOREARM AND HAND

Wick catheter in volar compartment

Volar incision

Radial a. and superficial branch of radial n.

Antebrachial (encircling) fascia

Antebrachial (encircling) fascia

Median n.

Radius

Ulnar a. and n.

Dorsal interosseous a. and n.

Anterior interosseous a. and n.

Deep branch of radial n.

Interosseous membrane

Wick catheter in dorsal compartment

Ulna

Dorsal incision

Section through midforearm

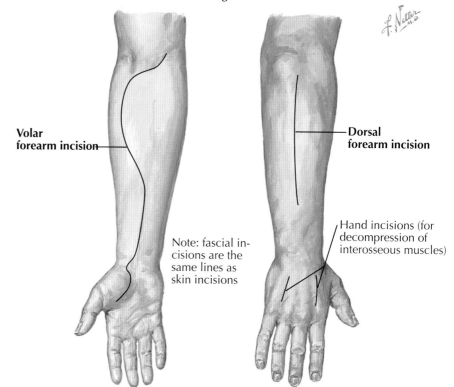

Volar forearm incision

Dorsal forearm incision

Note: fascial incisions are the same lines as skin incisions

Hand incisions (for decompression of interosseous muscles)

more challenging but provides the benefit of only having one skin incision requiring definitive closure/coverage.

The single-incision, or perifibular, approach is described through a single linear lateral incision just posterior to the fibula from the fibular head to the tip of the lateral malleolus. This exposure requires proximal identification and protection of the common peroneal nerve. The fasciotomy is made between the soleus and flexor hallucis longus distally and carried proximally to the soleus origin, allowing access to both posterior compartments. The anterior and lateral compartments are accessed by carefully retracting the anterior border of the incision (with care taken to avoid the superficial peroneal nerve), allowing the

fasciotomies in the lateral and anterior compartments to be made.

When the two-incision technique is used, the two skin incisions can be shorter (approximately one-third the length of the leg) if intraoperative pressure monitoring is performed. Decompression of the anterior and lateral compartments is performed through an incision placed halfway between the shaft of the fibula and the tibial crest. The incision is made approximately over the intermuscular septum dividing the anterior and lateral compartments, allowing easy access to both. When a slightly shorter incision is used, it is extremely important to undermine the skin incisions proximally and distally to allow wide exposure of the fascia. A

Plate 7-17

Musculoskeletal System: PART III

COMPARTMENT SYNDROME
(Continued)

transverse incision is made just through the fascia to identify the anterior intermuscular septum that separates the anterior and lateral compartments. This is important because the superficial peroneal nerve that lies in the lateral compartment next to the septum must be located. Fasciotomy of the lateral compartment is made in line with the shaft of the fibula posterior to the anterior intermuscular septum.

The posteromedial approach is used for decompression of the superficial and deep posterior compartments. This incision is made slightly distal to the anterolateral incision and 2 cm posterior to the posterior margin of the tibia to avoid injuring the saphenous nerve and vein located in this area. The skin edges are undermined and the saphenous nerve and vein retracted anteriorly. A transverse fascial incision allows identification of the septum between the deep and superficial posterior compartments. Usually, it is easier to decompress the superficial posterior compartment first. The fasciotomy is extended proximally under the bridge of the soleus muscle to allow proximal access to the deep posterior compartment. If the soleus muscle attaches to the tibia in the distal third, it should be released initially to allow visualization of the deep posterior compartment and to aid decompression. Distally, the deep posterior compartment is relatively subcutaneous and can be decompressed easily.

After the four-compartment fasciotomy, intraoperative monitoring of compartmental pressure should be performed to document the decompression. Very little muscle should be debrided at the time of initial decompression, because it is difficult to determine an infarcted muscle from an ischemic but recoverable muscle.

Postoperative care of the leg wounds is similar to that of the forearm wounds, but in compartment syndrome without associated fractures, closure in a week is often possible without skin grafting. Necrotic muscle is debrided once or twice a week until a satisfactory granulation bed is present. Skin grafting or closure before this may lead to infection and the need for subsequent amputation. To prevent the insidious development of contractures, the ankle is splinted posteriorly in neutral position.

Compartment syndrome associated with fractures of the tibia should be treated with internal fixation, using either intramedullary rods or plates, but open fractures may require external fixation. A major disadvantage of the external fixation device is that mobilization of skin for delayed primary closure is not feasible and thus skin grafting is nearly always required.

Prophylactic decompression of the leg should be performed after tibial osteotomy or use of the tibia as the donor site of a bone graft. During debridement of an open fracture of the tibia, compartments accessible through the exposed wound should also be opened if the anatomy is not distorted by the fracture and the location of the superficial nerves is apparent. Arterial injury, thrombosis, and arterial bypass surgery also predispose to compartment syndromes. If the period of ischemia lasts longer than 6 hours, prophylactic decompression of the four compartments should be considered.

INCISIONS FOR THIGH, BUTTOCK, AND FOOT

Compartment syndrome of the thigh and gluteus muscles is not common but may progress to a crush

INCISIONS FOR COMPARTMENT SYNDROME OF LEG

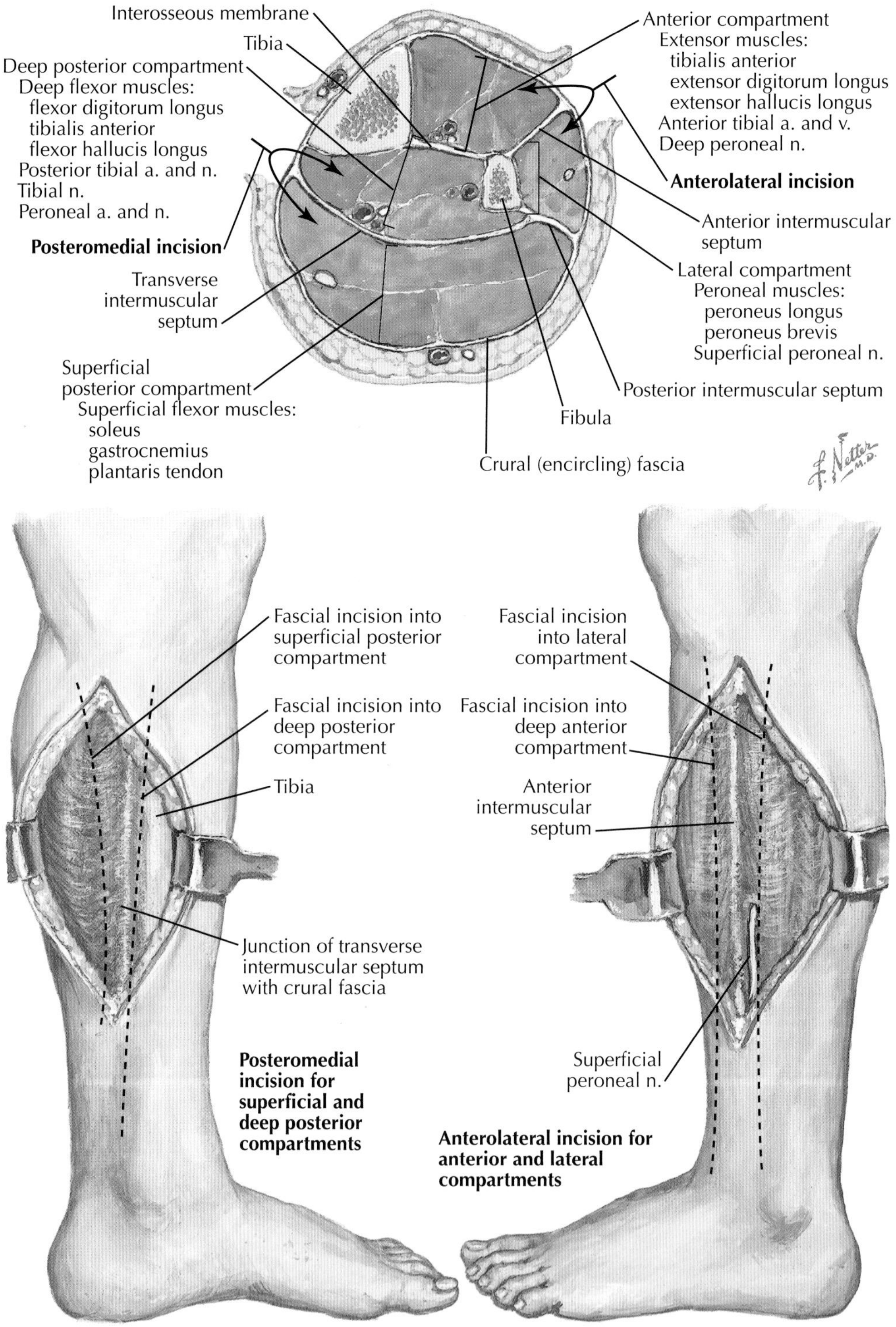

Interosseous membrane
Tibia
Deep posterior compartment
Deep flexor muscles:
flexor digitorum longus
tibialis anterior
flexor hallucis longus
Posterior tibial a. and n.
Tibial n.
Peroneal a. and n.
Posteromedial incision
Transverse intermuscular septum
Superficial posterior compartment
Superficial flexor muscles:
soleus
gastrocnemius
plantaris tendon

Anterior compartment
Extensor muscles:
tibialis anterior
extensor digitorum longus
extensor hallucis longus
Anterior tibial a. and v.
Deep peroneal n.
Anterolateral incision
Anterior intermuscular septum
Lateral compartment
Peroneal muscles:
peroneus longus
peroneus brevis
Superficial peroneal n.
Posterior intermuscular septum
Fibula
Crural (encircling) fascia

Fascial incision into superficial posterior compartment
Fascial incision into deep posterior compartment
Tibia
Junction of transverse intermuscular septum with crural fascia
Posteromedial incision for superficial and deep posterior compartments

Fascial incision into lateral compartment
Fascial incision into deep anterior compartment
Anterior intermuscular septum
Superficial peroneal n.
Anterolateral incision for anterior and lateral compartments

syndrome because of the large bulk of muscle involved. Longitudinal incisions are made over the thigh to decompress the adductor, quadriceps, or hamstring muscles. Measurement of pressure is helpful in the diagnosis of compartment syndromes in these areas because sensory deficits are rare. Gluteus compartment syndromes, most often due to limb compression after drug overdose, involve three separate compartments: the gluteus maximus, gluteus medius/gluteus minimus, and tensor fasciae latae muscles. The choice of approaches may vary based on surgeon familiarity, but one should be chosen that will allow adequate access to all three compartments. The fascia superficial to the

gluteus maximus muscle is relatively thin and blends with the epimysium, which sends septa into the muscle, forming multiple subdivisions. For adequate decompression, multiple incisions in this fascia-epimysium are required.

In the foot, the interosseous compartments are released via longitudinal incisions over the dorsum (medial to the second metatarsal and lateral to the fourth metatarsal), and the medial plantar structures are released using a separate medial incision or dissecting medially through the more medial dorsal incision. Again, measurement of intracompartmental pressure is helpful to ascertain the need for decompression.

Plate 7-18

Injury to Musculoskeletal System

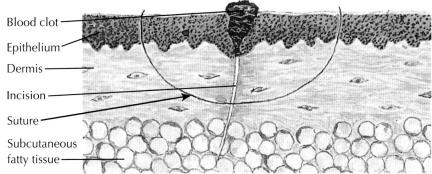

Blood clot

Epithelium

Dermis

Incision

Suture

Subcutaneous
fatty tissue

Immediately after incision
Blood clot with fine fibrin network forms in wound. Epithelium thickens at wound edges.

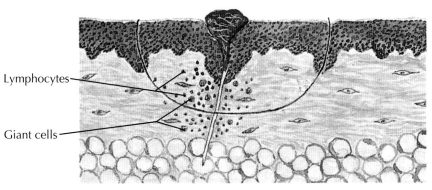

Lymphocytes

Giant cells

24-48 hours
Epithelium begins to grow down along cut edges and along suture tract. Leukocyte infiltration, chiefly round cells (lymphocytes) with few giant cells, occurs and removes bacteria and necrotic tissue.

HEALING OF INCISED, SUTURED SKIN WOUND

The healing of a typical incised wound can be divided into three phases: the inflammatory phase, the proliferation phase, and the maturation phase (see Plate 7-18).

The first step in the *inflammatory phase* is the formation of a blood clot, which controls bleeding and forms a thin fibrin network, bridging the wound margins. Simultaneously, an intense inflammatory reaction develops, with the arrival of a large number of leukocytes that remove bacteria, necrotic tissue, and other debris from the wound. Additionally, macrophages secrete growth factors important for the chemotaxis of fibroblasts, smooth muscle, and endothelial cells. Almost immediately after injury, fibroblasts begin to mobilize from the deeper dermal structures and migrate toward the wound edges. Simultaneously, the cut epithelial edges begin to proliferate, with new epithelial cells accumulating at the cut edges.

The proliferation phase begins 3 to 5 days after injury. Epithelialization of an incised wound starts immediately afterward with the epithelial cells at the edges loosening their connections to each other and the basement membrane. Epithelial cells are typically able to bridge an incised and approximated wound (≤1 mm) within 48 hours. New capillaries form, bringing oxygen and nutrients to the proliferating cells and a characteristic red color to the tissue. After approximately 5 days, the fibroblasts are synthesizing collagen precursors as well as mucopolysaccharides and other glycoproteins to form the wound matrix. Collagen is secreted into this matrix and quickly polymerizes to begin to add tensile strength to the wound. The production of collagen continues for 2 to 4 weeks. During this time, there is further fibroblastic proliferation into the depth of the wound.

The third phase of healing of an incised wound is the *maturation phase*, which begins about 3 weeks after injury and lasts as long as 9 months after injury. During this phase, the tensile strength of the wound continues to increase, owing to the further crosslinking of collagen fibers combined with the remodeling of collagen fibers along the lines of mechanical stress, producing a stronger and more durable matrix. Typically, the maximum tensile strength of the wound is achieved at approximately 60 days and is roughly 80% of the non-incised skin.

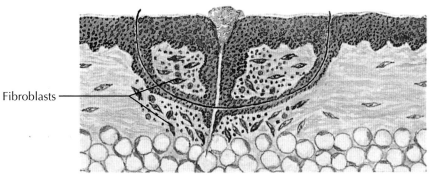

Fibroblasts

5-8 days
Epithelial downgrowth advances. Fibroblasts grow in from deeper tissues and add collagen precursors and glycoproteins to matrix. Cellular infiltration progresses.

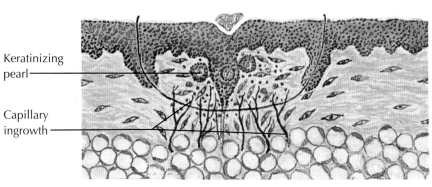

Keratinizing pearl

Capillary ingrowth

10-15 days
Capillaries grow in from subcutaneous tissue, forming granulation tissue. Epithelium bridges incision; epithelial downgrowths regress, leaving keratinizing pearls behind. Fibrosed clot (scab) is being pushed out. Collagen formation progresses and cellular infiltration abates.

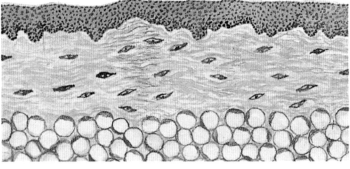

3 weeks–9 months
Epithelium is thinned to near normal. Tensile strength of tissue is increased owing to production and cross-linking of collagen fibers; elastic fibers reappear later.

Plate 7-19

Musculoskeletal System: PART III

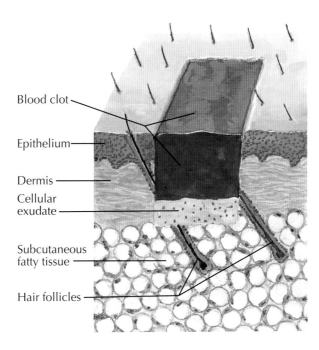

Blood clot

Epithelium

Dermis

Cellular exudate

Subcutaneous fatty tissue

Hair follicles

Immediately after excision. Wound gap filled with blood clot.

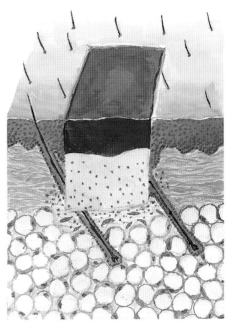

2-3 days after excision. Clot retracted somewhat, and cellular exudate beneath it increased. Surface epithelium begins to grow down along wound edges. Fibroblasts proliferate at base of wound.

HEALING OF EXCISED SKIN WOUND

The healing process of the excised skin wound is very similar to that of the incised wound (see Plate 7-19). A large blood clot immediately fills the excised defect. At the edges of the wound, epithelial cells rapidly proliferate and migrate downward into the edges of the wound. In 2 to 3 days after injury, the clot retracts somewhat and a large cellular exudate, composed mostly of leukocytes, begins to develop beneath the clot. Epithelium continues to advance from the edges of the wound as well as from any transected skin appendages such as hair follicles.

Fibroblasts begin to proliferate in the base of the wound. The fibroblastic proliferation is followed immediately by the development of new capillaries bringing nutrients and oxygen to the newly formed tissues. The blood clot is gradually elevated by the cellular exudate beneath it, allowing epithelial cells to grow across the base of the wound. Active contraction of the wound begins 8 to 10 days after injury as more collagen-rich connective tissue is laid down in the base of the wound. Eventually, the highly vascular granulation tissue disappears and a dense collagenous scar tissue persists underneath the new layer of epithelium. The new epithelium is devoid of normal skin appendages.

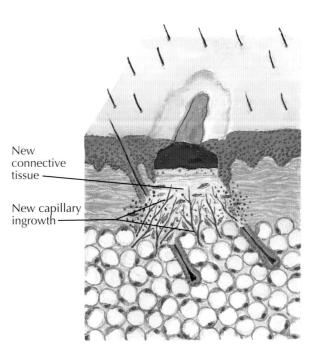

New connective tissue

New capillary ingrowth

6 days. Epithelium at surface and from severed skin appendages has grown partially across gap. Connective tissue at base increases, and new capillaries grow into it to form granulation tissue.

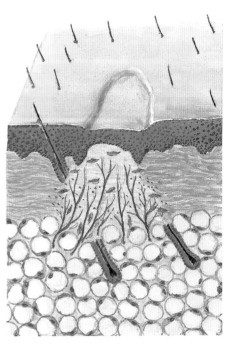

8-10 days. Any residual clot has been cast off or resorbed and epithelium grown completely across defect, which is being narrowed by contraction of surrounding connective tissue and filled by deposition of new tissue that is vascularized and collagen rich. Eventually, granulation tissue replaced with collagenous scar tissue devoid of skin appendages.

Plate 7-20

Injury to Musculoskeletal System

FRACTURES, DISLOCATIONS, AND SPRAINS

Injury to the musculoskeletal system takes many different forms, depending on the mechanism of injury, the amount and direction of deforming force applied to the skeleton, and the location at which the force is applied. Many terms and classification systems are used to define various patterns of musculoskeletal injury, including eponyms and colorful descriptions that are often misleading and incorrectly applied. The best and most accurate way to describe patterns of injury to the musculoskeletal system is to use specific and objectively definable terminology, which facilitates communication among health care providers and thus improves patient care.

TYPES OF JOINT INJURY

A *dislocation* is a complete and persistent displacement of the articular surfaces of the bones that make up a joint relative to one another, with disruption of at least part of the supporting capsule and/or ligaments (see Plate 7-20). After a dislocation, a muscle spasm locks the two displaced bone ends in an abnormal position, usually creating an obvious and significant deformity.

A *subluxation* is a partial dislocation of a joint; that is, the articular surfaces are partially separated from each other and are no longer congruent. Although not as severe as dislocations, subluxations usually also damage part of the joint capsule and some of the supporting ligaments. After subluxation, the patient may still be able to move the joint to some degree. Failure to recognize and treat a subluxation may result in permanent ligament laxity and joint incongruity. In both dislocations and subluxations the incongruent alignment of articular surfaces may cause abnormally high pressure to be placed on the articular cartilage, which can damage the cartilage. Because articular cartilage has limited capacity to regenerate, this predisposes to longer-term problems such as arthritis.

Joint injuries are often a combination of a fracture and a dislocation. In a *fracture-dislocation* or *fracture-subluxation*, there is a fracture with incongruency of the adjacent joint surfaces. A bimalleolar fracture of the ankle is a good example of a fracture subluxation. In this condition, fractures of the medial and lateral malleoli create instability of the ankle joint, resulting in subluxation of the tibiotalar articulation.

A *sprain* is a stretch and/or tear of a ligament resulting from force causing angulation, subluxation, or dislocation that may be seen even if the articular surfaces subsequently return to their normal alignment. Even though the displacement is transient, significant damage may occur to the joint capsule and ligaments. Except for swelling, sprains cause no significant deformity. Joint movement is limited only by pain and not by joint incongruity. A sprain should not be confused with a *strain*, which is the stretching of a musculotendinous unit (muscle and/or tendon).

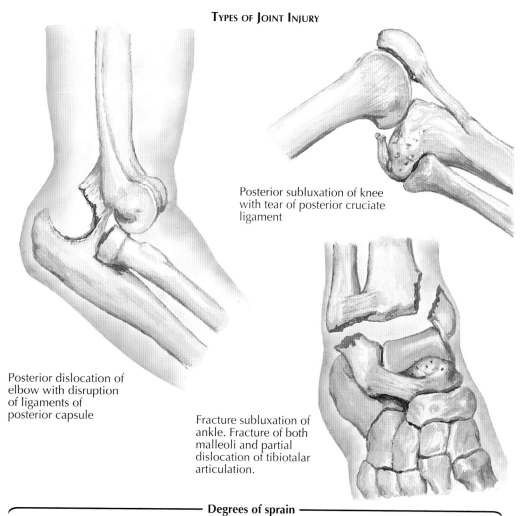

Posterior subluxation of knee with tear of posterior cruciate ligament

Posterior dislocation of elbow with disruption of ligaments of posterior capsule

Fracture subluxation of ankle. Fracture of both malleoli and partial dislocation of tibiotalar articulation.

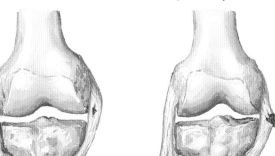

Degrees of sprain

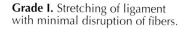

Grade I. Stretching of ligament with minimal disruption of fibers.

Grade II. Tearing of up to 50% of ligament fibers; small hematoma. Hemarthrosis may be present.

Grade III. Complete tear of ligament and separation of ends, hematoma, and hemarthrosis.

Sprains are graded into three categories according to the severity of damage to the joint capsule and some of the supporting ligaments. A grade I (mild) sprain is characterized by a slight stretching and damage to the fibers of a ligament with a firm end point still noted on physical examination. Grade I sprains usually heal in 3 to 4 weeks without significant loss of function. A grade II (moderate) sprain describes a partial disruption of the supporting ligaments and capsule that may demonstrate some laxity on physical examination. Most grade II sprains also heal in 3 to 4 weeks if the injured structures are protected from excessive loads or stretching and if appropriate rehabilitation and activity modification are provided. A grade III (severe) sprain refers to a complete rupture of the capsule and supporting ligaments. A grade III sprain is as severe an injury as a complete dislocation. The only difference between a grade III sprain and a dislocation is that in the sprain the articular

Plate 7-21

Musculoskeletal System: PART III

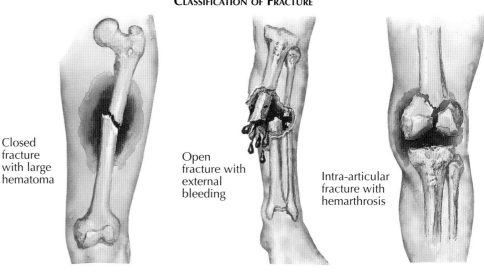

CLASSIFICATION OF FRACTURE

Closed fracture with large hematoma

Open fracture with external bleeding

Intra-articular fracture with hemarthrosis

FRACTURES, DISLOCATIONS, AND SPRAINS (Continued)

surfaces spontaneously return to their normal positions. In severe sprains, surgery may be required to repair the completely torn ligaments and capsule.

CLASSIFICATION OF FRACTURE

A fracture is a break in the surface of the bone, either across its cortex or through its articular surface. Fractures range in severity from a single crack to a complete disruption of the bone's architecture. A fracture through the cortex of a bone disturbs the normal load-bearing function of the bone. In addition, at the time of fracture, the overlying periosteum is torn, bleeding at the fracture site produces a hematoma, and electric and biochemical signals initiate the fracture healing process.

Proper management of all fractures and dislocations—regardless of location, extent, or severity—is based on three criteria: the integrity of the overlying skin and soft tissues (i.e., open or closed fracture), the specific location of the fracture within the bone, and the degree of displacement of the injured parts. Therefore, the initial evaluation must describe the musculoskeletal injury in terms of these variables.

Open and Closed Fracture

In a *closed* fracture, the overlying skin remains intact; in an *open* fracture, the integrity of the overlying skin and soft tissues has been violated (see Plate 7-21). Disruption of this envelope of soft tissue around the fracture site substantially increases the risk of complications. Open fractures result in greater blood loss, decreased healing rate, and increased risk of infection.

Bleeding occurs with every fracture because, at the time of injury, the periosteal vessels and the vessels supplying the soft tissues surrounding the fracture are disrupted, which leads to the formation of a large hematoma. In a closed fracture, the increased interstitial pressure within the hematoma compresses the blood vessels, limiting the accumulation of blood and thus the size of the hematoma. Nevertheless, the amount of bleeding in closed fractures remains substantial. For example, a closed fracture of the femoral shaft may result in blood loss of as much as 1 liter before the increased pressure within the hematoma tamponades the bleeding vessels. However, because the tamponade effect is lost in an open fracture, blood loss is even greater and may be life threatening.

Any open fracture can become infected because the hematoma that forms around the open fracture site is contaminated by contact with the external environment. The risk of infection is directly related to the severity of soft tissue damage. An infection that becomes established at a fracture site is much more resistant to treatment than a soft tissue infection and may be impossible to eradicate. Chronic purulent drainage from the

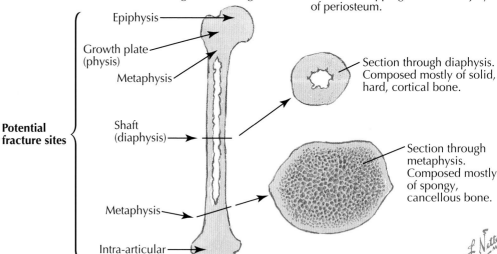

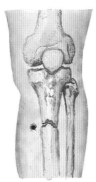 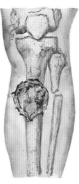 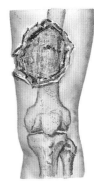 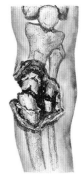 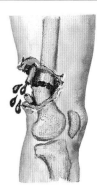

Gustilo and Anderson classification of open fracture

Type I. Wound <1 cm long. No evidence of deep contamination.

Type II. Wound >1 cm long. No extensive soft tissue damage.

Type IIIA. Large wound. Good soft tissue coverage.

Type IIIB. Large wound. Exposed bone fragments, extensive stripping of periosteum.

Type IIIC. Large wound with major arterial injury.

Potential fracture sites

Epiphysis

Growth plate (physis)

Metaphysis

Shaft (diaphysis)

Metaphysis

Intra-articular

Section through diaphysis. Composed mostly of solid, hard, cortical bone.

Section through metaphysis. Composed mostly of spongy, cancellous bone.

fracture site may persist for the rest of the patient's life. The chronic infection of the bone, called post-traumatic osteomyelitis, often cannot be cured or even controlled in spite of repeated and aggressive surgical debridement and appropriate antibiotic therapy (see Plate 7-21).

Because of the devastating nature of chronic post-traumatic osteomyelitis, all open fractures must be identified immediately and prompt treatment instituted to prevent infection in the fracture hematoma. The best means of managing the contaminated fracture is

through prompt and thorough surgical debridement combined with intravenous administration of broad-spectrum antibiotics immediately after the injury. The current standard of care is to administer antibiotic prophylaxis as soon as possible based on the work of Patzakis et al. A first-generation cephalosporin (e.g., cefazolin) should be given for all open fractures. For grossly contaminated fractures, an aminoglycoside may be added as well or a penicillin used in cases of organic contamination to protect against *Clostridium*.

Plate 7-22

Injury to Musculoskeletal System

FRACTURES, DISLOCATIONS, AND SPRAINS *(Continued)*

Debridement is usually repeated in the first few days after injury. Primary closure of the wound is delayed until there is no evidence of residual contamination at the fracture site.

Gustilo and Anderson Classification

This useful classification grades open fractures according to several factors, including the severity of soft tissue damage. In a type I open fracture, the wound is less than 1 cm long and there is no evidence of deep contamination. In a type II injury, the wound is greater than 1 cm long and there is no extensive soft tissue injury. A type IIIA open fracture has a large, open wound but the bone fragments remain adequately covered by soft tissues (periosteum). If the wound is large and open and the bone is stripped of periosteum and exposed, the fracture is classified as type IIIB. These injuries typically require additional soft tissue coverage such as grafts or flaps. The most serious open fracture is type IIIC, which comprises an open wound and an arterial injury that requires surgical repair.

Studies by Gustilo and associates documented a minimal risk of infection with type I open fractures if immediate surgical debridement is performed. However, in general, the greater the surrounding soft tissue injury, the higher the likelihood of infection and poor functional outcomes (even amputation). The classification system suffers from questionable interobserver reliability and from the fact that many surgeons believe the wound cannot be accurately staged until further debridements, because the extent of soft tissue damage may not be appreciated fully until the zone of necrosis is evident and debrided. Nevertheless, it is important to understand the grading system to facilitate communication between providers.

FRACTURE SITES

In the initial evaluation of any fracture, the examiner must identify the specific location of the fracture within the bone (see Plate 7-21). The different areas of bone heal with different mechanisms and at different rates. Fractures may occur in the shaft (diaphysis), metaphysis, joint (intra-articular fracture), growth plate (physis), or epiphysis. Fractures of the shaft and metaphysis heal in very dissimilar ways. Diaphyseal bone usually heals by the formation of an external bridging callus, whereas metaphyseal bone healing is dominated by intramembranous ossification. In addition, the cancellous metaphyseal bone heals much more rapidly than the cortical diaphyseal bone.

Intra-articular fractures involve the articular surface of the bone, and this involvement has important implications for both treatment and prognosis. The articular

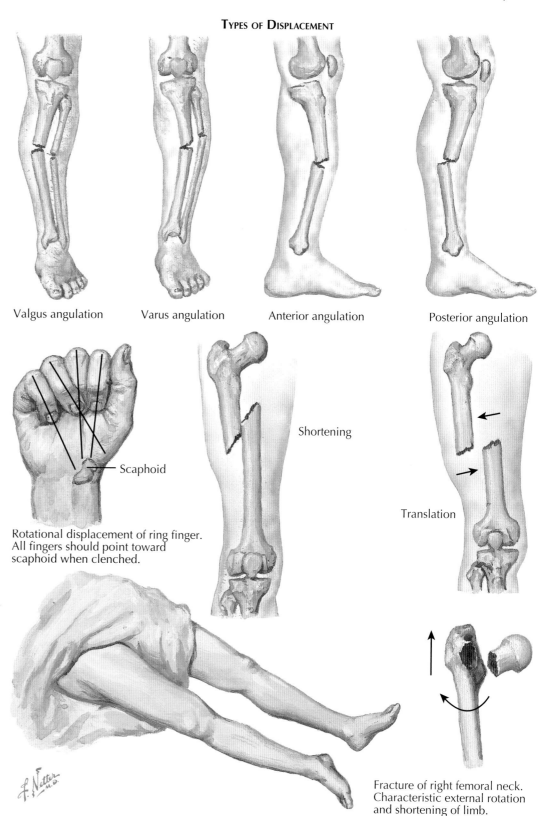

TYPES OF DISPLACEMENT

Valgus angulation

Varus angulation

Anterior angulation

Posterior angulation

Rotational displacement of ring finger. All fingers should point toward scaphoid when clenched.

Scaphoid

Shortening

Translation

Fracture of right femoral neck. Characteristic external rotation and shortening of limb.

surface must heal with anatomic congruity to minimize the risk of post-traumatic osteoarthritis. Epiphyseal (growth plate) fractures are quite common in children and heal more rapidly than fractures in adults.

TYPES OF DISPLACEMENT

The initial evaluation of any fracture, in addition to assessment of the degree of soft tissue injury and the location in the bone, must determine the degree of fracture displacement. All fractures must be described as nondisplaced or displaced (see Plate 7-22). *Nondisplaced* fractures are difficult to diagnose because there is no associated deformity except soft tissue swelling. Indeed, many nondisplaced fractures are overlooked or mistaken for a simpler injury such as a mild or moderate sprain. All patients with a musculoskeletal injury who complain of pain and exhibit swelling, ecchymosis, and point tenderness at the injury site should undergo radiographic evaluation to rule out disruption of the

Plate 7-23

Musculoskeletal System: PART III

TYPES OF FRACTURE

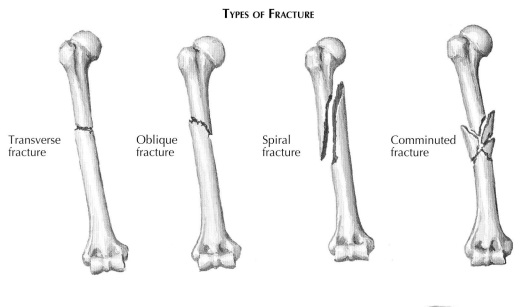

Transverse fracture

Oblique fracture

Spiral fracture

Comminuted fracture

FRACTURES, DISLOCATIONS, AND SPRAINS (Continued)

underlying bone architecture. If not appropriately treated, nondisplaced fractures often result in serious disability.

Displaced fractures are described by the type of deformity produced by the displacement: angulation, rotation, change in limb length, or translation. Angulation at the fracture site may be in the frontal or the sagittal plane or both. Frontal plane deformities are called varus or valgus depending on the angulation of the distal fragment at the point of the fracture. When the distal fragment is angulated toward the midline, a varus deformity is produced; when the distal fragment is angulated away from the midline, valgus deformity occurs. Sagittal plane deformities are described either as anterior or posterior angulation, depending on the direction in which the apex of the angulation points.

Fracture fragments can also be rotationally displaced. After fracture, the distal fragment is rotated along the long axis of the bone by muscle spasm or by the pull of gravity, resulting in either an internal rotation or an external rotation deformity.

A third type of displacement is a change in limb length. After a fracture, the surrounding muscles go into spasm, contracting to produce limb shortening.

Finally, translation occurs when the distal fragment shifts medially, laterally, anteriorly, or posteriorly in relation to the proximal fragment.

Frequently the displacement is a combination of several types of the patterns described. For example, a displaced intertrochanteric fracture of the hip due to a fall typically causes both shortening and external rotation of the limb. Often, a varus angulation is present as well.

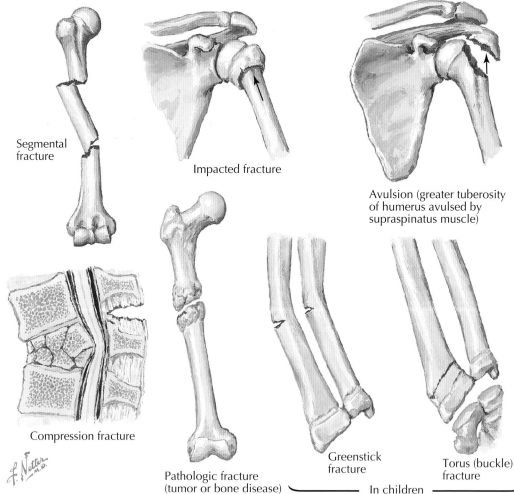

Segmental fracture

Impacted fracture

Avulsion (greater tuberosity of humerus avulsed by supraspinatus muscle)

Compression fracture

Pathologic fracture (tumor or bone disease)

Greenstick fracture

Torus (buckle) fracture

In children

TYPES OF FRACTURE

Many terms are used to describe the numerous fracture patterns (see Plate 7-23). *Transverse, oblique,* and *spiral* describe the pattern of fracture seen on the radiograph. A *comminuted* fracture has more than two fragments. A *segmental* fracture is a type of comminuted fracture in the shaft of a long bone in which there are three (or more) large, well-identified fragments. In an *impacted* fracture, two fracture fragments are telescoped on each other; usually, this pattern of injury is quite stable.

Avulsion fractures frequently occur at the site of attachment of a musculotendinous unit to bone; they are caused when a sudden muscular pull tears the bony attachment loose from the rest of the bone. *Compression* fractures are common in the cancellous flat bones, particularly the vertebrae. The cancellous trabeculae are compressed, or impacted, together. A *pathologic* fracture occurs at a site in a bone that is diseased or weakened, most commonly through areas weakened by tumor or by a metabolic bone disease such as osteoporosis.

Two specific terms are used to describe fractures that are unique to children. A *greenstick* fracture occurs in the shaft of the bone, with the cortex fractured on the convex side of the deformity but intact on the concave side. This pattern is identical to the way a green stick reacts when bent. A *torus,* or *buckle,* fracture occurs in the metaphysis of the long bones in response to compressive loading. Most frequently seen in the distal radius, the buckle fracture usually results from a fall on the outstretched hand.

Plate 7-24

Injury to Musculoskeletal System

HEALING OF FRACTURE

Inflammation

A hematoma forms as the result of disruption of intraosseous and surrounding vessels. Bone at the edges of the fracture dies. Bone necrosis is greater with larger amounts of soft tissue disruption. Inflammatory cells are followed by fibroblasts, chondroblasts, and osteoprogenitor cells. Low PO_2 at the fracture site promotes angiogenesis.

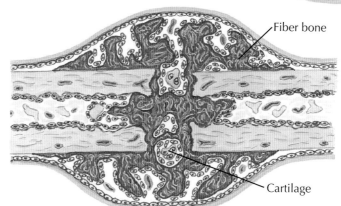

Repair of soft callus formation

Soft callus forms, initially composed of collagen; this is followed by progressive cartilage and osteoid formation.

Repair of hard callus formation

Osteoid and cartilage of external, periosteal, and medullary soft callus become mineralized as they are converted to woven bone (hard callus).

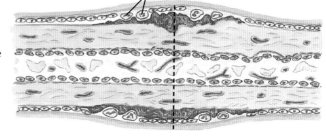

Remodeling

Osteoclastic and osteoblastic activity converts woven bone to lamellar bone with true haversian systems. Normal bone contours are restored; even angulation may be partially or completely corrected.

HEALING OF FRACTURE

Bone is unique among organs in its ability to heal a full-thickness injury by complete regeneration rather than by production of scar tissue. Although the biologic response of bone to a fracture can be modified by the method of treatment, it is useful to consider the typical biologic events that occur in the healing of a simple fracture in a nonimmobilized bone. The stages of fracture healing include inflammation, repair via soft callus and hard callus, and remodeling (see Plate 7-24). The blood supply, oxygen tension, and movement at the fracture site change as normal fracture healing progresses, and these changes have profound effects on subsequent events at the fracture site. At impact, periosteal and medullary blood vessels are ruptured, a hematoma forms, and inflammatory mediators accumulate at the fracture site.

STAGES OF HEALING

Inflammation

The stage of inflammation begins at the time of injury when bleeding at the fracture site from the bone and surrounding soft tissue causes hematoma formation. The organization of the fracture hematoma is one of the earliest stages of fracture repair. The damaged cells release inflammatory mediators that cause local edema and attract inflammatory cells. Inflammatory mediators promote local angiogenesis, and as the process progresses fibroblasts and chondrocytes are recruited that begin to form callus. The type of healing that occurs, and the rate at which it does, is dependent on intrinsic characteristics of the bone based on location and on extrinsic factors such as the method of treatment.

Repair—Formation of Soft Callus

The fracture hematoma is replaced with granulation tissue containing many of the cells responsible for healing at the fracture site. The development of soft callus involves the early formation of external bridging callus as well as the late formation of medullary callus. Soft callus formation is characterized by vigorous mitotic and metabolic activity and may at times be mistaken for a low-grade connective tissue malignancy.

Repetitive micromovement at the fracture site is an important mechanical stimulus for the formation of soft callus. The soft callus is composed of fibrous tissue, cartilage, and woven bone and provides mechanical scaffolding for the formation of hard bony callus, which stabilizes and eventually bridges the fracture gap. Despite the intense angiogenesis that accompanies soft callus formation, oxygen tension at the fracture site is low and pH is acidic. The callus formed at the periphery is harder and that formed in the central region is composed of more cartilage and fibrous tissue. The intense cellularity of the soft callus far outstrips the increased oxygen supply stimulated by angiogenesis. If the vascular supply is interrupted early in fracture healing, the regenerative response is impaired, preventing normal fracture repair.

Repair—Formation of Hard Callus

The transition from soft callus to hard callus occurs 3 to 4 weeks into the fracture healing process with the appearance of calcified cartilage, and it continues until

Plate 7-25   Musculoskeletal System: PART III

PRIMARY UNION

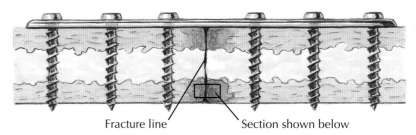

If fractured bone ends compressed securely so that no motion can take place between them, callus does not form. Dead bone at fracture site not resorbed but revitalized by ingrowth of haversian systems.

Fracture line   Section shown below

Mechanism of healing by primary union

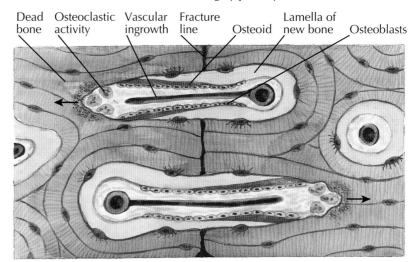

Dead bone Osteoclastic activity Vascular ingrowth Fracture line Osteoid Lamella of new bone Osteoblasts

Osteoclasts ream out tunnels through dead bone at fracture edges and across fracture line into opposite bone fragment. Osteoblasts line new tunnels and lay down new lamellae around them to form new osteons, restoring continuity of bone.

HEALING OF FRACTURE
(Continued)

the bone ends are firmly united. The process of hard callus formation mimics similar events in the normal growth plate. Calcified cartilage provides a scaffold for osteoblasts and for the subsequent deposition and mineralization of bone matrix. Primitive fiber bone at the fracture site is eventually transformed into normal lamellar bone in both medullary and external bridging callus. Blood supply and oxygen tension at the fracture site continue to increase during this stage.

Remodeling

The final stage of fracture healing, the stage of remodeling, begins about 6 weeks after fracture and may continue for weeks or months until the process is complete. During this stage, the abundant hard callus (external bridging callus and medullary callus) is slowly remodeled from immature woven bone into mature lamellar bone. During remodeling, the oxygen tension at the fracture site returns to normal.

Clinically, fracture healing is complete when bone strength at the fracture site has been restored to normal and the marrow space is re-formed. This may occur as soon as 6 weeks after fracture. Radiographic evidence of healing may also be seen as early as 6 weeks after fracture. Biologically, a fracture is considered healed when all regenerative processes at the fracture site have ceased. A bone scan may show increased metabolic activity at the fracture site for months or years while remodeling continues.

PRIMARY UNION

Primary union of bone does not occur normally in nature, but it can be induced artificially with internal fixation and rigid immobilization along with anatomic alignment (see Plate 7-25). Primary cortical union is not true bone regeneration but rather recruitment of normal remodeling processes to bridge the fracture gap. Compared with inductive callus healing, the process of primary union is extremely slow.

Complete immobilization inhibits the formation of inductive callus but promotes primary cortical union. When a rigid compression plate is affixed to a fracture, the necrotic cortical bone at the fracture site is not resorbed as in the normal process of inductive callus healing. Rather, the dead bone is recanalized by new

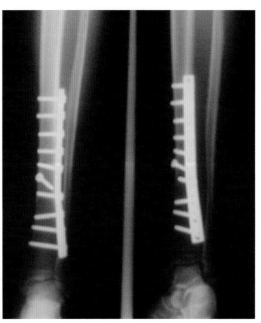

Fracture healing by primary union. Radiograph shows lack of callus formation.

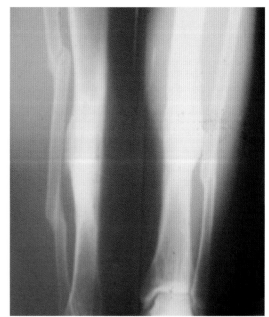

Fracture healing by inductive callus formation. Radiograph shows exuberant callus formation.

haversian systems with mature osteons, as occurs in normal bone remodeling. New bone also arises from endosteum to bridge the fracture gap. Revascularization occurs from adjacent medullary vessels.

Unlike inductive callus formation, which includes both external bridging callus and late medullary callus, primary union of cortical bone cannot effectively bridge gaps at a fracture site. For primary union to occur, the fracture gap must be obliterated by perfect apposition and compression of the fractured bone ends. In

addition, movement at the fracture site must be minimal. The bone's ability to heal by primary union depends on rigid immobilization, which enables the fragile medullary vessels to recanalize the necrotic bone and cross the fracture site. When the bone is healed, tolerance to total rigidity is excellent. The major disadvantages of primary union are its slowness compared with inductive callus formation and the need for artificial stability with rigid internal fixation to be maintained for a long period of time.

Plate 7-26

Injury to Musculoskeletal System

FACTORS THAT PROMOTE OR DELAY BONE HEALING

Factors that promote

Pituitary → Growth hormone

Thyroid → Thyroid hormones / Calcitonin

Pancreas → Insulin

Adrenal cortex   Gonads → Anabolic hormones

GI tract → Normal absorption of nutrients

Electric stimulation of bone

Vitamin D → Promotion of calcification

Vitamin C, retinoic acid, TGF-β, BMP

Exercise, weight bearing → Stimulation of physiologic bone growth

Youth → Rapid bone growth

Factors that delay

Corticosteroids / NSAIDs ← Adrenal cortex

Diabetes mellitus ← Pancreas

Deficiency of sex hormone ← Gonads

Poor oxygenation ← Anemia

Deficiency of vitamin D or its conversion to $1,25(OH)_2D$ / Osteomalacia ←

Excessive bone gap or motion ← Large bone defect or interposition of soft tissue

Impaired bone nutrition or vitality ← Loss of soft tissue, vascular injury, x-ray irradiation

Bone damage ← Infection, neoplasm

Synovial fluid fibrolysin ← Intra-articular fracture

Deficiency or abnormality of bone substance ← Osteoporosis, Paget disease of bone

Slow bone growth ← Advanced age

HEALING OF FRACTURE

(Continued)

FACTORS THAT PROMOTE BONE HEALING

Fracture healing is a complex regenerative process that begins at the moment of fracture and continues until all reparative events have ceased. Numerous endocrine, paracrine, autocrine, biochemical, and biophysical factors are involved in successful fracture healing, and an excess or deficiency of many of these factors impairs the regenerative response to fracture (see Plate 7-26). Although some factors play a role throughout healing, others are more critical at specific and limited times.

Peptide and steroid hormones help regulate fracture healing. Growth hormone, insulin, thyroid hormone, cortisol, and gonadal steroids all have important functions throughout the process of fracture healing; each of these hormones has cell membrane or nuclear receptors in the tissues involved in the regenerative response. Vitamin D and its active metabolites as well as parathyroid hormone are essential for normal mineralization of bone in the later stages of fracture healing.

Vitamin C is vital in fracture healing and in posttranslational modification of collage, the most abundant matrix component in both soft and hard callus. An adequate supply of amino acids, carbohydrates, fats, and trace elements is also critical for normal fracture healing.

Physical factors such as microenvironment and weight bearing are essential in the production of a normal inductive callus and are therefore essential in the promotion of bone healing.

FACTORS THAT DELAY BONE HEALING

Numerous factors are known to retard or inhibit bone repair. Glucocorticoid excess, for example, can lead to severe osteopenia, imperiling fracture healing; juvenile diabetes has the same potential effect. A deficiency of gonadal steroids in either men or women can also result in profound osteopenia, which slows the regenerative response after a fracture. Severe anemia can alter oxygen tensions at the fracture site. Deficiencies of vitamin D or its metabolites cause abnormal mineralization of the fracture callus, delaying fracture healing or causing nonunion.

The regenerative response is interrupted by large bone gaps due to the interposition of soft tissue and by devitalization of bone by irradiation, vascular loss, injury, loss of soft tissue, or denervation. Infections and neoplasm can retard fracture healing by some unknown mechanisms. The regenerative response can also be interrupted by components in the synovial fluid bathing the fragments of an intra-articular fracture, resulting in delayed union or nonunion. Severe osteoporosis from any cause, as well as metabolic diseases such as hyperparathyroidism, osteomalacia, Paget disease of bone, or fibrous dysplasia, can retard the regenerative response to a fracture.

Fractures heal more slowly in older persons than in children and young adults. Poor general nutrition and lack of vitamin C can have a direct inhibitory effect on the production of extracellular matrix, which can disrupt the formation of both soft and hard callus. Although movement can stimulate fracture healing, too little or too much movement disrupts endochondral callus formation, which may have important implications for fracture healing. Cigarette smoke has a negative effect on bone healing and increases the risk of nonunion. Nonsteroidal anti-inflammatory drugs have a negative impact on bone healing and should be avoided if possible during fracture healing as well.

SOFT TISSUE INFECTIONS

Plate 8-1

Musculoskeletal System: PART III

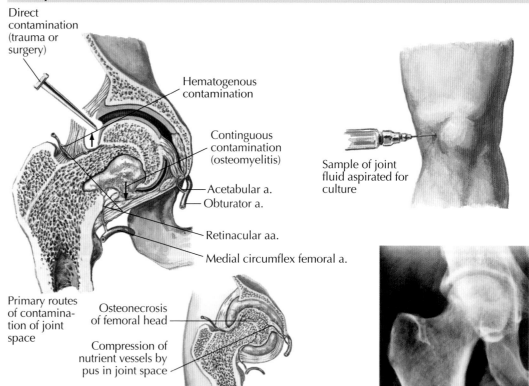

Septic bursitis

Tense, swollen prepatellar bursa

Normal joint space

Line of incision

Cellulitis and induration

Incision and drainage often necessary

JOHN A.CRAIG—AD

Repetitive trauma may cause small punctures in bursa. Bacterial contamination leads to septic bursitis, which may be confused with arthritis.

Septic arthritis

Direct contamination (trauma or surgery)

Hematogenous contamination

Continguous contamination (osteomyelitis)

Acetabular a.

Obturator a.

Retinacular aa.

Medial circumflex femoral a.

Sample of joint fluid aspirated for culture

Primary routes of contamination of joint space

Osteonecrosis of femoral head

Compression of nutrient vessels by pus in joint space

Some joints, such as hip, require prompt surgical decompression to avoid damage to vascular supply.

When vascular supply is damaged, osteonecrosis occurs, leading to collapse of femoral head.

SEPTIC JOINT

SEPTIC BURSITIS

The human body contains more than 150 bursae, which are sacs or potential spaces lined with a synovial membrane and containing synovial fluid. Bursae, located in the subcutaneous tissue over bony prominences, permit virtually friction-free movement of the skin over these prominences, minimizing irritation. With excessive irritation or use of a joint, a bursa can become inflamed and swollen as more synovial fluid is produced to lubricate the movement of adjacent tissues (see Plate 8-1). Excessive irritation can come from the outside of the bursa (knee rubbing on the floor) or from inside the bursa (bone spur). The bursal swelling becomes chronic and persistent, leading to conditions such as housemaid knee.

Direct trauma to the skin overlying the bursa can seed the fluid in an inflamed, swollen bursa with bacteria. The fluid is an excellent medium for bacterial growth, and the infection leads to extensive cellulitis (skin) or septic bursitis, characterized by heat, swelling, marked local tenderness, and loss of range of motion of the adjacent joint.

Treatment of septic bursitis consists of needle aspiration of the bursa to obtain fluid for culture, administration of appropriate antibiotics, and continuous application of warm, moist compresses to the area of inflammation. If the infected bursa does not respond quickly to such local treatment, it should be incised and drained.

SEPTIC ARTHRITIS

Septic arthritis occurs when a joint is seeded with an infective organism, either by direct contamination through traumatic or operative penetration of the joint, by contiguous spread of infection from osteomyelitis in an adjacent bone, or by hematogenous spread from bacteremia resulting from a distant focus of infection in the body. Hematogenous septic arthritis is particularly common in children, especially in the hip. Because of the unique blood supply to the femoral head, the accumulation of pus under pressure within the hip joint can compress the nutrient vessels to the femoral head. If the pressure persists for more than a few hours, osteonecrosis can develop. Therefore, in a child's hip, the

development of pus under pressure as a consequence of septic arthritis must be treated as an emergency. Immediate drainage of the fluid and pus is essential not only to treat the infection but also to avoid the devastating complication of osteonecrosis of the femoral head.

The general principles of the treatment of septic arthritis are similar to those of the treatment of septic bursitis. Aspirated joint fluid is cultured to determine appropriate antibiotics. Aspirations should be repeated

as needed to remove the infected and necrotic material from the joint. In most cases, the most effective way to remove the pus is by incision and drainage of the joint, followed by thorough irrigation. Aggressive early treatment usually results in complete resolution of the infection without residual joint problems. Persistent smoldering infections, however, will destroy the articular cartilage, leading to postinfection arthritis and sometimes complete destruction of the joint.

Plate 8-2

Soft Tissue Infections

ETIOLOGY AND PREVALENCE OF HEMATOGENOUS OSTEOMYELITIS

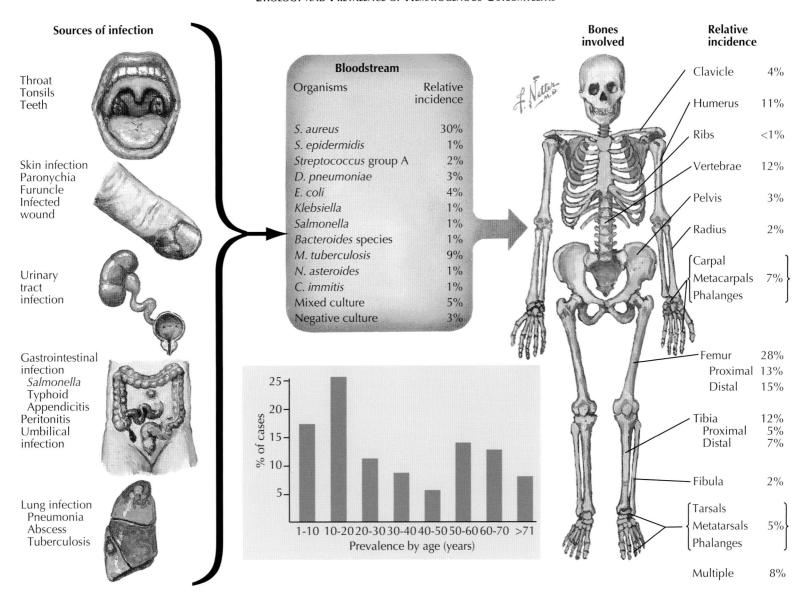

Sources of infection

Throat
Tonsils
Teeth

Skin infection
Paronychia
Furuncle
Infected
wound

Urinary
tract
infection

Gastrointestinal
infection
Salmonella
Typhoid
Appendicitis
Peritonitis
Umbilical
infection

Lung infection
Pneumonia
Abscess
Tuberculosis

Bloodstream	
Organisms	Relative incidence
S. aureus	30%
S. epidermidis	1%
Streptococcus group A	2%
D. pneumoniae	3%
E. coli	4%
Klebsiella	1%
Salmonella	1%
Bacteroides species	1%
M. tuberculosis	9%
N. asteroides	1%
C. immitis	1%
Mixed culture	5%
Negative culture	3%

Prevalence by age (years) — % of cases: 1-10, 10-20, 20-30, 30-40, 40-50, 50-60, 60-70, >71

Bones involved	Relative incidence
Clavicle	4%
Humerus	11%
Ribs	<1%
Vertebrae	12%
Pelvis	3%
Radius	2%
Carpal / Metacarpals / Phalanges	7%
Femur	28%
Proximal	13%
Distal	15%
Tibia	12%
Proximal	5%
Distal	7%
Fibula	2%
Tarsals / Metatarsals / Phalanges	5%
Multiple	8%

OSTEOMYELITIS

An infection of bone, osteomyelitis takes two forms, based on the source of the contamination. Hematogenous osteomyelitis results from an infection carried in the bloodstream. Exogenous (nonhematogenous) osteomyelitis is caused by spread from a nearby infection, open fractures, and surgical procedures in which the bone is penetrated and contaminated.

ETIOLOGY AND PREVALENCE OF HEMATOGENOUS OSTEOMYELITIS

In contrast to direct contamination of the bone from exogenous sources, hematogenous osteomyelitis results when the bone is seeded with bacteria from a distant site of infection in the body (see Plate 8-2). Common sources of infection are the throat, teeth, skin, urinary tract, gastrointestinal tract, and lungs. Infection in these locations can produce showers of bacteria in the bloodstream (bacteremia). Although the reticuloendothelial system clears most of these bacteria from the

bloodstream, occasionally a few settle in the bone, creating a focus of infection. The areas of bone particularly vulnerable to hematogenous infection are the metaphyses of the long bones—especially the humerus, femur, and tibia. The organisms that cause hematogenous osteomyelitis are the same as those responsible for the primary infection; the most common pathogen is *Staphylococcus aureus.* Gram-negative infections are commonly the results of seeding from a primary infection in the urinary tract, usually secondary to medical instrumentation or catheterization.

Hematogenous osteomyelitis is usually seen in children but may develop in adults (particularly those who are immunocompromised); a second, fairly high peak in occurrence is seen in persons between 50 and 70 years of age.

PATHOGENESIS OF HEMATOGENOUS OSTEOMYELITIS

Hematogenous osteomyelitis is particularly common in growing children for several reasons. Children are especially susceptible to bacterial infections in general and,

therefore, are likely to have frequent primary infectious foci and frequent episodes of bacteremia, which can lead to osteomyelitis. In addition, the peculiar anatomy of the growth plate may also play a substantial role in the development of hematogenous osteomyelitis in this age group. Virtually all cases of hematogenous osteomyelitis in children seem to originate in the metaphyseal bone, just beneath the growth plate. In this region, the terminal branches of the metaphyseal arteries form loops and enter afferent venous sinusoids, which are large and irregular (see Plate 8-3). The size of the vessels increases markedly from the metaphyseal artery to the venous sinusoids, and blood flow slows and becomes turbulent. The abrupt change in the dynamics of blood flow may allow bacteria to sludge and accumulate in this region, creating a focus of infection. Also, the cells in and around the venous sinusoids have little or no phagocytic activity, thus creating an ideal environment for bacterial growth.

After the bone is seeded with bacteria from the bloodstream, rapid bacterial duplication creates a localized abscess just beneath the growth plate. The developing abscess extends along the Volkmann canals to the

Plate 8-3   Musculoskeletal System: PART III

PATHOGENESIS OF HEMATOGENOUS OSTEOMYELITIS

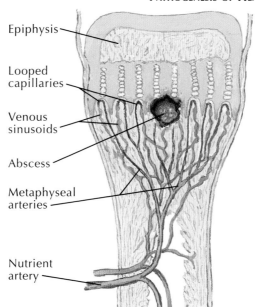

Epiphysis

Looped capillaries

Venous sinusoids

Abscess

Metaphyseal arteries

Nutrient artery

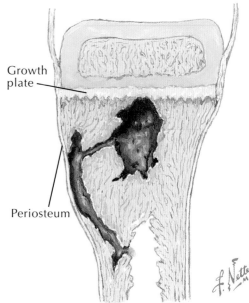

Growth plate

Periosteum

Terminal branches of metaphyseal arteries form loops at growth plate and enter irregular afferent venous sinusoids. Blood flow slowed and turbulent, predisposing to bacterial seeding. In addition, lining cells have little or no phagocytic activity. Area is catch basin for bacteria, and abscess may form.

Abscess, limited by growth plate, spreads transversely along Volkmann canals and elevates periosteum; extends subperiosteally and may invade shaft. In infants under 1 year of age, some metaphyseal arterial branches pass through growth plate, and infection may invade epiphysis and joint.

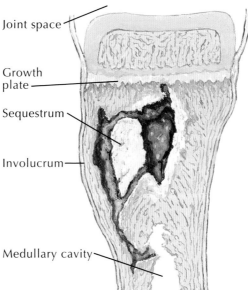

Joint space

Growth plate

Sequestrum

Involucrum

Medullary cavity

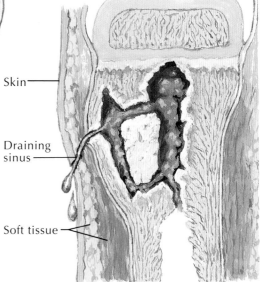

Skin

Draining sinus

Soft tissue

As abscess spreads, segment of devitalized bone (sequestrum) remains within it. Elevated periosteum may also lay down bone to form encasing shell (involucrum). Occasionally, abscess walled off by fibrosis and bone sclerosis to form Brodie abscess.

Infectious process may erode periosteum and form sinus through soft tissues and skin to drain externally. Process influenced by virulence of organism, resistance of host, administration of antibiotics, and fibrotic and sclerotic responses.

OSTEOMYELITIS (Continued)

subperiosteal region, where it elevates the thick periosteum. Elevation of the periosteum eventually stimulates the formation of new bone. Further extension of the abscess may cause it to rupture through the periosteum and extend to the subcutaneous tissue and then through the skin, creating a draining sinus. The infection may extend subperiosteally along the shaft of the bone; this extension strips a portion of the shaft of its blood supply and produces a dense, avascular piece of cortical bone called a sequestrum. The sequestrum, lacking a blood supply to deliver antibiotics or inflammatory cells to fight infection, acts as a nidus for the infection to persist.

In an attempt to wall off and isolate the infection, the elevated periosteum lays down new bone. This new bone, called an involucrum, is composed of new subperiosteal bone much like that found in a new fracture callus. Thus, histologically acute hematogenous osteomyelitis creates rarefaction in the metaphysis of the long bone due to the destruction of normal cancellous bone, forms sequestra, and creates an involucrum of new bone around the periphery of the infection.

Except in very young children, the infection rarely extends across the physical barrier of the growth plate. In children younger than 1 year of age, some branches of the metaphyseal arteries pass through the growth

plate to nourish the epiphysis. The passageways for these vessels allow the infection to spread into the epiphysis, then into the adjacent joint space itself.

Occasionally, the body's immune response can effectively eradicate a minor infection in the metaphysis. If the area of infection is walled off and the infecting bacteria are killed, the small, residual abscess cavity may persist indefinitely. The cavity, composed of fibrous tissue but containing no residual viable bacteria, is

called a Brodie abscess, even though there is no residual active infection present. In contrast, a more aggressive and virulent infection continues to destroy bone and eventually creates a draining sinus. The sinus will drain until the necrotic and infected tissue is completely removed and replaced with fibrous tissue or noninfected bone.

Early and aggressive diagnosis and treatment of hematogenous osteomyelitis can arrest the destruction

Plate 8-4

Soft Tissue Infections

CLINICAL MANIFESTATIONS OF HEMATOGENOUS OSTEOMYELITIS

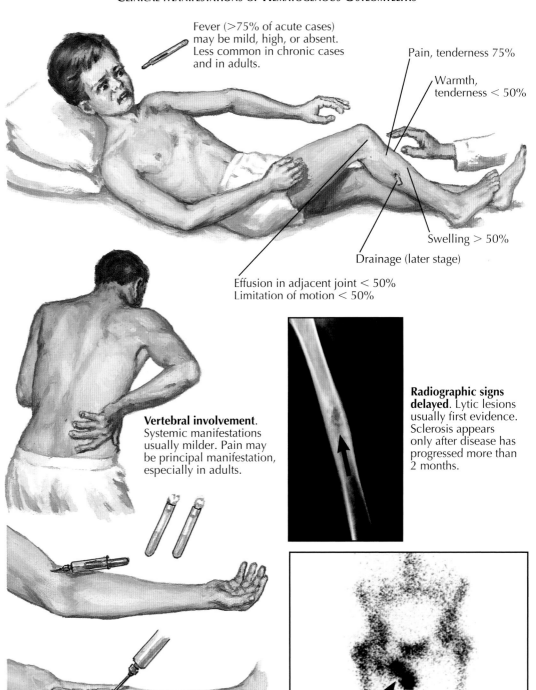

Fever (>75% of acute cases) may be mild, high, or absent. Less common in chronic cases and in adults.

Pain, tenderness 75%

Warmth, tenderness < 50%

Swelling > 50%

Drainage (later stage)

Effusion in adjacent joint < 50%
Limitation of motion < 50%

Vertebral involvement. Systemic manifestations usually milder. Pain may be principal manifestation, especially in adults.

Radiographic signs delayed. Lytic lesions usually first evidence. Sclerosis appears only after disease has progressed more than 2 months.

Indium-labeled leukocyte scintigram. Showing focal signal increase (arrow) and can be useful in early diagnosis

Blood culture and bone aspiration or open biopsy required to establish diagnosis and identify organism for choice of antibiotic therapy

OSTEOMYELITIS (Continued)

of normal, healthy bone by the extending abscess. Treatment includes administration of bacteria-specific antibiotics and surgical drainage of the infectious focus. Usually, antibiotics are administered intravenously over a period of at least 4 weeks, but they can be required for longer periods (months). Sometimes oral antibiotics can be used later in the treatment. Therefore, it is especially important to understand the early clinical manifestations of this disease so that appropriate therapy can be initiated promptly.

CLINICAL MANIFESTATIONS

Signs and symptoms of hematogenous osteomyelitis are fever, chills, malaise, and pain localized, to some degree, to the area of infection (see Plate 8-4). Fever is present in more than 75% of patients, although it is less common when the infection has been present for a long time. The patient usually reports malaise, decreased appetite, and generalized weakness. Point tenderness can be localized to the tissues around the infected area, and deep palpation also elicits tenderness. Osteomyelitis causes pain when the involved area is moved or used. For example, a child with acute hematogenous osteomyelitis of the distal femur appears reluctant to stand or walk on the infected limb. Generalized soft tissue

swelling develops about the area of infection, and, on palpation, the area feels warm to the touch. A so-called sympathetic effusion often develops in an adjacent joint. This reactive swelling of the joint occurs in response to the infection of the nearby bone, but the effusion contains no pathogenic bacteria. Active range of motion of a joint with sympathetic effusion is limited by the pain secondary to the bone infection. Drainage from the abscess is a manifestation of chronic infection only and

is not seen in the acute stages of hematogenous osteomyelitis.

Clinical manifestations of acute hematogenous osteomyelitis of the spine are more difficult to define. The patient may complain of a vague backache as well as generalized malaise, decreased appetite, and fever. Pain restricts the active range of motion of the back, and gentle percussion over the spinous processes often causes significant discomfort. This constellation of

Plate 8-5

Musculoskeletal System: PART III

DIRECT (NONHEMATOGENOUS) CAUSES OF OSTEOMYELITIS

Traumatic infections

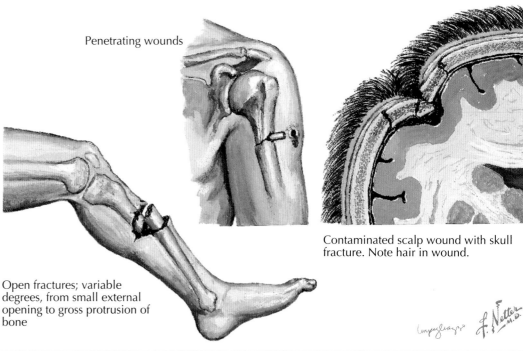

Penetrating wounds

Open fractures; variable degrees, from small external opening to gross protrusion of bone

Contaminated scalp wound with skull fracture. Note hair in wound.

Operative infections

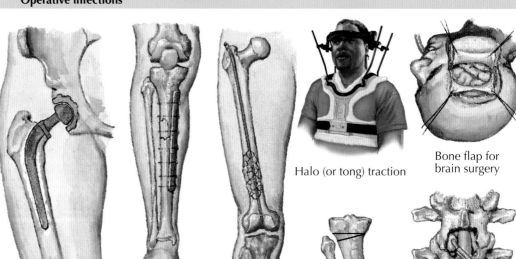

Total joint replacement (loosening of prosthesis usually occurs but does not necessarily indicate infection)

Internal fixation of fractures

Tumor resection with bone graft for limb salvage

Halo (or tong) traction

Bone flap for brain surgery

Osteotomy for limb alignment, limb lengthening, and other orthopedic procedures

Laminectomy for disc surgery or other spinal cord compression

OSTEOMYELITIS *(Continued)*

symptoms is not specific to osteomyelitis, and diagnosis of osteomyelitis may often be overlooked in the many patients who complain of backache. Frequently, osteomyelitis of the spine is secondary to a urinary tract infection. Therefore, a recent history of infection or surgical manipulation of the urinary tract should heighten the clinical suspicion of a secondary infection of the spine.

Diagnosis of hematogenous osteomyelitis requires a careful history, focusing on any recent infection at another site, such as the mouth and teeth, urinary tract, or throat. The physical examination should be thorough enough to identify any primary source of the infection. If the history and physical findings suggest hematogenous osteomyelitis, selected laboratory tests should be performed. A complete blood cell count often reveals an elevated leukocyte count with a shift to the left in the differential. Frequently, acute phase reactants, namely, the erythrocyte sedimentation rate and C-reactive protein, are elevated as well.

Radiographs of the painful area should be obtained, although radiographic signs are often minimal early in the infection. The earliest radiographic evidence of acute hematogenous osteomyelitis is swelling of soft tissue adjacent to the bone; within a few days of onset, lysis in the metaphyseal region becomes visible.

Periosteal elevation with its new bone formation and the creation of sequestra become obvious on radiographs after a couple of weeks. A technetium-99m bone scan is an extremely sensitive test for identification of areas of inflammation in the bone. However, the test is not particularly specific to bone infection, because it is also positive after fracture or any other condition that irritates the periosteum and causes new bone formation. Magnetic resonance imaging will reveal edema or

inflammation or show a collection of pus if present in the bone.

Recently, radioactively labeled leukocytes have been used to diagnose a focus of osteomyelitis. In this technique, a blood sample is drawn from the patient; the leukocyte cells are cultured and labeled with radioactive indium-111 and then reinjected into the patient. As leukocytes tend to accumulate at a focus of infection, the indium-labeled leukocytes also tend to focus in the

Plate 8-6

Soft Tissue Infections

DIRECT (NONHEMATOGENOUS) CAUSES OF OSTEOMYELITIS (CONTINUED)

Secondary to contiguous focus of infection

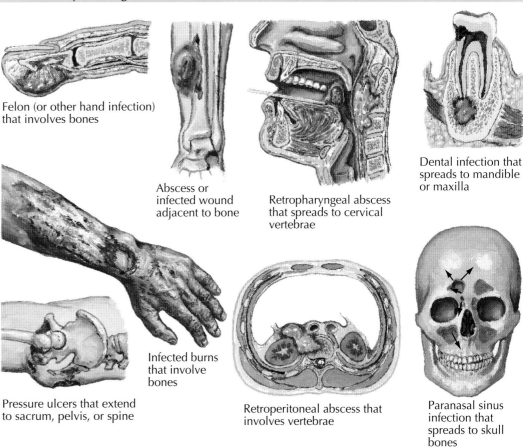

Felon (or other hand infection) that involves bones

Abscess or infected wound adjacent to bone

Retropharyngeal abscess that spreads to cervical vertebrae

Dental infection that spreads to mandible or maxilla

Pressure ulcers that extend to sacrum, pelvis, or spine

Infected burns that involve bones

Retroperitoneal abscess that involves vertebrae

Paranasal sinus infection that spreads to skull bones

Contributory or predisposing factors

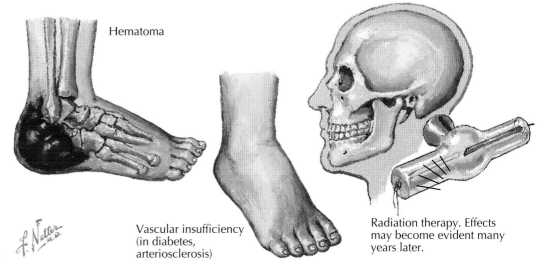

Hematoma

Vascular insufficiency (in diabetes, arteriosclerosis)

Radiation therapy. Effects may become evident many years later.

OSTEOMYELITIS *(Continued)*

infected area. The radioactivity can be identified on a scan performed 24 to 72 hours after reinjection.

The specific pathogen responsible for the osteomyelitis must be identified so that appropriate antibiotic therapy can be instituted. Although blood cultures often reveal the infecting organism, the most reliable way to identify the pathogen is direct aspiration of the osteomyelitic focus itself.

ETIOLOGY OF EXOGENOUS OSTEOMYELITIS

Exogenous (nonhematogenous) osteomyelitis results from the direct contamination of the bone by the infecting organism. The skin, subcutaneous tissue, and periosteum provide a protective barrier to contaminants; and as long as the skin and periosteum remain intact, the bone cannot be contaminated directly. These barriers can be violated by trauma (e.g., bullet wound, open fracture, direct blow) or by surgery, or they can be stripped away during displacement of fracture fragments (see Plate 8-5). When the protective skin is penetrated and the bone exposed, bacteria may invade the area, creating a focus of infection. Bone may also be contaminated during total joint replacement, application of traction-fixation devices, and implantation of fracture fixation devices. Even when careful surgical

dissection is combined with thorough debridement and prophylactic administration of antibiotics, infection occurs in about 1% of major surgical interventions.

During the implantation of artificial joints and fixation devices, the blood supply is often stripped from the bone, creating areas of dead bone. The dead bone acts as a sequestrum, allowing a bacterial infection to persist. Osteomyelitis may become chronic, persisting until the necrotic sequestrum is completely removed and the

foreign body, whether a fracture fixation device or total joint prosthesis, is removed.

Certain soft tissue infections may spread to adjacent bones (see Plate 8-6). For example, large soft tissue abscesses may erode the periosteum to infect the underlying bone. An infection of the pulp of the fingertip, called a felon, frequently extends to and infects the distal phalanx, to which the fibrous septa of the pulp of the finger are firmly attached. Retropharyngeal

Plate 8-7

Musculoskeletal System: PART III

OSTEOMYELITIS AFTER OPEN FRACTURE

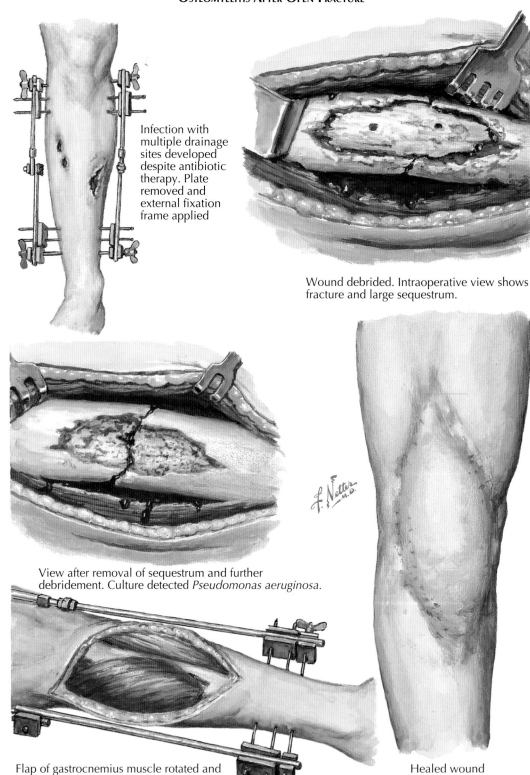

Infection with multiple drainage sites developed despite antibiotic therapy. Plate removed and external fixation frame applied

Wound debrided. Intraoperative view shows fracture and large sequestrum.

View after removal of sequestrum and further debridement. Culture detected *Pseudomonas aeruginosa.*

Flap of gastrocnemius muscle rotated and implanted into bone defect

Healed wound after skin graft

OSTEOMYELITIS (Continued)

abscesses tend to involve the cervical vertebrae, and periapical infections of the tooth frequently spread to the adjacent mandible or maxilla. Infection in the paranasal sinuses may extend to the adjacent bones of the skull.

Extensive soft tissue injury, such as pressure ulcers and third-degree burns, may erode through the periosteum, exposing the bone and leaving it vulnerable to infection. Similarly, radiation therapy destroys the adjacent soft tissue and damages the periosteum, making the bone and surrounding soft tissues more vulnerable to infection. One of the most common causes of bone infection in adults is the combination of vascular insufficiency and immunocompromise that occurs in diabetes mellitus. In diabetic patients, the foot is particularly susceptible to chronic skin ulcerations and secondary infection of the bone.

Although the many exogenous causes of osteomyelitis vary greatly, the resulting bone infections share some common characteristics. The bone becomes infected because the protective skin and periosteal barriers have been violated, allowing contamination of the bone. The infection usually persists because of the presence of necrotic soft tissue, necrotic bone, or a foreign body that serves as a nidus for continued bacterial proliferation.

Exogenous osteomyelitis can often be prevented immediately after an open fracture with early and thorough debridement of the contaminated and necrotic bone and administration of broad-spectrum antibiotics. Once established, exogenous osteomyelitis is very difficult to eradicate, and effective treatment requires surgical debridement of the infected necrotic bone, removal of infected foreign bodies (including implants),

and long-term intravenous administration of bacteria-specific antibiotics.

CHRONIC OSTEOMYELITIS

Bone infections are much more difficult to eradicate than soft tissue infections. Soft tissue cellulitis or abscess responds well to surgical drainage combined

Plate 8-8

Soft Tissue Infections

RECURRENT POSTOPERATIVE OSTEOMYELITIS

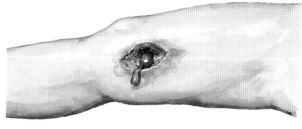

Closed fracture of femur due to skiing accident in 35-year-old woman. Fracture treated with intramedullary rod; drainage on medial side of distal thigh developed about 2 weeks after surgery. Blue staining of drainage fluid and around drainage site is due to methylene blue injected into sinus to track course.

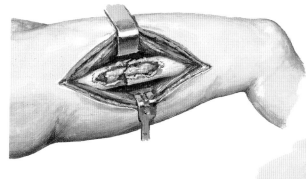

Intraoperative view. Primary problem found to be on lateral thigh even though drainage occurred on medial side. Large sequestrum revealed.

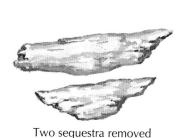

Two sequestra removed

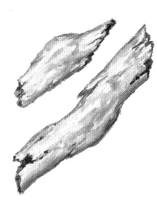

Additional sequestra surgically removed from lesion. Sinus tract excised, and all dead and infected tissue is thoroughly debrided.

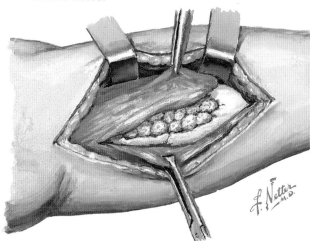

Bone defect after debridement and removal of sequestra. Wound closed.

Bone defect packed with cancellous bone autograft from ilium overlaid with muscle flap from vastus lateralis muscle. Patient remained free of pain and drainage.

OSTEOMYELITIS (Continued)

with the administration of appropriate antibiotics. However, simple surgical drainage combined with the administration of antibiotics may not eradicate chronic osteomyelitis. Bacteria become sequestered in the bone in areas where antibiotics cannot reach them in sufficient concentration owing to poor vascular penetration. A necrotic bone sequestrum or a fracture fixation device can act as a nidus for continued bacterial proliferation. Only removal of all of the necrotic bone and the foreign body can control the infection. This treatment often necessitates radical surgical debridement with removal of large segments of bone, creating significant mechanical instability and loss of function. In some patients, the infection can be fully eradicated only with amputation. Plates 8-7 and 8-8 depict two cases of chronic or recurrent osteomyelitis associated with unsuccessful plating of an open fracture and intramedullary rod fixation of a closed fracture.

Chronic osteomyelitis frequently manifests as one or more draining sinuses. The drainage is green or yellow, often thick, and usually foul smelling. Radiographs of the infected area show dense sclerotic bone characteristic of a sequestrum. Often, the fracture fixation devices loosen.

Treatment of chronic osteomyelitis requires removal of all infected, necrotic bone and all metal foreign bodies; debridement of all necrotic soft tissue; and marsupialization of the necrotic, infected bed. Stability of the limb can often be maintained with the use of an external fixation device that bridges the area of infection (see Plate 8-7). Repeated debridement is often necessary to ensure that all the infected, necrotic tissue is excised. Tissue samples should be obtained from the depths of the wound and cultured to determine the appropriate antibiotics. Antibiotics are then administered intravenously until the wound heals. Between debridements, the wounds are packed open; dressings are changed daily to remove any residual necrotic material while encouraging the development of granulation tissue in the base of the wound. Some researchers recommend the use of hyperbaric oxygen as a supplement to this treatment regimen. Hyperbaric oxygen therapy enhances the function of leukocytes and promotes the growth of granulation tissue.

Plate 8-9

Musculoskeletal System: PART III

DELAYED POSTTRAUMATIC OSTEOMYELITIS IN DIABETIC PATIENT

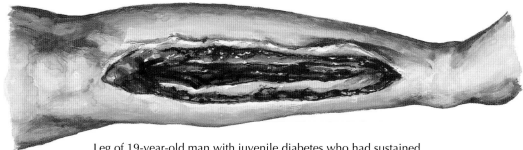

Leg of 19-year-old man with juvenile diabetes who had sustained closed fracture of tibia at age 7. Fracture healed, but hematogenous osteomyelitis later developed in area of decreased resistance. Drainage and tissue breakdown continued for many years, resulting in extensive, oozing wound.

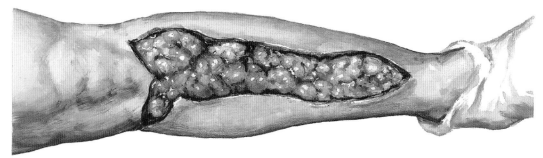

Leg after extensive debridement, removal of sequestra, and packing of cavity with omentum

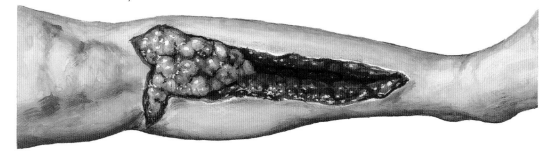

Proximal part of omentum transplant remained viable but distal section died, although good, clean granulation tissue developed there. Distal bone defect filled with cancellous bone graft, and wound healed uneventfully.

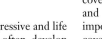

Limb healed with scarring despite skin graft; no drainage or pain

OSTEOMYELITIS *(Continued)*

When the base of the wound is fully covered with granulation tissue, a local muscle flap or a free vascularized myocutaneous flap can be transferred to the defect to provide soft tissue coverage. If the entire underlying bone architecture has been destroyed by the infection, bone grafts are needed to repair the bone after the infection is completely eradicated (see Plate 8-8).

The goal of treatment is to eliminate the draining sinuses and produce a functional limb that is free from pain. The complicated process just described to eradicate a focus of osteomyelitis is very expensive and time consuming. In some patients, amputation of the infected part may be the most reliable and effective way of restoring a pain-free and productive life.

DELAYED POSTTRAUMATIC OSTEOMYELITIS IN DIABETIC PATIENT

Infection in a diabetic patient can be aggressive and life threatening (see Plate 8-9). Infections often develop around skin ulcerations in the foot. The patient's impaired immune system allows the infection to ascend rapidly into the leg. Even after an aggressive soft tissue infection has been controlled, foot ulcers may persist.

The ulcers continue to drain, and the lack of soft tissue coverage over the bone exposes it to chronic irritation and the continued risk of infection. It is therefore important to try to achieve and maintain soft tissue coverage of such ulcerated areas.

The first step in the treatment of osteomyelitis associated with diabetes is extensive debridement of the necrotic tissue and removal of any underlying sequestra. When the necrotic, infected tissue has been removed, wet-to-dry dressings are applied to stimulate the formation of granulation tissue; hyperbaric oxygen therapy can further stimulate the development of a granulation tissue bed. Transplantation of vascularized tissue from other regions of the body (e.g., a vascularized omental graft) can also be performed to bring additional blood supply to the area to facilitate healing. Once a complete bed of granulation tissue develops, the defect can be covered with a split-thickness skin graft.

COMPLICATIONS OF FRACTURE

Plate 9-1

Musculoskeletal System: PART III

NEUROVASCULAR INJURY

Displacement of fracture fragments or bone ends at a dislocated joint carry the risk of producing compression or laceration of adjacent vessels and nerves (see Plate 9-1). Critical neurovascular structures (e.g., the brachial plexus) lie deep in the limb, close to the skeleton, which protects them from injuries. A fracture or dislocation makes nerves or vessels vulnerable to injury from sharp bone fragments or from entrapment in the fracture site.

Neurovascular complications must be identified by careful examination immediately after the injury and after any manipulation of the injured limb. Some complications are not immediately evident but appear 24 to 48 hours after injury. Re-examination and monitoring are essential both during this period and while circular compression dressings and casts are in place. Prompt and sometimes aggressive treatment is required to restore function and prevent permanent loss.

Radial Nerve Palsy. The radial nerve is the most commonly damaged nerve after fractures of the distal shaft of the humerus. Normally protected in the spiral groove of the humeral shaft, the nerve is susceptible to stretch, direct injury by a fracture fragment, or entrapment in the fracture site itself. Aggressive manipulation of the fracture during closed reduction may also result in nerve entrapment. Although wrist drop is the consequence of radial nerve injury, this is most often a neurapraxia, with nearly 100% recovery in low-energy trauma patients and over 33% recovery in high-energy trauma patients despite the method of treatment. Recovery of motor strength may take multiple months to occur, but radial nerve palsy in itself is usually not an indication for surgery.

Sciatic Nerve Palsy. Nerves and vessels at or near joints are particularly vulnerable to injury. The neurovascular structures are more securely tethered to the soft tissues around joints than elsewhere and are less likely to escape injury when significant joint displacement occurs. For example, the sciatic nerve is at risk in posterior dislocation of the hip, with injury occurring at a rate of approximately 13% in simple dislocations. Generally, the nerve is simply stretched or contused by direct impingement of the femoral head. The peroneal branch is most commonly affected, the sequela of which is foot drop. Immediate reduction of the dislocation relieves pressure on the nerve, and about two thirds of patients are likely to recover partial to full motor and sensory deficits. A possible indication for surgical exploration might be a patient in whom no neurologic deficits were present until after manipulation and reduction of the joint.

Neurovascular Injury About the Elbow. A musculoskeletal injury that is frequently associated with neurovascular injury is the supracondylar fracture of the humerus. It is most common in children between 3 and 10 years of age and usually results from a fall on the outstretched hand. In the most common type of fracture, hyperextension injury, the distal fracture fragment is displaced posteriorly, which can result in the critical neurovascular structures anterior to the elbow becoming tethered on the anterior edge of the fractured humeral shaft. The median nerve and the brachial artery are both particularly susceptible to direct injury

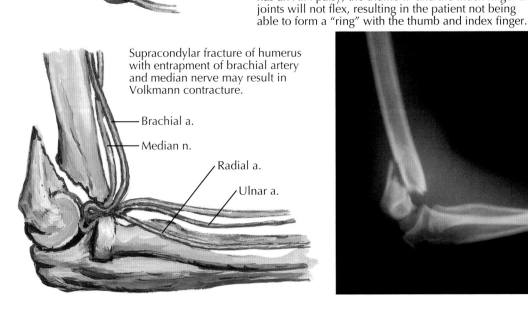

Fracture of shaft of humerus with entrapment of radial nerve in spiral groove

Wrist drop due to radial nerve injury

Foot drop due to sciatic (peroneal) nerve palsy

Posterior dislocation of hip. Femoral head may impinge on sciatic nerve, leading to nerve palsy (partial or complete).

Sciatic n.

In a patient with an intact anterior osseous nerve (AIN), the patient will form a normal "circle" or "ring" with the thumb and index finger. However, in a patient who has an AIN palsy, the thumb IP and the index finger DIP joints will not flex, resulting in the patient not being able to form a "ring" with the thumb and index finger.

Supracondylar fracture of humerus with entrapment of brachial artery and median nerve may result in Volkmann contracture.

Brachial a.

Median n.

Radial a.

Ulnar a.

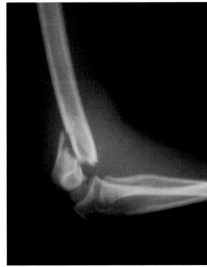

from the displaced fracture fragment and can be lacerated or entrapped in the fracture site at the time of injury or during the closed reduction. A common neurologic sequela is damage to a branch of the median nerve, the anterior interosseous nerve, which results in the inability to flex the interphalangeal joint of the thumb and the distal interphalangeal joint of the index finger. The anterior interosseous nerve is readily assessed by asking the patient to make an "OK sign" with the thumb and index finger. Distal neurovascular function must be assessed critically both before and

after any treatment, and manipulative reduction must be careful and gentle.

Compartment Syndrome. Direct damage to an artery or severe swelling in a muscle compartment can lead to development of compartment syndrome. This serious outcome is common after *any* fracture in which bleeding and swelling are extreme. Compartment syndromes can occur with open as well as with closed fractures and may also be caused by a circular cast. Failure to identify compartment syndrome early may lead to permanent loss of limb function.

Plate 9-2

Complications of Fracture

ADULT RESPIRATORY DISTRESS SYNDROME

Respiratory failure often develops 24 to 72 hours after severe musculoskeletal injury. The precise pathogenesis of the syndrome is not fully understood, and many etiologic factors play a role in its development, including pulmonary embolism, aspiration of gastric contents, pulmonary edema due to fluid overload or heart failure, atelectasis, and pneumonia. Although all these conditions may occur after trauma, a specific pattern of pulmonary deficit called adult respiratory distress syndrome (ARDS) results secondary to pulmonary edema. One possible trigger of ARDS is "fat embolism syndrome," which has been linked to fractures of long bones (see Plate 9-2). However, although fat embolism syndrome is more common after fractures of long bones, it has been reported after fracture in nearly every bone.

ARDS is characterized by the sudden onset of respiratory insufficiency and extreme arterial hypoxia in the immediate postinjury period. Clinical manifestations include fever, tachycardia, tachypnea, and mental confusion. Airway resistance increases, lung compliance progressively decreases, and pulmonary arteriovenous shunting becomes evident. If fat embolism syndrome is the cause of ARDS, petechiae often also develop, especially in the axillae, and arterial oxygen tension falls below 60 mm Hg.

Marrow emboli have been identified in the lungs of patients, leading to the term *fat embolism syndrome*, but ARDS may also develop in the absence of fracture marrow emboli. Studies have demonstrated the release of free fatty acids, cytokines, and other inflammatory cascade molecules into the blood stream, which produces characteristic pulmonary changes: congestion, atelectasis, venous and capillary engorgement, and interstitial edema. These pulmonary changes prevent the exchange of oxygen across the alveolocapillary membrane, resulting in profound systemic hypoxia. As a consequence, the patient becomes progressively more hypoxic and may die if the disorder is not treated aggressively. When ARDS is suggested, arterial oxygen tension should be determined. The severity of hypoxemia necessary to make the diagnosis of ARDS is defined by the ratio of the partial pressure of oxygen in the patient's arterial blood (Pao_2) to the fraction of oxygen in the inspired air (Fio_2). In ARDS, the Pao_2/Fio_2 ratio is less than 200.

Great debate exists among the trauma community regarding the best methods of reducing the incidence of ARDS that follows multiple-injury trauma. This has led to the term *damage control orthopaedics*, which refers to the theory that surgical management of patients should be staged to minimize the systemic effects of the patient sustaining subsequent iatrogenic trauma (i.e., surgery). Because patients with multiple injuries are already "primed" for systemic inflammation due to their injuries, clinicians must be mindful to not perform nonemergent procedures before medical optimization of the patient. Clinical evidence demonstrates that ARDS can be prevented, or at least minimized, by mobilizing the patient early and avoiding prolonged bed rest and traction. These precautions require immobilization of fractures as soon as possible after the injury. Intramedullary nailing of all long bone (especially femur) fractures should be performed in less than 24 hours from injury if possible. This reduces the risk of fat embolism syndrome, ARDS, and other medical complications such as large amounts of blood loss from unreduced fractures. This is particularly important in

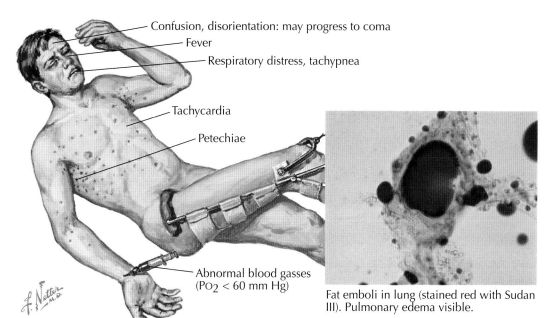

Confusion, disorientation: may progress to coma
Fever
Respiratory distress, tachypnea
Tachycardia
Petechiae
Abnormal blood gasses ($PO_2 < 60$ mm Hg)

Fat emboli in lung (stained red with Sudan III). Pulmonary edema visible.

Criteria for diagnosis of adult respiratory distress syndrome (ARDS) include an arterial partial pressure of oxygen/fraction of inspired oxygen (PaO_2/FIO_2) ratio less than 200 for 5 or more consecutive days, bilateral diffuse infiltrates on the chest radiograph in the absence of pneumonia, and absence of cardiogenic pulmonary edema. Associated findings of petechiae and confusion merge into systemic inflammatory response syndrome (SIRS).

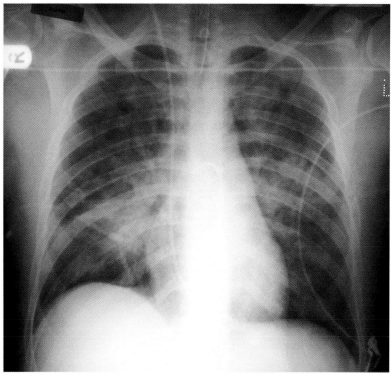

Chest radiograph in a patient with adult respiratory distress syndrome (ARDS) due to extrathoracic trauma. Bilateral airspace opacity is seen. *Reprinted with permission from Adam A, Dixon AK, Grainger RG, Allison DJ. Grainger & Allison's diagnostic radiology. 5th ed. Philadelphia: Elsevier; 2007.*

patients with multiple injuries. Intramedullary long bone fixation allows the patient to be mobilized immediately after fracture fixation, minimizing bed rest and eliminating the need for skeletal traction.

If promptly recognized and treated vigorously, the pulmonary changes of ARDS are possibly reversible. Failure to treat the patient aggressively may be fatal. Treatment focuses on correcting the hypoxemia and maintaining arterial oxygen tension greater than 70 mm Hg until the pulmonary lesions resolve. This essentially consists of improving oxygenation by way of utilizing

positive end-expiratory pressure (PEEP) to drive sufficient oxygen across the alveolocapillary membrane for adequate arterial oxygenation. Treatment may be required for 2 days to multiple weeks, depending on the severity of the pulmonary lesions. If oxygen delivered with a facemask does not restore the arterial oxygen tension to the desired level, mechanical ventilation with a closed system should be instituted. Even at this stage, fracture fixation to allow mobilization of the patient combined with vigorous respiratory therapy may help reverse the pulmonary insufficiency.

Plate 9-3

Musculoskeletal System: PART III

INFECTION

A fracture or dislocation becomes contaminated, and thus potentially infected, any time the protective layers of soft tissue enclosing the injury hematoma are violated. The hematoma is an excellent medium for the growth of bacteria, resulting in acute cellulitis or abscess or leading to a chronic deep infection of the bone (osteomyelitis). All skeletal injuries should be classified as open or closed immediately after injury. In an open fracture, the overlying skin and soft tissue have been penetrated; therefore, the fracture hematoma may be contaminated.

Classification of Open Fracture. Open fractures are graded by the severity of soft tissue damage, fracture pattern, and degree of contamination, as defined by Gustilo and Anderson (see Plate 9-3). In type I open fractures, the wound is less than 1 cm in length and is free of contamination. Type II fractures have a wound greater than 1 cm, but less than 10 cm, in length, and the soft tissues are not extensively stripped from the bone. In type IIIA fractures, the wound is larger than 10 cm but soft tissue coverage remains adequate. In type IIIB fractures, the wound is larger than 10 cm, the periosteum is stripped from the bone, and the bone is exposed. Type IIIC fractures have a large wound greater than 10 cm in length and have significant arterial injury that requires surgical repair. All type III injuries are generally considered contaminated and many times are the result of a high-energy gunshot, farm injury, or blast. Gustilo and colleagues noted that the incidence of infection was 1% for type I fractures, 1.8% for type II fractures, and 20.8% for type III fractures.

Contamination of Open Injury. The most important factors contributing to wound infection of an open fracture are the degree of contamination and the severity of the injury. However, even a type I wound may become infected if not adequately cleaned and treated. The potential for infection due to various strains of *Clostridium* (e.g., tetanus and gas gangrene, see Plate 9-5) always exists, because clostridia are ubiquitous and every contaminated wound may contain them.

Injuries at high risk for infection include wounds contaminated by manure or standing water (which often contains clostridia) and wounds caused by a high-velocity mechanism, such as a gunshot. An open fracture of the toe caused by a lawn mower blade, for example, is a very high-risk wound. The high velocity of the blade edge imparts tremendous energy, increasing soft tissue damage and the risk of contamination. Even in some wounds that appear trivial (e.g., a puncture in the sole of the foot caused by a rusty nail), particularly virulent organisms are inoculated deep into the wound, causing a significant infection. A puncture in the heel that penetrates the calcaneus would be classified as a type I wound; however, this type of puncture wound is notorious for becoming infected, in part because the initial treatment was inadequate. In addition, these puncture wounds are often contaminated by

Classification of open fractures

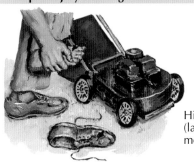

Type I. Wound <1 cm long with no evidence of contamination of deep tissues

Type II. Wound >1 cm long with no soft tissue stripped from bone

Type IIIA. Large wound with adequate soft tissue coverage of bone

Type IIIB. Large wound with periosteal stripping and exposed bone

Type IIIC. Open fracture with significant arterial injury that requires surgical repair

Open injury with high risk for infection

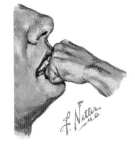

High-velocity trauma (laceration by lawn mower blade)

Penetration of metacarpophalangeal joint by tooth in fist fight

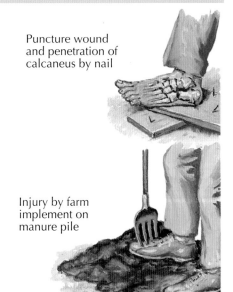

Puncture wound and penetration of calcaneus by nail

Injury by farm implement on manure pile

gram-negative organisms, such as *Pseudomonas*, which can cause a chronic infection that is very difficult to cure.

Puncture wounds resulting from human bites are also serious and are often initially overlooked by the patient. In a fist fight, a metacarpophalangeal joint may be punctured by a tooth and contaminated by anaerobic or microaerophilic bacteria contained in the mouth. These organisms can cause especially aggressive and destructive infections in the hand (see Section 8, Soft Tissue Infections, Plate 8-2). Because of this risk, the gold standard of treatment for all "fight bites" is surgical washout of the involved metacarpophalangeal joints.

Failure to remove contaminating organisms from an open fracture site may result in severe complications.

Acute infections with *Clostridium* species, as well as with streptococci and other bacteria, can lead to cellulitis, sepsis, and even death. Even if acute infections do not develop, osteomyelitis, a low-grade chronic infection of bone, may result (see Section 8, Soft Tissue Infections, Plates 8-2 to 8-9). This condition is distinguished from soft tissue infections by its persistence and severity. Once established, osteomyelitis is very difficult to eradicate. Although soft tissue infections are usually cured by incision and drainage, bacteria can become sequestered in bone, where perfusion is inadequate and bactericidal antibiotic levels cannot be achieved. Chronic osteomyelitis may not respond to surgical debridement and intravenous antibiotics, and purulent drainage often persists.

Plate 9-4

Complications of Fracture

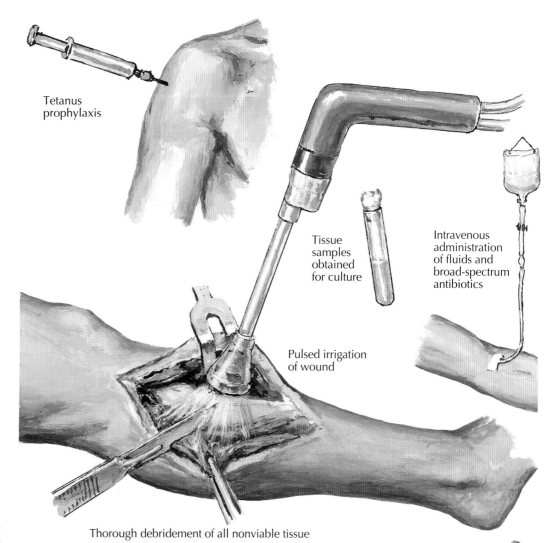

Tetanus prophylaxis

Tissue samples obtained for culture

Intravenous administration of fluids and broad-spectrum antibiotics

Pulsed irrigation of wound

Thorough debridement of all nonviable tissue

SURGICAL MANAGEMENT OF OPEN FRACTURES

All open fractures should undergo immediate and thorough debridement to remove all contaminating material (see Plate 9-4). Although nearly all open fractures will require surgical debridement in the operating room, this does not negate the need for immediate debridement in the emergency department. All foreign material (e.g., dirt, grass, metal fragments) should be removed as best possible by the clinician in the emergency department, and the wound should be copiously irrigated with sterile fluid. Surgical debridement should be done as soon as possible after the injury (typically within 6 to 8 hours). Tissue samples are taken from deep in the wound, and broad-spectrum antibiotics are administered intravenously for at least 48 hours thereafter. Depending on the extent of contamination, repeat washouts in 48-hour intervals may be necessary. To avoid sealing contaminants inside the wound, many wounds are left open after debridement. Delayed primary closure of the wound can be considered 3 to 5 days after the injury if the wound remains clean; however, some studies have found decreased infection rates in patients in which a "loose" closure was performed at the time of initial debridement. For all patients with an open fracture, the immunization record is checked and adequate tetanus prophylaxis provided, if needed.

If the fracture is accompanied by severe soft tissue injury, stabilization of the fracture with an external fixation device facilitates wound care. An external fixation device will many times need to remain in place until such time that infection has been eradicated, viable soft tissues have been maintained, and swelling has decreased enough to allow conversion to an internal fracture fixation and closure of soft tissue wounds.

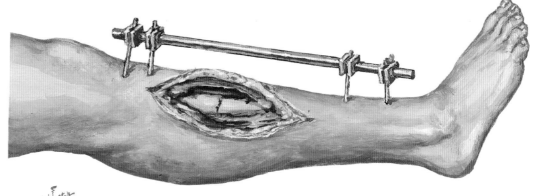

Wound left open. External fixation device allows access to wound for dressing. Delayed primary closure occurs after 3 to 5 days, if wound remains clean.

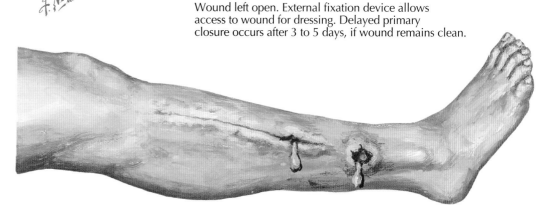

Despite good care, chronic osteomyelitis may develop with sequestra and drainage.

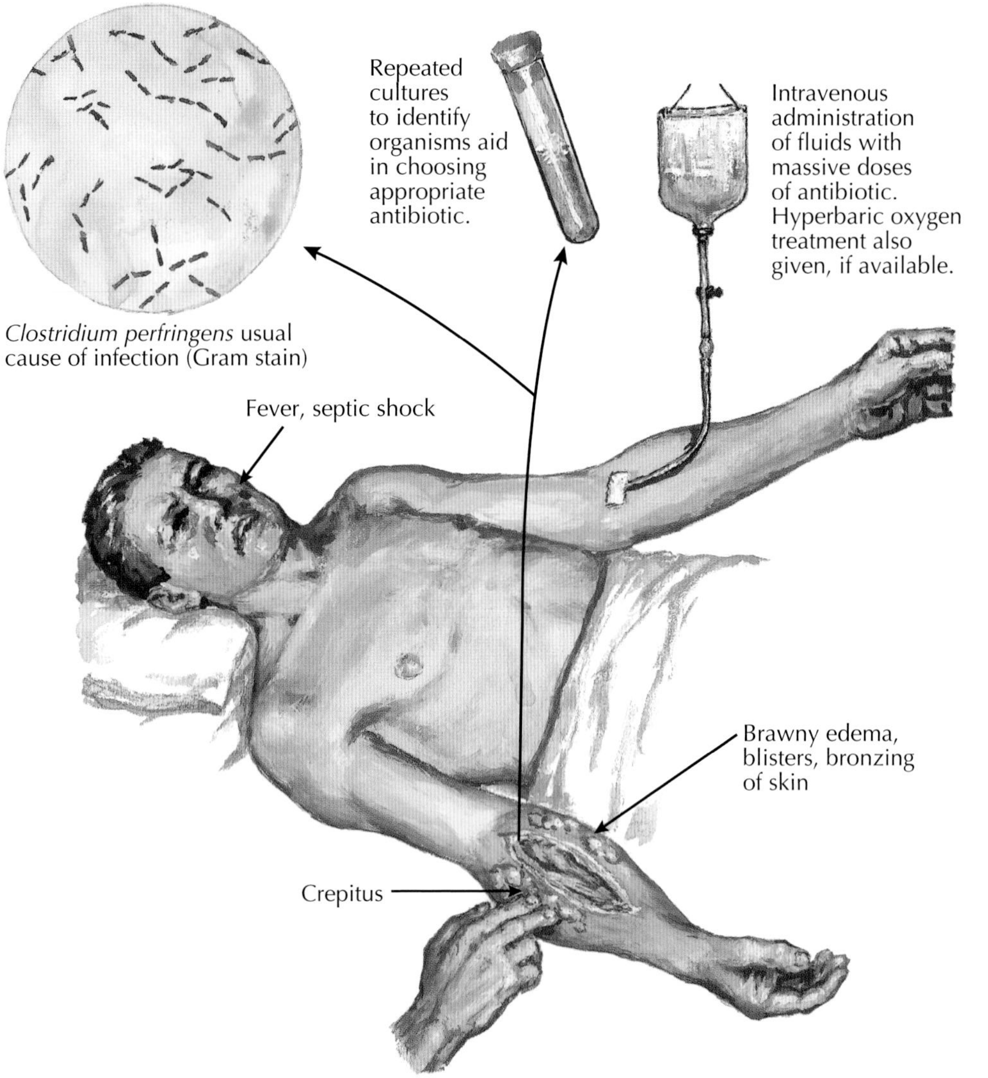

Plate 9-5

Musculoskeletal System: PART III

Repeated cultures to identify organisms aid in choosing appropriate antibiotic.

Intravenous administration of fluids with massive doses of antibiotic. Hyperbaric oxygen treatment also given, if available.

Clostridium perfringens usual cause of infection (Gram stain)

Fever, septic shock

Brawny edema, blisters, bronzing of skin

Crepitus

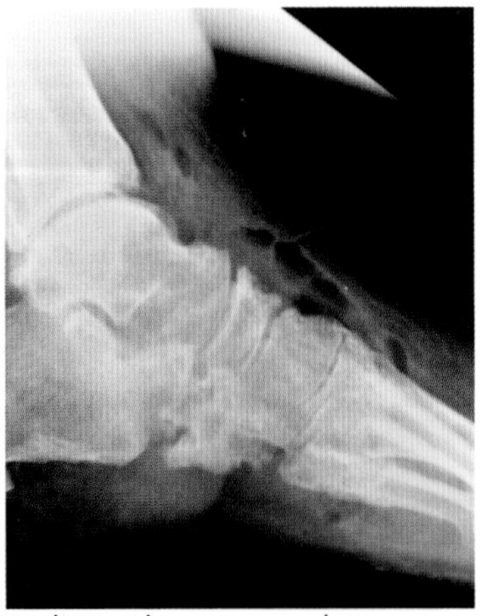

GAS GANGRENE

The most serious acute infection that can result from a contaminated open fracture is gas gangrene (see Plate 9-5), a form of myonecrotizing infection that progresses rapidly. Although the term *gas gangrene* is typically associated with the bacterial species *Clostridium*, many necrotizing soft tissue infections are caused by mixed aerobic and anaerobic gram-negative and gram-positive bacteria. Although this complication is rare, *Clostridium perfringens* is found virtually everywhere and should be considered a possible contaminant in every open wound. The reduced oxygen tension in the wound provides an excellent environment for the growth of clostridia.

Gas gangrene may develop when a contaminated open fracture is inadequately debrided. The infection tends to involve the subcutaneous tissue and muscles, sometimes sparing blood vessels, nerves, and bone. Once established, the infection may produce a localized cellulitis or extensive and aggressive myonecrosis. The onset of infection usually occurs within 72 hours after injury. Characteristic manifestations are localized pain, erythema, swelling, brawny edema, blister formation, and bronzing of the skin. Pockets of subcutaneous gas produce crepitus on palpation, and the wound often drains a thin, brownish, watery material. The extent of the infection will progress very quickly, with the erythematous edge of the infection spreading at a rate of up to 10 cm per hour. Severe systemic symptoms of fever, tachycardia, and lethargy may progress rapidly to septic shock and coma.

As with other wound infections, prevention is the keystone in the management of infections caused by *Clostridium*. The contaminated hematoma and all necrotic tissue should be debrided promptly after any open fracture. Antibiotics are administered to prevent infection, and the wound is left open. Primary closure is delayed until the wound is clean and there is no evidence of infection.

Gas gangrene is a true surgical emergency that demands immediate attention to preserve life and limb. Once gas gangrene, cellulitis, or myonecrosis develops,

Radiographs may reveal gas spaces between tissue layers.

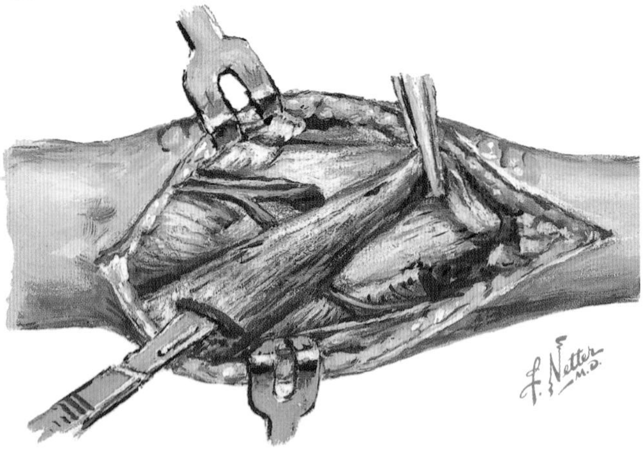

All nonviable tissue, especially muscle, debrided. Vessels and nerves sometimes spared.

treatment must be swift and aggressive. The decision to proceed with operative management must in some cases be made on clinical examination findings alone, because delay for computed tomography or magnetic resonance imaging may result in the loss of an extremity or even life. Intravenous administration of fluid and blood is performed as necessary to treat the systemic complications. Large doses of broad-spectrum antibiotics should be administered intravenously the instant gas gangrene is suggested. It is essential to open the infected

wound as soon as possible and perform a radical debridement of all necrotic and infected tissue. This precaution means that frequently the surgical procedures must be repeated every few hours because of the rapid and aggressive nature of the infection. Hyperbaric oxygen treatment may be considered if available; however, studies have shown mixed results with regard to benefit of this logistically difficult therapy. Intravenous antibiotics and immediate surgical debridement remain the absolute necessary treatment.

Plate 9-6

Complications of Fracture

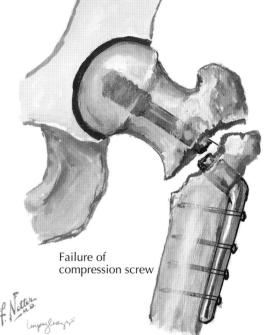

In above test, implant material will fracture with single stress of 140,000 psi. Material fatigues with repeated loading cycles, fracturing at 40,000 psi at 10 million cycles. In walking, estimated average of loading cycles on femur is 1 million/year.

Failure of compression screw

IMPLANT FAILURE

Implant devices used in the internal fixation of fractures may fail with normal use, either by breaking or by loosening (see Plate 9-6). After implantation of an internal fixation device, a race begins between the normal healing process and failure of the device due to metal fatigue. Normal, healthy bone has the ability to remodel, repair, and reinforce itself when subjected to repetitive loading forces, as in walking. However, metal fixation devices subjected to repetitive bending loads weaken and eventually fail, much as paper clips break with repeated bending. Metal fatigue of orthopaedic implants occurs only after many loading cycles, and the fracture usually heals long before the device would fail. If the fracture repair process is slow or inadequate, the body continues to depend on the implant to withstand mechanical stresses on the limb. All implants have a finite life span, and if the fracture fails to heal in the normal time frame, fatigue failure of the implant becomes more and more likely.

Bone mass deficiency may also contribute to implant failure, because stabilization of a fracture with plates and screws depends on the secure fixation of screws in the bone fragments. In bone weakened by osteoporosis or other metabolic bone diseases, the screws may pull out, resulting in loss of fracture fixation and loss of reduction. In these patients, when loads are applied to the fractured limb, screw fixation may not be secure if inappropriate implants are used. Advancements in fracture fixation methods, such as the use of locking plates, have improved our ability to fix osteoporotic or weakened bone; however, these newer methods still rely on the body's ability to eventually heal the fracture.

The risk of implant failure can be minimized by protecting the bone from excessive and repetitive stresses until full fracture healing has occurred. If the fixation is not secure, all loads must be avoided until radiographs clearly show evidence of fracture healing. Some devices, such as a dynamic compression screw, used in the treatment of certain intertrochanteric femur fractures, take advantage of the compression achieved across a fracture site when a patient bears weight on

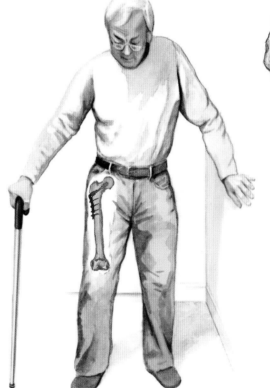

Crutches, brace, or cast provides external support to lessen stress on internal fixation implants during healing of bone.

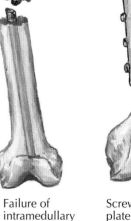

Failure of intramedullary rod

Screws of compression plate pulled loose from osteoporotic femur.

their injured limb. No matter what type of fracture or surgical treatment is performed, mobilization of patients as early as possible is of the utmost importance. If a patient remains immobilized in bed, the rate of multiple medical comorbidities such as respiratory insufficiency, pneumonia, deep venous thrombosis, pulmonary embolism, ileus, and overall deconditioning quickly elevates. Patients can usually begin protected weight bearing with crutches or a walker when fracture healing has been demonstrated. When delayed healing

increases the risk of fatigue failure in a metal fixation device, the stresses of weight bearing should be minimized by external support of the fracture through the use of crutches, casts, or braces until adequate healing is documented on radiographs.

If the implant fails, it is usually removed and replaced with another fixation device. Bone autografts are usually incorporated in the revision surgery to expedite the healing process and minimize the risk of repeat implant failure.

Plate 9-7

Musculoskeletal System: PART III

MALUNION OF FRACTURE

A malunion is a functional or cosmetic deformity that persists after fracture healing (see Plate 9-7). Essentially, a malunion is a failure of the fractured bones to heal in their normal, anatomic position. The deformity may be angular or rotational or may consist of a discrepancy in length (usually shortening).

Angular Malunion. Supracondylar fractures of the humerus are quite unstable, and reduction is difficult to maintain. Even an acceptable reduction may be lost, and the bone typically heals with a resulting varus deformity. The normal carrying angle of the elbow (5 to 20 degrees) is decreased or reversed. Despite the abnormal appearance of the elbow, function may not be compromised, even with a severe deformity. Closed reduction and percutaneous pinning, or even open reduction and pinning, of these unstable fractures is used to prevent or decrease the chances of deformity. Angular malunions that result in a significant loss of function or cosmetic deformity are best treated with a corrective osteotomy at the site of the original fracture. The alignment of the corrective osteotomy is maintained with a plate and screws or an intramedullary nail. The osteotomy is often supplemented with cancellous bone grafts to ensure healing.

Rotational Malunion. This complication can occur with fracture of any long bone and is very difficult to recognize on *standard* radiographs. After every fracture reduction, a clinical examination is essential to ascertain that there is no residual rotational malalignment. This is most easily accomplished by comparing the rotational alignment in the injured limb to that of the uninjured limb. Rotational malunions are common in spiral fractures of the second, third, or fourth metacarpal. Residual malalignment is frequently missed because the deformity can be detected only when the fingers are flexed. On flexion of the metacarpophalangeal joints, all four digits should point toward the scaphoid on the radial aspect of the wrist.

Change in Limb Length. Shortening of the limb is a particularly common complication of fractures of long bones, especially if the fracture is significantly displaced or comminuted. Loss of structural support of the skeleton allows the muscles to contract, causing the bone to overlap and the limb to shorten. Whereas shortening of long bones after a fracture was a more common occurrence in years past, the popularization of interlocking intramedullary nails has significantly decreased the rate of this complication. Moderate shortening of the upper limb does not significantly limit function, and mild shortening in the lower limb is usually well tolerated. A leg-length discrepancy greater than $\frac{1}{2}$ inch, however, often results in a limp. Simple shoe lifts compensate for leg-length discrepancies between $\frac{1}{2}$ inch and 1 inch, but discrepancies greater than 1 inch usually necessitate surgical treatment. Because the majority of fractures at risk for limb shortening are likely to undergo surgical fixation in the first place, the best way to avoid a limb-length inequality is simply achieving an

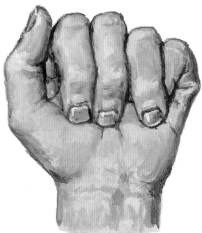

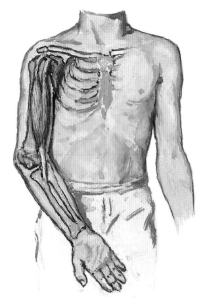

Cubitus varus deformity due to malunion of supracondylar fracture of humerus

Rotational malalignment of ring finger after fracture of proximal phalanx

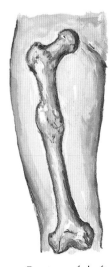

Fracture of shaft of femur with malunion (shortening)

Femoral shortening osteotomy

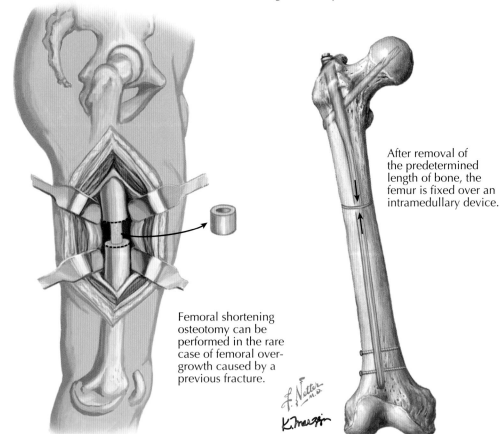

Femoral shortening osteotomy can be performed in the rare case of femoral overgrowth caused by a previous fracture.

After removal of the predetermined length of bone, the femur is fixed over an intramedullary device.

anatomic reduction and comparing the injured limb length to the unaffected limb at the time of initial surgery.

If limb shortening occurs in a growing child, growth of the longer limb should be arrested with fusion of the growth plate (epiphysiodesis) at the appropriate time, as determined with standardized growth charts. In a young child, a leg-length discrepancy of up to 1 inch can be corrected with epiphyseal arrest. In adults, the longer femur is usually shortened with osteotomy.

Although lengthening the shortened femur is also a possibility, this procedure carries a high risk of neurovascular complications owing to stretching of soft tissues, nerves, and vessels at the time of acute bone lengthening. If the decision is made to shorten the longer femur, an appropriately sized segment of the femoral shaft is removed by way of an open osteotomy and the two major fragments of the femoral shaft are reduced and held in anatomic alignment over an interlocking intramedullary nail.

Plate 9-8

Complications of Fracture

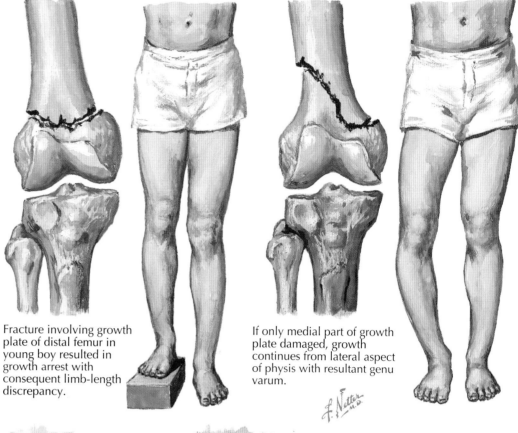

Fracture involving growth plate of distal femur in young boy resulted in growth arrest with consequent limb-length discrepancy.

If only medial part of growth plate damaged, growth continues from lateral aspect of physis with resultant genu varum.

GROWTH DEFORMITY

In children, fractures that involve the growth plate (physis) may require special treatment to prevent a deformity that develops with growth (see Plate 9-8). One of the most common causes of growth deformity is damage to the growth plate, which is responsible for the longitudinal growth of a limb. Particularly in younger children, damage to the growth plate (even though the fracture heals) can arrest limb growth, producing a shortened limb or an angular deformity.

Limb Shortening. Although limb shortening is a risk in virtually any growth plate fracture, it is particularly common in Salter-Harris type V injuries, in which the growth plate is crushed and destroyed (see Plate 9-8). Children with growth plate injuries require periodic re-examination to ascertain that normal bone growth is occurring. Radiographs taken 6 to 9 months after fracture should show an open growth plate and continued longitudinal growth. The physical examination must document that the limb lengths are remaining equal. This determination is most important because modest limb length discrepancies are best treated by stopping the growth of the uninjured limb with epiphysiodesis as soon as complete growth arrest is demonstrated in the injured limb.

Angular Deformity. Partial damage to the growth plate may produce a partial growth arrest. When a portion of the growth plate ceases to grow, an angular deformity results. This particular deformity is frequently seen in the distal femur after a Salter-Harris type II fracture in which the medial portion of the growth plate is damaged (see Plate 9-8). The medial portion of the physis stops growing while the lateral portion continues to grow, producing a varus deformity of the limb. A similar angular deformity can occur in the forearm or the leg when the growth plate of one bone is injured and fuses prematurely while the remaining bone continues to grow. For example, when a fracture of the tibia damages the entire proximal or distal growth plate, continued longitudinal growth of the fibula forces the limb into a varus position.

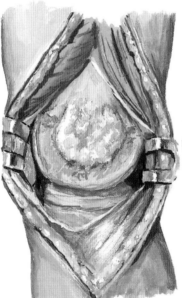

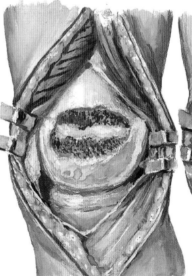

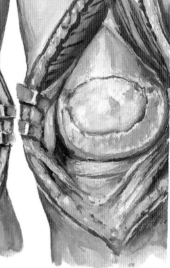

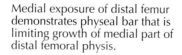

Medial exposure of distal femur demonstrates physeal bar that is limiting growth of medial part of distal femoral physis.

Bone bridge removed with dental burr, revealing normal growth plate underneath

Defect filled with cranioplast or autogenous fat to prevent re-formation of bone bridge

After some growth plate injuries, a bone bridge forms across a portion of the growth plate, arresting growth and creating a significant deformity. To prevent these complications, the bone bridge must be completely removed. Extensive preoperative planning is necessary to identify the extent of the bone bridge and is typically done with computed tomography and magnetic resonance imaging. After resection of the bone bridge, Silastic, autogenous fat, or even a physeal graft harvested from the iliac crest can be packed into the defect to prevent the bridge from re-forming. If this surgical procedure is effective in maintaining an open growth plate, longitudinal growth resumes, reducing the risk of further angular deformity. Despite the technique for bony bridge resection or what material is used for interposition, significant angular deformity is typically not corrected. However, resecting the bone bridge will likely decrease the number of osteotomies that need to be performed to fully correct a residual deformity when the child reaches skeletal maturity.

Plate 9-9

Musculoskeletal System: PART III

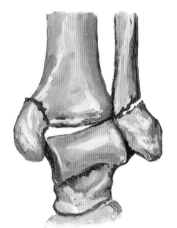

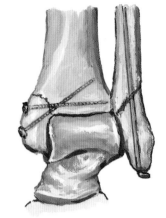

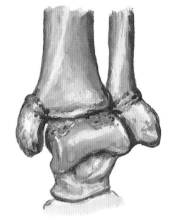

Intra-articular bimalleolar fracture with lateral displacement of talus

Open reduction to restore congruity of articular surfaces and fixation with screws and intramedullary rod

Inadequate closed reduction of bimalleolar fracture results in loss of congruity of articular surfaces and consequent post-traumatic arthritis.

Post-traumatic arthritis after acetabular fracture and repair may cause pain in hip joint. Total hip replacement may be needed to relieve pain.

POSTTRAUMATIC OSTEOARTHRITIS

Posttraumatic osteoarthritis is a common consequence of some fracture malunions and also frequently results from intra-articular fractures (see Plate 9-9). A malunion, especially in a lower limb, may create an angular deformity that produces excessive loading stresses on the adjacent joints. A varus deformity of the tibia, for example, puts excessive loads on both the ankle joint and the knee joint. The biomechanical imbalance concentrates the forces on one small area of the articular cartilage, increasing stress and wear on this area. With continued use of the limb, a degenerative process occurs in the articular cartilage and subchondral bone.

Intra-articular fractures are particularly likely to lead to post-traumatic osteoarthritis. Whenever a fracture line extends across the articular surface, the articular cartilage is permanently damaged. The amount of injury can be minimized by anatomic reduction of the articular surfaces. Therefore, virtually all displaced intra-articular fractures require open reduction and rigid internal fixation of the articular fragments to restore joint congruity. However, even if joint congruity is re-established, the cartilage injury does not fully heal. The smooth hyaline cartilage of the articular surface cannot regenerate, and a fracture through the hyaline articular cartilage is repaired with fibrocartilage. Fibrocartilage does not have the mechanical strength or durability of hyaline cartilage. When this reparative fibrocartilage is subjected to repeated stresses, it wears out, also leading to post-traumatic osteoarthritis. The arthritis may develop in the first few months after

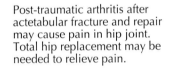

Successful definitive treatment of severe ankle arthritis can many times be obtained by arthrodesis (fusion) of the involved joints. One technique is arthrodesis of the tibiotalar and subtalar joints over a locked intramedullary nail.

fracture healing, or it may develop insidiously with time as the articular surface gradually wears away. Arthritic symptoms may appear 15 to 20 years after the injury.

Conservative management is adequate for mild post-traumatic osteoarthritis. These measures include limitation of activity, avoidance of stress, use of braces and other support devices for walking, and administration of nonsteroidal anti-inflammatory drugs (NSAIDs). Severe, disabling osteoarthritis of the hip, knee, or shoulder is treated with total joint replacement. With advancements in technology, total elbow and total ankle replacements are also becoming possibilities in select circumstances. Total joint replacement restores joint motion and relieves pain by replacing the articular surfaces with plastic and metal prostheses. Arthrodesis (fusion) of the joint is the preferred treatment of severe post-traumatic arthritis in other joints, particularly the ankle joint and the small joints of the foot and hand. However, although a successful arthrodesis eliminates pain in the arthritic joint, it also sacrifices joint motion.

Plate 9-10

Complications of Fracture

OSTEONECROSIS

Osteonecrosis, also called avascular necrosis, is an occasional but severe complication of certain fractures (see Plate 9-10). In healthy bone, a rich blood supply normally provides nourishment and enables the bone both to repair itself after fracture and to remodel when new stresses are applied to it. Osteonecrosis occurs when the blood supply to a segment of a bone is destroyed and the bone cells die. Extensive stripping of soft tissue away from bone, particularly in a high-velocity injury, may render any bone fragment avascular. When a large fragment at a fracture site loses its blood supply, it cannot participate in the normal reparative processes and delayed union or nonunion may result.

The blood supply to particular segments of certain bones is unique and one directional. Consequently, some specific fracture patterns are especially likely to create an avascular segment of bone. For example, the femoral head is particularly susceptible to osteonecrosis because virtually all the blood vessels to the femoral head traverse the femoral neck. A fracture of the femoral neck disrupts these blood vessels, leaving the femoral head with no blood supply. Because of this fact, displaced femoral neck fractures in children or young adults are surgical emergencies. Similarly, the body of the talus has very few soft tissue attachments and derives virtually all its blood supply from vessels that pass up through the talar neck in a retrograde fashion. A fracture of the neck disrupts these blood vessels and impairs the circulation. Another vulnerable area is the proximal pole of the scaphoid, because its circulation is supplied by blood vessels that enter the distal pole and waist of the bone, thus supplying the proximal pole in a retrograde fashion. A fracture of the waist of the scaphoid, therefore, leaves the proximal pole with inadequate circulation or none at all (see Plate 9-10).

Although the loss of circulation to a major bone segment impairs healing, healing does proceed, because the segment that retains its blood supply often generates sufficient callus to incorporate the avascular segment. Once healing occurs, the body removes the necrotic bone by a process called "creeping substitution." In this process, osteoclasts proliferate from the vascularized bone into the necrotic segment and remove the dead bone trabeculae. While this is happening, the necrotic segment is weakened and becomes susceptible to collapse. The process of creeping substitution is slow, taking as long as 3 years for the necrotic bone to be removed and replaced with new osteons. Stress applied to the weakened bone during this time causes it to collapse. This phenomenon, called late segmental collapse, removes the normal underlying support for the articular cartilage of the segment, disturbing the congruity of the adjacent joints surfaces and predisposing to osteoarthritis. If excessive stresses are avoided during the process of creeping substitution, the necrotic segment is eventually replaced with strong viable bone, late segmental collapse does not occur, and the risk of osteoarthritis is minimized.

In the early stage of osteonecrosis, when the dead bone is present and not yet replaced with new bone, the avascular segment is characterized by a very dense appearance on radiographs. This apparent increase in density is only relative because the surrounding bone, which is still alive, is undergoing disuse osteoporosis, a

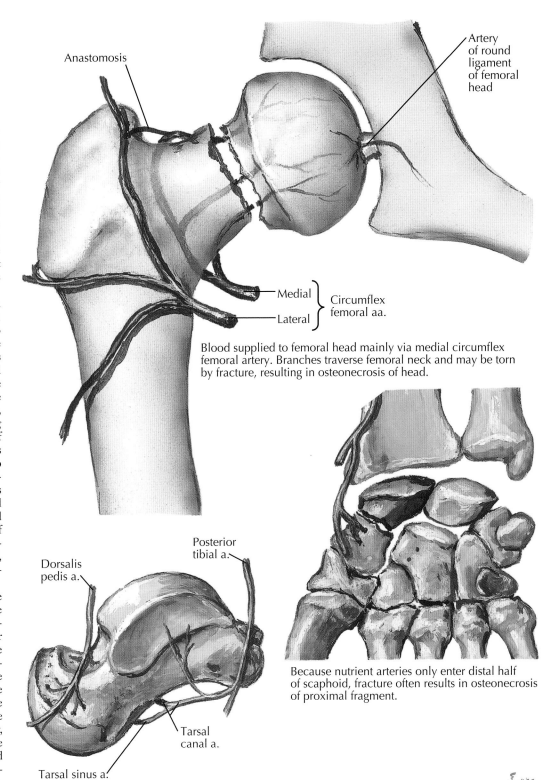

Anastomosis

Artery of round ligament of femoral head

Medial ⎫
Lateral ⎭ Circumflex femoral aa.

Blood supplied to femoral head mainly via medial circumflex femoral artery. Branches traverse femoral neck and may be torn by fracture, resulting in osteonecrosis of head.

Posterior tibial a.

Dorsalis pedis a.

Tarsal canal a.

Tarsal sinus a.

Disruption of nutrient arteries to talus may result in osteonecrosis of talar body.

Because nutrient arteries only enter distal half of scaphoid, fracture often results in osteonecrosis of proximal fragment.

normal phenomenon seen in the early stages of fracture healing. Without an adequate blood supply, the necrotic fragment does not become osteoporotic and thus appears relatively dense.

The absence of osteonecrosis can be inferred when Hawkins sign is seen on the radiograph. Hawkins sign is evidence of the resorption of subchondral bone as a consequence of disuse osteoporosis and suggests that the bone segment has adequate circulation, normal bone healing is occurring, and that osteonecrosis has not occurred.

Usually, osteonecrosis is a consequence of the pattern of injury and little can be done to prevent it besides stable anatomic fixation of the fracture. When osteonecrosis is detected, the bone must be protected from excessive stresses until it is fully reconstituted, a process that may take as long as 3 years. During this time, patients should wear a brace or use crutches until radiographs show evidence that the avascular segment has been replaced with new bone. These simple measures reduce the risk of late segmental collapse and the development of osteoarthritis.

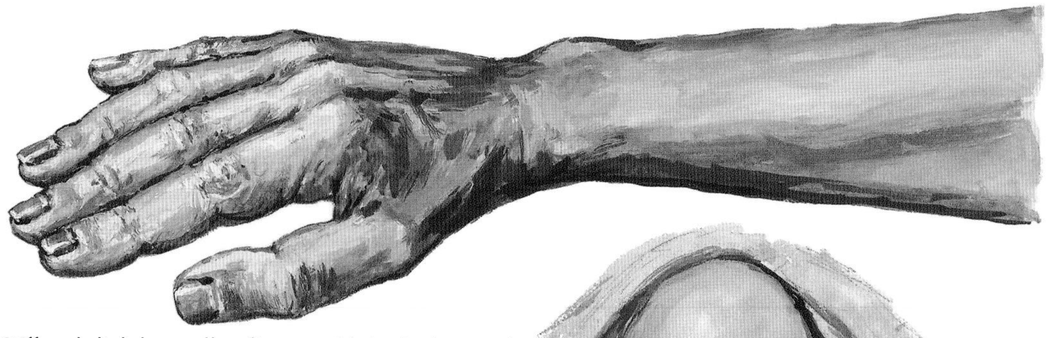

Plate 9-11

Musculoskeletal System: PART III

Stiff and slightly swollen fingers with intrinsic muscle atrophy evident 2 months after Colles fracture in elderly patient treated with prolonged casting.

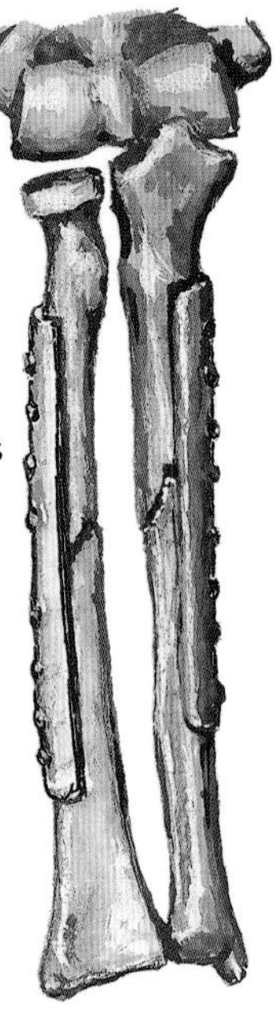

JOINT STIFFNESS

Effective immobilization of a fracture in a cast usually includes immobilization of the joints above and below the site of injury (see Plate 9-11). This extensive, prolonged immobilization frequently leads to joint stiffness, which may prove to be a bigger problem than the fracture itself. Immobilization lasting more than a few weeks leads to scarring of the joint capsule and contracture of the muscles, and it also impairs the nutrition of the articular surfaces. With prolonged immobilization, adhesions develop across the articular surfaces, even in joints that had not been injured directly. In addition, prolonged immobilization in a cast results in marked atrophy of the muscles in and around the site of injury.

One of the best examples of this problem is a Colles fracture of the distal radius in the older patient (see Plate 9-11). Although this fracture almost always heals, adequate healing takes 8 to 10 weeks. If the limb is immobilized in a cast for this amount of time, severe stiffness of the elbow and wrist may occur, and even the shoulder and finger joints may become stiff. Therefore, again, although the fracture heals, the resulting joint stiffness and muscle atrophy render the arm useless. Rehabilitation of the joints and muscles is a long and difficult process that may not restore full limb function.

Methods have been developed to ensure adequate fixation of the fracture fragments yet maintain joint motion and muscular activity to prevent the stiffness and atrophy that result from cast immobilization. If joint stiffness appears likely, the fracture is treated with early open reduction and internal fixation. A few days after surgery, the patient resumes gentle active range-of-motion exercises of the adjacent joints. Surgical stabilization and early rehabilitation are most effective in fractures of the shafts of both forearm bones in adults. Open reduction and internal fixation can restore a stable anatomic configuration of the bone architecture, which allows early restoration of motion in the elbow, wrist, and hand.

With certain fractures, such as a fracture of the shaft of the humerus, use of a functional brace accomplishes the same objectives. Traditional cast immobilization for a fracture of the humeral shaft requires immobilization of the shoulder and elbow joints in a shoulder spica cast. Such immobilization of both joints for 8 to 10 weeks would lead to a significant loss of function. Conversely, a functional brace allows active range of motion in the shoulder and elbow joints yet provides adequate support of the healing fracture. A functional brace can be applied at the time of injury, but the brace will likely

Open reduction and internal fixation of fracture of both forearm bones permits early muscle activity, minimizing joint stiffness.

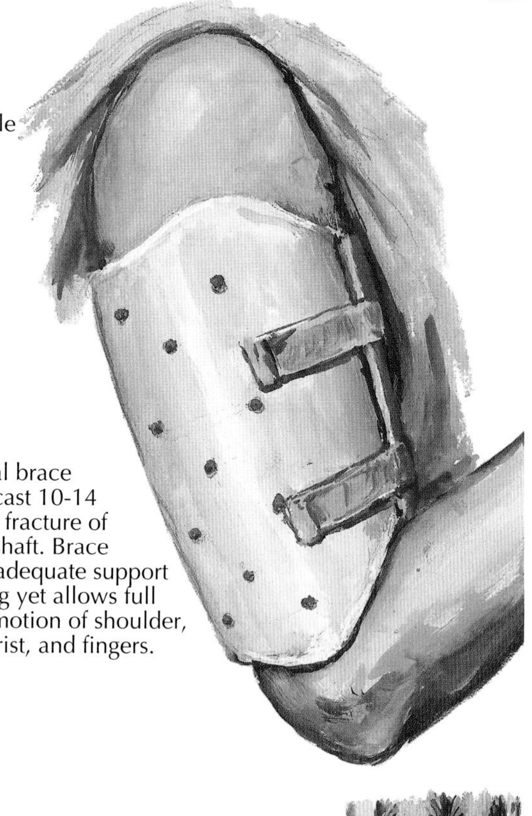

Functional brace replaces cast 10-14 days after fracture of humeral shaft. Brace provides adequate support for healing yet allows full range of motion of shoulder, elbow, wrist, and fingers.

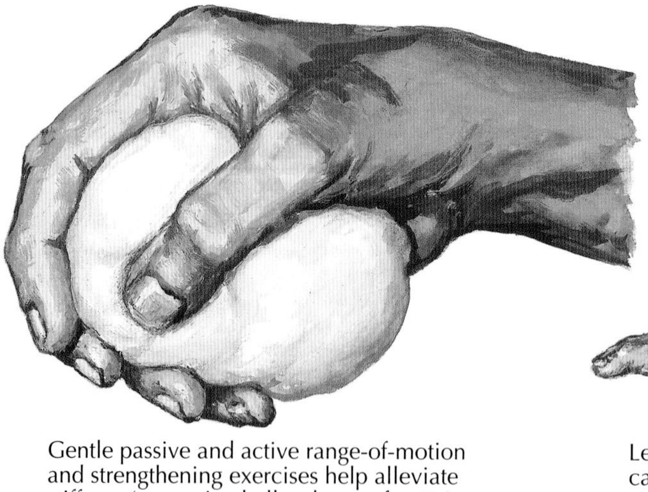

Gentle passive and active range-of-motion and strengthening exercises help alleviate stiffness (squeezing ball or lump of putty).

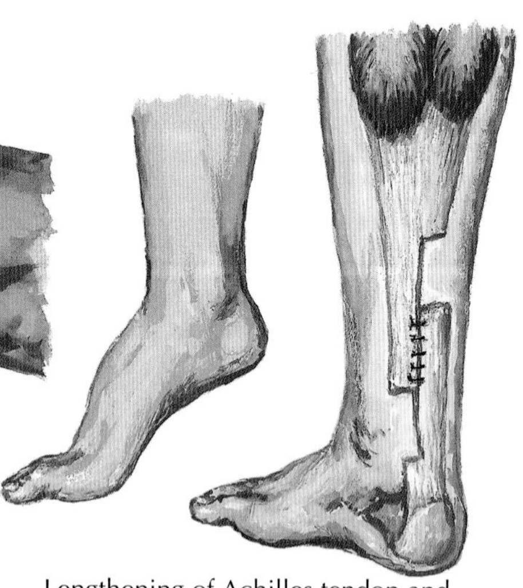

Lengthening of Achilles tendon and capsulotomy help correct severe equinus contracture deformity.

need to be adjusted 10 to 14 days after injury, once the initial swelling has subsided. The brace can be tightened to provide firm support about the arm and maintain acceptable alignment of the fracture.

When joint stiffness develops, restoring motion requires a long-term rehabilitation program, possibly lasting more than 1 year. After the patient regains joint motion with gentle passive range-of-motion exercises, active exercises are begun to strengthen the atrophied muscles. Manipulation under anesthesia, lysis of

adhesions, and capsulotomy is commonly required for a stiff shoulder or elbow joint that has not improved with aggressive physical therapy. When fixed muscle contractures fail to respond to aggressive and prolonged rehabilitation, surgical release of soft tissue may be necessary as a last resort. One of the most effective soft tissue releases is a Z-plasty lengthening of the Achilles tendon for persistent equinus contracture after injury to the ankle. A posterior capsulotomy may also be needed to restore full mobility of the ankle joint.

Plate 9-12

Complications of Fracture

COMPLEX REGIONAL PAIN SYNDROME

In 2% to 3% of patients with limb injuries, a persistent and severe pain develops shortly after the fracture or joint injury has healed. If severe pain continues in the context of a specific set of clinical symptoms, patients may be diagnosed with complex regional pain syndrome (CRPS), formerly known as reflex sympathetic dystrophy (see Plate 9-12). The pain is out of proportion to the severity of the initial injury and often involves the entire limb, not just the injured area. The precise pathophysiology of this disorder is not yet understood, but disinhibition of the sympathetic nervous system in the area of injury is one theory. The first clinical manifestations are redness, swelling, hyperhidrosis, and hyperesthesia of the limb at the injury site as well as proximally and distally. Frequently, the area affected follows the distribution of a specific cutaneous nerve. Severe disuse osteoporosis may be evident on radiographs. The initial phase of acute pain and hypersensitivity is eventually followed by brawny skin changes, limb stiffness, loss of function, and severe muscle atrophy.

Diagnosis of CRPS is based on clinical and radiographic manifestations, but other procedures may help confirm the diagnosis. Thermography may show asymmetry of skin temperature in a stocking or glove distribution, and skin temperature in the affected limb is often at least 1°F lower than in the opposite limb. Initial studies investigating elevated three-phase bone scans in the areas of pain revealed the test to be highly sensitive and specific; however, subsequent studies have shown wide variability in results. Besides clinical examination, the most reliable diagnostic tool, which is also therapeutic, includes local anesthetic nerve blocks and lumbar sympathetic ganglion blocks.

The most effective management of this potential complication is aggressive prevention. Because prolonged immobilization appears to be the most common

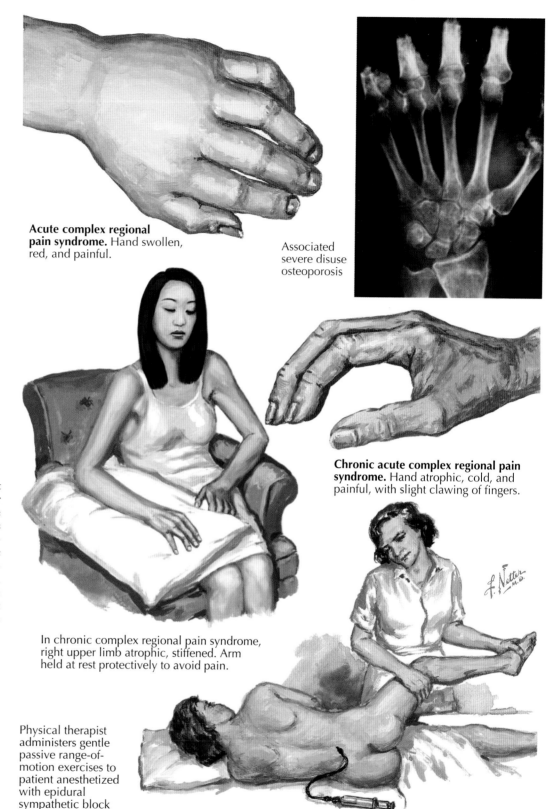

Acute complex regional pain syndrome. Hand swollen, red, and painful.

Associated severe disuse osteoporosis

Chronic acute complex regional pain syndrome. Hand atrophic, cold, and painful, with slight clawing of fingers.

In chronic complex regional pain syndrome, right upper limb atrophic, stiffened. Arm held at rest protectively to avoid pain.

Physical therapist administers gentle passive range-of-motion exercises to patient anesthetized with epidural sympathetic block

cause, the patient should be encouraged to begin active range-of-motion exercises as soon as possible after the injury. After immobilization, the patient should gradually resume normal activities, progressively increasing them as the injury heals. A very structured physical or occupational therapy program should be instituted.

Pain must be controlled with the administration of mild analgesics or NSAIDs. Use of transcutaneous electric stimulation (TENS) devices have shown mixed results. Avoidance of chronic narcotic medication use for CRPS is of utmost importance. Tricyclic antidepressants help decrease anxiety and apprehension. Some patients respond promptly to sympathetic blockade, and a series of sympathetic blocks provides at least temporary relief from pain, allowing the patient to begin a vigorous rehabilitation program. Restoring the limb to pain-free function takes a long time, and patients may need substantial psychological support during the long rehabilitation period.

Plate 9-13   Musculoskeletal System: PART III

Test for nonunion

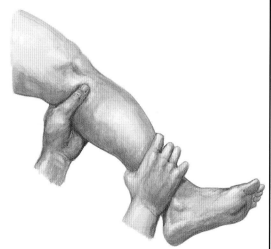

In clinical diagnosis of nonunion, examiner elicits pain and/or motion at old fracture site by exerting varus, valgus, or anteroposterior stress. Pain is absent in synovial pseudarthrosis.

Fibrous nonunion

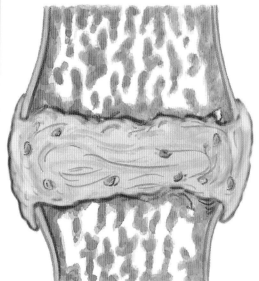

Hypertrophic nonunion:
Exorbitant callus formation but failure to unite

Synovial pseudarthrosis

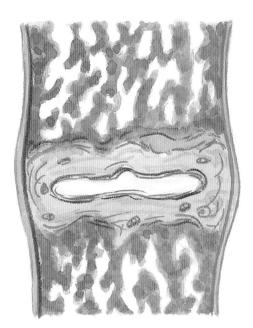

Histologic section shows false joint lined with synovial membrane and filled with fluid.

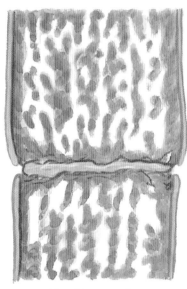

Atrophic nonunion:
Minimal to no callus formation and failure to unite

NONUNION OF FRACTURE

Normally, when a bone breaks, the fracture heals uneventfully to a solid bony union within a few months. In a typical long bone, such as the tibia, union usually takes about 3 months. Smaller bones heal faster. About 3% to 5% of fractures do not heal, however, and are called nonunions. In a nonunion, all of the reparative processes in the fractured bone have ceased but bone continuity has not been restored.

The diagnosis of nonunion is made both clinically and radiographically (see Plate 9-13). On clinical examination of a nonunion, the fracture fragments are still mobile after the appropriate healing time. Radiographs show no bony trabeculae spanning the fracture gap in the anteroposterior, lateral, or both oblique views. If the fracture was treated with an internal fixation device, diagnosis is based entirely on the radiographic evidence.

The causes of nonunion include inadequate reduction or immobilization of the fracture, interposition of soft tissue in the fracture gap, significant soft tissue loss or vascular damage at the time of the original injury, and osteomyelitis at the fracture site. In some cases, the cause remains unknown.

Several types of nonunion exist, and each nonunion must be classified to select the appropriate treatment. Three main types of nonunion include hypertrophic nonunion, atrophic nonunion, and pseudarthrosis. All three types of nonunion can additionally be described as infected if osteomyelitis is present. In most cases of nonunion, histologic examination shows a gap between the fracture fragments that is filled with a combination of fibrous, cartilaginous, and bony tissue. Because the fibrinous tissue usually dominates in hypertrophic nonunions, these were historically called a fibrous nonunion. Hypertrophic nonunions are characterized by excessive amounts of bony callus formation and occur when there is excessive fracture movement (due to inadequate fixation) in a healthy bone-healing environment. Atrophic nonunions are characterized by minimal to no bony callus formation but may also have small amounts of fibrous tissue present. Atrophic nonunions are the result of a poor healing environment devoid of proper biologic requirements of fracture healing, likely owing to soft tissue stripping and devascularization of the bone. Atrophic nonunions can actually also be the result of internal fracture fixation that is *too rigid*. Studies have shown that fractures require a small degree of "micromotion" to stimulate healing. Extremely rigid fixation devices such as locking plates may actually lead to atrophic nonunion in certain circumstances.

In about 12% of nonunions, however, the histologic composition of the fracture gap is quite different. The nonunion site is a cleft filled with fluid and lined with a synovial-like membrane. This type of nonunion, called synovial pseudarthrosis, can also be caused by excessive movement of the fracture fragment during the healing process.

Plate 9-14

Complications of Fracture

SURGICAL MANAGEMENT OF NONUNION

Bone graft surgery is the gold standard in the treatment of essentially all types of nonunion (see Plate 9-14). In the surgical management of nonunions, the type of nonunion and its cause must first be delineated. No matter which type of nonunion is present, the basic fracture treatment principle of achieving an anatomic reduction with regard to length, rotation, and angulation must be inherent. Surgical treatment of all nonunions should include thorough debridement of all fibrous or nonviable tissue interposing fracture fragments. In hypertrophic nonunions that are likely due to initial nonsurgical management or inadequate initial fixation, the patient's fracture should undergo revision internal fixation augmented with bone graft. Bone graft is ideally autologous and most commonly taken from the iliac crest. In atrophic nonunions, a healthy biologic environment supportive of fracture healing must be created. This is also performed by way of autologous bone grafting that may sometimes be in the form of a vascularized bone graft. When treating atrophic nonunions, it is essential to minimize stripping of soft tissue from bone in order to avoid further devascularization.

In the treatment of synovial pseudarthrosis, all of the synovial-like tissue is removed from between and around the nonunion fragments. If this tissue is not thoroughly removed, the synovial pseudarthrosis may recur. After complete excision of this material, bone autograft is packed in and around the nonunion fragments. Internal fixation is invariably required to secure a synovial pseudarthrosis because the fracture fragments are excessively mobile (which caused the synovial pseudarthrosis to form in the first place).

Another important factor in the treatment of nonunions is the need for compression across the fracture site. In nonunion of the tibia, some surgeons excise a short segment of the intact fibula to permit compression of the tibial fragments. Compression can be achieved either by specific plating technique or with an intramedullary device. The compression, which stimulates bone formation, results in slight shortening of the limb. However, once the nonunion has healed, a heel lift in the shoe easily compensates for the slight leg-length discrepancy.

A good example of a fracture with a higher incidence of nonunion (typically atrophic) than most other bones is the scaphoid. The nonunion is traditionally treated with a peg of autograft bone inserted in the medullary cavity of both fragments. With advancements in technology, small fragment compression screws augmented with bone graft have become the typical treatment of choice.

Severe injuries or open fractures in which large segments of bone are lost may create a large bone defect at the nonunion site. The routine method of bone grafting with autogenous bone may not be successful for large defects. A free vascularized bone graft is frequently used to heal this type of nonunion. The midshaft of the fibula with the accompanying arterial supply is typically used as the free vascularized graft, although iliac crest is an alternative donor site. An appropriate segment of the contralateral fibula is excised along with a cuff of muscle and vascular pedicle containing a nutrient artery. The vascularized fibular segment is secured between the nonunion fracture fragments, and the vessels are anastomosed using microsurgical technique. The nonunion containing the vascularized fibular graft must be protected with a cast or brace until a solid bony union develops between the host bone and both ends

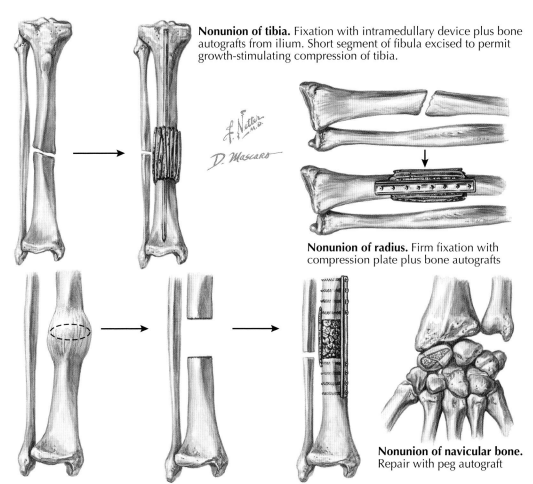

Nonunion of tibia. Fixation with intramedullary device plus bone autografts from ilium. Short segment of fibula excised to permit growth-stimulating compression of tibia.

Nonunion of radius. Firm fixation with compression plate plus bone autografts

Nonunion of navicular bone. Repair with peg autograft

Synovial pseudarthrosis of tibia. Bone margins, synovial-like tissue, and false joint cavity between bone ends excised. Gap filled with cancellous and cortical bone autografts. Fracture site rigidly secured with compression plate. Fibula osteotomized to allow compression of tibia.

Free vascularized bone graft in large bone defects

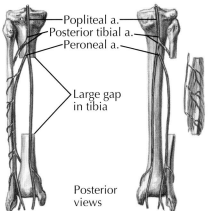

Popliteal a.
Posterior tibial a.
Peroneal a.

Large gap in tibia

Posterior views

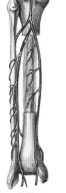

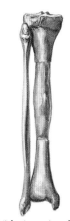

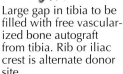

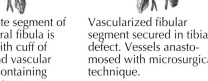

Large gap in tibia to be filled with free vascularized bone autograft from tibia. Rib or iliac crest is alternate donor site.

Appropriate segment of contralateral fibula is excised with cuff of muscle and vascular pedicles containing nutrient artery.

Vascularized fibular segment secured in tibial defect. Vessels anastomosed with microsurgical technique.

With time, implanted segment of fibula grows in diameter, eventually matching tibia in strength.

of the vascularized graft. The diameter of the free vascularized graft from the fibula is obviously smaller than that of the host tibia or femur. However, with time and use, the fibular graft tends to hypertrophy and its diameter may eventually approach that of the host tibia or femur. During this period of bone remodeling, however, the limb must be protected with a brace.

Infected nonunions of any type create a significant and difficult problem to fully treat. Elimination of infection must almost always occur before definitive

fixation and healing of a nonunion. Unfortunately, this may require all foreign material (i.e., fixation plates, screws, and rods) to be removed from the infected fracture while the patient undergoes multiple weeks of likely intravenous antibiotic treatment. Patients may need application of an external fixator device to provide some degree of stability while undergoing treatment of infection. After clinical evidence of infection clearance, the nonunion can then undergo definitive fixation by way of the methods just described.

Plate 9-15   Musculoskeletal System: PART III

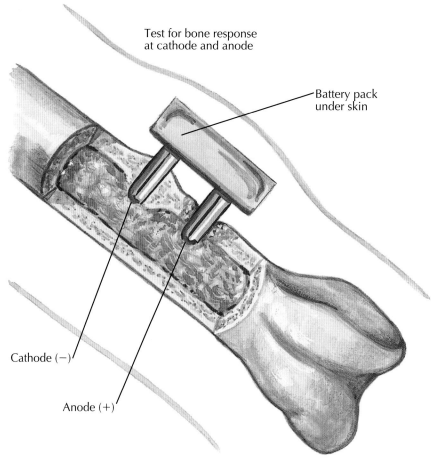

Test for bone response
at cathode and anode

Battery pack
under skin

Cathode (−)

Anode (+)

Cathode and anode electrodes inserted in drill holes in femur of rabbit, with battery pack under skin. Constant direct current applied for 18 days. At currents between 5 μA and 20 μA, new bone formed around cathode but only necrosis occurred around anode. Current under 5 μA produced no effect, and current over 20 μA caused necrosis around both cathode and anode.

ELECTRIC STIMULATION OF BONE GROWTH

The unique electric properties of bone were discovered in the 1950s. When bone is mechanically deformed, the side of bone under compression becomes electronegative and the side of bone under tension becomes electropositive. In the 1960s, researchers discovered that active areas of bone growth and repair were electronegative in relation to less active areas. These findings led to a series of experiments by different investigators (see Plate 9-15).

Another series of experiments was performed to determine if electricity could augment fracture repair in laboratory animals. The anode and cathode were placed in various configurations in relation to the fracture site in the fibula of a rabbit. Results showed that fracture healing increased only when the cathode was positioned directly in the fracture site. The augmentation of fracture healing by electricity was determined by testing the mechanical integrity of the fracture callus. Although the location of the cathode was critical for the stimulation of fracture healing, the location of the anode was not important; that is, as long as the anode made electric contact and completed the circuit, it made no difference whether it was placed in the bone, on the surface of the skin, or anywhere in between.

Based on these findings, clinical trials were performed in which cathodes delivering 20 μA each were inserted into the nonunion site by two different

Experiment for best location of cathode

1   2   3   4   5

Electrodes placed in various locations on fractured fibulas of rabbits, and 10-μA current applied for 18 days. Significantly greater healing occurred when cathode placed directly in fracture site (fibulas 3 and 5). Degree of healing was evaluated by measuring resistance to bending with apparatus at right.

methods: (1) percutaneous insertion under radiographic control or (2) surgical implantation, using an open procedure. In the percutaneous technique, a battery pack was connected to the portion of the cathodes that protruded externally through the skin. In the invasive method, a very small implantable battery pack was connected to the cathodes and placed into the subcutaneous tissue under the skin. The clinical trials demonstrated promising results that direct current could heal a

nonunion in about the same time and with the same rate of success as bone graft surgery.

Continued research over the past several decades on the benefit of electrical stimulation on bone healing has yielded mixed results; however, the overall data are mostly positive. Direct electrical stimulation for treatment of fracture nonunions is still seen, but the most common scenario in which this methodology is utilized is in the nonunion of spinal fusions.

Plate 9-16

Complications of Fracture

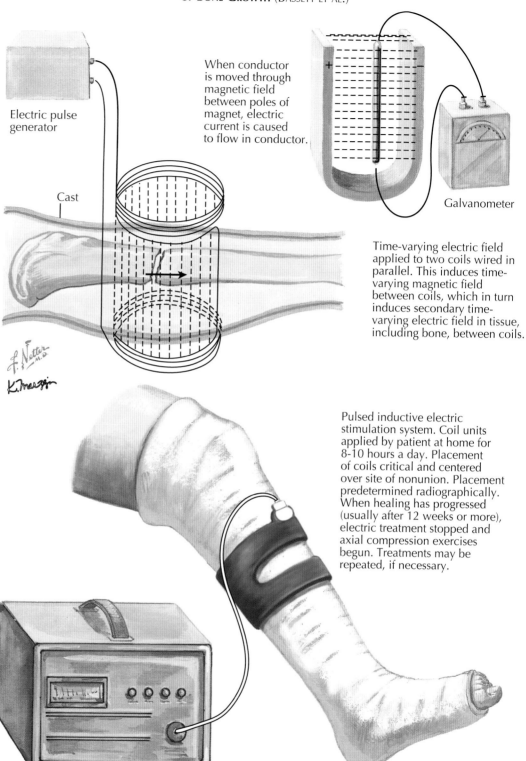

PULSED INDUCTIVE COUPLING METHOD OF ELECTRIC STIMULATION OF BONE GROWTH (BASSETT ET AL.)

Electric pulse generator

Cast

When conductor is moved through magnetic field between poles of magnet, electric current is caused to flow in conductor.

Galvanometer

Time-varying electric field applied to two coils wired in parallel. This induces time-varying magnetic field between coils, which in turn induces secondary time-varying electric field in tissue, including bone, between coils.

Pulsed inductive electric stimulation system. Coil units applied by patient at home for 8-10 hours a day. Placement of coils critical and centered over site of nonunion. Placement predetermined radiographically. When healing has progressed (usually after 12 weeks or more), electric treatment stopped and axial compression exercises begun. Treatments may be repeated, if necessary.

NONINVASIVE COUPLING METHODS OF ELECTRIC STIMULATION OF BONE

Two entirely noninvasive techniques can be used to apply electricity to bone (see Plate 9-16). Because these methods are noninvasive, they may be most beneficial in the case of an infected nonunion, in which all foreign material must be removed from a fracture until antibiotic treatment clears the infection. The first method, inductive coupling, takes advantage of the fact that an electric current is caused to flow in a conductor when the conductor is moved through a magnetic field between the poles of a magnet. When a time-varying electric field is applied to two coils placed on either side of a limb, a time-varied magnetic field is produced between the coils, which, in turn, induces a secondary time-varying electric field in the tissues, including bone, between the coils.

Pulsed Inductive Coupling Method. In the treatment of nonunion, coils are placed around the cast on the limb and, with radiographic guidance, are centered directly over the nonunion site. An asymmetric pulse signal is applied for 8 to 10 hours daily. Studies have shown significant difference in success rate in patients undergoing less than 3 hours of treatment day versus those undergoing treatment for a greater amount of time. The inductive coupling method heals a nonunion in about the same amount of time as direct current, and

the rate of successful healing is also about the same for both techniques.

Capacitive Coupling Method. In this second noninvasive method of applying electricity to nonunion, capacitor plates or electrodes are placed on the surface of the skin on either side of the underlying nonunion. A time-varying electric field is applied to the electrodes, which induces a secondary time-varying electric field in the tissues, including bone, between the electrodes.

This noninvasive treatment also takes approximately the same amount of time as the other electric treatments and has approximately the same degree of success.

Whereas all electrical and electromagnetic stimulation techniques have shown some promise of beneficence, none has proven superior to revision surgery with bone grafting techniques, which remains the gold standard of treatment for nonunion.

Section 1—Embryology

Glass 2nd DA, Karsenty G. In vivo analysis of Wnt signaling in bone. Endocrinology 2007;148(6):2630–4.

Kronenberg HM. Developmental regulation of the growth plate. Nature 2003;423:332.

Pacifici M, Koyama E, Iwamoto M. Mechanisms of synovial joint and articular cartilage formation: recent advances, but many lingering mysteries. Birth Defects Res C Embryo Today 2005;75(3):237–48.

Ralston SH, de Crombrugghe B. Genetic regulation of bone mass and susceptibility to osteoporosis. Genes Dev 2006;20: 2492–506.

Zelzer E, Olsen BR. The genetic basis for skeletal diseases. Nature 2003;423:343–8.

Section 2—Physiology

Skeletal Muscle

Brzeska H, Korn ED. Regulation of class I and class II myosins by heavy chain phosphorylation. J Biol Chem 1996;271: 16983–6.

Kamm KE, Stull JT. Signaling to myosin regulatory light chain in sarcomeres. J Biol Chem 2011;286:9941–7.

Krüger M, Linke WA. The giant protein titin: a regulatory node that integrates myocyte signaling pathways. J Biol Chem 2011;286:9905–12.

MacLennan DH, Rice WJ, Green NM. The mechanism of Ca^{2+} transport by sarco(endo)plasmic reticulum Ca^{2+}-ATPases. J Biol Chem 1997;272:28815–18.

Rayment I. The structural basis of the myosin ATPase activity. J Biol Chem 1996;271:15850–3.

Reisler E, Egelman EH. Actin structure and function: what we still do not understand. J Biol Chem 2007;282:36133–7.

Stull JT. Myosin minireview series. J Biol Chem 1996;271:15849.

Growth Plate

Beier F. Cell-cycle control and the cartilage growth plate. J Cell Physiol 2005;202(1):1–8.

Kronenberg HM. Developmental regulation of the growth plate. Nature 2003;423:332.

Tamamura Y, Otani T, Kanatani N, Koyama E, Kitagaki J, Komori T, et al. Developmental regulation of Wnt/β-catenin signals is required for growth plate assembly, cartilage integrity, and endochondral ossification. J Biol Chem 2005;280:19185–95.

Zelzer E, Olsen BR. The genetic basis for skeletal diseases. Nature 2003;423:343–8.

Composition and Structure of Cartilage

Cohen NP, Foster RJ, Mow VC. Composition and dynamics of articular cartilage: structure, function, and maintaining healthy state. J Orthop Sports Phys Ther 1998;28(4):203–15.

Dijkgraaf LC, de Bont LGM, Boering G, Liem RSB. Normal cartilage structure, biochemistry, and metabolism: a review of the literature. J Oral Maxillofac Surg 1995;53(8):924–9.

Huber M, Trattnig S, Lintner F. Anatomy, biochemistry, and physiology of articular cartilage. Invest Radiol 2000;35: 573–80.

Kuettner KE. Biochemistry of articular cartilage in health and disease. Clin Biochem 1992;25:155–63.

Poole AR, Kojima T, Yasuda T, Mwale F, Kobayashi M, Laverty S. Composition and structure of articular cartilage: a template for tissue repair. Clin Orthop Relat Res 2001;391:S26–33.

Composition and Structure of Bone

Downey PA, Siegel MI. Bone biology and the clinical implications for osteoporosis. Phys Ther 2006;86(1):77–91.

Harada S, Rodan GA. Control of osteoblast function and regulation of bone mass. Nature 2003;423:349–55.

Olszta MJ, Cheng Z, Jee SS, Kumar R, Kim YY, Kaufman MJ, et al. Bone structure and formation: a new perspective. Mater Sci Eng 2007;58(3–5):77–116.

Raggatt LJ, Partridge NC. Cellular and molecular mechanisms of bone remodeling. J Biol Chem 2010;285:25103–8.

Seeman E, Delmas PD. Bone quality—the material and structural basis of bone strength and fragility. N Engl J Med 2006;354: 2250–61.

Formation and Composition of Collagen

Fedorov AN, Baldwin TO. Cotranslational protein folding. J Biol Chem 1997;272:32715–18.

Khoshnoodi J, Cartailler J-P, Alvares K, Veis A, Hudson BG. Molecular recognition in the assembly of collagens: terminal noncollagenous domains are key recognition modules in the formation of triple helical protomers. J Biol Chem 2006;281: 38117–21.

Formation and Composition of Proteoglycan

Day AJ, Prestwich GD. Hyaluronan-binding proteins: tying up the giant. J Biol Chem 2002;277:4585–8.

Hardingham TE, Fosang AJ, Dudhia J. The structure, function and turnover of aggrecan, the large aggregating proteoglycan from cartilage. Eur J Clin Chem Clin Biochem 1994;32(4):249–57.

Bone Homeostasis

Boonen S, Bischoff-Ferrari HA, Cooper C, Lips P, Ljunggren O, Meunier PJ, Reginster J-Y. Addressing the musculoskeletal components of fracture risk with calcium and vitamin D: a review of the evidence. Calcif Tissue Int 2006;78(5):257–70.

Boonen S, Lips P, Bouillon R, Bischoff-Ferrari HA, Vanderschueren D, Haentjens P. Need for additional calcium to reduce the risk of hip fracture with vitamin D supplementation: evidence from a comparative metaanalysis of randomized controlled trials. J Clin Endocrinol Metab 2007;92(4):1415–23.

Parfitt AM. Bone and plasma calcium homeostasis. Bone 1987;8(Suppl 1):S1–8.

St. Arnaud R. Review: the direct role of vitamin D on bone homeostasis. Arch Biochem Biophys 2008;473(2):225–30.

Tang BM, Eslick GD, Nowson C, Smith C, Bensoussan A. Use of calcium or calcium in combination with vitamin D supplementation to prevent fractures and bone loss in people aged 50 years and older: a meta-analysis. Lancet 2007;370(9588): 657–66.

Regulation of Bone Mass

Glass 2nd DA, Karsenty G. In vivo analysis of Wnt signaling in bone. Endocrinology 2007;148(6):2630–4.

Karsenty G. Review: convergence between bone and energy homeostases: leptin regulation of bone mass. Cell Metab 2006;4(5):341–8.

Karsenty G, Oury F. The central regulation of bone mass, the first link between bone remodeling and energy metabolism. J Clin Endocrinol Metab 2010;95(11):4795–801.

Krishnan V, Bryant HU, MacDougald OA. Review series: regulation of bone mass by Wnt signaling. J Clin Invest 2006;116: 1202–9.

Ralston SH, de Crombrugghe B. Genetic regulation of bone mass and susceptibility to osteoporosis. Genes Dev 2006;20: 2492–506.

Rodan GA, Martin TJ. Review: therapeutic approaches to bone diseases. Science 2000;289(5484):1508–14.

Normal Calcium and Phosphate Metabolism

Heaney RP, Nordin BEC. Calcium effects on phosphorus absorption: implications for the prevention and co-therapy of osteoporosis. J Am Coll Nutr 2002;21(3):239–44.

Makoto K. Klotho as a regulator of fibroblast growth factor signaling and phosphate/calcium metabolism. Curr Opin Nephrol Hypertens 2006;15(4):437–41.

Walters JR. The role of the intestine in bone homeostasis. Eur J Gastroenterol Hepatol 2003;15(8):845–9.

Nutritional Calcium Deficiency

Cumming RG, Nevitt MC. Calcium for prevention of osteoporotic fractures in postmenopausal women. J Bone Miner Res 1997; 12(9):1321–9.

Ladhani S, Srinivasan L, Buchanan C, Allgrove J. Presentation of vitamin D deficiency. Arch Dis Child 2004;89:781–4.

Pettifor JM. Nutritional rickets: deficiency of vitamin D, calcium, or both? Am J Clin Nutr 2004;80(6):1725S–9S.

Effects of Disuse and Stress on Bone Mass

Dalsky GP. Effect of exercise on bone: permissive influence of estrogen and calcium. Med Sci Sports Exer 1990;22(3):281–5.

Stewart AF, Adler A, Byers CM, Segre GV, Broadus AE. Calcium homeostasis in immobilization: an example of resorptive hypercalciuria. N Engl J Med 1982;306:1136–40.

Uebelhartl D, Demiaux-Domenech B, Rothl M, Chantraine A. Bone metabolism in spinal cord injured individuals and in others who have prolonged immobilisation: a review. Paraplegia 1995;33:669–73.

van der Meulen MC, Globus RK. Progress in understanding disuse osteopenia. Curr Opin Orthop 2005;16(5):325–30.

Musculoskeletal Effects of Weightlessness (Spaceflight)

Carmeliet G, Vico L, Bouillon R. Space flight: a challenge for normal bone homeostasis. Crit Rev Eukaryot Gene Expr 2001;11(1-3):131–44.

Cavanagh PR, Licata AA, Rice AJ. Exercise and pharmacological countermeasures for bone loss during long-duration space flight. Grav Space Biol 2005;18:39–58.

Converino VA. Physiological adaptations to weightlessness: effects on exercise and work performance. Exer Sports Sci Rev 1990;18:119–66.

LeBlanc AD, Spector ER, Evans HJ, Sibonga JD. Skeletal responses to space flight and the bed rest analog: a review. J Musculoskelet Neuronal Interact 2007;7:33–47.

Physical Factors in Bone Remodeling

Layne JE, Nelson ME. The effects of progressive resistance training on bone density: a review. Med Sci Sports Exerc 1999;31(1):25–30.

Mosley JR. Osteoporosis and bone functional adaptation: mechanobiological regulation of bone architecture in growing and adult bone: a review. J Rehabil Res Dev 2000;37(2):189–99.

Robling AG, Castillo AB, Turner CH. Biomechanical and molecular regulation of bone remodeling. Annu Rev Biomed Eng 2006;8:455–98.

Zehnacker CH, Bemis-Dougherty A. Effect of weighted exercises on bone mineral density in post menopausal women: a systematic review. J Geriatr Phys Ther 2007;30(2):79–88.

Age-Related Changes in Bone Geometry

Ahlborg HG, Johnell O, Turner CH, Rannevik G, Karlsson MK. Bone loss and bone size after menopause. N Engl J Med 2003;349(4):327–34.

Akkus O, Adarb F, Schaffler MB. Age-related changes in physicochemical properties of mineral crystals are related to impaired mechanical function of cortical bone. Bone 2004; 34(3):443–53.

Brockstedt H, Kassem M, Eriksen EF, Mosekilde L, Melsen F. Age- and sex-related changes in iliac cortical bone mass and remodeling. Bone 1993;14(4):681–91.

Chan GK, Duque G. Age-related bone loss: old bone, new facts. Gerontology 2002;48:62–71.

Faibish D, Ott SM, Boskey AL. Mineral changes in osteoporosis: a review. Clin Orthop Relat Res 2006;443:28–38.

Fatayerji D, Eastell R. Age-related changes in bone turnover in men. J Bone Miner Res 1999;14(7):1203–10.

Seeman E. Periosteal bone formation—a neglected determinant of bone strength. N Engl J Med 2003;349:320–3.

Silva MJ, Gibson LJ. Modeling the mechanical behavior of vertebral trabecular bone: effects of age-related changes in microstructure. Bone 1997;21(2):191–9.

Section 3—Metabolic Diseases

Abelson A. A review of Paget's disease of bone with a focus on the efficacy and safety of zoledronic acid 5 mg. Curr Med Res Opin 2008;24(3):695–705.

Cundy T, Reid IR. Paget's disease of bone. Clin Biochem 2012;45:43–8.

Naot D. Paget's disease of bone: an update. Curr Opin Endocrinol Diabetes Obes 2011;18:352–8.

Ralston S, Albagha O. Genetic determinants of Paget's disease of bone. Ann NY Acad Sci 2011;1240:53–60.

Reid IR, Hosling DJ. Bisphosphonates in Paget's disease. Bone 2010;49:89–94.

Reid IR, Lyles K, Su G, Brown JP, Walsh JP, del Pino-Montes J, et al. A single infusion of zoledronic acid produces sustained remissions in Paget's disease—data to 6.5 years. J Bone Miner Res 2011;26:2261–70.

Shore EM, Meiqu X, Feldman GJ, Fenstermacher DA, Cho TJ, Choi IH, et al. A recurrent mutation in the BMP type I receptor ACVR1 causes inherited and sporadic fibrodysplasia ossificans progressiva. Nat Genet 2006;38:525–7.

Silverman S. Bisphosphonate use in conditions other than osteoporosis. Ann NY Acad Sci 2011;1218:33–7.

Singer F. The etiology of Paget's disease of bone: viral and genetic interactions. Cell Metab 2011;13(1):5–6.

Section 4—Congenital and Developmental Disorders

Benacerraf BB. The Sherlock Holmes approach to diagnosing fetal syndromes by ultrasound. Clin Obstet Gynecol 2012;55(1): 226–48.

Blackmur JP, Murray AW. Do children who in-toe need to be referred to an orthopaedic clinic? J Pediatr Orthop B 2010;19(5):415–17.

Carlisle ES, Ting BL, Abdullah MA, Skolasky RL, Schkrohowsky JG, Yost MT, et al. Laminectomy in patients with achondroplasia: the impact of time to surgery on long-term function. Spine 2011;36(11):886–92.

Fabry G, MacEwen GD, Shands A Jr: Torsion of the femur: a follow-up study in normal and abnormal conditions. J Bone Joint Surg Am 1973;55:1726.

Farsetti P, Weinstein SL, Caterini R, De Maio F, Ippolito E. Sprengel's deformity: long-term follow-up study of 22 cases. J Pediatr Orthop B 2003;12(3):202–10.

Fernandez DL. Corrective osteotomy for symptomatic increased ulnar tilt of the distal end of the radius. J Hand Surg Am 2001;26:722–32.

Grogan DP, Love SM, Guidera KJ, Ogden JA. Operative treatment of congenital pseudoarthrosis. J Pediatr Orthop 1991;11(2): 176–80.

Guven O, Tekin U, Hatipoglu M. Surgical and prosthodontic rehabilitation in a patient with Freeman-Sheldon syndrome. J Craniofac Surg 2010;21(5):1571–74.

Hart ES, Grottkau BE, Rebello GN, Albright MB.The newborn foot: diagnosis and management of common conditions. Orthop Nurs 2005;24(5):313–21; quiz 322–3.

Hoffmeister E. Exploring gait abnormalities in children with cerebral palsy. Bone & Joint 2006;12(11):121, 123–4.

Johnston II CE. Simultaneous open reduction of ipsilateral congenital dislocation of the hip and knee assisted by femoral diaphyseal shortening. J Pediatr Orthop 2011;31(7): 732–40.

Laederich MB, Horton WA. Achondroplasia: pathogenesis and implications for future treatment. Curr Opin Pediatr 2010; 22(4):516–23.

Mackenzie W, Bassett GS, Mandell GA, Scott Jr CI. Avascular necrosis of the hip in multiple epiphyseal dysplasia. J Pediatr Orthop 1989;9:666–71.

Martirosyan NL, Cavalcanti DD, Kalani M, Yashar S, Maughan PH, Theodore N. Aplasia of the anterior arch of atlas associated with multiple congenital disorders: case report. Neurosurgery. 2011;69(6):E1317–20.

Martus JE, Griffith TE, Dear J, Cuyler B, Rathjen KE. Pediatric cervical kyphosis: a comparison of arthrodesis techniques. Spine 2011;36(17):E1145–53.

McKay SD, Al-Omari Ali, Tomlinson LA, Dormans JP. Review of cervical spine anomalies in genetic syndromes. Spine 2012; 37(5):E269–77.

Muntoni F, Torelli S, Wells DJ, Brown SC. Muscular dystrophies due to glycosylation defects: diagnosis and therapeutic strategies. Curr Opin Neurol 2011;24(5):437–42.

O'Sullivan R, Walsh M, Hewart P, Jenkinson A, Ross LA, O'Brien T. Factors associated with internal hip rotation gait in patients with cerebral palsy. J Pediatr Orthop 2006;26(4):537–41.

Porreco RP. Noninvasive prenatal diagnosis. Postgrad Obstet Gynecol 2010;30(23):1–5.

Rao S, Dietz F, Yack HJ. Kinematics and kinetics during gait in symptomatic and asymptomatic limbs of children with myelomeningocele. J Pediatr Orthop 2012;32(1):106–12.

Savva N, Ramesh R, Richards RH. Supramalleolar osteotomy for unilateral tibial torsion. J Pediatr Orthop B 2006;15(3): 190–3.

Shah HH, Doddabasappa SN, Joseph B. Congenital posteromedial bowing of the tibia: a retrospective analysis of growth abnormalities in the leg. J Pediatr Orthop B 2009;18(3):120–8.

Shalom A, Khermosh O, Wientroub S. The natural history of congenital pseudarthrosis of the clavicle. J Bone Joint Surg Br 1994;76(5):846–7.

Sprenger J. The epiphyseal dysplasias. Clin Orthop Relat Res 1976;114:46.

Teitge RA. Osteotomy in the treatment of patellofemoral instability. Tech Knee Surg 2006;5(1):2–18.

Wall JJ. Congenital pseudoarthrosis of the clavicle. J Bone Joint Surg Am 1970;52(5):1003–9.

Wang Y, Caggana M, Sango-Jordan M, Sun M, Druschel CM. Long-term follow-up of children with confirmed newborn screening disorders using record linkage. Genet Med 2011; 13(10):881–6.

Section 5—*Rheumatic Diseases*

ACR Subcommittee on Osteoarthritis Guidelines. Recommendations for the medical management of osteoarthritis of the hip and knee. Arthritis Rheum 2000;43:1905–15.

Deng J, Younge BR, Olshen RA, Goronzy JJ, Weyand CM. Th17 and Th1 T-cell responses in giant cell arteritis. Circulation 2010;121:906–15.

Goekoop-Ruiterman YP, de Vries-Bouwstra JK, Allaart CF, van Zeben D, Kerstens PJ, Hazes JM, et al. Clinical and radiographic outcomes of four different treatment strategies in patients with early rheumatoid arthritis (the BeSt study): a randomized, controlled trial. Arthritis Rheum 2005;52(11):3381.

Grigor C, Capell H, Stirling A, et al. Effect of a treatment strategy of tight control for rheumatoid arthritis (the TICORA study): a single-blind randomised controlled trial. Lancet 2004;364(9430): 263.

Hoffman GS, Cid MC, Hellmann DB, Guillevin L, Stone JH, Schousboe J, et al. A multicenter, randomized, double-blind, placebo-controlled trial of adjuvant methotrexate treatment for giant cell arteritis. Arthritis Rheum 2002;46:1309–18.

Jover JA, Hernandez-Garcia C, Morado IC, Vargas E, Banares A, Fernandez-Gutierrez B. Combined treatment of giant-cell arteritis with methotrexate and prednisone: a randomized, double-blind, placebo-controlled trial. Ann Intern Med 2001;134:106–14.

Lee MS, Smith SD, Galor A, Hoffman GS. Antiplatelet and anticoagulant therapy in patients with giant cell arteritis. Arthritis Rheum 2006;54:3306–9.

Maksimowicz-McKinnon K, Clark TM, Hoffman GS. Takayasu arteritis and giant cell arteritis: a spectrum within the same disease? Medicine 2009;88:221–6.

Moskowitz RW, Hooper M. State-of-the-art disease-modifying osteoarthritis drugs. Curr Rheumatol Rep 2005;7:15–21.

Nesher G, Berkun Y, Mates M, Baras M, Rubinow A, Sonnenblick M. Low-dose aspirin and prevention of cranial ischemic complications in giant cell arteritis. Arthritis Rheum 2004;50:1332–7.

Nuenninghoff DM, Hunder GG, Christianson TJ, McClelland RL, Matteson EL. Mortality of large-artery complication (aortic aneurysm, aortic dissection, and/or large-artery stenosis) in patients with giant cell arteritis: a population-based study over 50 years. Arthritis Rheum. 2003;48:3532–37.

Ostberg G. On arteritis, with special reference to polymyalgia rheumatica. Acta Pathol Microbiol Scand Suppl 1973;1–59.

Rantalaiho V, Korpela M, Hannonen P, et al. The good initial response to therapy with a combination of traditional disease-modifying antirheumatic drugs is sustained over time: the eleven-year results of the Finnish rheumatoid arthritis combination therapy trial. Arthritis Rheum 2009;60(5):1222.

Saag KG, Teng GG, Patkar NM, et al. American College of Rheumatology 2008 recommendations for the use of nonbiologic and biologic disease-modifying antirheumatic drugs in rheumatoid arthritis. Arthritis Rheum 2008;59(6):762.

Smolen JS, Aletaha D, Bijlsma JW, et al. Treating rheumatoid arthritis to target: recommendations of an international task force. Ann Rheum Dis 2010;69(4):631.

Smolen JS, Landewé R, Breedveld FC, et al. EULAR recommendations for the management of rheumatoid arthritis with synthetic and biological disease-modifying antirheumatic drugs. Ann Rheum Dis 2010;69(6):964.

Weyand CM, Hicok KC, Hunder GG, Goronzy JJ. Tissue cytokine patterns in patients with polymyalgia rheumatica and giant cell arteritis. Ann Intern Med 1994;121:484–91.

Weyand CM, Hunder NN, Hicok KC, Hunder GG, Goronzy JJ. HLA-DRB1 alleles in polymyalgia rheumatica, giant cell arteritis, and rheumatoid arthritis. Arthritis Rheum 1994;37:514.

Zhang W, Moskowitz RW, Nuki G, Abramson S, Altman RD, Arden N, et al. OARSI recommendations for the management of hip and knee osteoarthritis, part II: OARSI-evidence-based, expert consensus guidelines. Osteoarthritis Cartilage 2008;16: 137–62.

Section 6—*Tumors*

Lietman SA. Soft-tissue sarcomas: overview of management, with a focus on surgical treatment considerations. Cleve Clin J Med 2010;77(Suppl 1):S13–17.

Lietman SA, Joyce MJ. Bone sarcomas: overview of management, with a focus on surgical treatment considerations. Cleve Clin J Med 2010;77(Suppl 1):S8–12.

Link MP, Goorin AM, Miser AW, Green AA, Pratt CB, Belasco JB, et al. The effect of adjuvant chemotherapy on relapse-free survival in patients with osteosarcoma of the extremity. N Engl J Med 1986;314:1600–6.

Newcomer AE, Dylinski D, Rubin BP, Joyce MJ, Hoeltge G, Bershadsky B, Lietman SA. Prognosticators in thigh soft tissue sarcomas. J Surg Oncol 2011;103:85–91.

Rosen G, Marcove RC, Caparros B, Nirenberg A, Kosloff C, Huvos AG. Primary osteogenic sarcoma: the rationale for preoperative chemotherapy and delayed surgery. Cancer 1979; 43:2163–77.

Weiss RB, DeVita Jr VT. Multimodal primary cancer treatment (adjuvant chemotherapy): current results and future prospects. Ann Intern Med 1979;91:251–60.

Weiss SW, Goldblum JR, Enzinger FM. Enzinger and Weiss' soft tissue tumors. 5th ed. Philadelphia: Mosby Elsevier; 2008.

Wold LE. Atlas of orthopedic pathology. Philadelphia: Saunders; 1990.

Section 7—*Injury*

Achauer and Sood's burn surgery: reconstruction and rehabilitation. Philadelphia: Saunders; 2006.

American Burn Association White Paper. Surgical management of the burn wound and use of skin substitute.

Bucholz RW, Heckman JD, editors. Rockwood and Green's fractures in adults. Philadelphia: Lippincott Williams & Wilkins; 2009.

Olson SA, Glasgow RR. Acute compartment syndrome in lower extremity musculoskeletal trauma. J Am Acad Orthop Surg 2005;13:436–44.

Remaley D, Jaeblon T. Pressure ulcers in orthopaedics. J Am Acad Orthop Surg 2010;18:568–75.

Romanelli M, Clark M, Cherry GW, Colin D, Defloor T, editors. Science and practice of pressure ulcer management. 2006.

Webb LX. New techniques in wound management: vacuum-assisted wound closure. J Am Acad Orthop Surg 2002;10: 303–11.

Whitesides TE, Heckman MM. Acute compartment syndrome: update on diagnosis and treatment. J Am Acad Orthop Surg 1996;4:209–18.

Section 8—*Soft Tissue Infections*

Gordon A, Jeffery HE. Antibiotic regimens for suspected late onset sepsis in newborn infants. Cochrane Database Syst Rev 2005;(3):CD004501.

Gosselin RA, Roberts I, Gillespie WJ. Antibiotics for preventing infection in open limb fractures. Cochrane Database Syst Rev 2004;(1): CD003764.

John J, Chandran L. Arthritis in children and adolescents. Pediatr Rev 2011;32(11):470–9; quiz 480. Erratum in: Pediatr Rev 2012;33(3):109.

Pääkkönen M, Kallio PE, Kallio MJ, Peltola H. Management of osteoarticular infections caused by *Staphylococcus aureus is* similar to that of other etiologies: analysis of 199 staphylococcal bone and joint infections. Pediatr Infect Dis J 2012;31(5): 436–8.

Section 9—*Complications of Fracture*

Allgower M, Durig M, Wolff G. Infection and trauma. Surg Clin North Am 1980;60:133–44.

Bosse MJ, Riemer BL, Brumback RJ, et al. Adult respiratory distress syndrome, pneumonia and mortality following thoracic injury and a femoral fracture treated with intramedullary nailing with reaming or with a plate. J Bone Joint Surg Am 1997;79: 799–809.

Brinker M. Nonunions: evaluation and treatment. In: Browner B, editor. Skeletal trauma. 3rd ed. Philadelphia: Elsevier; 2003.

Cleveland K. Delayed union and nonunion of fractures. In: Canale S, Beaty J, editors. Campbell's operative orthopaedics. 11th ed. Philadelphia: Elsevier; 2008.

Chalidis B, Sachinis N, Assiotis A, Maccauro G. Stimulation of bone formation and fracture healing with pulsed electromagnetic fields: biologic responses and clinical implications. Int J Immunopathol Pharmacol 2011;24(1 Suppl 2):17–20.

Gellman H, et al. Gunshot wounds to the musculoskeletal system. In: Browner B, editor. Skeletal trauma. 3rd ed. Philadelphia PA: Elsevier; 2003.

Griffin XL, Costa ML, Parsons N, Smith N. Electromagnetic field stimulation for treating delayed union or non-union of long bone fractures in adults. Cochrane Database Syst Rev 2011;(4):CD008471.

Johnson KD, Cadambi A, Seibert GB. Incidence of adult respiratory distress syndrome in patients with multiple musculoskeletal injuries: effect of early operative stabilization of fractures. J Trauma 1985;25:375–84.

Murray DW, Kambouroglou G, Kenwright J. One-stage lengthening for femoral shortening with associated deformity. J Bone Joint Surg Br 1993;75:566.

Papakostidis C, Kanakaris NK, Pretel J, Faour O, Morell DJ, Giannoudis PV. Prevalence of complications of open tibial shaft fractures stratified as per the Gustilo-Anderson classification. Injury 2011;42(12):1408–15.

Perron AD, Miller MD, Brady WJ. Orthopedic pitfalls in the ED: fight bite. Am J Emerg Med 2002;20(2):114–17.

Roberts C, et al. Diagnosis and treatment of complications. In: Browner B, editor. Skeletal trauma. 3rd ed. Philadelphia PA: Elsevier; 2003.

Schurmann M, et al. Early diagnosis in post-traumatic complex regional pain syndrome. Orthopedics 2007;30(6):450–6.

Stannard J. Trauma. In: Miller M, editor. Review of orthopaedics. 5th ed. Philadelphia: Elsevier; 2008.

Whittle AP. Malunited fractures. In: Canale S, Beaty J, editors. Campbell's operative orthopaedics. 11th ed. Philadelphia: Elsevier; 2008.
